AF602066

Medicinal Plants: Phytochemistry, Pharmacology and Therapeutics

Medicinal Plants: Phytochemistry, Pharmacology and Therapeutics

– Volume 1 –

– Editor-in-Chief –
V.K. Gupta

– Editors –
G.D. Singh
Surjeet Singh
A. Kaul

Daya Publishing House®
A Division of
Astral International Pvt. Ltd.
New Delhi – 110 002

© EDITORS

First Published, 2010
Reprinted, 2021

ISBN: 978-93-5124-105-8 (International Edition)

Publisher's Note:

Every possible effort has been made to ensure that the information contained in this book is accurate at the time of going to press, and the publisher and author cannot accept responsibility for any errors or omissions, however caused. No responsibility for loss or damage occasioned to any person acting, or refraining from action, as a result of the material in this publication can be accepted by the editor, the publisher or the author. The Publisher is not associated with any product or vendor mentioned in the book. The contents of this work are intended to further general scientific research, understanding and discussion only. Readers should consult with a specialist where appropriate.

Every effort has been made to trace the owners of copyright material used in this book, if any. The author and the publisher will be grateful for any omission brought to their notice for acknowledgement in the future editions of the book.

All Rights reserved under International Copyright Conventions. No part of this publication may be reproduced, stored in a retrieval system, or transmitted in any form or by any means, electronic, mechanical, photocopying, recording or otherwise without the prior written consent of the publisher and the copyright owner.

Published by : **Daya Publishing House®**
A Division of
Astral International Pvt. Ltd.
– ISO 9001:2008 Certified Company –
4736/23, Ansari, Road, Darya Ganj,
New Delhi-110 002
Ph. 011-43549197, 23278134
E-mail: info@astralint.com
Website: www.astralint.com

Dedicated to

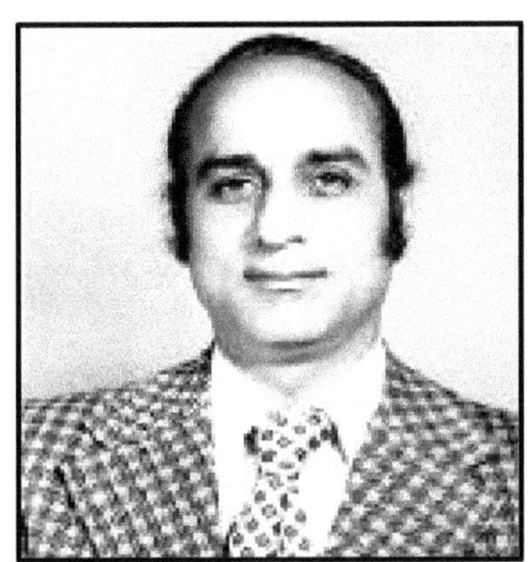

Prof. C. K. Atal

Former Director, Indian Institute of Integrative Medicine, Jammu
(Erstwhile, Regional Research Laboratory, Jammu)

Foreword

The twenty-nine chapters of the book *Medicinal Plants: Phytochemistry, Pharmacology and Therapeutics, Volume 1,* edited by Dr. V. K. Gupta, Dr. G. D. Singh, Dr. Surjeet Singh and Dr. A. Kaul (2009) represent enormous progress, as they cover themes currently under discussion in all of these research fields. Some of the contributions are still based on Ayurvedic herbs and medicine, but most are of general interest, addressing herbs with antioxidant, antilipedemic, vasodilatory, opioid, antiinflammatory, antisickling, antimicrobial, antidiabetic antiparasitic, antimalaria or antiaging activities. This wide spectrum of themes may be of great value for research in natural products chemistry and biology, and to medical doctors as well.

I congratulate the editors and appreciate their efforts in bringing out such an excellent book which will give all round readers an exciting and serious reading material and also continuing the outstanding works for which Indian Institute of Integrative Medicine (CSIR), Jammu (Formerly Regional Research Laboratory, Jammu) has been known.

It is a pleasure for me to recommend this volume without reservation to all researches in the field of phytomedicine. I wish the book much success and a broad distribution.

I do hope that this book will be followed by second volume in the next years.

Dr. H. Wagner

Professor Emeritus
Centre of Pharma Research, Department Pharmacy,
University of Munich, Germany

Preface

Plants have been used for alleviating human suffering from the very beginning of human civilization, and records of the use of plants are available since about 5000 years ago. The active principles isolated, have provided leads in the development of several life saving drugs, which are in use today. Different civilizations developed their own indigenous system of medicines. Historically, about two centuries ago, our medicinal practices were largely dominated by plant-based medicines. However, the medicinal use of herbs went into decline in the West when more predictable synthetic drugs were made commonly available. In contrast, many developing nations continued to benefit from the rich knowledge of medical herbalism. For example Ayurvedic medicine in India, Kampo medicine in Japan, Traditional Chinese Medicine and Unani Medicine in the Middle East and South Asia are still used by a large majority of people.

All around the world there is talk about 'health for all' but it has been realized that modern pharmaceuticals are and will remain out of reach of a large proportion of the human population for the foreseeable future. This necessitates the use of other sources of human knowledge to provide common health benefits. Thus, herbal medicine is now regarded as important but underutilized tool against disease. The World Health Organization (WHO) recognized this fact in the early 1970s and encouraged governments to effectively utilize local knowledge of herbal medicines for disease prevention and health promotion.

There is now a popular belief that allopathic drugs have serious side effects on human body. As against the same, herbal medicines work better and provide long lasting healing effect and are without any side effects. As such there is now a growing demand of herbal medicines and herbal therapeutic applications. The primary health care of 70-80 per cent of the world's population is based on the use of medicinal plants derived from traditional systems of medicine and local health practices. During the past few decades public interest in traditional, complementary and alternative medicine (TCAM) and use of herbal medicines has increased dramatically in industrialized countries. Traditional medicine has a bright future and an immense potential to extend medical relief to millions, who for lack of resources remain deprived of it. When undesirable side effects of certain drugs have unnerved the patients, herbal medicine is the only hope in India where 60 per cent of the population lives below the poverty line.

This has increased the international trade in herbal medicine enormously. WHO said in 2003 that the global market for herbal medicines stood at US $ 60 billion and was growing steadily. Global sales of herbal products including herbal medicine has already crossed 100 billion in the last five years and is expected to exceed one trillion in the next 20 years at the present growth rate. In India, the herbal drug market is about $ one billion and the export of plant based crude drugs is around $ 80 million.

Many pharmaceutical companies are showing interest in the production and marketing of herbal medicines. The sales for herbal medicine products have plateaued to such an extent that these products have become available to consumers as positive healthcare just like vitamins. Herbal medicines are in great demand in the developed as well as developing countries for primary healthcare because of their wide biological activities, higher safety margins and lesser costs.

Out of 20,000 plants recognized of medicinal value, only a very few are in use. Their use is not scientifically validated much with the scientific data. Plant extracts of therapeutic relevance are of paramount importance as reservoirs of structural and chemical diversity. A recent report reveals that at least 120 distinct chemical substances from different plants have utility as lifesaving drugs. This has been achieved through chemical and pharmacological screening of only 6 per cent of the total plant species.

It is for their world wide and a sustained effort of scientist's that an enormous information is being generated and there has been a series of publications on medicinal plant researches. Based on this rational, the present book "Medicinal Plants: Phytochemistry, Pharmacology and Therapeutics - Vol. 1" presents information on review/research communications received from eminent scientists from India and abroad, providing recent and present state of the art data on therapeutic properties, action and uses of medicinal plants in combating a number of diseases and condition for which there is lesser satisfactory treatment in modern medicine.

It is hoped that the present volume will attract wide acceptance of phytochemists, pharmacologists, medical personals in particular and a host of other scientists and biologists to facilitate further research on medicinal plants.

V.K. Gupta

G.D. Singh

Surjeet Singh

A. Kaul

Contents

Medicinal Plants: Phytochemistry, Pharmacology and Therapeutics, Vol. 1 *Pages* 1–31
Editors: V.K. Gupta, G.D. Singh, Surjeet Singh and A. Kaul
Published by: DAYA PUBLISHING HOUSE, NEW DELHI

Chapter 1

Resveratrol: A Natural Polyphenol, that Prevents Illness and Increases Longevity–An Overview

Mahesh Masna, Gottumukkala V. Subbaraju* and Modukuri V. Ramani
Aptuit Laurus Pvt. Ltd., ICICI Knowledge Park, Hyderabad – 500 078, India

ABSTRACT

Resveratrol, a natural polyphenol that occurs widely in several plants and foods, was found to be a strong antioxidant, cardioprotective agent, antidiabetic, antiinflammatory compound and anticancer agent. Resveratrol is one of the polyphenolic constituents in wines and is believed to be the basis for 'French Paradox'. Its importance has grown further after it was recognized that it acts as calorie restriction mimic and increases longevity.

Keywords: *Polyphenol, Resveratrol, Red wine, Cardioprotective, Anticancer, Longevity.*

Introduction

Polyphenols, a group of naturally occurring compounds, are characterized by chemical structures with aromatic rings possessing number of hydroxyl groups. These compounds are responsible for the colors observed in flowers and fruits of many plants. Polyphenols are strong antioxidants and offer potential health benefits. Among the group of naturally occurring polyphenols (tannins, flavonoids, stilbenes and lignans), stilbenes are gaining increasing importance, recently.

* Corresponding Author: E-mail: subbaraju.gv@aptuitlaurus.com.

Stilbenes are low molecular weight (200-300 amu) naturally occurring compounds and occur in a wide range of plant sources. It is believed that these compounds are produced by the plants as a response to environmental stress or threat and are called phytoalexins. Stilbenes act as natural protective agents to defend the plant against viral and microbial attack, excessive ultraviolet exposure and the disease.

Stilbenes exist in two (*trans*–and *cis*-) stereoisomeric forms, depending on the orientation of aryl groups with respect to double bond (Figure 1.1).

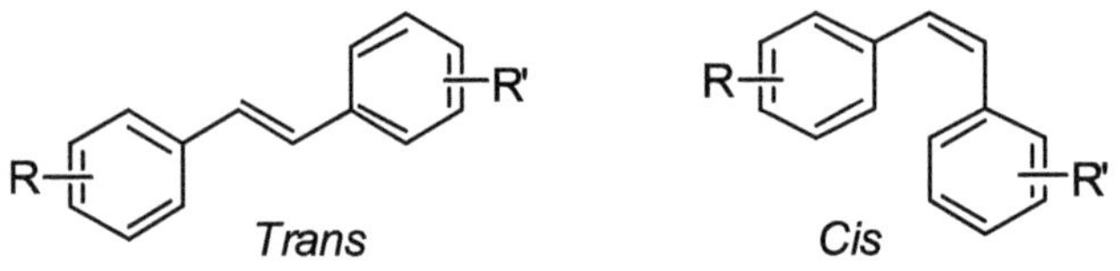

Figure 1.1: Stereoisomeric Forms of Stilbenes

Naturally occurring stilbenes (Table 1.1) exist overwhelmingly in the *trans* form. It has been observed that the *trans* and *cis* forms of stilbenes elicit different pharmacological activities. For example, *trans*-resveratrol was found to be ten times more potent in its ability to induce apoptosis in the HL 60 leukaemia cell line compared to *cis*-resveratrol (Roberti *et al.*, 2003). Additional research has shown that *trans*-stilbene compounds to be significantly more potent in their ability to inhibit cyclooxygenase I (COX-I) activity compared to *cis*-stilbene compounds (Waffo-Teguo *et al.*, 2001).

Table 1.1: Naturally Occurring Stilbenes

Name of the Stilbene and Structure	*Str.No.*	*Source*	*Activity*	*Reference*
Resveratrol 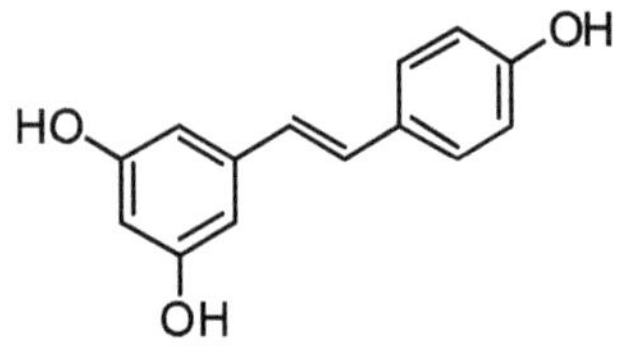 (HO, OH, OH)	1	*Polygonum cuspidatum*; *Vitis* spp.; *Vaccinum* spp.; *Morus* spp.; *Veratrum* spp.; *Arachis hypogaea;* etc.,	Antioxidant; Anticancer; Cardioprotectant; Antiinflammatory; Antiaging; Antidiabetic.	Bagchi 2000
Dihydroresveratrol 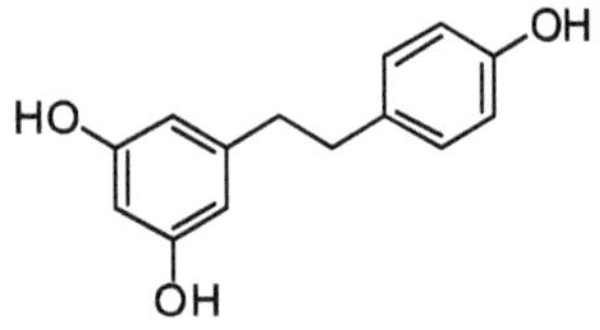 (HO, OH, OH)	2	*Dioscorea* spp.; *Bulbophyllum triste*	Murine tyrosinase activity	Kittisak 2008
Piceatannol or astringinin 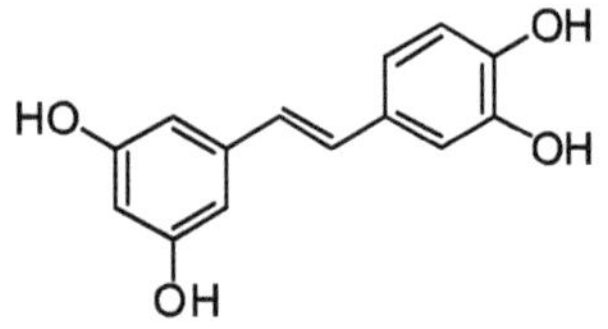 (HO, OH, OH, OH)	3	*Melaleuca leucadendron*; *Cassia garretitana* *Vaccinium* berries	Antileukaemic; tyrosine kinase inhibitor; anti inflammatory anti proliferative; anti cancer and anti Epstein-Barr virus drug	Potter *et al.*, 2002; Wung *et al.*, 2006; Swanson-Mungerson, *et al.*, 2003

Contd...

Table 1.1–Contd...

Name of the Stilbene and Structure	*Str.No.*	*Source*	*Activity*	*Reference*
Dihydropiceatannol 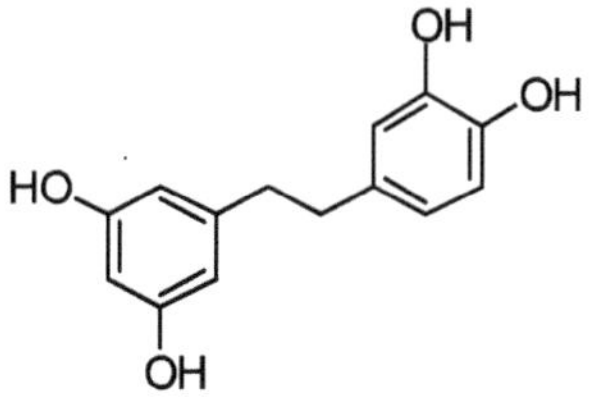	4	*Cassia garretitana*	—	Cunningham *et al.*, 1963; Erdtman and Ronlán, 1969
Gnetol 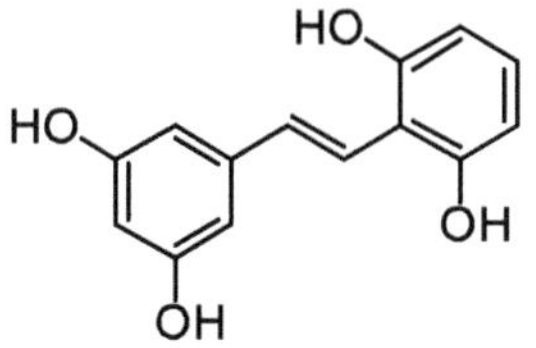	5	*Gnetum* spp.	Potent tyrosinase inhibitor	Ohguchi *et al.*, 2003
Oxyresveratrol 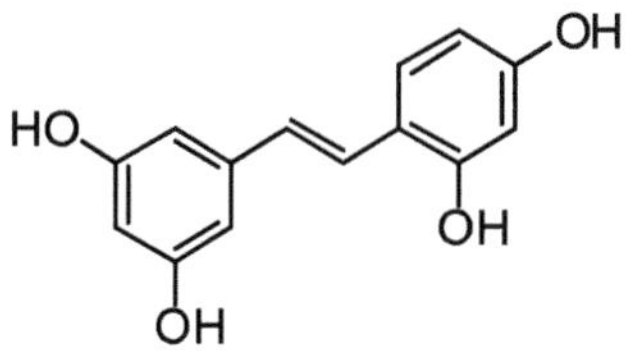	6	*Morus* spp.; *Maclura pomifera*; *Artocarpus gomezianus*	Neuroprotective, dopa oxidase activity of tyrosinase	Andrabi *et al.*, 2004 Shin *et al.*, 1998
Hydroxyresveratrol 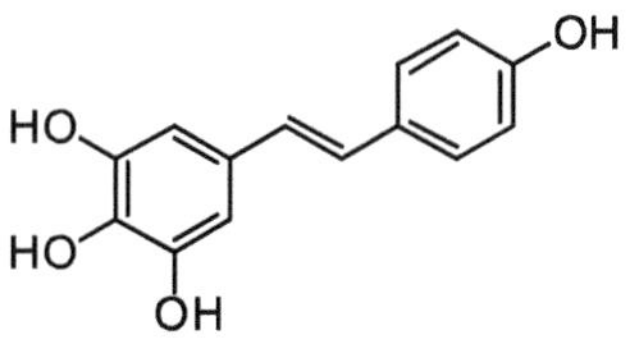	7	*Polygonum cuspidatum*	—	Sovak, 2001
Trans-3,3',4',5,5'-pentahydroxystilbene 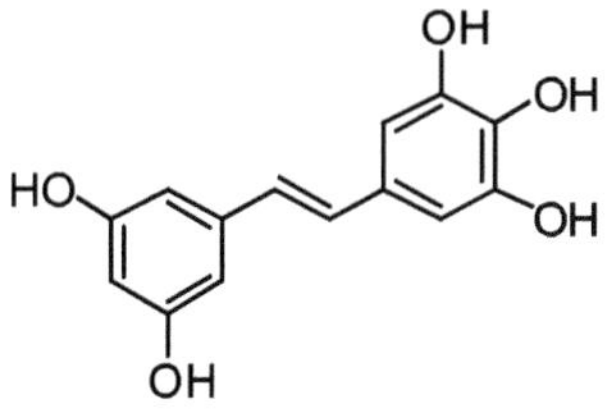	8	*Eucalyptus wandoo*	—	Castro *et al.*, 1986
Pinosylvin 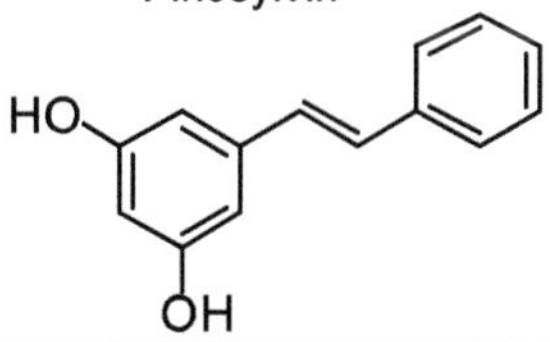	9	*Gnetum cleistostachyum; Polygonum nodosum*	Antifungal, Antibacterial	Lee *et al.*, 2005

Contd...

Table 1.1–Contd...

Name of the Stilbene and Structure	*Str.No.*	*Source*	*Activity*	*Reference*
Dihydropinosylvin 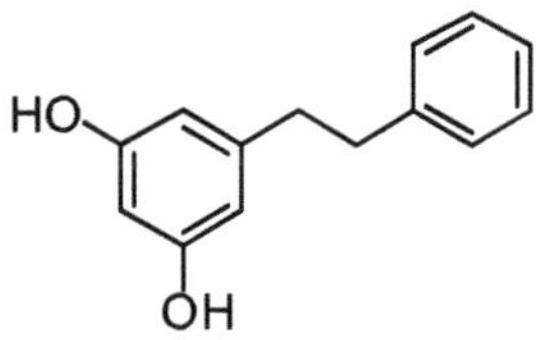	10	*Dioscorea batatas*	Antifungal; antibacterial	Harborne *et al.*, 1999
Rhapontigenin 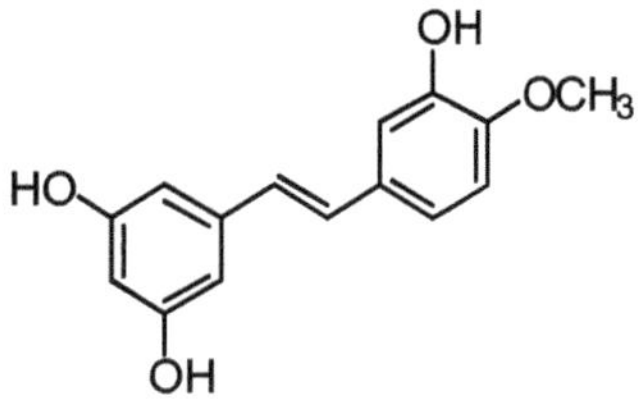	11	*Rheum* spp. (incl. *R. rhaponticum, R. undulatum*); *Scilla nervosa*	Antioxidant	Zhang *et al.*, 2007
Isorhapontigenin 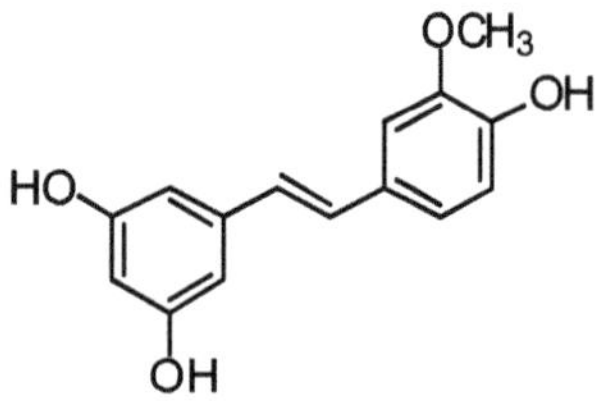	12	*Gnetum* spp.; *Belamcanda chinensis*;	Antioxidant	Wang *et al.*, 2001
Desoxyrhapontigenin 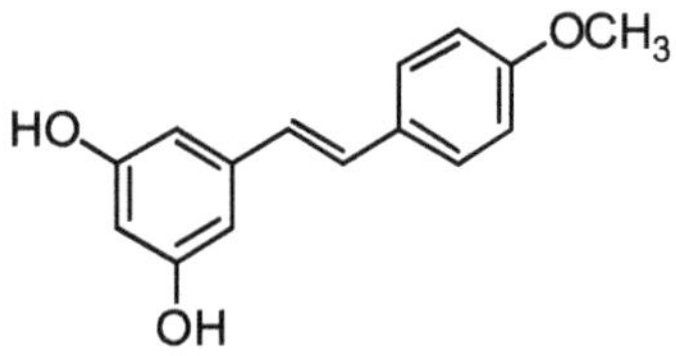	13	*Gnetum cleistostachyum; Rheum undulatum Knema austrosiamensis; Rumex bucephalophorus*	Potent inhibitor of CYP1A1 catalytic activity	Mikstacka *et al.*, 2007
Pinostilbene 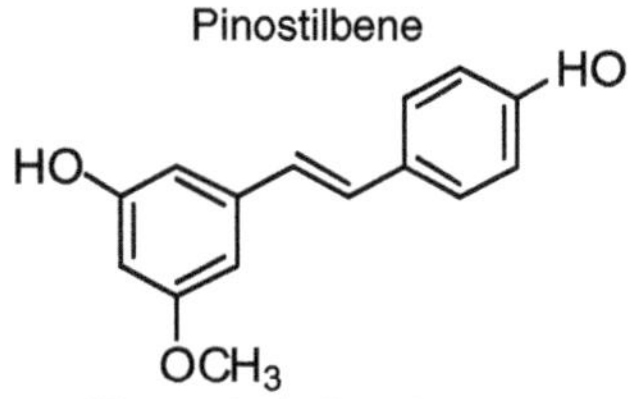	14	*Rumex bucephalophorus*; *Pinus koraiensis*	Potent inhibitor of CYP1A1 catalytic activity	Mikstacka *et al.*, 2007
Trans-3,4'-dimethoxy-5-hydroxystilbene 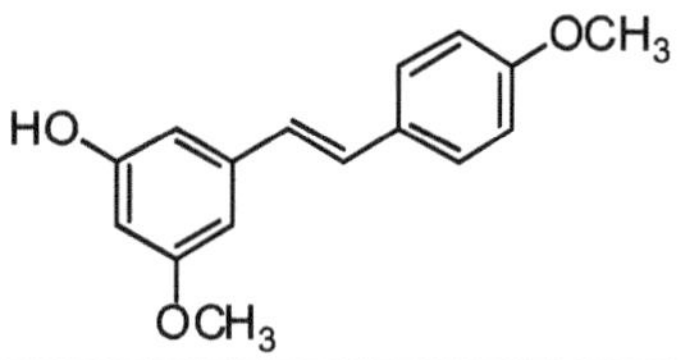	15	*Knema austrosiamensis*	Apoptosis	Chun *et al.*, 2001

Contd...

Table 1.1–Contd...

Name of the Stilbene and Structure	*Str.No.*	*Source*	*Activity*	*Reference*
Trimethylresveratrol 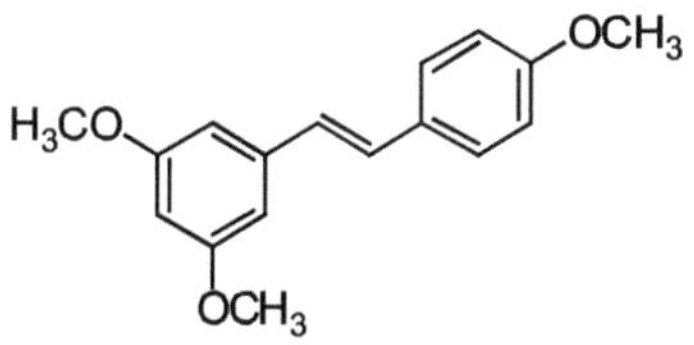	16	*Pterolobium hexapetallum*	Antiallergic	Matsuda *et al.*, 2004
Trans-5,4'-dihydroxy-3-methoxystilbene 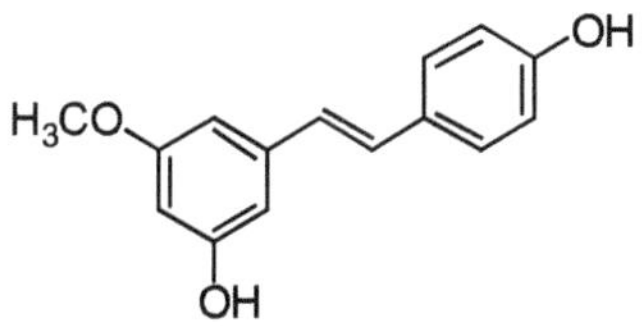	17	*Rumex bucephalophorus*	Antioxidant	Kerem *et al.*, 2003
Pterostilbene 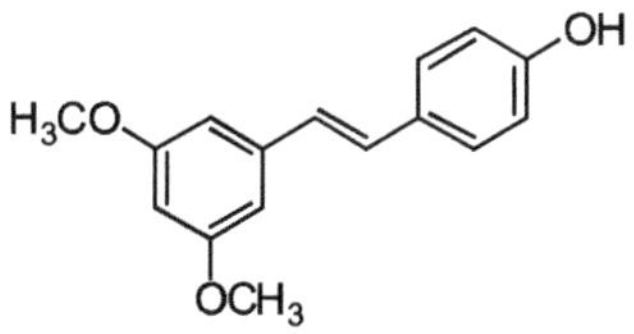	18	*Dracena cochinchinensis; Pterocarpus* spp. (incl. *P. santalinus, P. marsupium*); *Vitis vinifera*; *Pterolobium hexapetallum*;	Antioxidant, anticancer, antihypercholesterolemia, anti hypertriglyceridemia, antidiabetic; antifungal, lowers cholesterol	Amorati *et al.*, 2004 Rimando *et al.*, 2002
Trans-3,4,3',5'-tetra methoxystilbene 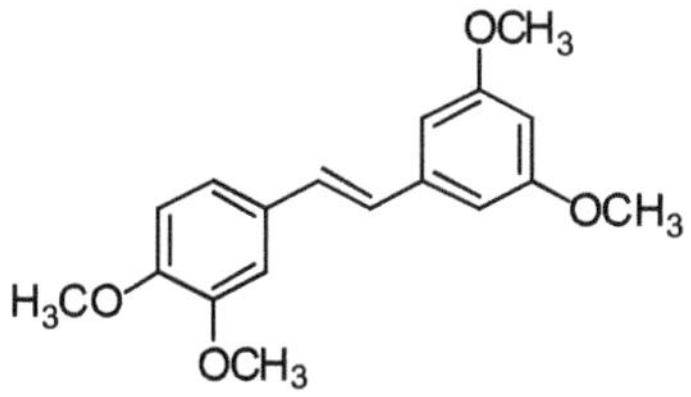	19	*Crotalaria madurensis*	—	Bhakuni and Chaturvedi, 1984
Trans-and cis-3,3',5,5'-tetrahydroxy-4-methoxystilbene 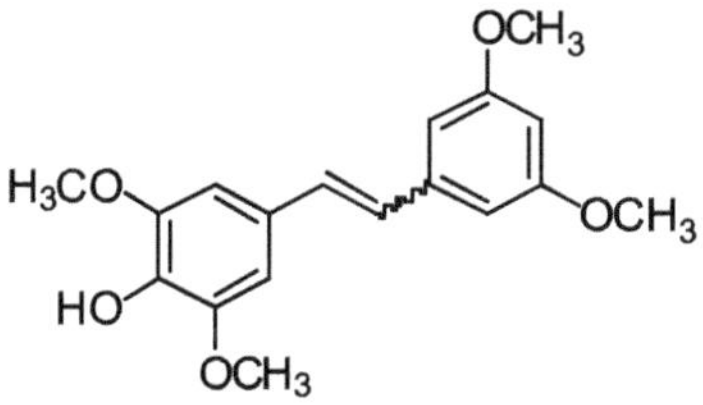	20	*Yucca periculosa, Y. schidigera; Cassia pudibunda*	Antioxidant	Torres *et al.*, 2003

Contd...

Table 1.1–Contd...

Name of the Stilbene and Structure	*Str.No.*	*Source*	*Activity*	*Reference*
Trans-4,4'-dihydroxystilbene 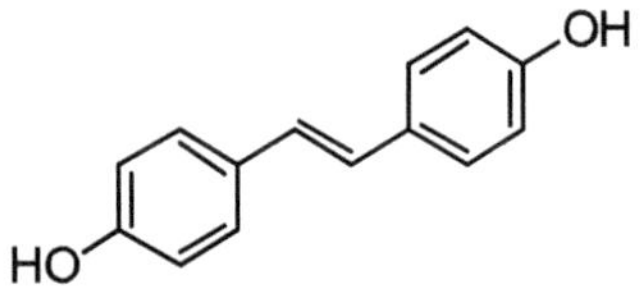	21	*Yucca periculosa*	—	Torres *et al.*, 2003
Trans-3-hydroxy-5-methoxystilbene 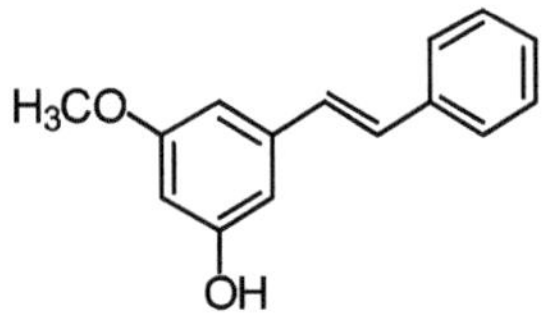	22	*Cryptocarya idenburgensis*	—	Juliawaty *et al.*, 2000
Trans-4,3'-dihydroxy-5'-methoxystilbene 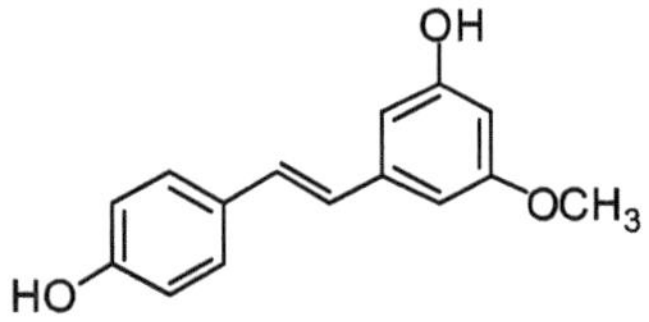	23	*Dracaena loureiri*	—	Kittisak *et al.*, 2002
Piceid 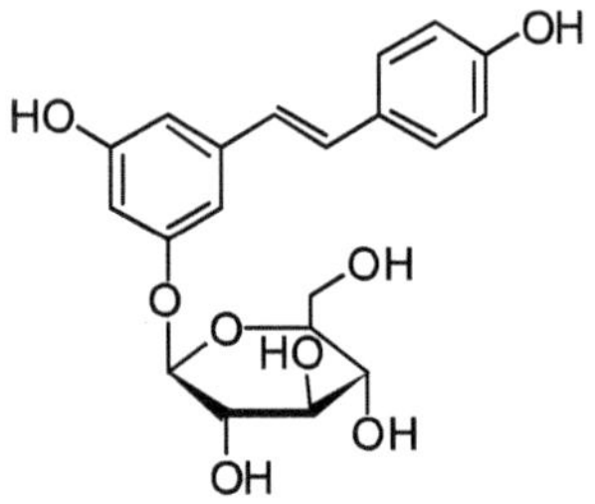	24	*Polygonum cuspidatum*; *Rheum* rhaponticum *Picea* spp.; Lentils (*Lens culinaris*)	—	Romero-Pérez *et al.*, 1999
Rhapontin 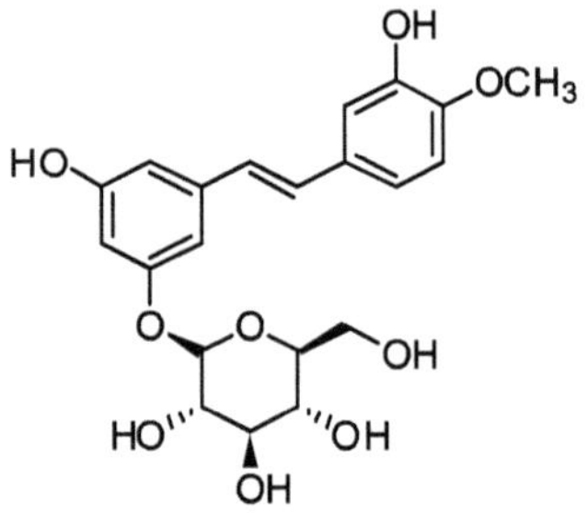	25	*Rheum* spp.; Eucalyptus	Induction of apoptosis	Hibasami *et al.*, 2007

Contd...

Table 1.1–Contd...

Name of the Stilbene and Structure	*Str.No.*	*Source*	*Activity*	*Reference*
Deoxyrhapontin 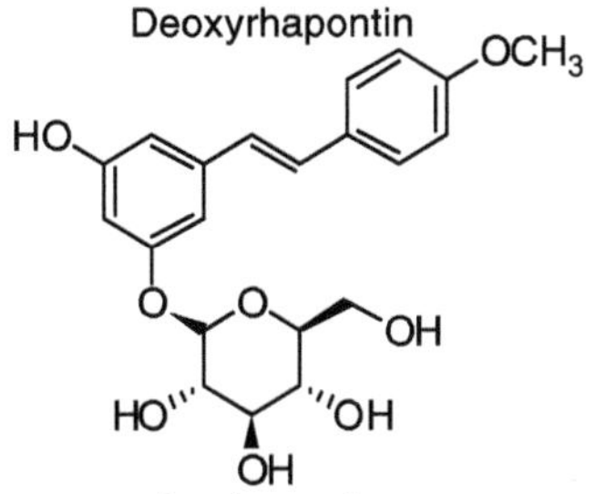	26	*Rheum rhaponticum*	—	Aaviksaar *et al.*, 2003
Isorhapontin 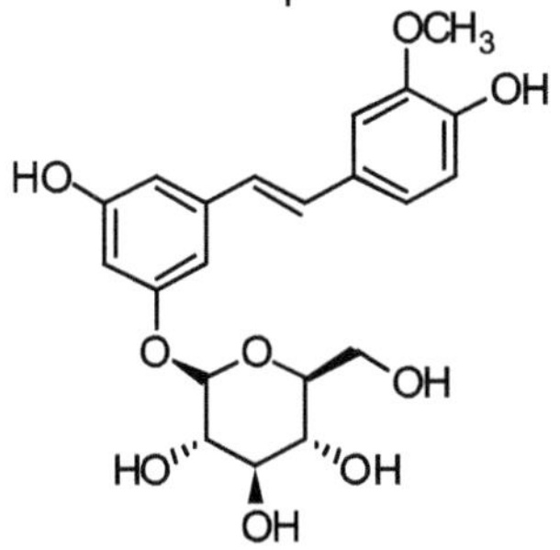	27	*Pinus sibirica*; *Picea* spp.	Hydrolytic activity of Trichoderma cellobiohydrolase	Shibutani *et al.*, 2001
Piceatannol glucoside (3,5,3',4'-tetrahydroxy stil bene-4'-O-β- 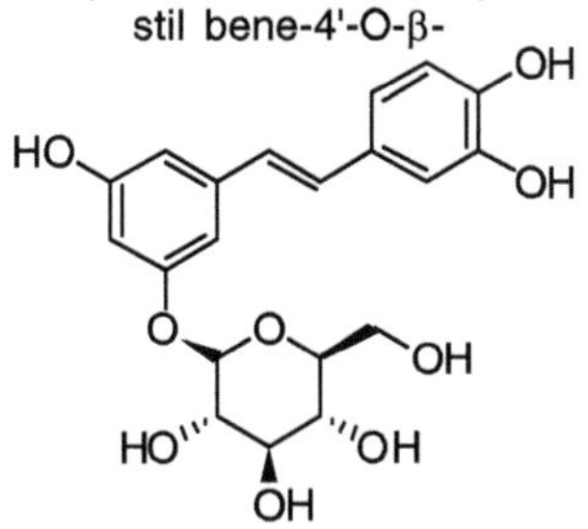	28	*Rheum rhaponticum* D-gluco pyran oside) *Polygonum cuspidatum*; Spruce	—	Vastano *et al.*, 2000
Resveratroloside 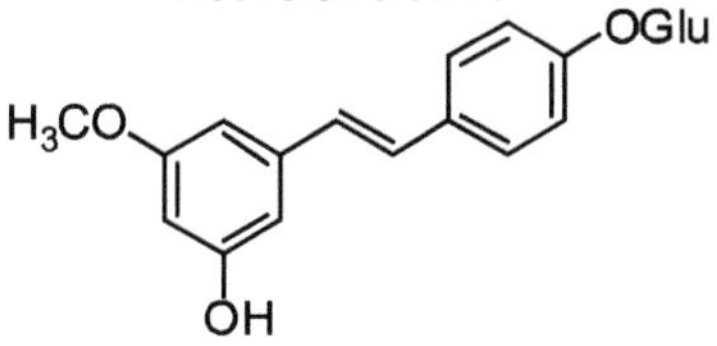	29	*Polygonum cuspidatum*; *Pinus* spp.; *Vitis vinifera*	Antioxidant	Gromova *et al.*, 1975
Rhaponticin-2''-O–gallate and–6''-O-gallate 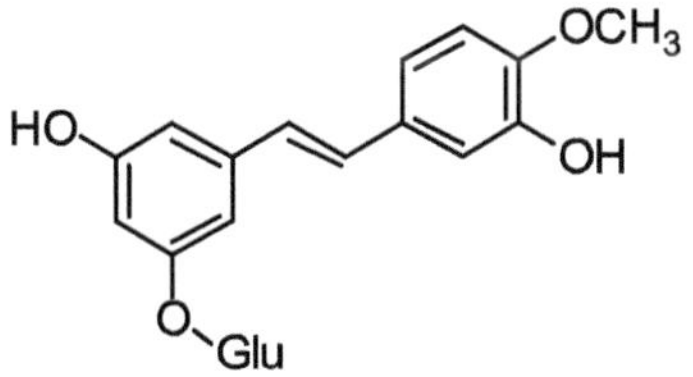	30	Rhubarb (*Rheum undulatum*)	Inhibitory activity of NO production in lipopolysaccharide-activated macrophages	Matsuda, 2000

Resveratrol

In the group of stilbenes, the celebrity is resveratrol. Resveratrol (3, 4', 5-trihydroxystilbene) is a natural polyphenol known to occur widely in plant sources (Figure 1.2). Resveratrol is found in at least 72 species of plants distributed among 31 genera and 12 families (Jang *et al.*, 1997). Foods are also known to contain resveratrol and are limited to grapes, grape juice, cranberries, cranberry juice, peanuts and peanut products. In addition, it is also known to be present in various wines and maximum concentration was found in red wine (Table 1.2).

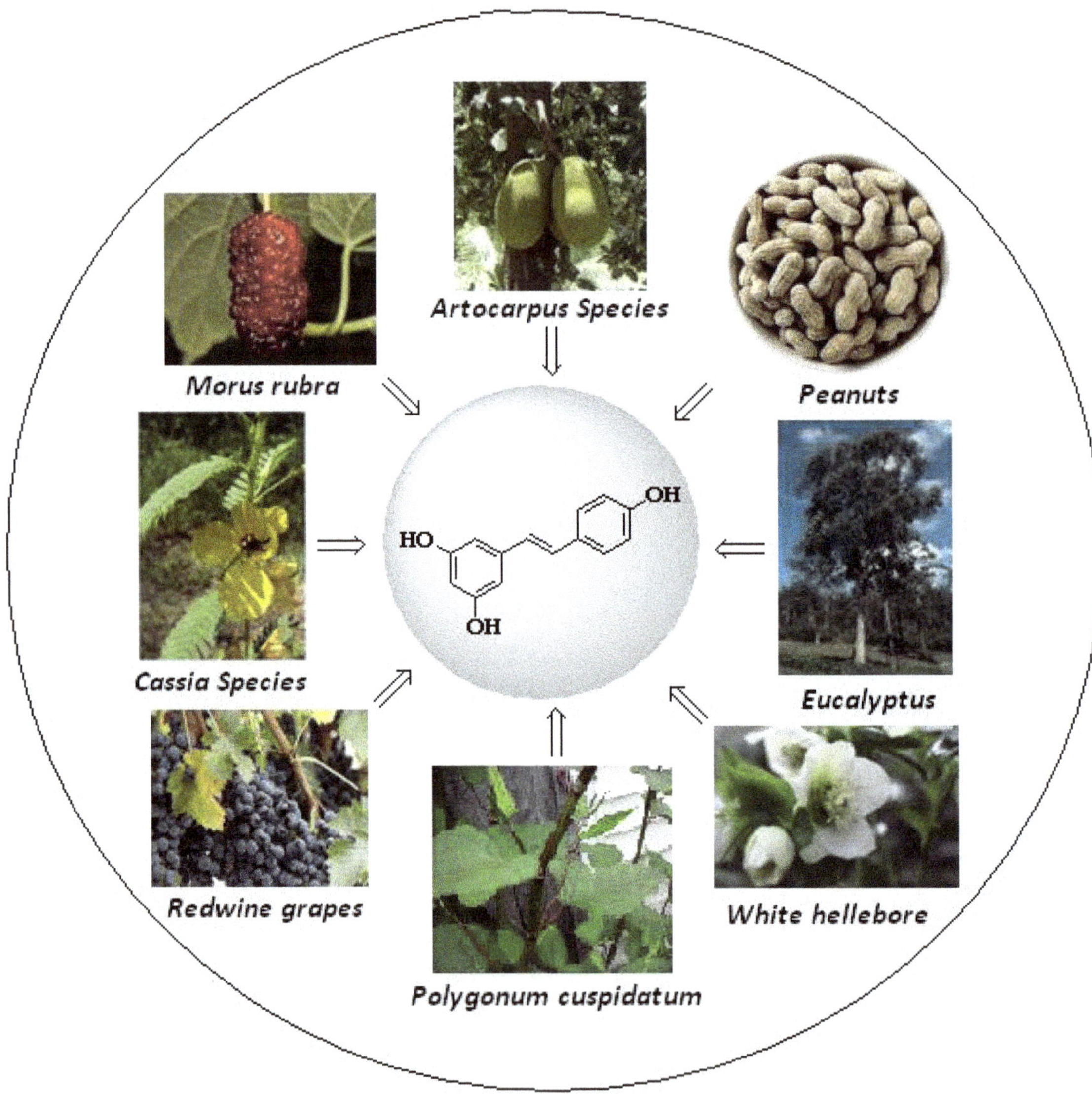

Figure 1.2: Source of Resveratrol

Table 1.2: Concentration of Resveratrol in Wines and Other Beverages (Baur and Sinclair, 2006)

Source	*Conc. of trans-Resveratrol*
Red wines	0.1–14.3 mg/l
White wines	0.1–2.1 mg/l
Grapes	0.16–3.54 μg/g
Dry grape skins	24.06 μg/g
Red grape juices	0.50 mg/l
White grape juices	0.05 mg/l
Cranberry raw juice	~0.2 mg/l
Blueberries	~0.32 ng/g
Peanuts (raw)	0.01–0.26 mg/146 g
Roasted peanuts	0.02–1.92 μg/g
Boiled peanuts	5.1 μg/g
Peanut butters	0.3–0.4 μg/g
100% Natural peanut butters	0.65 μg/g
Polygonum cuspidatum	0.524 mg/g

Natural Source of Resveratrol

Resveratrol is a polyphenolic compound found in plants of many families. It can inhibit fungi pathogens of plants and regulate plants–parasite interaction (Sato *et al.*, 1997). It was first reported in the peel of grape berries for disease resistance and later, in wines as one of the health promoting phenolic components. It was found to be the major polyphenol in the roots of *Polygonum cuspidatum*. The roots of this plant were traditionally used in Korea, China, and Japan as a folk medicine for the treatment of atherosclerosis and other therapeutic purposes. Resveratrol generated further interest after it was discovered to inhibit the copper-catalyzed oxidation of low density lipoprotein (Frankel *et al.*, 1993), the platelet aggregation, arachidonic acid metabolism, reducing liver injury from peroxidized oil (Jang *et al.*, 1997) and having cancer-chemopreventive activities (Jayatilake *et al.*, 1993). Recent discovery that it acts as calorie restriction mimic and can extend life span of organisms, epitomized the interest in this molecule.

Technical Information on *Polygonum cuspidatum*

Japanese knotweed (*Polygonum cuspidatum*) is a perennial herb with spreading rhizomes and numerous reddish-brown, freely branched stems. The plant can reach four to eight feet in height and is often shrubby. The petioled leaves are four to six inches long and generally ovate with an abrupt point. The whitish flowers are borne in open, drooping panicles. The plant is dioecious, so male and female versions of the inconspicuous flowers are produced on separate plants. The approximately 1/8 inch long fruits are brown, shiny, triangular achenes (Hitchcock and Cronquist,1964; Hickman, 1993).

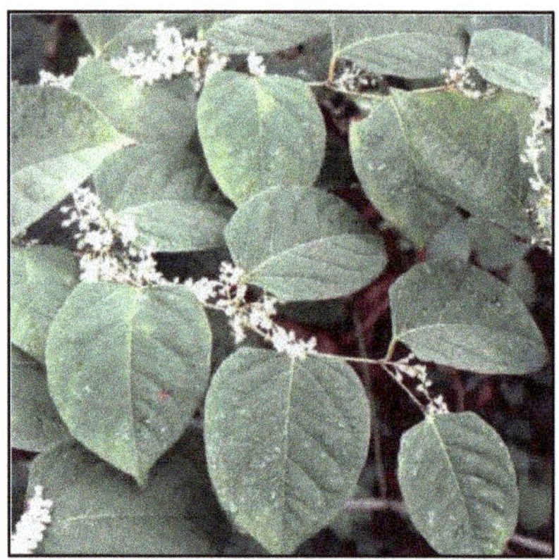

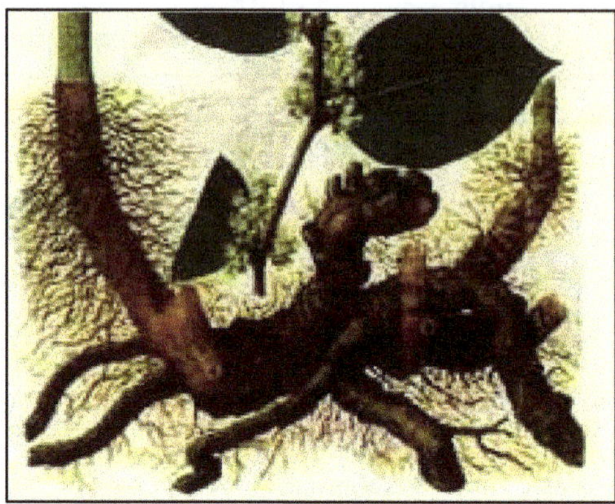

Figure 1.3: Leaves and Roots of *Polygonum cuspidatum*

Isolation of Resveratrol

Typical Process

The dried and crushed roots were extracted with methanol three times under reflux, and the extract was concentrated by reduced pressure to give a dark brown residue. The residue was chromatographed over silica gel column using mixtures of chloroform/methanol (3:1 to 1:1, v/v) for elution or chromatography over polyamide column using methanol for elution to give resveratrol and pieced as individual pure compounds.

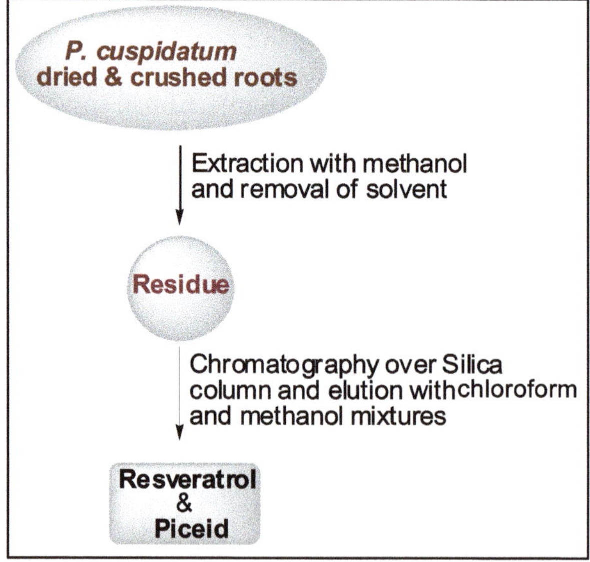

Synthetic Approaches to Resveratrol

Many synthetic routes were developed to obtain resveratrol and a summary is given in Figure 1.4.

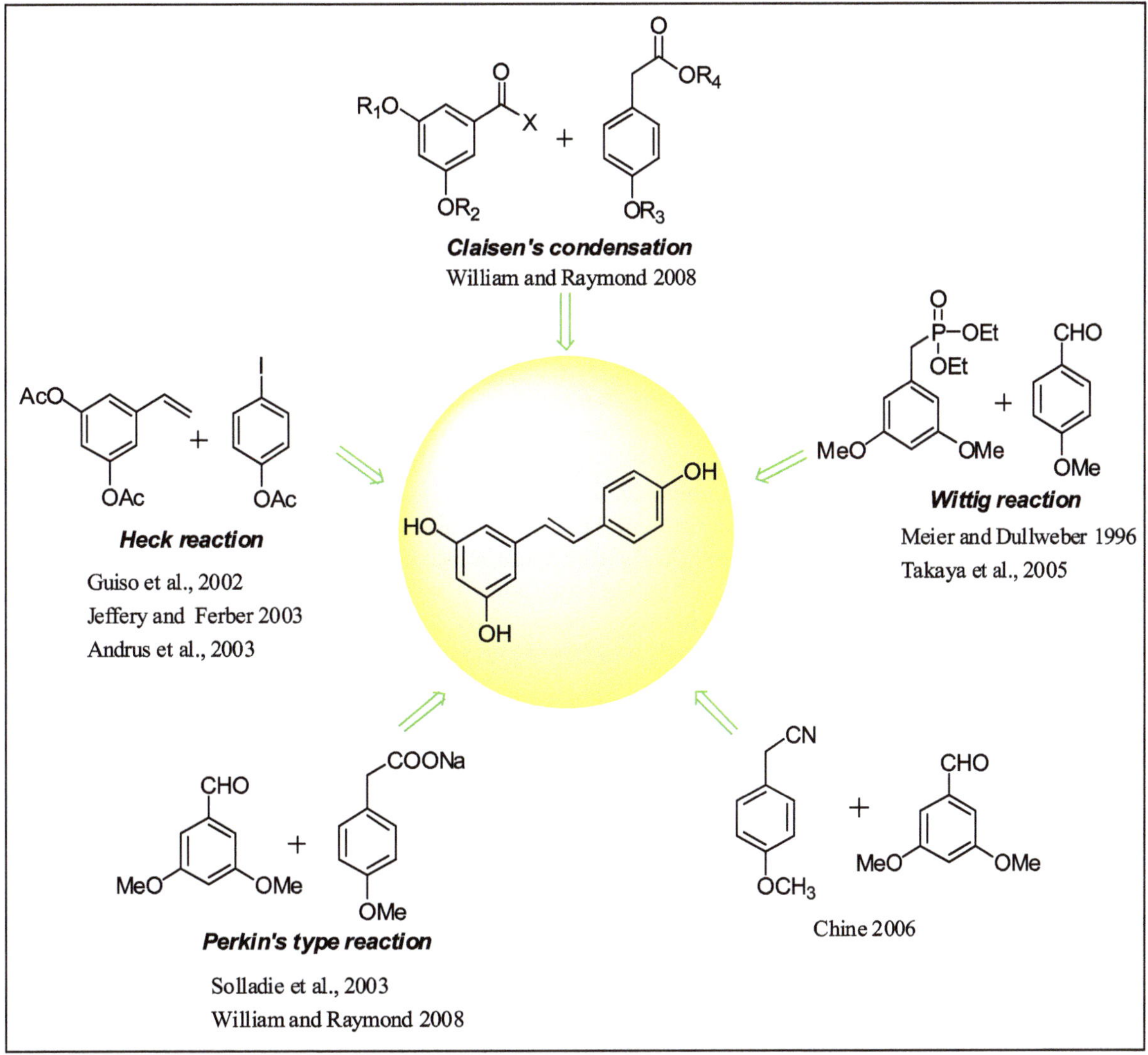

Figure 1.4: Synthetic Approaches to Resveratrol

Biological Activities of Resveratrol

Resveratrol has acquired lot of importance, because of its diverse biological activity and therapeutic profile. There is ongoing debate about the exact mechanism of action by which the desired effects of resveratrol take place. Important biological activities are listed below.

1. A strong free-radical scavenger and antioxidant
2. An antiinflammatory agent
3. Anticancer agent
4. Cardioprotectant

5. Antidiabetic
6. Antiobese
7. Phytoestrogen
8. A neuroprotectant
9. Calorie Restriction Mimic

Free-radical Scavenger and Antioxidant Activity

Resveratrol is a strong free radical scavenger and potent antioxidant, because of its ability to promote the activities of a variety of antioxidative enzymes. The antioxidant activity of polyphenolic compounds depend on the redox properties due to their phenolic hydroxyl groups and the potential electron delocalization across the chemical structure. Oxidation is the transfer of electrons from one atom to another and represents an essential part of aerobic life and in our metabolism, since oxygen is the ultimate electron acceptor in the electron flow system that produces energy in the form of ATP (Adenosine triphospate). The oxygen molecule is very stable in the ground state, but it is changed into reactive oxygen species (ROS), namely, superoxide ion (O_2^{-1}), peroxide radical (?OOH), hydroxyl radical (?OH) and nitric oxide (NO?) by the environmental pollutants, radiolysis, UV and the reduction pathway to H_2O in the living tissues. These free radicals play a major role in the initiation and progression of a wide range of pathological diseases like cancer, Alzheimer's, Parkinson's and cardiovascular diseases. In view of this, considerable attention has been given to the addition of antioxidants in foods and supplementation of antioxidants to biological systems to scavenge free radicals.

The aging process exemplifies the cumulative result of deterioration of individual cells, tissues and organs, promoted by free radicals. The human body has built-in mechanisms to counteract free radicals. These mechanisms are collectively known as the body's antioxidant defense mechanism. Unfortunately, in most instances, the antioxidant defense is gradually overwhelmed by the aging process, or a disease, or both. The inflammatory processes associated with microbial or viral infections and the progression of cancer are just a few disease conditions which contribute to depletion of the antioxidant defense system of the body. Therefore, it is important to preserve the body's defenses against damages by free radicals. Some vitamins, minerals, and natural compounds such as phenolics, flavonoids and carotenoids, have the ability to counteract free radical damage by scavenging or neutralizing the free radicals. These diversified groups of biologically important substances are known as "antioxidants'.

Phenolic compounds exert their antioxidant activity by acting primarily as hydrogen atom donators, thereby inhibiting the propagation of radical chain reactions. Antioxidant potential of the phenolics depends on the number and arrangement of phenolic hydroxyl groups, as well as the nature of the other substituents on the aromatic rings.

Losa, 2003 studied the radical scavenging property of resveratrol using peripheral mononuclear cells from healthy humans which are incubated with the oxidant 2-deoxy-d-ribose and found that resveratrol scavenged O_2 generated by 2-deoxy-d-ribose. The research group at the university of California, Davis (Frankel *et al.*, 1993) have observed that an *ex vivo* system whereby conjugated dienes were generated from native LDL during Cu^{2+} mediated oxygen, and showed that the phenolic constitutes of red wine prevented these oxidative changes and were several fold more potent than α–tocopherol in this respect and the same team extended their studies using pure quercetine, epicatechin and trans-resveratrol. The later was not as potent as quercetine, epicatechin in blocking Cu^{2+}induced oxidation of human LDL, but it was superior to α-tocopherol on a molar basis.

Amorati *et al.*, 2004, investigated recently a series of compounds, *cis*-resveratrol and *trans*–resveratrol and their derivatives to understand the effect of the geometry of the olefinic double bond on their antioxidant activity. These authors have evaluated antioxidant activity quantitatively by measuring two parameters, *i.e.*, the rate constant for the reaction with peroxyl radicals and the bond dissociation enthalpy (BDE) of the phenolic O-H bond. The results revealed higher activity for the *trans* resveratrol compared to cis-isomer, but, such a significant difference was not observed in other pairs of *trans* and *cis* isomers (Figure 1.5).

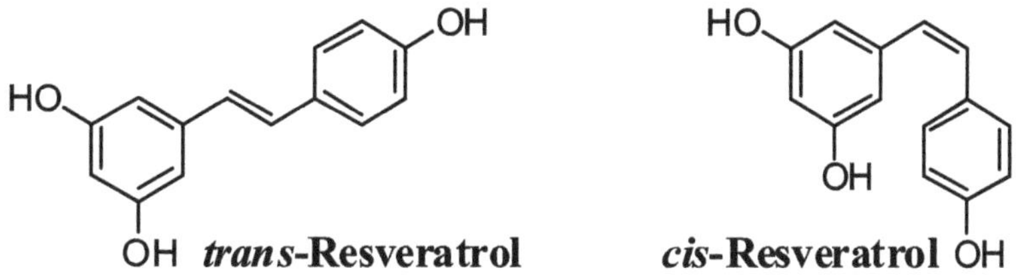

HO OH OH ***trans*-Resveratrol** HO OH ***cis*-Resveratrol** OH

Figure 1.5

Zhou and Liu 2005, have studied antioxidant activity by kinetic and mechanistic studies in micelles, in red blood cells, in low-density lipoprotein (LDL) and in microsomes on resveratrol and related *trans*-stilbene analogs such as, *trans*-3, 5-dihydroxystilbene (9), *trans*-4,4'-dihydroxystilbene (21), *trans*-4-hydroxystilbene (31),, *trans*-3,4-dihydroxystilbene (34), *trans*-3,4,5-trihydroxystilbene (35), and *trans*-3,4,4'-trihydroxystilbene (36) and found that all of these resveratrol analogs exhibit significant antioxidant activity. It is worth noting that the antioxidative activities of stilbenes bearing *ortho*-dihydroxyl functionality (34, 35 and 36) are appreciably higher than those of resveratrol. The antioxidant activity was found to correlate with the electrochemical behavior. Molecules with lower oxidation potentials and reversible cyclic voltammograms, that is, compounds, 21, 34, 35 and 36, exhibit higher activity, while molecules with higher oxidation potentials and irreversible cyclic voltammograms, that is, 9 and 31, and resveratrol are less active. The data suggest that electron-transfer antioxidation might take place simultaneously with a direct hydrogen-abstraction reaction.

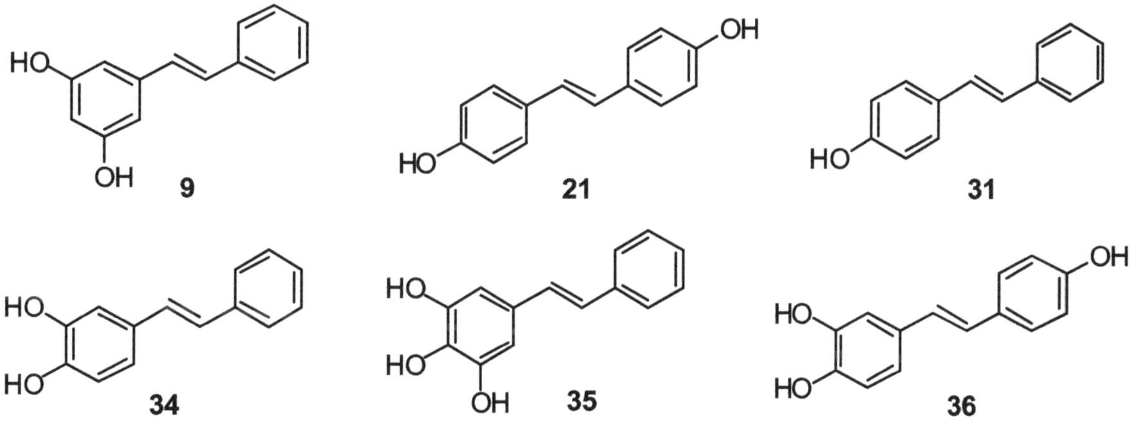

HO OH **9** OH HO **21** HO **31**

HO HO **34** HO HO OH **35** OH HO HO **36**

A team at New York Medical College (Ungvari *et al.*, 2007) found in their study in blood vessels, that resveratrol i) attenuates oxidative stress-induced cell death and ii) exerts antioxidant effects, in part, by up regulating vascular antioxidant systems. However, the mechanisms by which resveratrol exerts its vasculoprotective effects are not completely understood. Because oxidative stress and endothelial cell injury play a critical role in vascular aging and atherogenesis, they evaluated whether resveratrol inhibits oxidative stress-induced endothelial apoptosis and found that oxidized LDL and TNF-α elicited significant increases in caspase-3/7 activity in endothelial cells and cultured rat aortas, which were prevented by resveratrol pretreatment. The protective effect of resveratrol was attenuated by inhibition of glutathione peroxidase and heme oxygenase-1, suggesting a role for antioxidant systems in the antiapoptotic action of resveratrol. Indeed, resveratrol treatment protected cultured aortic segments and/or endothelial cells against increases in intracellular H_2O_2 levels and H_2O_2-mediated apoptotic cell death induced by oxidative stressors (exogenous H_2O_2, paraquat, and UV light). Resveratrol treatment upregulated the expression of glutathione peroxidase, catalase, and heme oxygenase-1 in cultured arteries, whereas it had no significant effect on the expression of superoxide dismutase (SOD) isoforms. Resveratrol also effectively scavenged H_2O_2 *in vitro*. Thus, resveratrol seems to increase vascular oxidative stress resistance by scavenging H_2O_2 and preventing oxidative stress-induced endothelial cell death. The prevention of oxidative stress-induced apoptotic cell death, the dual H_2O_2-lowering effects of resveratrol (both direct scavenging of H_2O_2 and up regulation of antioxidant enzymes) are likely to contribute to its inhibitory effect on H_2O_2-induced endothelial activation and NF-κB induction.

A team from Rutgers University (Wang *et al.*, 1999) have synthesized resveratrol (1) and five other polyhydroxystilbenes, namely, *trans*-3,3',4,5'-tetrahydroxystilbene (3); *trans*-3,4,4',5-tetrahydroxystilbene (7), *trans*-3,3',4,5,5'-pentahydroxystilbene (8); *trans*-3,5-dihydroxystilbene (9), and *trans*-3,3',5,5'-tetrahydroxystilbene (41) and evaluated their antioxidative properties using Rancimat method in pure lard and by 2, 2-diphenyl-1-picryhydrazyl (DPPH). All these compounds exhibited free radicals scavenging ability at the concentration of 20 μM, specially, 7 and 8 exhibited 92.9 per cent inhibition. It is well known that the DPPH radical scavenging ability of phenolic compounds is due to their hydrogen-donating ability, the more the number of hydroxyl groups, the higher the possibility of free radicals scavenging ability and pentahydroxystilbene is the most active antioxidant in this model. Phenolic compounds possessing with *o*-dihydroxy or *p*-dihydroxy phenyl units, exhibit strong antioxidant activity.

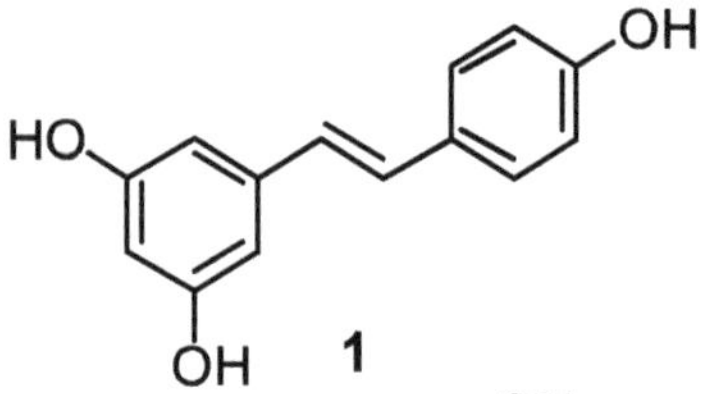

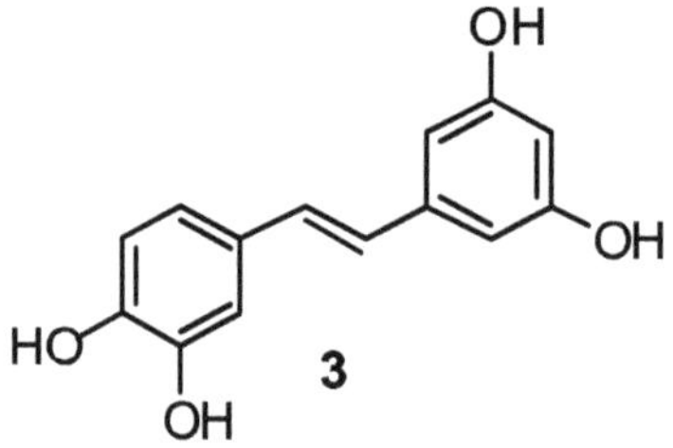

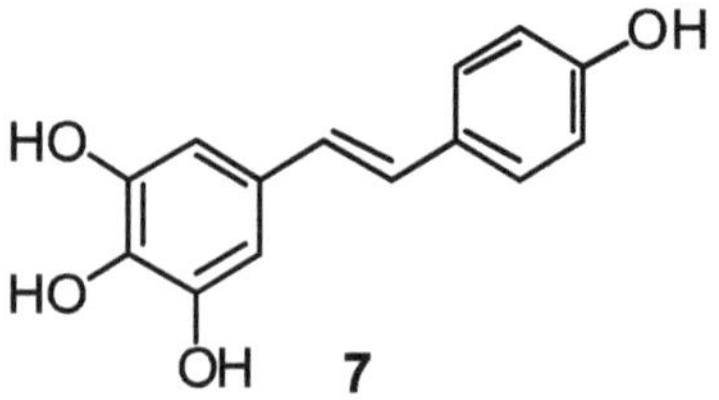

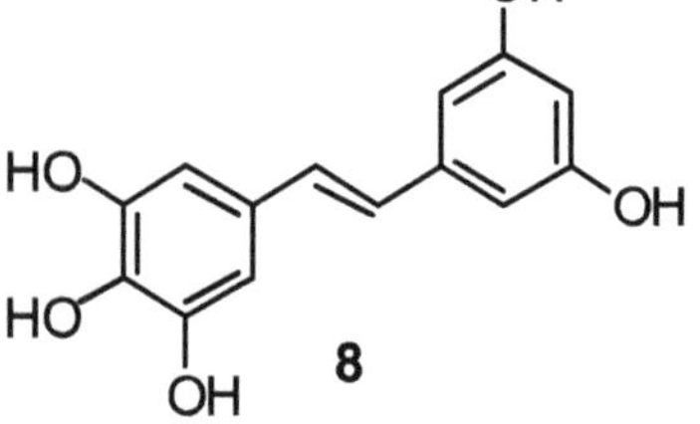

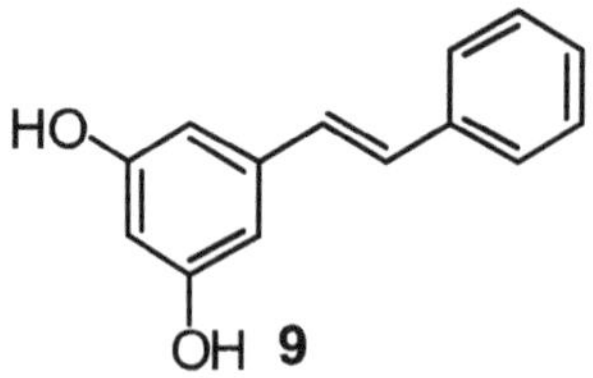

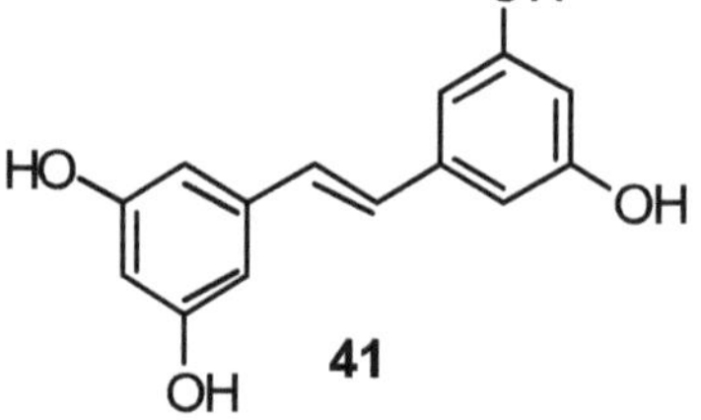

The researchers from Laila Impex, India (Gangaraju *et al.*, 2006) have synthesized novel analogs of resveratrol and established superoxide scavenging activity by McCord and Fridovich method. The percentage value of inhibition of superoxide production by the above invented compounds was compared with control experimental data and the invented compound are found to show better antioxidant activity compare to resveratrol and out of these novel analogs compound 44 (3,3',4,4',5,5'-hexahydroxystilbene) shown higher value of antioxidant activity.

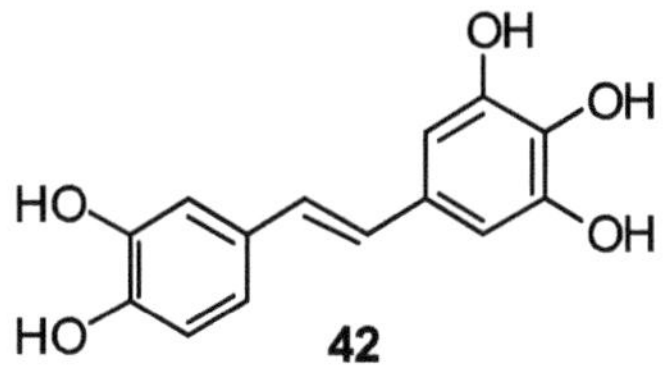
42

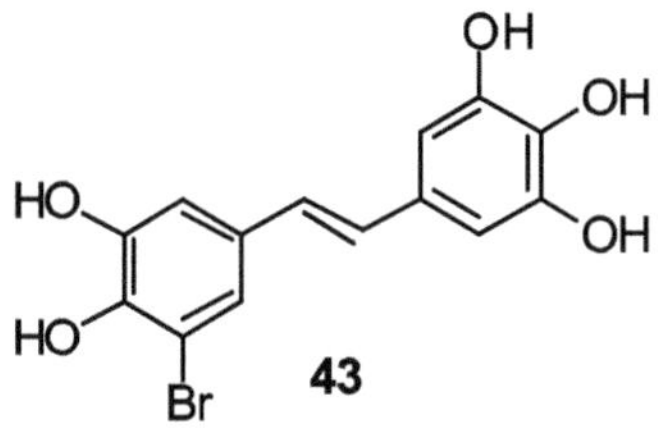
43

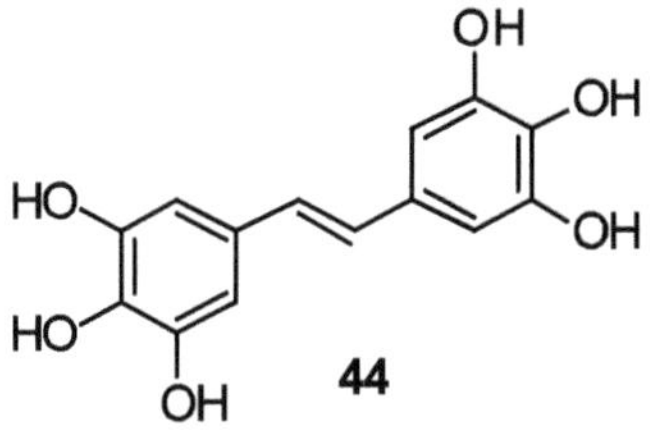
44

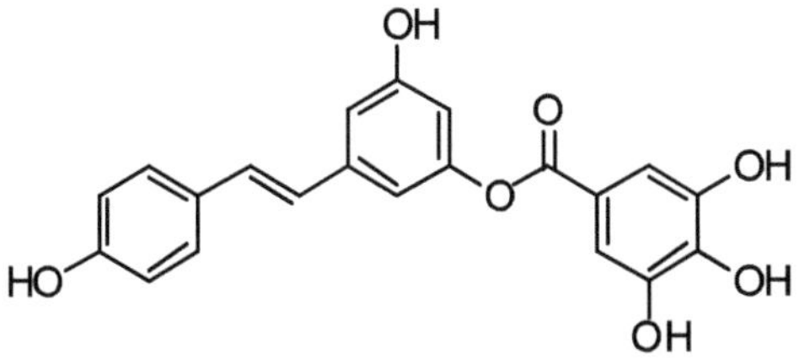
45

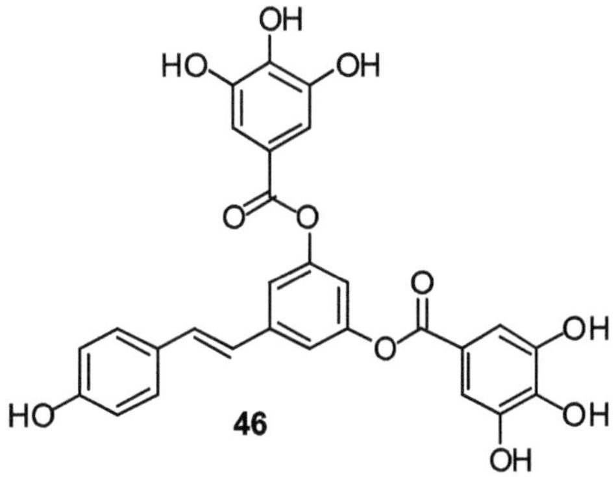
46

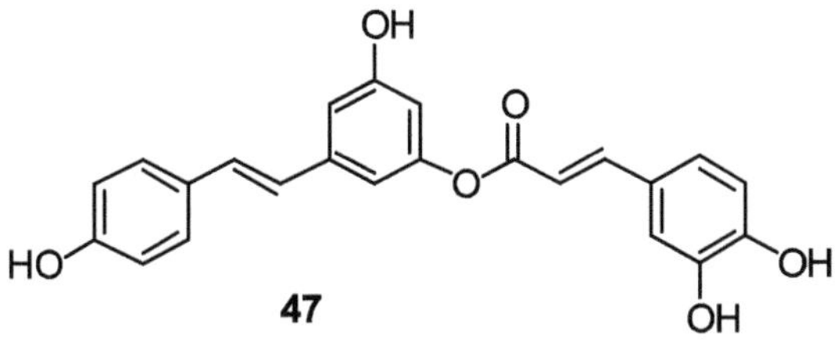
47

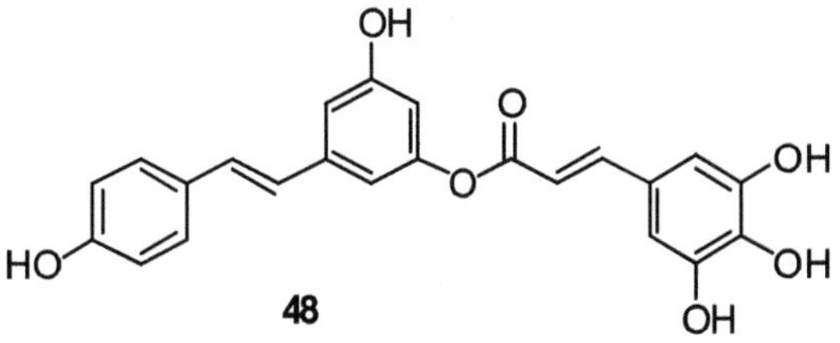
48

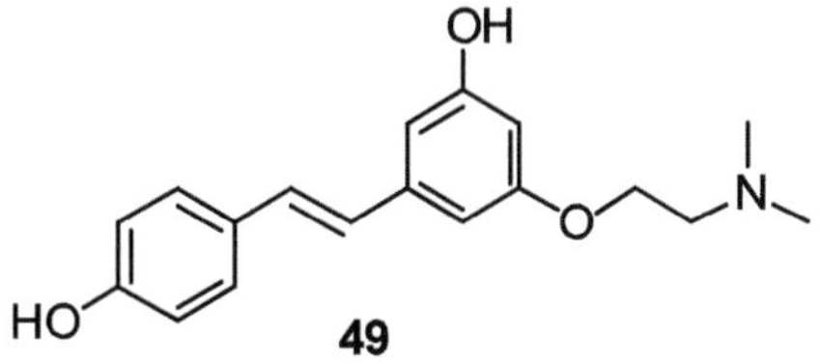
49

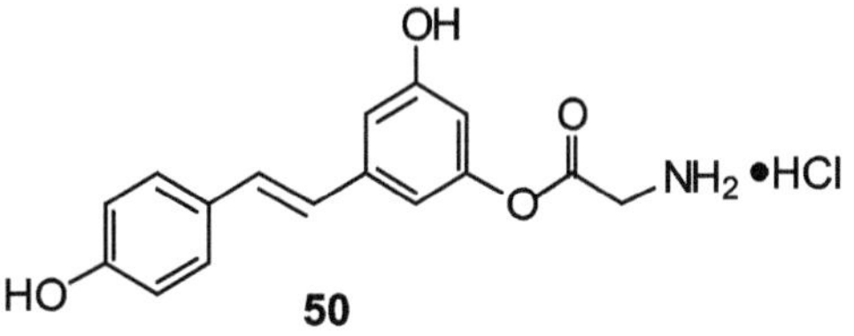
50

Antiinflammatory Activity

Inflammation results from the complex series of actions and reactions triggered by the body's immunological response to tissue damage. Many diseases as well as physical trauma, including surgery, induce inflammatory reactions. These reactions, although necessary to start the healing process, too often create an unbearably painful condition, which may even perpetuate the disease. Several inflammatory mediators, such as, histamine, eicosanoids, platelet activating factor, TNF etc are involved in the inflammation process.

Inflammation is an active part of many chronic disease states. Steroidal drugs like cortisone, and non-steroidal antiinflammatory drugs (NSAID) like phenylbutazone and indomethacin, are used in clinical practice to subdue the inflammation. Some of the antiinflammatory drugs inhibit the lipoxygenase pathway, and the other by cyclooxygenase pathway resulting in different potency and clinical applications for the antiinflammatory drugs. Two of the factors that are very active mediators in the inflammatory process are both derived from the fatty acid, arachidonic acid. These are the leukotrienes, produced by 5-lipoxygenase (5-LOX) and the prostaglandins, produced by cyclooxygenase (COX).

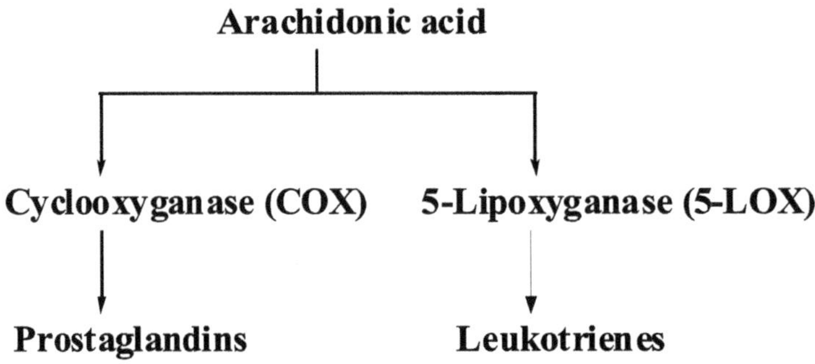

Figure 1.6: Important Mediators of Inflammation

The enzyme cyclooxygenase (COX) catalyzes the first two steps in the biosynthesis of prostaglandins (PGs) from the substrate arachidonic acid. At least two forms of this enzyme exist (Xie *et al.*, 1991). One of these forms, cyclooxygenase-1 (COX-1), is constitutively expressed and is responsible for maintaining normal physiologic function and the prostaglandins produced by this enzyme play a protective role. The second form of the enzyme, cyclooxygenase-2 (COX-2), is an inducible form and its expression is affected by various stimuli such as mitogens, oncogenes, tumor promoters, and growth factors (Fournier and Gordon, 2000). COX-2 is the principal isoform that participates in inflammation, and induction of COX-2 is responsible for the production of PGs at the site of inflammation. Consequently, selective inhibition of COX-2 should have therapeutic actions similar to those of non-steroidal antiinflammatory drugs (NSAIDs), but without gastrointestinal side effects, which are being caused as a consequence of COX-1 inhibition. Several selective COX-2 inhibitors are currently used in the clinics which provide effective treatment of inflammatory disease states such as rheumatoid arthritis and osteoarthritis. Several lines of evidence suggest that selective COX-2 inhibitors may also provide an opportunity for both cancer prevention and therapy. Furthermore, promising *in vitro* data also indicate that treatment with selective COX-2 inhibitors may also reduce the risk of Alzheimers (Giovannini *et al.*, 2003) and Parkinsons disease (Hunot *et al.*, 2004) and may also be effective in the treatment of asthma (Profita *et al.*, 2003).

The antiinflammatory properties of resveratrol (Wadsworth and Koop, 1999) have been attributed to the inhibition of cyclooxygenase (COX-2) (Martinez and Moreno, 2000) and COX-1 enzymes (Jang *et al.*, 1997) via a peroxidase-mediated mechanism (Vayssiere *et al.*, 1997). Resveratrol has been shown to bind to the peroxisome proliferator activated receptor–α (PPAR-α) in murine brain. More recently, the antiinflammatory effects of resveratrol have been associated with inhibition of the transcription factor NF-κB (Manna *et al.*, 2000), possibly mediated via the inhibition of IκB kinase (Holmes-McNary *et al.*, 2000). A second transcription factor, activator protein-1 (AP-1), may also be inhibited by Resveratrol (Manna *et al.*, 2000). NF-κB and AP-1 may be important in the regulation of many genes that are induced via oxidative stress and might in part explain some of the antioxidative properties of resveratrol. The interesting aspect of resveratrol is that, although it inhibits COX-2 and Prostoglandin E-2, it does so by suppressing the action of NF κB, the supreme controller of the inflammatory war.

Anticancer Activity

Cancer is the largest single cause of death in both men and women, claiming over 7 to 8 million lives each year worldwide. Cancer is a group of diseases in which cells are aggressive (grow and divide without respect to normal limits), invasive (invade and destroy adjacent tissues), and sometimes metastatic (spread to other locations in the body). These three malignant properties of cancers differentiate them from benign tumors, which are self-limited in their growth and don't invade or metastasize (although some benign tumor types are capable of becoming malignant). Cancer may affect people at all ages, even fetuses, but risk for the more common varieties tends to increase with age. Cancer causes about 13 per cent of all deaths. According to the American Cancer Society, 7.6 million people died from cancer in the world during 2007. Apart from humans, forms of cancer may affect other animals and plants. Nearly all cancers are caused by abnormalities in the genetic material of the transformed cells. These abnormalities may be due to the effects of carcinogens, such as tobacco smoke, radiation, chemicals, or infectious agents. Other cancer-promoting genetic abnormalities may be randomly acquired through errors in DNA replication, or are inherited, and thus present in all cells from birth. Complex interactions between carcinogens and the host genome may explain why only some develop cancer after exposure to a known carcinogen. New aspects of the genetics of cancer pathogenesis, such as DNA methylation, and micro-RNAs are increasingly being recognized as important.

Chemoprevention, the prevention of cancer by ingestion of chemical agents that reduce the risk of carcinogenesis, is one of the most direct ways to reduce mortality. Epidemiological evidence suggests that long-term inhibition of cyclooxygenase significantly reduces the risk of developing many cancers, and deletion of the gene that encodes COX-2 is protective in a mouse model of colorectal cancer (Oshima *et al.*, 1996). Jang *et al.* (1997) originally proposed that resveratrol inhibits the enzymatic activity of both cylooxygenase enzymes COX-1 and COX-2. An extract derived from *Cassia quinquangulata* Rich. (Leguminosae), collected in Peru, was identified as a potent COX-2 inhibitor, and on the basis of bioassay-guided fractionation, Resveratrol (3, 5, 4'-trihydroxy-*trans*-stilbene) was identified as the active principle. Resveratrol inhibited the tumour-induced neovascularisation required to support solid tumour growth, illustrating its antiangiogenic properties. Resveratrol can modulate the expression and activity of multiple drug-metabolising enzymes. It inhibited various cytochrome P450s (Chan and Delucchi, 2000) and induced expression of phase II drug detoxifying enzymes (Cao and Li, 2004). These activities suggest that resveratrol may reduce the exposure of cells to carcinogens by decreasing carcinogen formation and/or increasing their detoxification. Resveratrol possesses also antiproliferative and pro-apoptotic effects in tumour cell lines (Clement *et al.*, 1998). These effects may be mechanistically linked to its abilities to down-regulate cell cycle proteins and increase apoptosis (Garvin *et al.*, 2006) in tumor models *in vivo*. Resveratrol sensitised tumor cells to apoptosis induced by Tumor necrosis factor-related apoptosis-inducing ligand and this property may explain its pro-apoptotic effects *in vivo*.

Resveratrol has been found to inhibit the proliferation of a variety of human cancer cell lines when added to cells cultured outside the body, including those from breast, prostate, stomach, colon, pancreatic and thyroid cancer. In animal models, oral administration of resveratrol inhibited the development of esophageal, intestinal, and mammary (breast) cancer induced by chemical carcinogens. It is not known whether high intakes of resveratrol can help prevent cancer in humans. Studies on human metabolism of resveratrol suggest that even very high dietary intakes of resveratrol may not result in tissue levels that are high enough to realize most of the protective effects demonstrated in cell culture studies.

Resveratrol has been shown to decrease an elevated prostate-specific antigen in cancer cells. In one study, only four days of treatment with resveratrol reduced prostate-specific antigen levels in prostate cancer cells by 80 per cent (Hsieh *et al.*, 2000; Narayanan *et al.*, 2002). In addition, resveratrol has multiple, antiprostate cancer effects, it can halt the growth of hormone-positive and negative cancers; it works via multiple mechanisms to stop cancer cells from multiplying; it is effective from the earliest to the latest stages of cancer; it can protect DNA from damage; and it may inhibit cancer metastasis. Taking resveratrol in addition to key dietary recommendations can mean a decisive difference in the prognosis for prostate cancer.

Cardio-protectant

Coronary heart disease (CHD) has been and remains a major contributor to mortality in developed countries. The most common form of CHD in the western world is atherosclerosis (AS), especially of the major coronary arteries. Failure to maintain an intact endothelium, as a result of episodic and/or persistent injury and perturbation of the vascular endothelium, promotes formation of fatty streaks which are considered initiation events of atherosclerosis. Cellular constituents contributing to endothelial injury include endothelial cells, monocytes, platelets, and smooth muscle cells. Individuals diagnosed with atherosclerosis face complex, enduring clinical complications and enormous medical costs. Simple and easily compliant prevention and treatment measures are therefore strategic considerations in the management of this vascular disease. Based on known risk factors for CHD, priorities in atherosclerosis prevention should include smoking cessation, blood pressure control, and diet modification.

In recent years, the possible benefits of low to moderate consumption of alcoholic beverages, particularly of red wine, in the prevention of heart disease has received increasing attention and debate in the popular media as well as in the scientific community. Such attention has been prompted by research findings supporting a relationship between red wine consumption and the French paradox. This phenomenon refers to people residing in certain parts of France where red wine is customarily consumed during meals having a low CHD mortality, despite living a lifestyle considered to have comparably high CHD risks, as those in the US and many other developed countries. Studies have reported that the cardioprotective effects of red wine are greater than those attributed solely to ethanol and other types of alcoholic beverages. Epidemiological studies suggest that Mediterranean diets rich in resveratrol are associated with reduced risk of coronary artery disease.

Resveratrol has been found to exert a number of potentially cardioprotective effects *in vitro* (Bays *et al.*, 2005), including the inhibition of platelet aggregation, promotion of vasodilation by enhancing the production of NO and inhibition of inflammatory enzymes. However, the concentrations of resveratrol required to produce these effects are often higher than those that have been measured in human plasma after oral consumption of resveratrol. The results of some animal studies suggest that high oral doses of resveratrol could decrease the risk of thrombosis (clot formation) and atherosclerosis, but at least one study found increased atherosclerosis in animals fed resveratrol. Although its presence in red wine has stimulated a great deal of interest in the potential for resveratrol to prevent cardio–vascular disease.

The effect of free radicals on the arteries is to help, along with cholesterol, to promote the thickening and hardening of the artery walls. Damage to the arteries by free radicals, and the resulting scar tissue, causes the production of even more free radicals and a vicious circle of damage and even more free radical production occurs. The antioxidant action of resveratrol is in the enhancement of the nitric oxide content of the blood. Free radicals can reduce the levels of blood nitric oxide that in turn increases blood pressure. An increase in nitric oxide by appropriate antioxidants can help to reduce blood pressure closer to normal. Resveratrol is more effective in achieving this than any of the vitamin antioxidants, A, C or E. It does so by opening up the arteries and reducing the resistance to blood flow through them. It also helps to prevent blood cells from sticking together and forming clots that can lead to serious cardiovascular problems, and has been found to be effective against a much wider range of chemicals that promote blood clotting than any other anticlotting components of wine.

Antidiabetic Activity

Human body has to maintain the blood glucose level at a very narrow range, which is achieved with the release of insulin and glucagon. The function of glucagon is causing the liver to release glucose from its cells into the blood, for the production of energy. On the other hand, insulin, a hormone that is required to convert sugar, starches, and other food into energy and there by reduces the sugar levels in the blood. Diabetes mellitus is a metabolic disorder wherein the body does not produce or properly uses insulin and it is characterized by constant high levels of blood sugar.

Diabetes is rapidly reaching epidemic proportions and eventually leads to diseases of the coronary arteries, the cerebrovascular system, renal failure, blindness, neurological complications, and premature death. Two forms of Diabetes mellitus, type 1 and type 2, have been identified. Type 1 is primarily due to the autoimmune-mediated destruction of pancreatic cells of the islets, resulting in absolute insulin deficiency. People with type 1 must rely on exogenous insulin to prevent the development of ketoacidosis for survival. Type 2 is characterized by a failure of normal insulin levels to stimulate glucose uptake by tissue cells. People with type 2 are not dependent on exogenous insulin but may eventually become dependent because the pancreatic islet cells fail to compensate for insulin resistance. The incidence of type 1 is low relative to type 2, which accounts for more than 90 per cent of the Diabetes cases globally.

Su *et al.* (2006) have found that resveratrol having significant hypoglycemic and hypolipidemic effects in their experiments on streptozotocin-induced diabetic rats. Silan (2008) has observed that the protective effects of long term Resveratrol treatment on vascular bed of streptozotocin induced diabetic rats. Thus, Resveratrol treatment for 42 days improved blood glucose levels, body weight gain and partially vascular contraction responses against vasoactive agents in Streptozotocin diabetic rats. The mechanism of resveratrol, like glibenclamide, inhibits K^+ channels in the cells of insulinoma cell-lines, leading to an increase in insulin secretion *in vitro*. Resveratrol increased insulin secretion associated with a decline in plasma glucose in normal rats, but not in streptozotocin diabetic rats. Additionally, it was shown that resveratrol increased glucose uptake to tissues without increasing the insulin level in streptozotocin diabetic rats. The antioxidant effect of resveratrol decreased the oxidative-stress related damage in diabetic tissues and made cells function normally.

Antiobese Property

Obesity means excess accumulation of fat in the body. During the past few decades, the prevalence of obesity has risen substantially in developed countries. Across the world obesity is becoming one of the most preventable and modifiable metabolic disorders. There is evidence linking obesity to an increased health risk, raising an appropriate concern that this alarming trend will have major health consequences. Serious conditions such as increased risk of type 2 diabetes mellitus, coronary heart disease, hypertension, and cancer, higher overall mortality rate and decreased lifespan have been associated with obesity. Morbid obesity can cause a decrease in life expectancy among young adults by as much as 5–20 years. In addition to being a primary health concern, obesity is also becoming a major economic problem with significant consequences for health services worldwide. During the last 20 years beneficial trends have been evident in many cardiovascular disease risk factors including smoking, relative saturated fat intakes and cholesterol levels. Unfortunately, the parallel increase in adverse factors such as increased energy density of foods and reduced exercise, resulting in obesity, has counter balanced or may have overwhelmed these benefits causing a growing prevalence of obesity-associated syndrome X. The awareness of the health consequences of overweight and obesity, the benefits of modest weight loss and the frequent failure of lifestyle interventions for both weight loss and weight loss maintenance has led to the search for effective antiobesity treatment.

Evidence suggests that most obese individuals have an inappropriate control of their food intake rather than a metabolic defect in energy expenditure. This concept has turned attention toward drugs which reduce appetite and so decrease energy intake as compared to thermoregulatory agents which increase energy expenditure.

Researchers have found that resveratrol protected laboratory mice fed a high fat diet from having health problem associated with obesity by mimicking the effects of calorie restriction. University of Ulm in Germany researchers Fischer-Posovszky *et al.* (The endocrine society News, Friday June 10, 2005) wanted to know if resveratrol exert its antiobesity effects by changing the size or function of the fat cells. For the study, the German team used a strain of human fat cell precursors known as pre-adipocytes which in the body go on to develop into mature fat cells. The researchers found that Resveratrol prevented the pre-fat cells from increasing in the number and being converted into mature fat cells and it also hindered fat storage and also resveratrol reduced cytokines which may be linked to the development of obesity-related disorders such as diabetes and clogged coronary arteries and increased the production of a protein called adiponectin, which is known to decrease risk of heart attack and unfortunately its production is reduced by obesity. Fischer-Posovszky *et al.* (2005) found that resveratrol has antiobesity properties by exerting its effects directly on the fat cells, thus, resveratrol might help to prevent development of obesity or might be suited to treating obesity.

A Phytoestrogen

Epidemiological data and clinical studies provide compelling evidence to indicate that oestrogen therapy after the menopause offers protection from cardiovascular disease and osteoporosis, improves cognitive function and relieves menopausal symptoms associated with acute ovarian oestrogen loss. However, postmenopausal women are faced with a dilemma: oestrogen use may protect against CHD and osteoporosis but may increase the risk of breast and endometrial cancer. These lingering concerns about the potential long-term risks associated with hormone replacement therapy (HRT) preparations have stimulated interest in estrogen-like compounds. These compounds would offer all the benefits of oestrogen therapy without the accompanying risks. Phytoestrogens are compounds found in various plants and foods that have similar effects as estrogen. Phytoestrogens are dietary nonsteroidal compounds that have been speculated to offer protection against estrogen-dependent cancers or heart disease. Most phytoestrogens bind to estrogen receptors with much lower affinity than 17 β-estradiol and are weakly estrogenic. The decreased incidence of breast cancer in Asian women who consume a high soy diet containing a significant amount of isoflavones has been associated with phytoestrogens capable of antagonizing the effects of 17 β-estradiol. Dietary consumption of phytoestrogens has become a common treatment for menopausal symptoms (Umland *et al.*, 2000)

The researchers (Henry and Witt, 2002) from Department of Psychology, Binghamton University demonstrated that resveratrol affects reproductive physiology in female Sprague–Dawley rats. Resveratrol exposure reduced overall body weight, increased ovarian weight, and disrupted estrous cyclicity. However, in ovariectomized females resveratrol (10–1000 mg) did not induce estrous behaviors, such as those typically observed with exogenous 17 β-estradiol benzoate treatment, but subtly affected other aspects of social behavior. Furthermore, resveratrol preexposure in ovariectomised females had no detectable effect on subsequent 17 β-estradiol benzoate-induced sociosexual behaviors. These studies suggest that resveratrol may act as an estrogen agonist in gonadally intact females, but has little effect on 17 β-estradiol benzoate inducible behaviors at doses tested in ovariectomized females.

Gehm *et al.* (1997) of Northwestern University Medical School, Chicago have found that resveratrol is a phytoestrogen and it is chemically very similar to the synthetic estrogenic agent, diethylstilbestrol. These similarities in the chemical structures of these two agents are the key to recognizing the usefulness of products containing resveratrol in the relief of menopausal symptoms. Recently, resveratrol was shown to compete with 17β-estradiol for estrogen receptors *in vitro* (Gehm *et al.*, 2004). Bhat and Pezzuto (2001) of University of Illinois at Chicago explored that resveratrol exhibits antiestrogenic property with Human Endometrial adenocarcinoma (Ishikawa) Cells.

Neuroprotectant

Due to the high rate of oxygen consumption in the brain, and especially low levels of antioxidant defense enzymes, this organ is particularly susceptible of free radical damage. Most of the protective biological actions associated with resveratrol have been associated with its intrinsic radical scavenger properties and also investigated the possibility of other indirect pathways by which resveratrol can exert its neuroprotective abilities. The researchers (Tredici *et al.*, 1999), have specifically tested whether heme oxygenase neuroprotective enzyme could be stimulated after resveratrol treatment. Using primary neuronal cultures, resveratrol was able to significantly induce heme oxygenase 1, whereas vehicle control showed no effect. No detectable toxicity was quantified. It is well established that after stroke significant levels of intracellular heme levels increase. The source of free heme comes mainly from several heme-containing enzymes. Heme (iron-protoporphyrin IX) is a pro-oxidant and its rapid degradation by heme oxygenase is believed to be protective. Moreover, the generation of heme metabolites can also have their own intrinsic cellular properties. All together, increased heme oxygenase activity by resveratrol is a unique pathway by which this compound can exert its neuroprotective actions (Tredici *et al.*, 1999)

Parkinson's disease (PD) is a common progressive neurodegenerative disease which is characterized by muscle rigidity, akinesia, and resting tremor. The characteristic pathological and biochemical changes are severe loss of dopamine (DA) cell bodies in the substantia nigra (SN) and a severe decrease of dopamine concentration in the striatum (nigrostriatal pathway). Accumulating evidence indicates that multiple factors, including genetic and environmental ones, contribute to acceleration of dopaminergic neurodegeneration in this neurological disorder. Free radical damage has been shown to have a significant impact on the pathogenesis of parkinson's disease. Dopamine is a relatively unstable molecule, subject to hydroxyl radical attack, that can induce free radicals both from within the cell as well as from outside the cell. At present, the most useful neurotoxin used to induce Parkinsonism is 1-methyl-4-phenyl-1, 2, 3, 6-tetrahydropyridine (MPTP). MPTP is metabolically converted to 1-methyl-4-phenyl pyridinium (MPP+) which interferes with mitochondrial respiration via inhibition of mitochondrial complex I, thereby triggering dopaminergic neurodegeneration that leads to Parkinsonism.

A new indication of resveratrol's neuroprotective capacity comes from a study by researchers in Quebec (Blanchet *et al.,* 2008), who investigated its effects on mice in which a condition similar to Parkinson's disease had been induced. In mice, a Parkinson-like condition can be induced by a neurotoxic compound called MPTP (1-methyl-4-phenyl-1, 2, 3, 6-tetrahydropyridine) which reduces dopamine levels and the numbers of dopaminergic neurons in the *substantia nigra*. Because resveratrol is a phytoestrogen and the researchers wanted to observe its effects independently of those of other phytoestrogens, which are known to modify the course of Parkinson's disease. What they found, when they examined the mouse brains at autopsy 5 days after the MPTP treatment, was that the resveratrol pretreatment maintained normal dopamine levels in the *substantia nigra* and that it provided substantial (but not complete) protection against the loss of neurons. This indicates a strong neuroprotective effect, in line with the results of other studies. Overall, resveratrol is an efficient protective molecule against MPTP-induced brain lesions and may serve as a complementary and/or preventive therapy in neurodegenerative diseases. (Blanchet *et al.,* 2008). Karlsson *et al.* (2000) have investigated the potential neuroprotective properties of the resveratrol by electron paramagnetic resonance (EPR) spin-trapping technique. The ability of resveratrol to protect rat embryonic mesencephalic tissue, rich in dopaminergic neurones, from the prooxidant *tert*butyl hydroperoxide. The main radicals detected in cell suspensions were the *tert*-butoxyl radical and the methyl radical, indicating the one-electron reduction of the peroxide followed by a β-scission reaction. The appearance of EPR signals from the trapped radicals preceded the onset of cytotoxicity, which was almost exclusively necrotic in nature. The inclusion of resveratrol in incubations resulted in the marked protection of cells from *tert*-butyl hydroperoxide. In parallel spin-trapping experiments, they were able to demonstrate the scavenging of radicals by resveratrol, which involved direct competition between resveratrol and the spin trap for reaction with the radicals (Karlson *et al.,* 2000).

Studies show that resveratrol may be a key compound that can halt this relentless, neurodegenerative process, especially for those with Alzheimer's disease or those at risk. (Jang and Surh, 2003). Resveratrol has been shown to protect the brain against oxidative stress, and in conjunction with other antioxidants like vitamins C and E, has been proven to provide an even greater measure of brain cell protection than with any single antioxidant alone (Chanvitayapongs *et al.,*1997).

Calorie Restriction Mimic

Caloric restriction (CR) retards several aspects of the aging process in mammals, including age-related mortality, tumorigenesis, physiological decline and the establishment of age-related transcriptional profiles. Caloric restriction has been shown in several studies to lower fasting plasma glucose concentration and serum low-density lipoprotein cholesterol, to decrease insulin resistance, fat mass and the levels of inflammatory markers. The wide scope of these actions, and the profound metabolic and hormonal shifts induced by caloric restriction has led to efforts at identifying natural or synthetic compounds that mimic the effects of caloric restriction in the absence of over metabolic and endocrine disturbances or reduced caloric intake. Because most age-related diseases are likely to be secondary to the aging process itself, the discovery of such compounds could have a profound public health impact by reducing disease incidence and possibly extending the quality and length of the human lifespan. Therefore, one major interest is to develop caloric restriction mimics to provide all of the healthy physiological, metabolic and hormonal effects of caloric restriction without the need to reduce food intake.

Dr. Guarente decided to study the basis of aging, and then considered an unpromising field of research. He spent four years searching for strains of yeast, a common laboratory organism that lived longer than others. By 1997, he and Sinclair, who worked in his laboratory at the time, had discovered the reason for the new strains' longevity. It centered on a gene called sir2, for silent information regulator 2. Dr. Guarente had found that the yeast which live longer, because of starvation, it is the sir2 gene that modulates the response. His research then started to fuse with longstanding work on caloric restriction as he and others showed that starvation is sensed by sir2, which triggers the cellular changes that lead to increased life span.

The Sir2 family of proteins (sirtuins) are NAD^+-dependent protein deacetylases that couple the cleavage of NAD^+ and deacetylation of protein substrates to form nicotinamide, the deacetylated product, and a novel metabolite, 2_-*O*-acetyl-ADP-ribose (*O*AADPr)1 (Imai *et al.*, 2000; Tanner *et al.*, 2000; Jackson and Denu, 2002). This family of proteins is evolutionarily conserved, with five homologs in yeast (ySir 2 and HST 1–4) and seven in humans (SIRT 1–7) (Frye, 2000). The founding member of this family, y Sir 2, is essential for gene silencing at the three silent loci in yeast (Aparicio *et al.*, 1991; Strahl-Bolsinger *et al.*, 1997; Gottschling *et al.*, 1990; Rine and Herskowitz, 1987; Shou *et al.*, 1999, 2001; Bryk *et al.*, 1997; Fritze *et al.*, 1997; Smith and Boeke, 1997; Loo and Rine, 1995). Besides gene silencing, Sir2 proteins are important for many processes, such as cell cycle regulation (Dryden *et al.*, 2003), fatty acid metabolism and life span extension (Starai *et al.*, 2002; Tissenbaum and Guarente, 2001; Sinclair and Guarente, 1997). SIRT 1, the most extensively studied human homolog, mediates p53-dependent processes (Luo *et al.*, 2001; Langley *et al.*, 2002), transcription regulation (Motta *et al.*, 2004) muscle differentiation, adipogenesis (Picard *et al.*, 2004), protection from axonal degeneration (Araki *et al.*, 2004), and life span extension (Howitz *et al.*, 2003; Wood *et al.*, 2004)

Howitz *et al.* (2003) took the human version of sirtuin, the enzyme produced by the sir2 gene, and devise a test to identify when the enzyme was activated. Then the authors have screened a large group compounds to explore that any compound promotes the activity of sirtuins. The results of the experiments revealed that two polyphenolic compounds, both having similar chemical structure. Further screening of polyphenols for sirtuin modulation led to the discovery of resveratrol as the most active compound. Sinclair said he was amazed "that in an unbiased screen we pulled out something already associated with health benefits."

Recent studies show that resveratrol activates molecular pathways involved in life-span extension. Extension of longevity has now been demonstrated in yeast, worms, flies, fish, and mice. While this effect has not yet been demonstrated in humans, research is ongoing and looks promising. Research with mice also demonstrates that resveratrol mitigates the harmful effects of high calorie diets, including metabolic changes resembling diabetes, liver and heart damage, and premature death. Resveratrol may enhance health and support longevity via multiple mechanisms, including potent antioxidant effects, enhancement of cellular energy production and influence of gene expression pattern in a manner similar to caloric restriction.

Conclusions

Resveratrol, a commonly available polyphenol in various foods and beverages, has been found to play a vital role in regulating the cellular processes that maintains the health and prevents the disease. As a constituent of redwine, resveratrol was attributed as one of the factors of 'French Paradox'. Resveratrol exhibits strong antioxidant, anticancer, antiinflammatory and cardioprotective properties. Resveratrol modulates the sirtuin family of proteins and mimics the advantages of calorie restriction and thus offering the potential of extending the life span and healthy aging. It is a phytoestrogen and reduces the menopausal problems in women. In a society that is habituated to eat fatty foods and lack of exercise, the impending problems of obesity can be partly avoided by the supplementation with resveratrol. It is non-toxic and large quantities can be made available by chemical synthesis. The ongoing research on resveratrol worldwide is set to unravel further the advantages of resveratrol, the wonder molecule.

Acknowledgements

The authors thank Dr C. Satyanarayana and the other members of management of Aptuit Laurus for the interest in nutraceuticals and encouragement.

References

Aaviksaar,A., Haga, M., Kuzina, K., Pussa, T., Raal, A., and Tsoupras, G. (2003). Hydroxystilbenes in the roots of *Rheum rhaponticum*. *Proceedings of the Estonian Academy of Sciences*, 52: 99-107.

Amorati, R., Lucarini M., Mugnaini, V., Pedulli, G.F., Roberti, M., and Pizzirani, D. (2004). Antioxidant activity of hydroxystilbene derivatives in homogeneous solution. *Journal of Organic Chemistry*, 69: 7101-7107.

Andrabi, A. S., Spina, G. M., Lorenz, P., Ebmeyer, U., Wolf, G., and Horn, T. F. W. (2004). Oxyresveratrol (trans-2,3',4,5'-tetrahydroxystilbene) is neuroprotective and inhibits the apoptotic cell death in transient cerebral ischemia. *Brain Research*, 1017: 98-107.

Andrus, M.B., Liu, J., Meredith, E.L., and Nartey, E. (2003). Synthesis of resveratrol using a direct decarbonylative Heck approach from resorcylic acid. *Tetrahedron Letters*, 44: 4819-4822.

Aparicio, O.M., Billington, B.L., and Gottschling, D.E. (1991). Modifiers of position effect are shared between telomeric and silent mating-type loci in *S. cerevisiae*. *Cell*, 66: 1279-1287.

Araki, T., Sasaki, Y., and Milbrandt, J. (2004). Increased nuclear NAD biosynthesis and SIRT1 activation prevent axonal degeneration. *Science*, 305: 1010-1013.

Baur, A. J., and Sinclair, A.D. (2006). Therapeutic potential of resveratrol: the *in vivo* evidence. *Nature Reviews-Drug Discovery*, 5: 493-506

Bays, H., Abate, N., and Chandalia, M. (2005). Adiposopathy: sick fat causes high blood sugar, high blood pressure and dyslipidemia. *Future Cardiology*, 1: 39-59.

Bhat, K.P.L., and Pezzuto, J.M. (2001). Resveratrol exhibits cytostatic and antiestrogenic properties with human endometrial adenocarcinoma (Ishikawa) cells. Cancer Research, 61: 6137-6144.

Bhakuni, D.S., and Chaturvedi, R. (1984). Chemical constituents of *Crotalaria madurensis*. *Journal of Natural Products*, 47: 585-591.

Blanchet, J., Longpre, F., Bureau, G., Morissette, M., DiPaolo, T., Bronchti, G., and Martinoli, M.G. (2008). Resveratrol, a red wine polyphenol, protects dopaminergic neurons in MPTP-treated mice. *Progress in neuropsychopharmacology and biological psychiatry*, 32: 1243-1250.

Bryk, M., Banerjee, M., Murphy, M., Knudsen, K.E., Garfinkel, D. J., and Curcio, M.J. (1997).

Transcriptional silencing of Ty1 elements in the RDN1 locus of yeast. *Genes Development*, 11: 255-269

Castro, O.; Lopez, J., Vergara, A., Stermitz, F.R., Gardner, D.R. (1986). Isoflavones and a Stilbene from Wood of the Decay-Resistant Tropical Tree *Diphysa robinioides*. *Journal of Natural Products*, 49: 680-683.

Cao, Z., and Li, Y. (2004).Potent induction of cellular antioxidants and phase 2 enzymes by resveratrol in cardiomyocytes: protection against oxidative and electrophilic injury. *European Journal of Pharmacology*, 489: 39-48.

Chanvitayapongs, S., Draczynska-Lusiak, B., and Sun, A.Y. (1997). Amelioration of oxidative stress by antioxidants and resveratrol in PC12 cells. *Neuro Report*, 8: 1499-1502

Chan, W.K., and Delucchi, A.B. (2000). Resveratrol, a red wine constituent, is a mechanism-based inactivator of cytochrome P450 3A4. Life Sciences, 67: 3103-3112.

Chine, G.C.I. (2006). Methods for preparing Resveratrol. CN 1775721.

Chun, Y. J., Ryu, S.Y., Jeong, T. C., and Kim, M. Y. (2001). Mechanism-based inhibition of human cytochrome P450 1A1 by Rhapontigenin. *Drug Metabolism and Disposition*, 29: 389-393.

Clement, M.V., Hirpara, J.L., Chawdhury, S.H., and Pervaiz, S. (1998). Chemopreventive agent resveratrol, a natural product derived from grapes, triggers CD95 signaling-dependent apopotosis in human tumor cells. Blood, 92: 996-1002.

Cunningham, J., Haslam, E., and Haworth, R.D. (1963). The Constitution of piceatannol. *Journal of Chemical Society*, 2875-2883.

Debasis Bagchi (2000). *Resveratrol and Human Health*; Keats Publishing, NTC/Contemporary Publishing Group Inc., Illinois, USA.

Dryden, S.C., Nahhas, F.A., Nowak, J.E., Goustin, A.S., and Tainsky, M.A. (2003). Role for humar SIRT2 NAD-Dependent deacetylase activity in control of mitotic exit in the cell cycle. *Molecular and Cellular Biology*, 23: 3173-3185.

Erdtman, H.; and Ronlán, A. (1969). Phenol Dehydrogenation. Part 11. Intramolecular Oxidative Coupling of Dihydropiceatannol. *Acta Chemica Scandinavica*, 23: 249-254

Fischer-Posovszky, (2005). Red wine's resveratrol may help battle obesity.

The Endocrine Society Newsroom (Friday, June 10, 2005).

Frankel, E. N., Waterhouse, A.L., and Kinsella, J.E. (1993). Inhibition of human LDL oxidation by resveratrol. *The Lancet*, 341: 1103-1104.

Fournier, D.B., and Gordon, G.B. (2000). COX-2 and colon cancer: potential targets for chemoprevention. *Journal of Cellular Biochemistry. Supplement*, 34: 97-102.

Fritze, C.E., Verschueren, K., Strich, R., and Esposito, R.E.(1997). Direct evidence for *SIR2* modulation of chromatin structure in yeast rDNA. *The EMBO Journal*, 16 : 6495–6509.

Frye, R. A. (2000). Phylogenetic Classification of Prokaryotic and Eukaryotic Sir2-like Proteins. *Biochemical and Biophysical Research Communications*, 27: 793-798.

Gangaraju, G., Ramaraju, G., Subbaraju, G.V., and Venkateswarlu, S. (2006). Resveratrol Analogues. *US 7026518 B2*, April 11.

Garvin, S., Ollinger, K., and Dabrosin, C. (2006). Resveratrol induces apoptosis and inhibits angiogenesis in human breast cancer xenografts *in vivo*. *Cancer Letters*, 231: 113-122.

Gehm, B.D., McAndrews, J.M., Chien, P,Y., and Jameson, J.L. (1997). Resveratrol, a polyphenolic compound found in grapes and wine, is an agonist for the estrogen?receptor. *Proceedings of the National Academy of Sciences of the United States of America*, 94: 14138-14143.

Gehm, B.D., Levenson, A.S., Liu, H., Lee, E.J., Amundsen, B.M., Cushman, M., Jordan, V.C., and Jameson, J.L. (2004). Estrogenic effects of resveratrol in breast cancer cells expressing mutant and wild-type estrogen receptors: role of AF-1 and AF-2. *Journal of steroid biochemistry and molecular biology*, 88: 223-234.

Giovannini, M.G., Scali C., Prosperi, C., Bellucci, A., Pepeu, G., and Casamenti, F. (2003). Experimental brain inflammation and neurodegeneration as model of Alzheimer's disease: protective effects of selective COX-2 inhibitors. *International Journal of Immunopathology and Pharmacology*, 16: 31-40.

Gottschling, D.E., Aparicio, O.M., Billington, B.L., and Zakian, V. A. (1990). Position effect at *S. cerevisiae* telomeres: Reversible repression of Pol II transcription. *Cell*, 63: 751–762.

Gromova, A.S., Tyukavkina, N.A., Lutskii, V.I., Kalabin, G.A., and Kushnarev, D.F. (1975). Hydroxystilbenes of the inner bark of *Pinus sibirica*. *Chemistry of Natural Compounds*, 11: 715-719.

Guiso, M., Marra, C., and Farina, A. (2002). A new efficient resveratrol synthesis. *Tetrahedron Letters*, 43: 597-598.

Harborne, J. B., Baxter, H., Moss, G. P., 1999: Phytochemical dictionary. A handbook of bioactive compounds from plants. 2nd edn., Taylor and Francis, London, UK.

Henry, L.A., and Witt, D.M. (2002). Resveratrol: Phytoestrogen effects on reproductive physiology and behavior in female rats. *Hormones and Behavior*, 41: 220-228.

Hibasami, H., Takagi, K., Ishii, T., Tsuiikawa, M., Imai, N., and Honda, I. (2007). Induction of apopotosis by rhapontin having stilbene moiety, a component of rhubarb (*Rheum officinale* Baillon) in human stomach cancer Kato III cells. *Oncology Reports*, 18: 347-351.

Hickman, J.C., ed. (1993). The Jepan Manual: Higher Plants of California, University of California Press, Berkeley.

Hitchcock, C. L. and Cronquist. A. (1964). Vascular Plants of the Pacific Northwest. Part 2: Salicaceae to Saxifragaceae, University of Washington Press, Seattle.

Holmes-McNary, M., and Baldwin, A.S. Jr. (2000). Chemopreventive properties of *trans*-Resveratrol are associated with inhibition of activation of IκB kinase. *Cancer Research*, 60 : 3477-3483.

Howitz, K. T., Bitterman, K.J., Cohen, H.Y., Lamming, D.W. Lavu, S., Wood, J.G., Zipkin, R.E., Chung, P., Kisielewski, A., Zhang, L.L., Scherer, B., and Sinclair, D.A. (2003). Small molecule activators of sirtuins extend *Saccharomyces cerevisiae* life span, *Nature*, 425: 191-196.

Hsieh, T.C., and Wu, J.M. (2000). Grape-derived chemopreventive agent resveratrol decreases prostate-specific antigen (PSA) expression in LNCaP cells by an androgen receptor (AR)-independent mechanism. *Anticancer Research*, 20: 225–228.

Hunot, S., Vila, M., Teismann, P., Davis, R.J., Hirsch, E.C., Przedborski, S., Rakic, P., and Flavell, R.A. (2004). JNK-mediated induction of cyclooxygenase 2 is required for neurodegeneration in a mouse model of Parkinson's disease. *Proceedings of the National Academy of Sciences of the United States of America*, 101: 665-670.

Imai, S., Armstrong, C. M., Kaeberlein, M., and Guarente, L. (2000). Transcriptional silencing and longevity protein Sir2 is an NAD-dependent histone deacetylase p795. *Nature*, 403: 795–800

Jackson, M.D., and Denu, J.M. (2002). Structural identification of 2'–and 3'-*O*-Acetyl-ADP-ribose as novel metabolites derived from the Sir2 family of β-NAD$^+$-dependent histone/protein deacetylases. *Journal of Biological Chemistry*, 277: 18535-18544

Jang, J.H., and Surh, Y.J. (2003). Protective effect of resveratrol on β-amyloid-induced oxidative PC12 cell death. *Free radical biology and Medicine*, 34: 1100-1110.

Jang, M., Cai, L., Udeani, G. O., Slowing, K.V., Thomas, C.F., Beecher, C.W., Fong, H.H., Farnsworth, N.R., Kinghorn, A.D., Mehta, R.G., Moon, R.C., and Pezzuto, J.M. (1997). Cancer chemopreventive activity of resveratrol, a natural product derived from grapes. Science, 275: 218-220.

Jayatilake, G.S., Jayasuriya, H., Lee, E.S., Koonchanok, M.N., Geahlen, L.R., Ashendel, C.L., McLaughlin, J.L., and Chang, C.J. (1993). Kinase inhibitors from *Polygonum cuspidatum*. *Journal of Natural Products*, 56: 1805-1810.

Jeffery, T., and Ferber, B. (2003). One-pot palladium-catalyzed highly chemo-, region-, and stereoselective synthesis of trans-stilbene derivatives. A concise and convenient synthesis of resveratrol. *Tetrahedron Letters*, 44 : 193-197.

Juliawaty, L.D., Kitajima, M., Takayama, H., Achmad, S.A., and Aimi, N. (2000). A new type of stilbene-related secondary metabolite, idenburgene, from *Cryptocarya idenburgensis*. *Chemical and Pharmaceutical Bulletin*, 48: 1726-1728.

Karlson, J., Emgard, M., Brundin, P., and Burkitt, M.J. (2000). *Trans*-resveratrol protects embryonic mesencephalic cells from tert-butyl hydroperoxide : electron param. *Journal of Neurochenistry*, 75:141-150.

Kerem, Z., Regev-Shoshani, G., Flaishman, M.A., and Sivan, L. (2003). Resveratrol and two monomethylated stilbenes from Israeli *Rumex bucephalophorus* and their antioxidant potential. *Journal of Natural Products*, 66: 1270-1272.

Kittisak, L., Kanokporn, S. and Kanyawim, K. (2002). Flavonoids and stilbenoids with COX-1 and COX-2 inhibitory activity from *Dracaena loureiri*. *Planta Medica*, 68: 841-843.

Kittisak Likhitwitayawuid, (2008). Stilbenes with tyrosinase inhibitory activity. *Current Science*, 94 : 44-52.

Langley, E., Pearson, M., Faretta, M., Bauer, U.M., Frye, R.A., Minucci, S., Pelicci, P.G., and Kouzarides, T. (2002). Human SIR2 deacetylates p53 and antagonizes PML/p53-induced cellular senescence. *The EMBO Journal*, 21: 2383-2396.

Lee, S.K., Lee, H. J., Min, H. Y., Park, E. J., Lee, K. M., Ahn, Y. H., Cho, Y.J., and Pyee, J. H. (2005). Antibacterial and antifungal activity of pinosylvin, a constituent of pine. *Fitoterapia*, 76: 258-260.

Loo, S., and Rine, J.(1995). Silencing and heritable domains of gene expression. *Annual Review of Cell and Developmental Biology*, 11: 519-548.

Losa, G. A. (2003). Resveratrol modulates apoptosis and oxidation in human blood mononuclear cells. *European Journal of Clinical Investigation*, 33: 818-823.

Luo, J., Nikolaev, A.Y., Imai, S., Chen, D., Su, F., Shiloh, A., Guarente, L., and Gu W. (2001). Negative control of p53 by SIR-2 α promotes cell survival under stress. *Cell*, 107: 137-148.

Manna,S.K. Mukhopadhyay, A., and Aggarwal, B.B. (2000). Resveratrol suppresses TNF-induced activation of nuclear transcription factors NF-κB, activator protein-1, and apoptosis: potential role of reactive oxygen intermediates and lipid peroxidation. *Journal of Immunology*, 164: 6509-6519.

Martinez, J., and Moreno, J.J. (2000). Effect of resveratrol, a natural polyphenolic compound, on reactive oxygen species and prostaglandin production. *Biochemical Pharmacology*, 59: 865-870.

Matsuda, H., Kageura, T., Morikawa, T., Toguchida, I., Harima, S., and Yoshikawa, M. (2000). Effects of stilbene constituents from rhubarb on nitric oxide production in lipopolysaccharide-activated macrophages. *Bioorganic and Medicinal Chemistry Letters*, 10: 323-327.

Matsuda, H., Tewtrakul, S., Morikawa, T., and Yoshikawa, M. (2004). Antiallergic activity of stilbenes from Korean rhubarb (*Rheum undulatum* L.): structure requirements for inhibition of antigen-induced degranulation and their effects on the release of TNF-α and IL-4 in RBL-2H3 cells. *Bioorganic and Medicinal Chemistry*, 12: 4871-4876.

Meier, H., and Dullweber, U. (1996). Bis(stilbenyl)squaraines-Novel pigments with extended conjugation. *Tetrahedron Letters*, 37: 1191-1194.

Mikstacka, R., Przybyiska, D., Rimando, A. M., and Baer-Dubowska, W. (2007). Inhibition of human recombinant cytochromes P450 CYP1A1 and CYP1B1 by *trans*-resveratrol methyl ethers. *Molecular Nutrition and Food Research*, 51: 517-524.

Motta, M.C., Diyecha, N., Lemieux, M., Kamel, C., Chen, D., Gu, W., Bultsma, Y., McBurney, M., and Guarente, L. (2004). Mammalian SIRT1 represses forkhead transcription factors. *Cell*, 116: 551-563.

Narayanan, B..A., Narayanan, N..K., Stoner, G..D., and Bullock, B..P. (2002). Interactive gene expression pattern in prostate cancer cells exposed to phenolic antioxidants. *Life Sciences*, 70: 1821-1839.

Ohguchi, K., Tanaka, T., Iliya, I.,Ito, T.,Iinuma, M., Matsumoto, K., Akao, Y., and Nozawa, Y. (2003). Gnetol as a potent tyrosinase inhibitor from genus gnetum. *Bioscience, Biotechnology and Biochemistry*, 67: 663-665.

Oshima, M., Dinchuk, J.E., Kargman, S.L., Oshima, H., Hancock, B., Kwong, E., Trzaskos, J.M., Evans, F.J., and Taketo, M.M. (1996). Suppression of intestinal polyposis in *Apc*^{D716} knockout mice by inhibition of Cyclooxygenase 2 (COX-2). *Cell*, 87: 803-809.

Picard, F., Kurtey, M., Chung, N., Topark-Ngram,A., Senawong, T., Machado de Oliveira, R., Leid, M., McBurney, M.W., and Guarente, L. (2004). Sirt1 promotes fat mobilization in wihite adipocytes by repressing PPAR-γ. *Nature*, 429: 771-776.

Potter, G.A., Patterson, L.H., Wanogho, E., Perry, P.J., Butler, P.C., Ijaz, T., Ruparelia, K.C., Lamb, J.H., Farmer, P.B., Stanley, L.A., and Burke, M.D. (2002). The cancer preventative agent resveratrol is converted to the anticancer agent piceatannol by the cytochrome P450 enzyme. *British Journal of Cancer*, 86: 774-778.

Profita, M., Sala, A., Bonanno, A., Riccobono, L., Siena, L., Melis, R.M., Giorgi, D.R., Mirabella, F., Gjomarkaj M., Bonsignore, G., and Vignola, M.A. (2003). Increased prostaglandin E2 concentrations and cyclooxygenase-2 expression in asthmatic subjects with sputum eosinophilia. *Journal of Allergy and Clinical Immunology*, 112: 709-716.

Rimando, A.G., Cuendet, M., Desmarchelier, D., Mehta, R.G., Pezzuto, J.M., and Duke, S.O. (2002). Cancer chemopreventive and antioxidant activities of Pterostibene, a naturally occurring analogue of resveratrol. *Journal of Agricultural And Food Chemistry*, 50: 3453-3457.

Rine, J., and Herskowitz, Ira. (1987). Four Genes Responsible for a Position Effect on Expression From *HML* and *HMR* in *Saccharomyces cerevisiae. Genetics*,116: 9-22.

Roberti, M., Pizzirnai, D., Simoni, D., Rondanin, R., Baruchello, R., Bonora, C., Buscemi, F., Grimaudo, S., and Tolomeo, M. (2003). Synthesis and Biological Evaluation of Resveratrol and Analogues as Apoptosis-Inducing Agents. *Journal of Medicinal Chemistry*, 46: 3546-3554.

Romero-Perez, A.I., Ibem-gomez, M., Lamuela-Raventos, R.M., and Torre-Boronat, M.C. (1999). Piceid, the major resveratrol derivative in grape juices. *Journal of Agricultural and Food Chemistry*, 47: 1533-1536.

Sato, M., Suzuki, Y., Okuda, T., amd Yokotsuka, K. (1997). Contents of Resveratrol, Piceid, and their isomers in commercially available wines made from Grapes cultivated in Japan. *Bioscience, Biotechnology and Biochemistry*, 61:1800-1805.

Shibutani, S., Igarashi, K., Samejima, M., and Saburi, Y. (2001). Inhibition of Trichoderma cellulose activity by a stilbene glucoside from *Picea glehnii* bark. *Journal of Wood Science*, 47: 135-140.

Shin, N.H., Ryu, S.Y., Choi, E.J., Kang, S.H., Chang, I.M., Min, K.R., and Kim, Y. (1998). Oxyresveratrol as the potent inhibitor on dopa oxidase activity of mushroom tyrosinase. *Biochemical and Biophysical Research Communications*, 243: 801-803.

Shou, W., Seol, J.H., Shevchenko, A., Baskerville, C., Moazed, D., Chen, Z.W. S., Jang, J., Shevchenko, A., Charbonneau, H., and Deshaies, R.J. (1999). Exit from mitosis is triggered by Tem 1-Dependent release of the protein phosphatase Cdc14 from nucleolar RENT complex. *Cell*, 97: 233-244.

Shou, W., Sakamoto, K.M., Keener, J., Morimoto, K.W., Traverso, E.E., Azzam, R., Hoppe, G.J., Renny Feldman, R M., DeModena, J., Moazed, D., Charbonneau, H., Nomura, M., and Deshaies, R.J. (2001). Net1 stimulates RNA polymerase I transcription and regulates nucleolar structure independently of controlling mitotic exit. *Molecular Cell*, 8: 45-55.

Silan, C. (2008). The Effects of Chronic Resveratrol Treatment on Vascular Responsiveness of Streptozotocin-Induced Diabetic Rats. *Biological and Pharmaceutical Bulletin*, 31: 897-902.

Sinclair, D.A., and Guarente, L. (1997). Extrachromosomal rDNA circles-A cause of aging in yeast. *Cell*, 91: 1033-1042.

Smith, J. S., and Boeke, J.D. (1997). An unusual form of transcriptional silencing in yeast ribosomal DNA. *Genes Development*, 11: 241-254.

Solladie, G., Pasturel-Jacope, Y., and Maignan, J. (2003). A reinvestigation of resveratrol synthesis by Perkins reaction. Application to the synthesis of aryl cinnamic acids. *Tetrahedron*, 59: 3315-3321.

Sovak, M. (2001). Grape Extract, Resveratrol, and Its Analogs: A Review. *Journal of Medicinal Food*, 4: 93-105.

Starai, V. J., Celic, I., Cole, R. N., Boeke, J. D., and Escalante-Semerena, J. C. (2002). SIR 2-Dependent activation of acetyl-CoA synthetase by deacetylation of active lysine. *Science*, 298: 2390-2392.

Strahl-Bolsinger, S., Hecht, A., Luo, K., and Grunstein, M. (1997). SIR2 and SIR4 interactions differ in core and extended telomeric heterochromatin in yeast. *Genes Development*, 11: 83-93.

Su, H.C., Hung, L.M., and Chen, J.K. (2006). Resveratrol, a red wine antioxidant, possesses an insulin-like effect in streptozotocin-induced diabetic rats. *American Journal of Physiology-Endocrinology and Metabolism*, 290: 1339-1346.

Swanson-Mungerson, M., Ikeda, M., Lev, L., Longnecker, R., and Portis, T. (2003). Identification of latent membrane protein 2A (LMP2A) specific targets for treatment and eradication of Epstein-Barr virus (EBV)-associated diseases. *Journal of Antimicrobial Chemotheraphy*, 52: 152–154.

Takaya, Y., Terashima, K., Ito, J., He, Y.H., Tateoka, M., Yamaguchi, N., and Niwa, M. (2005). Biomimic transformation of resveratrol. *Tetrahedron*, 61: 10285-10290.

Tanner, K.G., Landry, J., Stemglanz, R., and Denu, M.J. (2000). Silent information regulator 2 family of NAD–dependent histone/protein deacetylases generates a unique product, 1-O-acetyl-ADP-ribose. *Proceedings of the National Academy of Sciences of the United States of America*, 97: 14178–14182.

Thirunavukkarasu M., Penumathsa, S.V., Koneru, S., Juhasz, B., Zhan, L., Otani, H., Bagchi, D., Das, D.K., and Maulik, N. (2007). Resveratrol alleviates cardiac dysfunction in streptozotocin-induced diabetes: Role of nitric oxide, thioredoxin, and heme oxygenase. *Free Radical biology and Medicine*, 43: 720-729.

Tissenbaum, H. A., and Guarente, L. (2001). Increased dosage of a SIR-2 gene extends lifespan in *Caenorhabditis elegans*. *Nature*, 410: 227-230.

Torresa, P., Avilab, J.G., Romo de Vivarc, A., Garcia, A.M., Marin, J.C., Arandad, E., and Cespedesc, C.L. (2003). Antioxidant and insect growth regulatory activities of stilbenes and extracts from *Yucca periculosa*. Phytochemistry, 64: 463-473.

Tredici, G., Miloso, M., Nicolini, G., Galbiati, S., Cavaletti, G., and Bertelli, A. (1999). Resveratrol, map kinases and neuronal cells: might wine be a neuroprotectant? *Drugs under experimental and clinical research*, 25: 99-103.

Umland, E.M., Cauffield, J.S., Kirk, J.K., and Thomason, E. T. (2000). Phytoestrogens as therapeutic alternatives to traditional hormone replacement in postmenopausal women. *Pharmacotherapy*, 20: 981-990.

Ungvari, Z., Orosz, Z., Rivera, A., Labinskyy, N., Xiangmin, Z., Olson, S., Podlutsky, A., and Csiszar, A. (2007). Resveratrol increases vascular oxidative stress resistance. American Journal of Physiology–Heart and Circulatory Physiology, 292 : 2417-2424.

Vastano, B.C., Cen, Y., Zhu, N., Ho, C.T., Zhou, Z., and Rosen, T.R. (2000). Isolation and identification of stilbenes in two varieties of *Polygonum cuspidatum*. *Journal of Agricultural and Food Chemistry*, 48: 253-256.

Vayssiere, M. B., Dupont, S., Choquart, A., Petit, F., Garcia, T., Marchandeau, C., Gronemeyer, H., and Resche-Rigon, M. (1997). Synthetic glucocorticoids that dissociate transactivation and AP-1 transrepression exhibit antiinflammatory activity *in vivo*. *Molecular Endocrinology*, 11: 1245-1255.

Wadsworth, T.L., and Koop, D.R. (1999). Effects of the wine polyphenolics quercetin and resveratrol on pro-inflammatory cytokine expression in RAW 264.7 macrophages. Biochemical Pharmacology, 57: 941-949.

Wang, M., Jin, Y., and Ho, C.T. (1999). Evaluation of resveratrol derivatives as potential antioxidants and identification of a reaction product of resveratrol and 2,2-diphenyl-1-picryhydrazyl radical. *Journal of Agricultural and Food Chemistry*, 47: 3974-3977.

Wang, Q. L., Lin, M., and Liu, G.T. (2001). Antioxidative Activity of Natural Isorhapontigenin. *Japanese Journal of Pharmacology*, 87: 61-66.

Waffo-Teguo, P., Hawthorne, M. E., Cuendet, M., Merillon, J. M., Kinghorn, A.D., Pezzuto, J.M., and Mehta, R.G. (2001). Potential Cancer-Chemopreventive Activities of Wine Stilbenoids and Flavones Extracted From Grape (Vitis vinifera) Cell Cultures. *Nutrition and Cancer*, 40: 173-179.

William, W.J., and Raymond, M. (2008). Process for the preparation of polyhydroxylated stilbenes via claisen condensation. EP 1884508.

Wood, G. J., Rogina, B., Lavu, S., Howitz, K., Helfand, S.L., Tatar, M., and Sinclair, D. (2004). Sirtuin activators mimic caloric restriction and delay ageing in metazoans. *Nature*, 430: 686-689.

Wung, B., Ming-Chun Hsu, Chun-Ching Wu, and Chia-Wen Hsieh, (2006). Piceatannol upregulates endothelial heme oxygenase-1 expression via novel protein kinase C and tyrosine kinase pathways. *Pharmacological Research*, 53: 113-122.

Xie, W.L., Chipman, J.G., Robertson, D.L., Erikson, R.L., and Simmons, D.L. (1991). Expression of a mitogen-responsive gene encoding prostaglandin synthase is regulated by mRNA splicing. *Proceedings of the National Academy of Sciences of the United States of America*, 88: 2692-2696.

Zhang, R., Kang, K. A., Piao, M. J., Lee, K.H., Jang, H.S., Park, M. J., Kim, B.J., Kim, J.S., Kim, Y.S., Ryu, S.Y., and Hyun, J.W. (2007). Rhapontigenin from *Rheum undulatum* Protects against Oxidative-Stress-Induced Cell Damage through Antioxidant Activity. *Journal of Toxicology and Environmental Health, Part A*,70: 1155-1166.

Zhou, B and Liu, Z.L. (2005). Bioantioxidants: From chemistry to Biology. *Pure and Applied Chemistry*, 77: 1887-1903.

Medicinal Plants: Phytochemistry, Pharmacology and Therapeutics, Vol. 1 *Pages 32–50*
Editors: **V.K. Gupta, G.D. Singh, Surjeet Singh and A. Kaul**
Published by: **DAYA PUBLISHING HOUSE, NEW DELHI**

Chapter 2

Ethnobotany, Chemistry and Pharmacology Studies of the Medicinal Specimen *Ixora coccinea* Linn.

Maria Aparecida M. Maciel[1]*, Aurea Echevarria[2], Silvana A.F.A. Monteath[2], Valdir F. Veiga Jr.[3], Carlos R. Kaiser[4], Fabiano E.S. Gomes[1], Joao Walter S. Silveira[5], Ricardo H. Costa e Sousa[5] and Frederico A. Vanderlinde[5]

[1]Departamento de Química, Universidade Federal do Rio Grande do Norte, Campus Universitário, 59078-970, Natal, RN, Brazil
[2]Departamento de Química, Instituto de Ciências Exatas, Universidade Federal Rural do Rio de Janeiro, 23890-000, Seropédica, RJ, Brazil
[3]Departamento de Química, Universidade Federal do Amazonas, 60077-000, Manaus, AM, Brazil
[4]Instituto de Química, Universidade Federal do Rio de Janeiro, 21941-972, Rio de Janeiro, RJ, Brazil
[5]Departamento de Ciências Fisiológicas, IB, Universidade Federal Rural do Rio de Janeiro, Rio de Janeiro, RJ, Brazil

ABSTRACT

The goal of this article is to emphasize the relevance of multidisciplinary studies with the medicinal plant *Ixora coccinea* Linn. (Rubiaceae) involving ethnobotany, chemistry and pharmacology. Phytochemical investigations on the methanolic extract obtained from flowers (ME-F), showed the presence of the bioactive ursolic acid, which was presented in this extract as

* Corresponding Author: E-mail: mammaciel@hotmail.com.

major component. The pentacyclic triterpenoid ursolic acid was isolated from ME-F by phytochemical procedures (classical chromatographic procedure using silica gel and eluents in gradienty of polarity) and also by specific methodology for acids isolation in which silica gel was impregnated with basis leading to the selective isolation of this terpenoid. Additionally, steroids and the sugar mannitol were isolated from ME-F. GC-MS analysis of this extract pointed out the presence of several non-polar constituents. The hydroalcoholic extract obtained from the leaves of *Ixora coccinea* (HE-L) showed by CG-MS analyzes a mixture of hydrocarbons, sesquiterpenes, heavy acids, steroids and alcohols. From this extract a triterpene mixture of lupeol, α–and β-amirin were isolated. Analytical study by prospection was performed for the hidroalcoholic extracts obtained from branches (HE-B) and roots (HE-R). Pharmacological evaluations were performed with those hydroalcoholic extracts (HE-L, HE-R, and HE-B) and methanolic extracts [ME-F (flowers) and ME-B (branches)] in order to investigate their antinociceptive activity. Treatment with ME-B, HE-B, HE-R and HE-L significantly reduced the total number of writhes in the acetic acid-induced abdominal constriction in mice. Meanwhile, ME-F lacked efficacy. In formalin assay, HE-B showed significant antinociception in the second phase of the test. These results confirmed the specificity of antinociceptive activity of *Ixora coccinea*.

Keywords: *Antinociceptive activity, Ethnopharmacological approach, Ixora coccinea Linn., Phytochemical investigations.*

Introduction

Ixora coccinea Linn. (Rubiaceae) a native specimen from western India, is also known as its synonymous *Ixora bandhuca* Roxbg and *Ixora grandiflora* Ker-Gaw. Its compact habit, evergreen foliage, and abundance of bright red to orange blooms make it a very favorite for hedge and foundation plantings. During the past several years, new *Ixora* hybrids have appeared on the market. These varieties (obtained in white, pink, yellow, orange, salmon, rose, and red) are the result of cross-breeding, importing, and hybridizing. There are about 150 species of *Ixora*, the most common being *Ixora coccinea* Linn., which is popularly known as 'ixora, flame-of-the-woods, or west india jasmine'. In Brazil its common names are 'ixora, ixora coral and equisósea', where it was introduced early two centuries ago. Since then, this plant has been found growing in gardens and fields of the Northern and Northeastern regions of Brazil, mainly due to its characteristic to be flowered during almost all year. The medicinal uses of *Ixora coccinea* includes diarrhea (medicinal benefits of leaves and flowers); hiccough, fever, sores, chronic ulcers and skin diseases (roots); bronchitis, leucorrhoea, dysmenorrhoea, haemoptysis and scabies (flowers) (Sivarajan and Balachandran, 1941; Latha and Panikkar, 1998).

The *Ixora* genus has been well documented in many works involving its propagation, acquisition of new species, plant pathology (plague control), and inorganic chemical evaluations. The pharmacological benefits of *Ixora coccinea* has long been reported (Sivarajan and Balachandran, 1941; Reena *et al.*, 1994; Sasidharan, 1997; Latha and Panikkar, 2001; Annapurna *et al.*, 2003). The antitumoral activity for an active fraction (AF) obtained of the hexane extract obtained from flowers of *Ixora coccinea* was reported by Latha and Panikkar (1998; 1999; 2001). This active fraction was identified by phytochemical methods as the triterpenoid ursolic acid. Among other pharmacological results, the non-toxic effect of AF in mice was confirmed. Moreover, AF prevented a decrease in body weight, haemoglobin levels and leucocyte counts of mice. According to the authors, these results were not surprising since the *Ixora coccinea* flowers constitute an important ingredient of several Ayurvedic formulations used for a variety of ailments (Latha and Panikkar, 1998; 1999; 2001). However, concerning to its phytochemical studies only few works was evidenced. In this context, *Ixora coccinea* roots and leaves were the most studied, from which were identified heavy acids; $\Delta^{9,11}$ octadecadienoic, palmitic, stearic, oleic and linoleic acids; the triterpenes lupeol and ursolic acid; anthocyanins; saponins, and tannins (Kartha and Menom, 1943; Latha and Pannikkar, 1998; 1999; Annapurna *et al.*, 2003).

Taking in account the ethnopharmacological importance of *Ixora coccinea* Linn., this present work focuses on the phytochemical investigations of a specimen collected in Brazil, as well as analyze its pharmacological effectiveness evaluating several polar extracts obtained from all parts of this plant. For that the antinociceptive effect of different hydroalcoholic extracts [obtained from leaves (HE-L), roots (HE-R) and branches (HE-B)], as well as methanolic extracts (ME-F/flowers and ME-B/branches) were evaluated.

Materials and Methods

Botanical Description

Ixora coccinea Linn. (Rubiaceae) is a woody, erect, and poor-branched shrub that can reach heights of 1.5-2.5 m, with clustered branches and broad flowering. It possesses light greenish leaves, long and erect terminal inflorescence with large clusters of tiny orange flowers.

Plant Material

Plant material was collected in botanical garden at Universidade Federal Rural do Rio de Janeiro, and identified by Botanic Department of this institution, where a voucher specimen (no. 4243e.) has been deposited.

Phytochemical Approach

The hydroalcoholic extract (HE-L; 55.2 g; 6.3 per cent) was obtained from leaves and methanolic extracts (ME-F; 26.3 g; 8.4 per cent) from flowers of *Ixora coccinea*. These extracts were prepared by percolation (at room temperature extracting solvent). Each extraction was repeated twice for flowers and four times for leaves. HE-L was obtained from dried and powdered vegetable material (865 g of leaves) and ME-F from flowers (315 g) without dryness. The obtained crude extracts (HE-L and ME-F) were submitted to chromatographic separations by classical phytochemical procedures (Maciel *et al.*, 2002; 2005). ME-F extract afforded 340 mg (0.12 per cent) of a rich mixture of several non-polar constituents (hydrocarbons and steroids), which was obtained from the fractions group F1-19 (eluted with Hexane:EtOAc 10:0–9:1); 570 mg (0.18 per cent) of ursolic acid [from F20-39 eluted with Hexane:EtOAc (8:2–5:5)] and 143 mg (0.04 per cent) of the sugar mannitol [from F40-46 eluted with EtOAc:MeOH (100:0–50:50)]. The ursolic acid was selectively isolated using silica gel column/potassium hydroxide chromatography methodology (Pinto *et al.*, 2000). In that, 280 mg (0.14 per cent) of ursolic acid was obtained from 200 g of flowers (without dryness). The hydroalcoholic extract HE-L afforded 5.56 g (0.64 per cent) of a rich mixture of several non-polar constituents (hydrocarbons, sesquiterpenes, heavy acids, steroids and alcohols) which was obtained from the fractions group F1-5 [Hexane:EtOAc (10:0–9:1) and 1.33 g (0.15 per cent) of a triterpenoidic mixture containing lupeol, α- and β-amirin [F6-10/eluted with Hexane:EtOAc (8:2–7:3)].

Pharmacological Procedures

Plant Material

The hydroalcoholic extracts HE-L (leaves), HE-R (roots), and HE-B (branches) and the methanolic extracts ME-F (flowers) and ME-B (branches) were evaluated in order to investigated their antinociceptive effects.

Animals

Adult male albino mice (20-35g) were housed in plastic cages, with food and tap water available *ad libitum* in the colony room. Mice were acclimatized in the laboratory for at least 60 min. prior to the test procedure and left without food for 12 to 18 h before the gavages. All experiments were carried out in accordance with current guide lines for the care of laboratory animals and the ethical guidelines on the use of animals in pain research (CIOMS, 1985; Zimmermann, 1986).

Chemicals

Acetic acid, Tween 80 (Merck AG, Darmstadt, Germany), indomethacin, silica gel (Sigma Chemical Co., St. Louis, MO, USA), fentanyl, formaldeyde (Janssen Pharmaceutical), diethyl ether (Unilab, Brazil), ethanol, methanol, dichloromethane, and *n*-hexane (Labsynth, Brazil). Extracts and drugs were diluted in water (p.o.) or saline solution (*s.c.* or *i.p*).

Acetic Acid-induced Abdominal Constriction Assay

The methodology described by Koster *et al.* (1959) was employed to evaluate the antinociceptive potency of *Ixora coccinea* in mice. Groups of animals (n=6) were pretreated orally with vehicle (10µL/g), indomethacin (10 mg/kg, *i.p.*, positive control), or HE-L, HE-B, HE-R, ME-F, ME-B extracts (0.3 up 2.0 g/kg). A 1.2 per cent saline solution of acetic acid (100 µL/10 g, *i.p.*) was given to mice 60 min. later. The acetic acid-induced abdominal constrictions were cumulatively counted during 30 min. (Vacher *et al.*, 1964) and expressed as mean±S.D., or as percentage of constriction inhibition compared to the control group.

Hot-plate Assay

Groups of mice (n=8) were treated with water (vehicle, *p.o.*), HE-B (1 g/kg *p.o.*), or phenthanyl (500 mg/kg *s.c.*) as positive control. The mice were placed on a hot plate maintained at 55±1.0 °C (Woolfe and McDonald, 1944; Sietsema *et al.*, 1988), and their response to thermal stimuli (in seconds) were evaluated at 60 and 30 min. before treatment, and after treatment it was 0, 30, 60, 90 and 120 minutes. Twenty five seconds was taken as cut-off time to avoid mouse tissue damage. The results were expressed as mean±S.D., and the parameters evaluated as thermal stimulus was licking, biting, or grooming one of the paws.

Formalin-induced Nociception

Groups of 8 mice were orally treated with water, HE-B (2 g/kg) or indomethacin (10 mg/kg), 60 min. prior to injection of the formalin solution (3 per cent; 20 µL/paw; *s.c.*) into the plantar surface of the hind paw (*i.pl.* injection). The time that animals spent licking the injected paw was measured with a chronometer and was considered as an index of pain.

From the formalin injection, the initial nociceptive response peaked at about 5 min. (first phase) and was followed by a second peak (second phase) that occurred at 15 to 30 min. post injection (Hunskaar *et al.*, 1986; Hunskaar and Hole, 1987).

Rota Rod Assay

The rota rod test described by Duham and Myia (1957) is commonly used to predict motor incoordination, mainly caused by sedation and/or muscle relaxation in mice. The apparatus used in test consists of a rotated bar (2.5 cm in diameter) subdivided into 5 compartments revolving at 9 rpm at a height of 35 cm.

The mice were divided in groups (n=6) and pretreated with HE-L, HE-B, or HE-R (2 g/kg *p.o.*). After that, the mice were placed into the rotarod apparatus and the time spent upon the rotating bar was recorded up to 60 seconds.

Open-field Assay

An acrylic arena with transparent walls and dark floor (dimensions of 30 x 30 x 15 cm), subdivided into 9 squares with 10 cm of side each one, was employed in order to evaluate both locomotor activity and exploratory behavior of mice. Groups of mice (n=6) pretreated orally one hour before the test with HE-L, HE-B, and HE-R (2 g/kg) were placed into the mouse arena, and then the behavior of the mice were evaluated in a period of 5 min. in terms of number of square and central square crossings, rearing behavior, duration of grooming, and defecation frequency (Archer, 1973; Siegel, 1946). Due the fact that an animal placed in a new ambience has the natural tendency to explore it regardless any negative emotions like fear, the open-field test provides a manner to evaluate both depressive and stimulant activities in the central nervous system.

Statistical Analysis

Data were presented as mean±S.D., and the statistical significance between groups was assessed by one way analysis of variance (ANOVA) followed by Scheffé's and Student's test, with significance difference set at $p < 0.05$ (Sokal and Rohlf, 1981).

Results

The species *Ixora coccinea* Linn. may found in different countries around the world, resulting in possible chemical changes which may take place due to different environmental factors such as fertility, humidity, solar radiation, wind temperature, herbivores, air/soil pollution, and seasonality. According to Maciel *et al.* (2000; 2002; 2005) these variations may account for different results in the pharmacological action of the plant. Other factors such as the plants age and time for gathering may also bring changes into the chemical components contents as well as pharmacological results. Since secondary metabolites represent a chemical interface between plants and surrounding environment, their biosyntheses are frequently affected by environmental conditions. Thus, variations in the total content and/or of the relative proportions of secondary metabolites in plants can take place. Recently, Maciel *et al.* (2000; 2002; 2005), Munné-Bosch *et al.* (2000), Raffo *et al.* (2006), Gobbo-Neto and Lopes (2007), and also Kowalski (2007) have shown how environmental conditions influenced on the content of bioactive secondary metabolites.

This present work links phytochemistry and pharmacology investigations of the specimen *Ixora cocinea* Linn. collected in Rio de Janeiro (Brazil) in order to improve its biological importance, analyze its chemical constituents and confront these obtained results to those data previously reported (from plants collected in other countries). Taking in account the importance of *Ixora cocinea* flowers as human diet (Latha and Panikkar, 2001; Annapurna *et al.*, 2003), we first focused the phytochemistry studies with hydrated flowers of this plant. In that, the phytochemical approach comprised the following sequence: preparation of the methanolic extract (ME-F), chromatographic fractioning of this extract, purification of the obtained fractions (a total of 46), identification of non-polar compounds by GC-MS analyses, isolation of the other chemical constituents by classical chromatographic procedure (and its characterization by spectroscopy data). From the ME-F crude extract were obtained hydrocarbons, functionalized hydrocarbons, steroids, one bioactive triterpene, and one carbohydrate. The GC-MS analysis of the non-polar fractions (F1-19) revealed the presence of a mixture containing the steroids b-sitosterol, stigmasterol, clionasterol, fucosterol, cholesterol and ergosterol, in which the two first were the major constituents. Another mixture containing hydrocarbons long chain (ranging from 20 to 31 carbon atoms) such as: icosane, henicosane, docosane, tricosane, tetracosane, pentacosane, hexacosane, heptacosane, octacosane, nonacosane, triacontane, and hentriacontane were identified. In the hydrocarbon mixture, the most abundant were heptacosane, followed by pentacosane and icosane. From the functionalized hydrocarbon mixture were found palmitic acid, isopropyl tetradecanoate, methyl palmitate, methyl stearate and hexahydrofarnesyl acetone, as well as fatty acids (ranging from 14 to 23 carbon atoms) detected through their methylated derivatives: methyl heptadecanoate, methyl hexadecanoate, methyl pentadecanoate, methyl henicosanoate, methyl tetracosanoate, and methyl tricosanoate.

The presence of the steroids β-sitosterol and stigmasterol was confirmed after purification of the F1-19 fractions group. Fractions F20-39 afforded the triterpene ursolic acid. From the polar fractions F40-46 was obtained the carbohydrate mannitol. These isolated constituents were characterized by infrared (IR) and NMR (^{1}H and ^{13}C) spectroscopic data; being the triterpene characterized by its methylated derivative.

Pharmacological Results

Acetic Acid-induced Abdominal Constrictions Assay

The oral treatment with HE-B at 0.3, 1 or 2 g/kg reduced 51.5 per cent (21.2±9.3), 72.5 per cent (12.0±8.4) and 83.7 per cent (7.1±2.7 writhes) respectively, the number of cumulative writhes when compared to the control group (water), which presented 43.7±3.7 writhes. Similar results were obtained in treatment with indomethacin (positive control) which showed 68.2 per cent the number of cumulative writhes (13.9±2.6) (Figure 2.1).

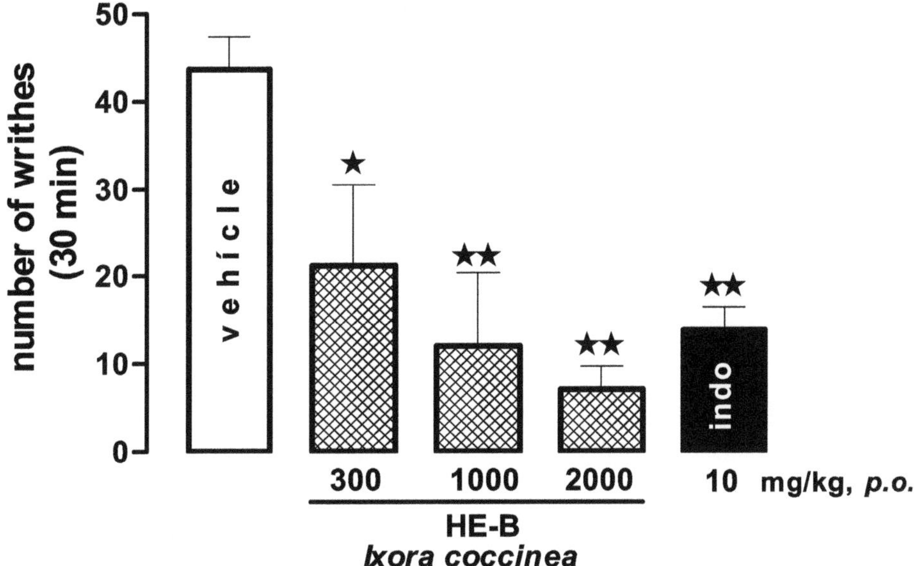

Figure 2.1 Acetic Acid-induced Abdominal Writhes (1.2 per cent saline, 100 µL/10 g, *i.p.*) in Mice Previously Treated (60 min., *p.o.*) with Vehicle (water, 100 µL/10 g), Indomethacin (indo.; 10 mg/kg), or Hydroalcoholoic Extracts Obtained from Branches (HE-B) of *Ixora coccinea* (0.3, 1 or 2 g/kg). The columns and vertical bars represent the mean±S.D. of six animals in each experimental group. Statistical significances: *p<0.05; **p<0.01.

The treatment (*p.o.*) with HE-L (2 g/kg) and HE-R (2 g/kg) reduced in 36 per cent (36.4±4.2 writhes) and 57 per cent (24.4±4.4), respectively, the number of cumulative writhes. The experimental group (water) presented 57.2±2.2 writhes and the treatment with the positive control, indomethacin (10 mg/kg, *p.o.*) inhibited 59 per cent the total number of cumulative writhes (23.4±1.3) (Figure 2.2).

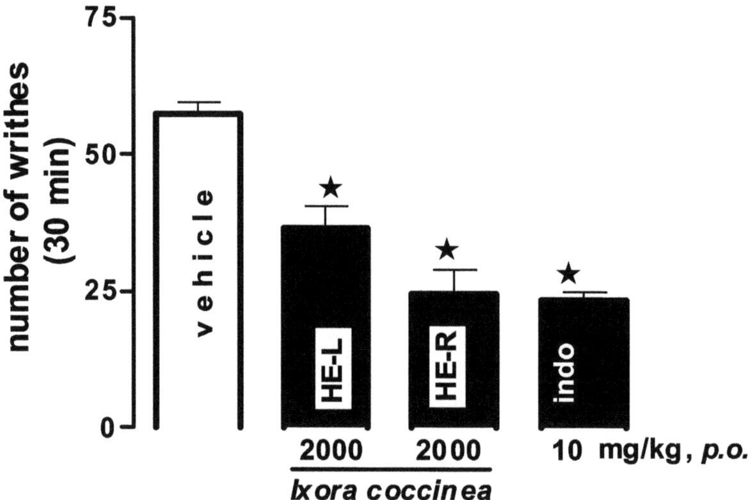

Figure 2.2: Acetic Acid-induced Abdominal Writhes (1.2 per cent saline, 10 µL/g, *i.p.*) in Mice Previously Treated (60 min., *p.o.*) with Vehicle (water, 100 µL/10 g), Indomethacin (indo., 10 mg/kg), or Hydroalcoholoic Extracts Obtained from the Leaves (HE-L) and Roots (HE-R) of *Ixora coccinea* (2 g/kg). The columns and vertical bars represent the mean±S.D. of six animals in each experimental group. Statistical significance: *p<0.01.

The total number of acetic acid-induced abdominal writhes in the mice group treated with the vehicle (DMSO 0.5 per cent, *p.o.*) was 55.3±8.3 (Figure 2.3).

The administration of ME-B (2 g/kg, *p.o.*) reduced in 61 per cent (21.3±4.7 writhes) the total number of cumulative writhes. The group treated with indomethacin (10 mg/kg, *p.o.*) showed 72 per cent writhing inhibition (15.3±7.0 writhes). However, the treatment at the same dose (2 g/kg, *p.o.*) with ME-F did not show significant changes in the total number of cumulative writhes (52.7±8.1), when compared to the control group (Figure 2.3).

Hot-plate Assay

The treatment with HE-B (1 g/kg, *p.o.*) did not cause significant changes in thermal nociception, while the treatment with the positive control phentanyl (500 µg/kg, *s.c.*) increased substantially the thermal response time at 0 (23.2±1.8 s), 30 (15.8±2.6 s), and 60 min. (13.0±2.3 s), when compared to control group (water) (7.0±0.7, 8.5±1.1, and 7.9±1.1 s, respectively) (Figure 2.4).

Formalin Assay

In the formalin assay, the treatment with HE-B (2 g/kg, *p.o.*) reduced in 69 per cent (40.4±21.1 s) the inflammatory nociception (second phase), when compared to control group (130.1±30.6 s) (Figure 2.5). In similar manner, the positive control (indomethacin 10 mg/kg, *p.o.*) reduced in 79 per cent (27.0±12.0 s) the pain reactivity associated to the second phase. However, at the early phase of the test

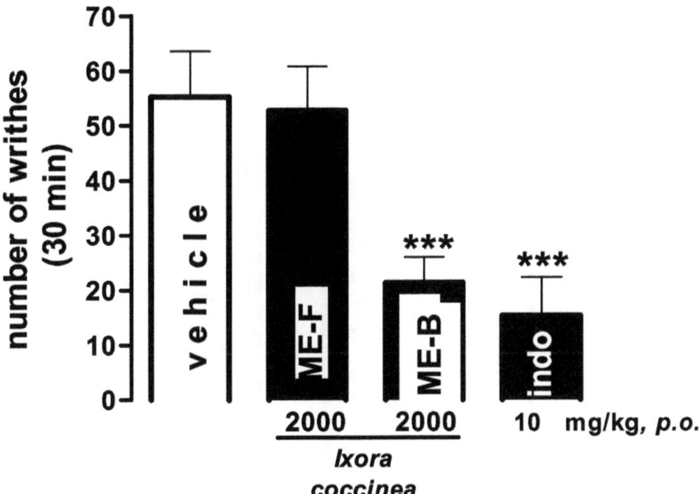

Figure 2.3: Acetic Acid-induced Abdominal Writhes (1.2 per cent saline, 10 µL/g, *i.p.*) in Mice Previously Treated (60 min., *p.o.*) with Vehicle (DMSO 0.5 per cent), Indomethacin (indo.; 10 mg/kg), and Methanolic Extracts Obtained from the Flowers (ME-F) and Branches (ME-B) of *Ixora coccinea* (2 g/kg). The columns and vertical bars represent the mean±S.D. of six animals in each experimental group. Statistical significance: ***p<0.001.

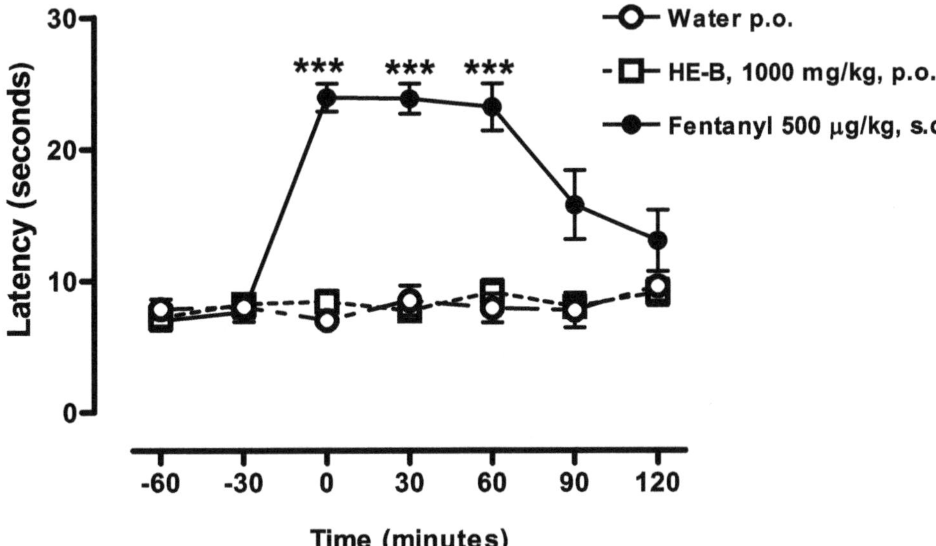

Figure 2.4: Thermal Antinociceptive Effect of Hydroalcoholic Extracts Obtained from the Branches (HE-B) of *Ixora coccinea* (□–1 g/kg *p.o.*), in Terms of Time Interval in which the Mouse Stands on Hot Plate P55.0±1.0 ºC). Phentanyl (●–500 µg/kg *s.c.*) was the positive control while the negative control group was treated with water (o–10 mL/g, *p.o.*). The results shown herein represent the mean±S.D. of eight animals in each experimental group. Statistical significance: ***p<0.001.

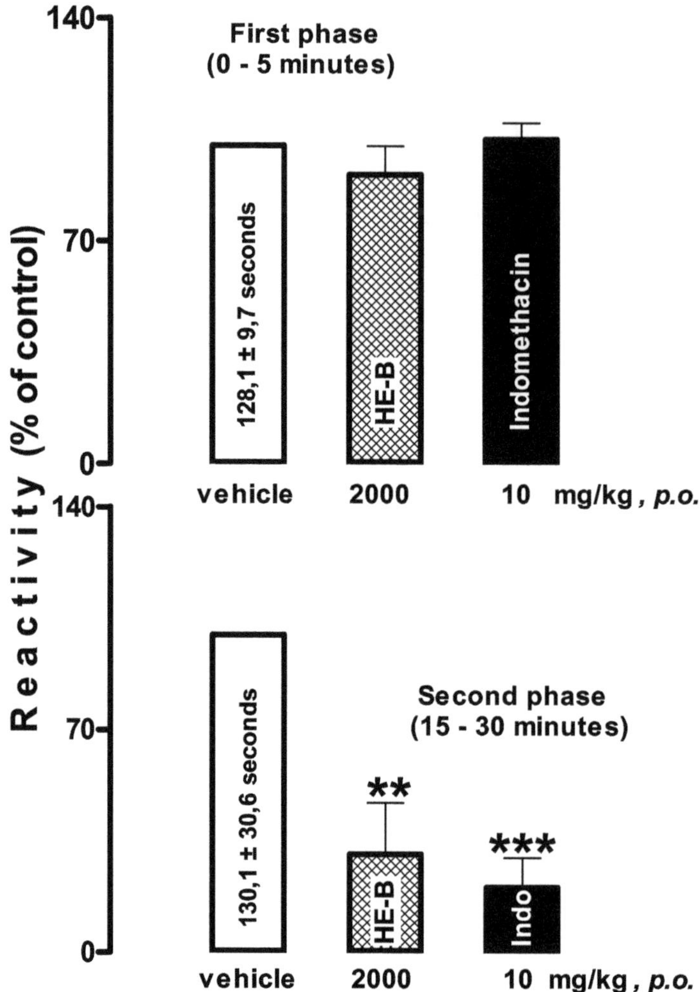

Figure 2.5: Reactivity (control per cent) to Sub-plantar Application of Formalin (20 μL saline formaldehyde 1.2 per cent) in Mice Right Hind Paw Previously Treated (60 min., *p.o.*) with Vehicle (10 μL/g), HE-B (2 g/kg), Or indomethacin (indo.; 10 mg/kg). The columns and vertical bars represent the mean of phase I (0 to 5 min., neurogenic pain) and phase II (15 up 30 min., inflammatory pain)±S.D. of twelve animals in each experimental group. Statistical significance: **p<0.01, ***p<0.001.

(first 5 min), none of the treatments showed results statistically different from control group (128.1±9.7 s) (Figure 8.5).

Rota Rod Assay

The control group (vehicle) remained on the rota rod apparatus for 60.0±0.0 s, with 1.6±0.5 falls down over a period of 1 minute. This performance was not affected by the oral administration (2 g/kg, *p.o.*) of HE-L, HE-B, and HE-R (60.0±0.0, 57.5±1.8, and 53.5±6.4 s, respectively) (Figure 2.6).

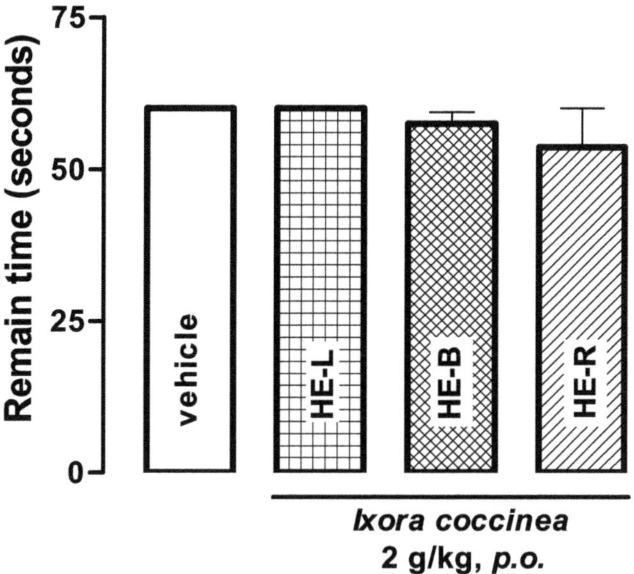

Figure 2.6: Evaluation of Remain Time on the Rota Rod Apparatus. Experimental groups of six animals were submitted to oral treatment with vehicle (water), hydroalcoholic extracts obtained from the leaves (HE-L), branches (HE-B), and roots (HE-R) of *Ixora coccinea* (2 g/kg). The columns and vertical bars represent mean±S.D.

Open-field Assay

The results obtained for locomotors activity and exploratory behavior of mice from open-field test corroborate those obtained from rota rod test. After treatment with HE-R, HE-B, and HE-L (2 g/kg, *p.o.*), the number of square crossings observed was 75.4±9.8, 67.6±6.1, and 58.4±10.6, respectively. These results do not differ from the control group result (71.7±14.1 crossings). Similar results were observed for the number of central square crossings 6.0±1.1 (HE-R), 5.1±1.1 (HE-B), 2.7±1.1 (HE-L), and 6.4±1.4 crossings (vehicle); rearing behavior 44.4±4.7 (HE-R), 40.4±4.2 (HE-G), 24.3±4.6 (HE-L), and 28.1±7.5 (vehicle); time consuming of grooming 21.3±5.8 (HE-R), 23.3±4.5 (HE-B), 19.4±5.5 (HE-L) and 12.3±2.9 s (vehicle).

Dicussion and Conclusions

The phytochemical study on the methanolic extract obtained from the flowers of *Ixora coccinea* (ME-F) resulted in the identification of 40 compounds, including the triterpene ursolic acid, the carbohydrate mannitol, and the steroids β-sitosterol and stigmasterol, in which this triterpene was the major compound (0.18 per cent). The triterpene lupeol was isolated from HE-L, as a mixture containing also the two terpenoids α–and β-amirin. This triterpene, previously isolated from *Ixora coccinea* leaves, a specimen collected in Thiruvanathapuram (India) that showed antiinflammatory and antimicotic activities (Reena *et al.*, 1994). In this present work those isolated constituents were confirmed by spectroscopic analyzes, including NMR ^{1}H, ^{13}C, DEPT and HMQC data). Additionally, analytical study by prospection suggested the presence of organic acids, steroids, triterpenes, anthocyanins, carbohydrates, and saponins in the hydroalcoholic extracts of flowers (HE-F), leaves (HE-L), branches

(HE-B), and roots (HE-R), as well as tannins in HE-R. Comparing the GC-MS analysis of the non-polar fractions (F1-19 obtained from ME-F) and (F1-5 obtained from HE-L) to those previously results reported to *Ixora coccinea* roots, which was rich in palmitic, stearic, oleic and linoleic acids (Latha and Panikkar, 1998), only heavy acids, stearic and palmitic acids are present in both flowers and leaves of the specimen collected in Brazil. Those phytochemical results confirmed that Brazil climatic conditions do not affect the occurrence of the chemical constituents of *Ixora coccinea*, which was collected in Botanical Garden of Universidade Federal Rural do Rio de Janeiro (Brazil), been in agreement with those previously reported phytochemical data. In other hand, this present work improves its chemical data, since other compounds were cited to be isolated or detected by GC-MS analyzes, in flowers and leaves of *Ixora coccinea*.

Previously pharmacological results pointed out special features for a bioactive fraction obtained from the methanolic extract obtained from the flowers of *Ixora coccinea* Linn. (AF-ME-L) from which a non-toxic effect and antitumoral activity were detected (Latha and Panikkar, 1998). The triterpene ursolic acid was isolated from this extract and its antiviral activity was reported (Latha, 1999). Concerning to ursolic acid (3b-hydroxy-urs-12-en-28-oic acid) and its position isomer oleanolic acid (3b-hydroxy-olean-12-en-28-oic acid), belong respectively to the ursane and the oleanane groups, they share many common pharmacological properties and are included among the most notable bioactive triterpenoid compounds (Liu, 1995). During the last decades over 900 research articles have been published on ursolic acid (UA) as well as oleanolic acid (OA), reflecting tremendous interest and progress in their pharmacological importance, including in those studies UA and OA chemical modifications to make this natural products more effective and water soluble derivatives. Pharmacological research of both UA and OA, includes pre-clinical and toxicity evaluations, and human clinical uses. Among the many important pharmacological effects anticancer chemotherapies, hypolipidemic, hypoglycemic, and hepatoprotective effects; antiatherosclerotic and antidiabetogenic properties; cardiovascular protective effect; gastrointestinal transit modulating activity; antiulcer, antiinflammatory, antibacterial, and antifungal activities; additionally to immunomodulatory, and diuretic properties were confirmed, as well as their insecticidal property (Shatilo *et al.*, 1973; Kowalewski *et al.*, 1976; Parfentieva, 1979; Gupta *et al.*, 1981; Vasilenko *et al.*, 1981; 1982; Yamahara *et al.*, 1981; Kosuge *et al.*, 1985; Wrzeciono *et al.*, 1985; Ma, 1986; Collins and Charles, 1987; Liu *et al.*, 1987; Lee *et al.*, 1988; Hao *et al.*, 1989; Hirota *et al.*, 1990; Huang *et al.*, 1994; Liu *et al.*, 1994; 1998; 1999; Liu, 1995; 2005; Sattar *et al.*, 1995; Hsu *et al.*, 1997; Jeong *et al.*, 1999; Latha and Panikkar, 1999; 2001; Li *et al.*, 1999; 2002; Mizushina *et al.*, 2000; Tang *et al.*, 2000; Yoshikawa *et al.*, 2000; Marquina *et al.*, 2001; Mix *et al.*, 2001; Alvares *et al.*, 2002; Murakami *et al.*, 2004; Somova *et al.*, 2003). Additionally, the potent inhibitory effect of ursolic acid against HIV-1 protease (with IC_{50} values of 8.0 μM) was reported by Min *et al.* (1999) and confirmed by Ma *et al.* (2000). Kashiwada *et al.* (2000) confirmed antiHIV effect for its derivatives. Moreover, ursolic acid has been shown to possess antiarthritic (Iwu and Ohiri, 1980).

Both ursolic acid and oleanolic acid exist widely in plant kingdom, medicinal herbs, and also are integral part of the human diet. These two triterpenes may occur in the form of free acids or aglycones of saponins (Li *et al.*, 1999; Marquina *et al.*, 2001; Janicsák *et al.*, 2006; Kowalski, 2007; Razboršek *et al.*, 2008), which represent a source of materials for the pharmaceutical industry. The fruiting spikes of *Prunella vulgaris* L. (Labiatae), known as "Hsia ku Tsao" in Chinese folklore, are used as herbal remedies for human tuberculosis, jaundice, infectious hepatitis, bacillary dysentery, pleuritis with effusion, and cancer (Zurcher *et al.*, 1954; Lee *et al.*, 1988). The triterpenoids UA and OA among other constituents, were isolated from the whole herb. From this other herbal remedies "Khin Piah Leng" obtained from *Psychotria serpens* (Rubiaceae) and/or *Hyptis capitata* (Labiatae) a specific bioassay-directed fractionation led to the isolation and characterization of ursolic acid as one of the bioactive principle of this herbal remedies (Zurcher *et al.*, 1954; Lee *et al.*, 1988). Reinforcing its uses, Oguro *et al.* (1998) reported the inhibitory effect of oleanolic acid on 12-*O*-tetradecanoylphorbol-13-acetate-induced gene expression in mouse skin. Because of its biological efficacy and apparent low side effects, oleanolic acid has been patented in Japan as additive to health drinks (Okudo *et al.*, 1990).

Taking in account that Paracelsus pointed out in the 16th century that "All substances are poisons; there is none which is not poison. The right dose differentiates a poison from a remedy". Thus, it should be kept in mind that the dose of any natural product determines the mode of action and the doses makes a poison. As an example, low-doses of oleanolic acid showed hepatoprotective effect [60-90 mg/day, for 30 days/in 70 cases of clinical trial or long-term use (more than 3 months)/in 188 cases of chronic hepatitis] (Xu and Wan, 1980; Xu, 1985). Meanwhile, the high-dose could produce cholestasis and hepatotoxicity (Liu, 2005). Because of this notably hepatoprotection oleanolic acid was marketed in China for human liver disorders (Liu, 1995).

The overall chronic and acute toxicity of ursolic acid, is generally known to be low. In the early studies Wenzel and Koff (1956) reported that this terpenoid has a marked effect on the electrolytic balance of the adrenalectomized rat. Concerning to its derivative ursolic acid acetate, 3 mg of subcutaneously injected dose produce the same retention of sodium ions as 3 μg of desoxycorticosterone and a much higher level of potassium elimination. According to these authors, since ursolic acid acetate is absorbed very slowly, these are significant results (Wenzel and Koff, 1956; Mezzetti *et al.*, 1971). In the other hand the widely use of both UA and OA in cosmetics and health products has long been reported, justifying their relatively non-toxic effect. Among their largely uses without significant adverse effect, UA and OA as antiinflammatory agents is supported by Gupta (1981) and Singh *et al.* (1992) who showed that these terpenoids in comparison to aspirin exerts antiinflammatory effects without causing ulcerogenic effect. These two triterpenoids was reported by Gbaguidi *et al.* (2005) as active agents against dermatophilosis in African animals. Additionally, the specimen *Mitracarpus scaber* which is a reach source of UA and OA, has been used to treat various human skin diseases including eczema and ring-worm (Gbaguidi *et al.*, 2005; Ependu *et al.*, 1994).

Reports on the natural occurrence of both ursolic and oleanolic acids furnishes numerous data. In this context, Liu (1995), Janicsák *et al.* (2006), Kowalski (2007), and Razboršek *et al.* (2008) showed partial survey on medicinal plants containing these triterpenes, been evidenced that their occurrence were simultaneous in almost of the studied plants. However, similarly as for other chemotaxonomic markers, there are significant quantitative differences among subfamilies. With few exceptions, the content of UA was always higher than those observed to OA. In this present work using classical column chromatograph procedures the free ursolic acid was isolated from the flowers of *Ixora coccinea* Linn. (Rubiaceae) in great amount (0.18 per cent). When a specific methodology for acids isolation (Pinto *et al.*, 2000) was performed (in which silica gel was impregnated with basis aim the selective isolation of the target compound, reducing experimental time consuming and costs), the triterpene UA was also isolated in good amount (0.14 per cent). This contents was considered to be satisfactory since other Rubiaceae specimens presents low amount of UA and OA, such as *Gardenia saxatilis* (0.001 per cent of OA and 0.0009 per cent of UA) and *Mitracarpus scaber* (0.004 per cent of OA and 0.01 per cent of UA) (Suksamrarn *et al.*, 2003 and Gbaguidi *et al.*, 2005, respectively). These other Rubiaceae specimens *Coussarea paniculata*, *Chiococca braquiata*, and *Morinda lucida* Benth. also presented these bioactive triterpenes (Chaturvedula *et al.*, 2003; Lopes *et al.*, 2004; Cimanga *et al.*, 2006). Similar to the *Ixora coccinea* Linn., these two Rubiaceae specimens *Galianthe brasiliensis* (Spreng.) E.L.Cabral and Bacigalupo

(De Moura *et al.*, 2006) and *Psychotria serpens* (Zurcher *et al.*, 1954; Lee *et al.*, 1988) produced only ursolic acid.

Pharmacological Discussions for the Tested Extracts

The aim of the abdominal constriction test is evaluate the presence of analgesic activity. This method has the advantage to evaluate even weak analgesic activities, but is also unspecific, since drugs like non-steroidal antiinflammatory or opioids are writhing inhibitors (Hendershot and Forsaith, 1959; Chernov *et al.*, 1967; Loux *et al.*, 1978).

In this work the treatment with the hydroalcoholic extracts HE-B, HE-L, HE-R, and the methanolic extract ME-B significant reduced the number of cumulative writhing.

Meanwhile, the treatment with ME-F was ineffective in writhing inhibition, suggesting absence of antinociceptive compounds in this extract. Since the ursolic acid is the major compound in this extract, this result is in agreement with the wide-ranging pharmacological data for this natural product, in which non-analgesic effect was cited.

In order to confirm the antinociceptive activity and its mechanism of action, other assays were carried out. In that the hydroalcoholic extract HE-B extract was assessed in hot-plate test, sensitive to opioid drugs (Janssen *et al.*, 1963), whose analgesic activity is measured by m, k and δ receptors dispersed either in peripherical as in central nervous system (Besson and Chaouch, 1987; Stein and Shippenberg, 1989). In this test, HE-B showed ineffective in suppressing thermal-induced pain, restricting some possibilities of mechanism of action in central nervous system upon the detected antinociceptive.

In formalin assay, the sub-plantar injection of formalin 3 per cent in mice produces a biphasical behavioral response, where the early phase (0 to 5 min.) results essentially in a direct stimulation on nociceptors, while the last phase (15 to 30 min.) involves the inflammatory sensitization period (Hunskaar *et al.*, 1985, 1986, 1987). Confirming the initial hypothesis, HE-B showed accentuated antinociception only in the second phase, suggesting the existence in this extract of compounds that exerts analgesic activity through antiinflammatory mechanisms. Considering that the previous methodologies utilized to evaluate antinociceptive activity suffer influence from motor behavior of animals, the utilization of rota rod and open-field tests had as objective exclude the possibility of false results due motor incoordination caused by sedation or muscle relaxation. In both tests, these effects were not observed demonstrating the specificity of antinociceptive activity evidenced in acetic acid-induced abdominal constriction, hot-plate and formalin assays.

In conclusion, HE-B when administered orally, showed antinociceptive properties probably through antiinflammatory activity. Further assays for specific pharmacological activity are needed to complement this characterization as well as elucidate the mechanism of action involved in the antinociception effect of HE-L and HE-R. The antinociception effect of HE-L (evidenced by acid-induced abdominal constriction test) could be correlated to the presence of the terpenoid mixture lupeol, α-amirin and b-amirin, additionally to a mixture of sesquiterpenes (confirmed in this work to be present in the leaves of *Ixora coccinea*). As a continuing work, new phytochemical analyzes will be performed with the bioactive extracts HE-B and HE-R to confirm the presence of steroids, triterpenes, anthocyanins, carbohydrates, and saponins in both HE-B and HE-R extracts, as well as tannins in HE-R, which were detected to be present in these extracts by prospection analytical study.

Acknowledgement

The authors are grateful to Conselho Nacional de Desenvolvimento Científico e Tecnológico (CNPq) for financial support.

References

Álvarez, M.E., María, A.O.M., and Saad, J.R. (2002). Diuretic activity of *Fabiana patagonica* in rats. *Phytotherapy Research*, 16: 71-73.

Annapurna, J., Amarnath, P.V.S., Kumar, D.A., Ramakrishna, S.V., and Raghavan, K.V. (2003). Antimicrobial activity of *Ixora coccinea* leaves. *Fitoterapia*, 74: 291-193.

Archer, J. (1973). Tests for emotionality in rats and mice: a review. *Animal Behavior*, 21:205-235.

Besson, J.M., and Chaouch, A.J. (1987). Peripheral and spinal mechanisms of nociception. *Physiological Reviews*, 67: 67-186.

Chaturvedula, V.S.P., Schilling, J.K., Johnson, R.K., and Kingston, D.G.I. (2003). New cytotoxic lupane triterpenoids from the twigs of *Coussarea paniculata*. *Journal of Natural Products*, 66: 419-422.

Chernov, H.I., Wilson, D.E., Fowler, W.F., and Plummer, A.J. (1967). Non-specificity of the mouse writhing test. *Archives Internationales de Pharmacodynamie et de Therapie*, 167: 171-178.

Cimanga, R.K., Tona, G.L., Mesia, G.K., Kambu, O.K., Bakana, D.P., Kalenda, P.D.T., Penge, A.O., Muyembe, J.J.T., Totté, J., Pieters, L., and Vlietinck, A.J. (2006). Bioassay-guided isolation of antimalarial triterpenoid acids from the leaves of *Morinda lucida*. *Pharmaceutical Biology*, 44: 677-681.

CIOMS (1985). Council for International Organization of Medical Sciences. *International Guiding Principles for Biomedical Research Involving Animals*, <http://http://www.cioms.ch/frame_1985_texts_of_guidelines.htm>, accessed 26 July 2007.

Collins, M.A., and Charles, H.P. (1987). Antimicrobial activity of carnosol and ursolic acid: Two antioxidant constituents of *Rosimarinus officinalis* L. *Food Microbiology*, 4: 311-315.

De Moura, V.M., Dos Santos, V.P., Santin, S.M.O., De Carvalho, J.E., and Foglio, M.A. (2006). Chemical constituents of *Galianthe brasiliensis* (Spreng.) E.L.Cabral and Bacigalupo (Rubiaceae). *Química Nova*, 29: 452-455.

Duham, N.W., and Miya, T.S. (1957). A note on a simple apparatus for detecting neurological deficit in rats and mice. *Journal of the American Pharmacists Association*, 46: 208-209.

Ependu, T.O., Akah, P.A., Adesomoju, A.A., and Okogun, J.I. (1994) Antiinflammatory and antimicrobial activities of *Mitracarpus scaber* extracts. *International Journal of Pharmacognosy*, 32: 191-196.

Gbaguidi, F., Accrombessi, G., Moudachirou, M., and Quetin-Leclercq, J. (2005). HPLC quantification of two isomeric triterpenic acid isolated from *Mitracarpus scaber* and antimicrobial activity on *Dermatophilus congolensis*. *Journal of Pharmaceutical and Biomedical Analysis*, 39: 990-995.

Gobbo-Neto, L., and Lopes, N. P. (2007) Medicinal Plants: factors of influence on the content of secondary metabolites. *Química Nova*, 30: 374-381.

Gupta, M.B., Nath, R., Gupta, G.P., and Bhargava, K.P. (1981). Antiulcer activity of some plant triterpenoids. *Indian Journal of Medical Research*, 73: 51-52.

Hao, Z. Hang, B., and Wang, Y. (1989). Hypoglycemic effect of oleanolic acid. *Zhougguo Yaoke Daxue Xuebao*, 22: 210-212.

Hendershot, L.C., and Forsaith, J. (1959). Antagonism of the frequency of phenylquinone-induced writhing in the mouse by weak analgesic and nonanalgesics. *Journal of Pharmacology and Experimental Therapeutics*, 125: 237-240.

Hirota, M., Mori, T., Yoshida, M., and Iriye, R. (1990). Supression of tumor promoter-induced inflammation of mouse ear by ursolic acid and 4,4-dimethylcholestane derivatives. *Agricultural and Biological Chemistry*, 54: 1073-1075.

Hsu, H.Y., Yang, J.J, and Lin, C.C. (1997) Effects of oleanolic acid and ursolic acid on inhibiting tumor growth and enhancing the recovery of hematopoietic system postirradiation in mice. *Cancer Letters*, 111: 7-13.

Huang, M.T., Ho, C.T., Wang, Z.Y., Ferraro, T., Lou, Y.-R., Stauber, K., Ma, W., Georgiadis, C., Laskin, J.D., and Conney, A.H. (1994). Inhibition of skin tumorigenesis by rosemary and its constituents carnosol and ursolic acid. *Cancer Research*, 54: 701-708.

Hunskaar, S., Fasmer, O.B., and Hole, K. (1985). Formalin test in mice, a useful technique for evaluating mild analgesia. *Journal of Neuroscience Methods*, 14: 69-76.

Hunskaar, S., Berger, O.G. and Hole, K. (1986). Dissociation between antinociceptive and antiinflammatory effects of acetylsalicylic acid and indomethacin in the formalin test. *Pain*, 25: 125-132.

Hunskaar, S., and Hole, K. (1987). The formalin test in mice: dissociation between inflammatory and non-inflammatory pain. *Pain*, 30: 103-114.

Iwu, M.M., and Ohiri, F.C. (1980). Antiarthritic triterpenoids of *Lonchocarpus cyanescens* Benth. *Canadian Journal of Pharmaceutical Sciences*, 15: 39-42.

Janicsák, G., Veres, K., Kakasy, A.Z., and Máthé, I. (2006). Study of the oleanolic and ursolic acids contents of some species of the Lamiaceae. *Biochemical Systematics and Ecology*, 34: 392-396.

Janssen, P.A.J., Niemegeers, C.J.E., and Dony, J.G.H. (1963). The inhibitory effect of fentanyl and other morphine-like analgesics on the warm water induced tail withdrawal reflex in rats. *Arzneimittelforschung*, 6: 502-507.

Jeong, H.G. (1999). Inhibition of cytochrome P450 2E1 expression by oleanolic acid: Hepatoprotective effects against carbon tetrachloride-induced hepatic injury. *Toxicology Letters*, 105: 215-222.

Kartha, A.R.S., and Menon, K.N. (1943). The isolation and constitution of an acid from the root bark of *Ixora coccinea*. *Proceedings of the Indian Academy of Sciences*, 17A: 11-15.

Kashiwada, Y., Nagao, T., Hashimoto, A., Ikeshiro, Y., Okabe, H., Cosentino, L.M., and Lee, K.H. (2000). AntiHIV activity of 3-*O*-acyl ursolic acid derivatives. *Journal of Natural Products*, 63: 1619-1622.

Koster, R., Anderson, M., and De Beer, E.J. (1959). Acetic acid for analgesic screening. *Federation Proceedings*, 18: 412-416.

Kosuge, T., Yokota, M., and Sugiyama, K. (1985). Studies on bioactive substances in crude drugs used for arthritic diseases in traditional Chinese medicine. III. Isolation and identification of antiinflammatory and analgesic principles from the whole herb of *Pyrola rotundifolia* L. *Chemical and Pharmaceutical Bulletin*, 33: 5355-5357.

Kowalewski, Z., Kortus, M., Kedzia, W., and Koniar, H. (1976). Antibiotic action of β-ursolic acid. *Archivum Immunologiae et Therapiae Experimentalis*, 24: 115-119.

Kowalski, R. (2007). Studies of selected plant raw materials as alternative sources of triterpenes of oleanolic and ursolic acid types. *Journal of Agricultural and Food Chemistry*, 55: 656-662.

Latha, P.G., and Panikkar, K.R. (1998). Cytotoxic and antitumor principles from *Ixora coccinea* flowers. *Cancer Letters*, 130: 197-202.

Latha, P.G., and Panikkar, K.R. (1999). Modulatory effects of *Ixora coccinea* flower on cyclophosphamide-induced toxicity in mice. *Phytotherapy Research*, 13: 517-520.

Latha, P.G., and Panikkar, K.R. (2001). Chemoprotective effect of *Ixora coccinea* L. flowers on cisplatin induced toxicity in mice. *Phytotherapy Research*, 15: 364-366.

Lee, K.H., Lin, Y.M., Wu, T.S., Zhang, D.C., Yamagishi, T., Hayashi, T., Hall, I.H., Chang, J.J., Wu, R.Y., and Yang, T.H. (1988). The cytotoxic principles of *Prunella vulgaris*, *Psychotria serpens*, and *Hyptis capitata*: Ursolic acid and related derivatives. *Planta Medica*, 54: 308-311.

Li, Y., Matsuda, H., and Yoshikawa, M. (1999). Effects of oleanolic acid glycosides on gastrointestinal transit and ileus in mice. *Bioorganic and Medicinal Chemistry*, 7: 1201-1205.

Li, J., Guo, W.J., and Yang, Q.Y. (2002). Effects of ursolic acid and oleanolic acid on human colon carcinoma cell line HCT15. *World Journal of Gastroenterology*, 8: 493-495.

Liu, J., Chen, X.F., Xia, L., Geng, X.Z., and Li, Z.S. (1987). Effect of oleanolic acid on serum glyceride cholesterol and β-lipo-proteins in normal and experimental hyperlipedermia rats. *Chinese Pharmacological Bulletin*, 4: 14-15.

Liu, J., Liu, Y., and Klaassen C.D. (1994). The effect of Chinese hepatoprotective medicines on experimental liver injury in mice. *Journal of Ethnopharmacology*, 42: 183-191.

Liu, J. (1995). Pharmacology of oleanolic acid and ursolic acid. *Journal of Ethnopharmacology*, 49: 57-68.

Liu, Y., Hartley, D.P., and Liu, J. (1998). Protection against carbon tetrachloride hepatotoxicity by oleanolic acid is not mediated through metallothionein. *Toxicology Letters*, 95: 77-85.

Liu, J., Liu, Y.P., Klaassen, C.D., Waalkes, M.P., Park, R.T., Anderson, S., and Corton, C. (1999). Gene expression pattern in mice and rats produced by the hepatoprotectant oleanolic acid. *Hepatology*, 30: 948-948.

Liu, J. (2005). Oleanolic acid and ursolic acid: Research perspectives. *Journal of Ethnopharmacology*, 100: 92-94.

Lopes, M.N., Oliveira, A.C., Young, M.C.M., and Bolzani, V.D.S. (2004). Flavonoids from *Chiococca braquiata* (Rubiaceae). *Journal of the Brazilian Chemical Society*, 15: 468-471.

Loux, J.J., Smith, S., and Salem, H. (1978). Comparative analgesic testing of various compounds in mice using writhing techniques. *Arzneimittelforschung*, 28: 1644-1647.

Ma, X.H., Zhao, Y.C., Yin, L., Xu, R.L., Han, D.W., and Wang, M.S. (1986). Studies on the preventive and therapeutic effects of ursolic acid (UA) on acute hepatic injury in rats. *Acta Pharmaceutica Sinica*, 21: 332-335.

Ma, C.M., Nakamura, N., Hattori, N., Kakuda, H., Qiao, J.C., and Yu, H.L. (2000). Inhibitory effects on HIV-1 protease of constituents from the wood of *Xanthoceras sorbifolia*. *Journal of Natural Products*, 63: 238-242.

Maciel, M.A.M., Pinto, A.C., Arruda, A.C., Pamplona, S.G.S.R., Vanderline, F.A., Lapa, A.J., Echevarria, A., Grynberg, N.F., Côlus, I.M.S., Farias, R.A.F., Luna Costa, A.M., and Rao, V.S.N. (2000). Ethnopharmacology, phytochemistry and pharmacology: a successful combination in the study of *Croton cajucara*. *Journal of Ethnopharmacology*, 70: 41-55.

Maciel, M.A.M., Pinto, A.C., and Veiga JR., V.F. (2002). Plantas Medicinais: a necessidade de estudos multidisciplinares. *Química Nova*, 25: 429-438.

Maciel, M. A. M., Dantas, T. N. C., Pinto, A.C., Veiga Jr., V. F., Grymberg, N. F., and Echevarria, A. (2005). Medicinal Plants: the need for multidisciplinary scientific studies. Part II. *Current Topics in Phytochemictry*, 7: 73-88.

Marquina, S., Maldonado, N., Garduño-Ramírez, M.L., Aranda, E., Villarreal, M.L., Navarro, V., Bye, R., Delgado, G., and Alvarez, L. (2001). Bioactive oleanolic acid saponins and other constituents from the roots of *Viguiera decurrens*. *Phytochemistry*, 56: 93-97.

Mezzetti, T., Orzalesi, G., and Bellavita, V. (1971). Chemistry of ursolic acid. *Planta Medica*, 20: 244-252.

Min, B.S., Jung, H.J., Lee, J.S., Kim, Y.H., Bok, S.H., Ma, C.M., Nakamura, N., Hattori, M., and Bae, K. (1999). Inhibitory effect of triterpenes from *Crataegus pinatifida* on HIV-I protease. *Planta Medica*, 65: 374-375.

Mix, K.S., Mengshol, J.A., Benbow, U., Vincenti, M.P., Spom, M.B., and Brinckerhoff, C.E. (2001). A synthetic triterpenoid selectively inhibits the induction of matrix metalloproteinases 1 and 13 by inflammatory cytokines. *Arthritis Reumatology*, 44:1096-1104.

Mizushina, Y., Iida, A., Ohta, K., Sugawara, F., and Sakaguchi, K. (2000). Novel triterpenoids inhibit both DNA polymerase and DNA topoisomerase. *Biochemical Journal*, 350: 757-763.

Munné-Bosch, S., Alegre, L., and Schwarz, K. (2000). The formation of phenolic diterpenes in *Rosmarinus officinalis* L. under Mediterranean climate. *European Food Research Technology*, 210: 263-267.

Murakami, S., Takashima, H., Sato-Watanabe, M., Chonan, S., Yamamoto, K., Saitoh, M., Saito, S., Yoshimura, H., Sugawara, K., Yang, J., Gao, N., and Zhang, X. (2004). Ursolic acid, an antagonist for transforming growth factor (TGF)-β1. *FEBS Letters*, 566: 55-59.

Oguro, T., Liu, J., Klaassen, C.D., and Yoshida, T. (1998). Inhibitory effect of oleanolic acid on 12-*O*-tetradecanoylphorbol-13-acetate-induced gene expression in mouse skin. *Toxicological Sciences*, 45: 88-93.

Okudo, T., Koshimizu, K., Daito, H., Kin, B., Nishimoto, K., and Yamazaki, N. (1990). Health drinks containing ursolic acid and/or oleanolic acid. *Chemical Abstracts*, 112, P54097m.

Parfentieva, E.P. (1979). Effect of ursolic acid and its derivatives on lipid-metabolism in experimental atherosclerosis. *Khimiko-Farmatsevticheskii Zhurnal*, 13: 10-16.

Pinto, A.C., Braga, W.F., Rezende, C.M., Garrido, F.M.S., Veiga Jr., V.F., Bergter, L., Patitucci, M.L., and Antunes, A.O.C. (2000). Separation of acid diterpenes of *Copaifera cearensis* Huber ex Ducke by flash chromatography using potassium hydroxide impregnated silica gel. *Journal of the Brazilian Chemical Society*, 11: 355-360.

Raffo. A., La Malfa, G., Fogliano, V., Maiani, G., and Quaglia, G. (2006) Seasonal variations in antioxidant components of cherry tomatoes (*Lycopersicon esculentum* cv. Naomi F1). *Journal of Food Composition Analysis*, 19: 11-19.

Razborsek, M.I, Voncina, D.B., Dolecek, V., and Voncina, E. (2008). Determination of oleanolic, betulinic and ursolic acids in Lamiaceae and mass spectral fragamentation of their trimethylsilylated derivatives. *Chromatographia*, 67: 433-440.

Reena, Z., Sudhakaran, N.C.R., and Velayudha, P.P. (1994). Antiinflammatory and antimitotic activities of lupeol isolated from the leaves of *Ixora coccinea* Linn. *Indian Journal of Pharmaceutical Sciences*, 56: 129-132.

Sasidharan, V.K. (1997). Search for antibacterial and antifungal activity of some plants of Kerala. *Acta Pharmaceutica*, 47: 47-51.

Sattar, A.A., Bankova, V., Kujumgiev, A., Galabov, A., Ignatova, A., Todorova, C., and Popov, S.S. (1995). Chemical composition and biological activity of leaf exudates from some Lamiaceae plants. *Pharmazie*, 50: 62-65.

Siegel, P.S. (1946). A simple electronic device for the measurement of gross bodily activity of small animals. *Journal of Psychology*, 21: 227-236.

Sietsema, W.K., Berman, E.F., Farmer, R.W., and Maddin, C.S. (1988). The antinociceptive effect and pharmacokinetics of olvanil following oral and subcutaneous dosing in the mouse. *Life Sciences*, 43: 1385-1391.

Singh, G.B., Singh, S., Bani, S., Gupta, B.D., and Banerjee, S.K. (1992). Antiinflammatory activity of oleanolic acid in rats and mice. *Journal of Pharmacy and Pharmacology*, 44: 456-458.

Sivarajan, V.V., and Balachandran, I. (1941). Ayurvedic drugs and their plant sources. New Delhi: Oxford and IBH Publishing Co. (P) Ltd, p.1941.

Shatilo, V.V., Gerashchenko, G.I. and Semenchenko, V.F. (1973). Antiinflammatory properties of ursolic acid and its effect on biochemical indices of carbohydrate metabolism in albino rats. *Biologicheskie Nauki*, 120: 41-44.

Sokal, R.R., and Rohlf, F.J. (1981). Biometry: The principles an Practice of Statistics, 2nd. Ed., W. H. Freemann, New York, p. 859.

Somova, L.O., Nadar, A., Rammanan, P., and Shode, F.O. (2003). Cardiovascular, antihyperlipidemic and antioxidant effects of oleanolic and ursolic acids in experimental hypertension. *Phytomedicine*, 10: 115-121.

Stein, C., Millan, M.J., Shippenberg, T.S., Peter, K., and Herz, A. (1989). Peripheral opioids receptors mediating antinociception in inflammation. Evidence for involvement of mu, delta and kappa receptors. *Journal of Pharmacology and Experimental Therapeutics*, 248: 1269-1275.

Suksamrarn, A., Tanachatchairatana, T., and Kanokmedhakul, S. (2003). Antiplasmodial triterpenes from twigs of *Gardenia saxatilis*. *Journal of Ethnopharmacology*, 88: 275-277.

Tang, H.Q., Hu, J., Yang, L., and Tan, R.X. (2000). Terpenoids and flavonoids from *Artemisia* species. *Planta Medica*, 66: 391-393.

Vacher, P.J., Duchêne-Marullaz, P., and Barbot, P. (1964). A propos de quelques produits usuels. Comparaison de deux méthodes d'étude des analgésiques. *Medicina Experimentalis (International Journal of Experimental Medicine)*, 11: 51-58.

Vasilenko, Y.K., Ponomarev, V.D., and Oganesyan, E.T. (1981). Comparative study of the hypolipidemic properties of triterpenoids. *Khimiko-Farmatsevticheskii Zhurnal*, 15: 50-53.

Vasilenko, Y.K., Lisevitskaya, L.I., and Frolova, L.M. (1982). Hypolipidaemic properties of triterpenoids. *Russian Pharmacology and Toxicology*, 45: 162-168.

Wenzel, D.G., and Koff, G.Y. (1956). The effect of triterpenes on the excretion of sodium and potassium by rats. *Journal of the American Pharmaceutical Association*, 45: 372-373.

Woolfe, G., and Macdonald, A.D. (1944). The evaluation of the analgesic action of pethidine hydrochloride (Demerol). *Journal of Pharmacology and Experimental Therapeutics*, 80: 300-307.

Wrzeciono, U., Malecki, I., Budzianowski, J., Kierylowicz, H., Zaprutko, L., Beimvik, E., and Kostepska, H. (1985). Nitrogenous triterpene derivatives. Part 10: Hemisuccinates of some derivatives of the oleanolic acid and their antiulcerous response. *Pharmazie*, 40: 542-544.

Xu, L.Z., and Wan, Z.X. (1980). The effect of oleanolic acid on acute hepatitis (70 cases). *Human Medicine*, 7: 50-52.

Xu, S.L. (1985). Effects of oleanolic acid on chronic hepatitis: 188 case reports. *Symposium on oleanolic acid*, 23-25.

Yamahara, J., Mibu, H., Sawada, T., Fujimura, H., Takino, S., Yoshikawa, M., and Kitogawa, I. (1981). Biologically-active principles of crude drugs: Antidiabetic principles of corni fructus in experimental diabetes induced by streptozotocin. *Yakugaku Zasshi*, 101: 86-90.

Yoshikawa, M., and Matsuda, H. (2000). Antidiabetogenic activity of oleanolic acid glycosides from medicinal foodstuffs. *BioFactors*, 13: 231-237.

Zimmermann, M. (1986). Ethical considerations in relation to pain in animal experimentation. *Acta Physiologica Scandinavica*, 128: 221-233.

Zurcher, A., Jerger, O., and Ruzicka, L. (1954). Zur kenntnis der triterpene. 180. Uberfuhrung der chinovasaure in phyllanthol und uvaol: Urber die konstitution der ursolsaure und des uvaols. *Helvetica Chimica Acta*, 37: 2145-2152.

Medicinal Plants: Phytochemistry, Pharmacology and Therapeutics, Vol. 1 *Pages* **51–74**
Editors: **V.K. Gupta, G.D. Singh, Surjeet Singh and A. Kaul**
Published by: **DAYA PUBLISHING HOUSE, NEW DELHI**

Chapter 3

A Review on Phytochemistry, Pharmacology and Therapeutic Uses of *Wrightia tinctoria* R. Br.

Papiya Bigoniya[1]* and A.C. Rana[2]**
[1]Department of Pharmacology, Radharaman College of Pharmacy, Fatehpur Dopra, Ratibad, Bhopal – 462 002, M.P. India
[2]Department of Pharmacology, B.N College of Pharmacy, B.N Group of Colleges, Udaipur, Rajastna, India

ABSTRACT

Natural products have served mankind as a source of drugs and higher plants provide most of these therapeutic agents. Undoubtedly, the plant kingdom still holds many species of plants containing substances of medicinal value, which have yet to be discovered. India is a land of immense biodiversity in which two (Eastern Himalayas and The Western Ghats of India) out of twenty five hot spots of the world are located.

Wrightia tinctoria (Roxb.) R.Br. is a small deciduous tree of the family Apocynaceae distributed in Central India, Burma and Timor. This plant is extensively used in the Indian system of medicine. The seeds resemble the seeds of Jau (Barley), this is the reason it is known as Indrajau. Fresh leaves are pungent and are chewed for relief from toothache. Bark and seeds are antidysenteric, carminative, astringent, aphrodisiac and diuretic, used in flatulence, stomach pain and bilious affections. The plant is very useful as stomachic, in the treatment of abdominal pain, skin diseases, as antidiarrhoeal and antihaemorrhagic. Traditional healers of Chhattisgarh use Indrajau both internally and externally in the treatment of about 16 diseases. The bark is used externally in skin

* Corresponding Author: E-mail: p_bigoniya2@hotmail.com; **E-mail: acrana4@rediffmail.com.

troubles. Oil emulsion of *W. tinctoria* pods is used to treat psoriasis. *W. tinctoria* bark showed antinociceptive, immunomodulatory and wound healing effect.

The stem bark of *W. tinctoria* contains β-amyrin, lupeol, β-sitosterol. Triacontanol and tryptanthrin have been isolated from *W. tinctoria* leaves. Immature seed pod of *W. tinctoria* gives cycloartenone, b-amyrin, cycloeucalenol, β-sitosterol and wrightial. A new sterol 14α-methylzymosterol in addition to four rare plant sterols, desmosterol, clerosterol, 24-methylene-25-methylcholesterol and 24-dehydropollinastanol have been isolated from *W. tinctoria* seeds.

Keywords: *Antimicrobial, Antinociceptive, Apocynaceae, Ethnopharmacology, Psoriasis, Seed oil, Triterpenes, Wrightia tinctoria (Roxb.) R.Br.*

Introduction

The Apocynaceae includes 155 genera and about 1700 species, which are almost equally shared by the two subfamilies, Apocynoideae and Plumerioideae. The family is easily recognized by the opposite leaves, the white latex and the sympetalous actinomorphic flowers with contorted aestivation. The family also is well known for the numerous medicinal plants it contains, *e.g.* in the genera *Rauwolfia, Strophanthus, Tabernaemontana* and *Voacanga.* The areas of distribution of most genera are mainly within the tropics and some species reach southern China. These species have areas either covering south-eastern continental Asia, the whole of continental tropical Asia, plus the area of the Malaysia and tropical Australia.

Apocynaceae family plants are chiefly tropical trees, shrubs or herbs having milky juice. Leaves evergreen, alternate or opposite or whorled, when whorled 3 per whorl, simple or decussate. Flowers are 5-merous, with androecium and gynoecium fused to form a gynostegium, pollen sacs fused to form pollinia and a corona. Inflorescences are a single flower to cymes, hypogynous or perigynous. Flowers aggregated in 'inflorescences', color white, yellow, red, pink, purple or blue. Fruits are follicles, dehiscent along the adaxial suture and filled with seeds that each has a tuft of long, silky hairs (a coma). Fruit is a berry, drupe, two follicles or a schizocarp. Seeds are often with hairs at one end.

Wrightia Genus

Wrightia is a genus of tropical shrubs and trees belonging to the family Apocynaceae. They usually have slender branches, and bear cymes of yellow, red or white flowers with salver-shaped corollas. *Wrightia* is named after a Scottish physician and botanist William Wright (1740–1827). Wrightia was first proposed as a genus by Brown in honor of Dr. William Wright who spent 18 years on the island of Jamaica. The genus at that time includes four species and out of which two (*W. antidysenterica* and *W. zeylanica*) had previously being included within Nerium by Linnaeus. Between 1809 and 1844 Wrightia was established as a genus based on its clear diagnostic characters like structure of seeds and embryo but still several species were described from flowering specimen under the genera *Nerium, Strophanthus, Cameraria, Chonemorpha, Anasser* and *Hunteria* (Ngan, 1965).

Species and Varieties of *Wrightia* Common in India

- *Wrightia arborea* (Dennst.) Mabb.
- *Wrightia coccinea* Sims. Parts used: wood has non medicinal use.
- *Wrightia cunninghamiis*

- *Wrightia hainanensis* Merr. var.
- *Wrightia indica*
- *Wrightia laevis* J. D. Hooker
- *Wrightia laniti* (Blanco) Merr.
- *Wrightia mollissima*
- *Wrightia pubescens* R. Br. subsp.
- *Wrightia religiosa* (Teijsm. and Binn.) Benth.
- *Wrightia saligna*
- *Wrightia schlechteri* H. Leveille
- *Wrightia sikkimensis* Gamble
- *Wrightia tomentosa* (Roxb.) Roem. and Schult. (Dudhi, Dharauli, Daira), Parts used: leaf, bark, seed, fruit and latex.
- *Wrightia wallichii*
- *Wrightia zeylanica* R. Br.

Wrightia tinctoria (Roxb.) R. Br.

Wrightia tinctoria (Roxb.) R.Br. is a small deciduous tree with light gray, scaly smooth bark of the family Apocynaceae (Chary, 1980). Plant is native to India, Burma and Timor. This plant grows in abandance in dry, hilly, rocky and desarted areas of Tamil Nadu, Andrapradesh, Madhya Pradesh and Rajasthan This plant is extensively used in the Indian system of medicine. Detailed taxonomical classification is given in Table 3.1.

Synonym(S)

Nerium tinctorium Roxb., *Nerium tinctorium* Roxb. ex Rottler,

Vernacular Name

Ayurveda: Dhudi/Mitha Indrajao/Strikutaja

English: Sweet Indrajao/Black indrajau/Pala indigo

Sanskrit : Hyamaraka/Asit kutaj

Hindi: Indrajau/Mitha-indrajau/Dudhi/Kuraiya

Bengali: Indrajau

Gujarati: Runchallodudhlo/Dudhlo/Dudheli kado

Marathi: Kala Kuda/Indrajau

Telugu: Tedlapaala/Amkuda/Jeddapaala

Tamil: Veypale/Irumpalai/Thonthapalai/Paalai

Kennard: Kodamurki/Bepalle/Kodesige

Malayalam: Kotakappalla/Aiyapala

Oriya: Pita Karuan/Dudho Kriya/Krya

Table 3.1: Taxonomical Classification of *Wrightia tinctoria* (Roxb.) R.Br.

Taxonomy	*Wrightia tinctoria (Roxb.) R.Br.*
Kingdom	Plantae
Subkingdom	Tracheobionta
Division	Magnoliophyta
Superdivision	Spermatophyta
Class	Magnoliopsida
Subclass	Asteridae
Order	Gentianales
Family	Apocynaceae
Subfamily	Apocynoideae
Tribe	Wrightieae
Genus	*Wrightia*
Species	*Wrightia tinctoria* ☆ Wrightia (RITE-ee-a)–Named for William Wright, 19th century Scottish physician and botanist. ☆ Tinctoria (tink-TOR-ee-uh)–Indicates a plant used in dyeing or has a sap which can stain.
Author	William Wright (1740–1827); Standard form R.Br.
Duration	Perennial
Growth habit	Small deciduous Tree or shrub

Parts Used

Leaf, bark, seed and pods.

Morphological Description

W. tinctoria is a small deciduous tree of 10–15 meter tall with milky latex, bark scaly, smooth, yellow or light brown, glabrous or puberulous branchlets. The tree is covered by a pale, smooth bark. The wood is white, grained and amenable for carving. Bark pale grey, tasteless and gives gray powder after milling. The plant has slender cord like branches. Leaves are variable, 7.5-15 by 2.5-5.7 cm, simple, opposite, elliptic lanceolate or oblong-lanceolate, obtusely acuminate and glabrous. The young leaves are bluish with reddish nerves, puberulous beneath, base acute or rounded, main nerves 6-12 pairs, petioles 3-4 mm long. Leaves on piercing would cause a flow of milky latex, characterize the vegetative phase of the tree. The leaves of this tree yield a blue dye called Pala Indigo. Flowering occurs during dry season from the second week of April to the first week of June and fruiting cold season to greater part of the year. From a distance, the white flowers may appear like snow flakes on a tree. It shows sparse flowering occasionally during the rainy season from the second week of July to the second week of August. It produces bisexual flowers on terminal panicles (Anonymous, 2005). The flowers are creamy-white, fragrant, actinomorphic and hypogynous. The calyx consists of five small, green-coloured sepals. Flowers are in lax terminal cymes which are sometimes 12.5 cm diameter with slender spreading dichotomous, branches bracts minute, ovate, calyx glabrous glandular inside segment 2.5 mm long, oblong, rounded at the apex and with membranous margins. Corolla tube short

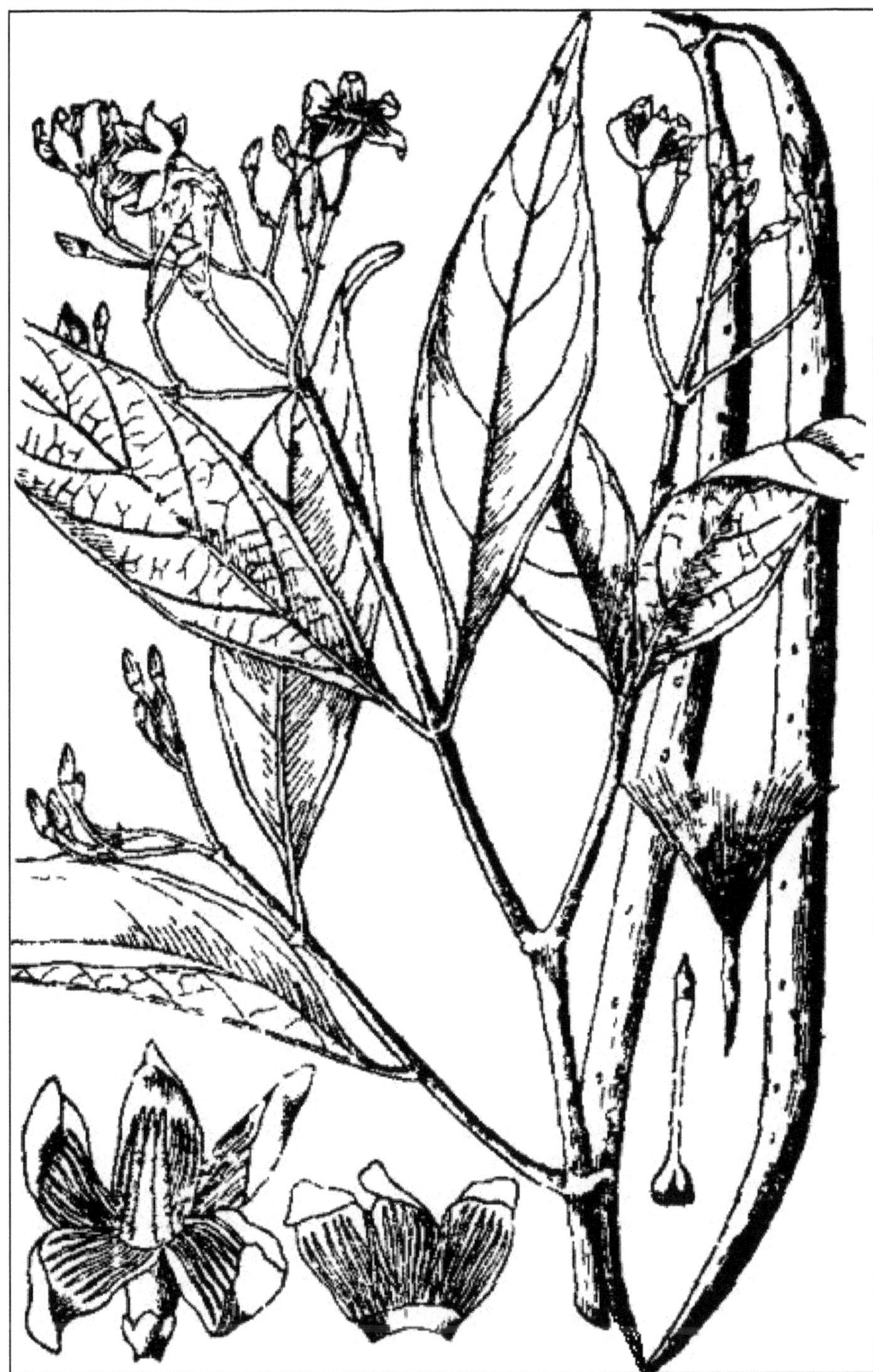

Figure 3.1: ***Wrightia tinctoria*** **(Roxb.) R. Br.**
(A) Flowering twig, (B) Fruit, (C) Flower

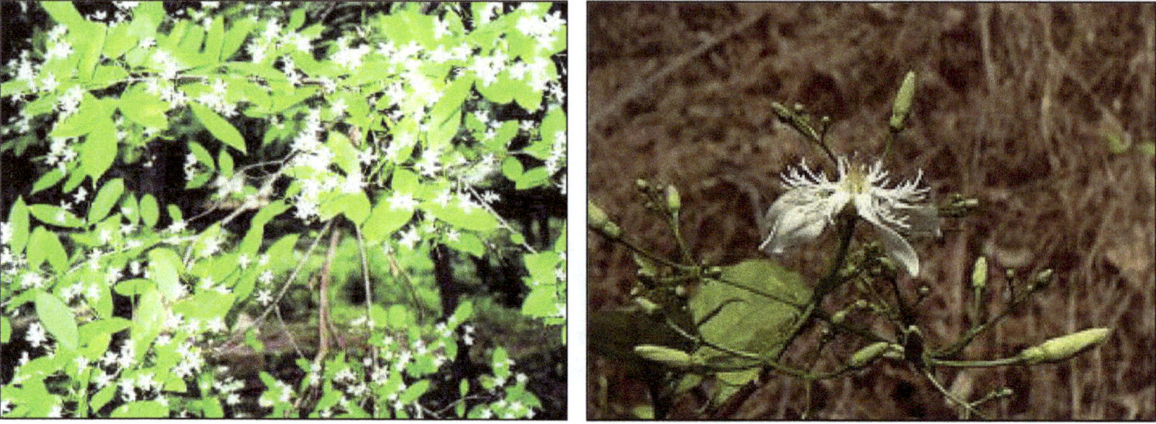

Figure 3.2: Photographs of *Wrightia tinctoria* (Roxb.) R. Br. Flowers

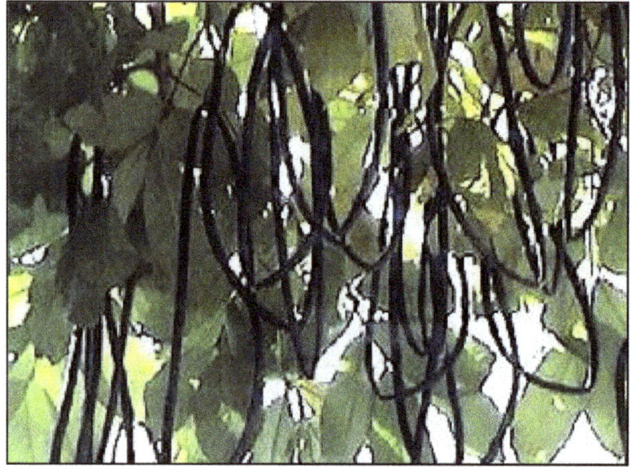

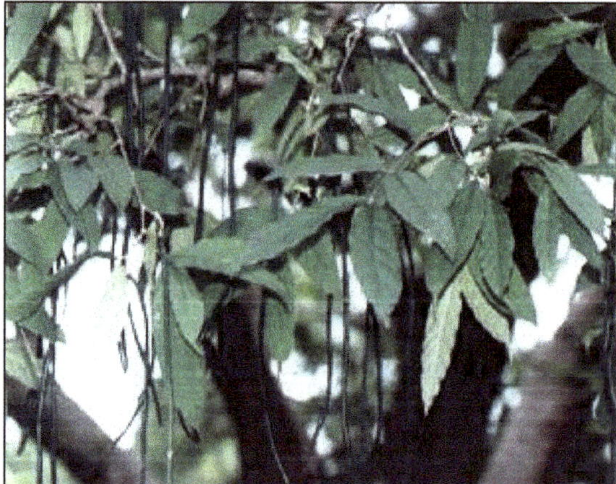

Figure 3.3: Photographs of *Wrightia tinctoria* (Roxb.) R. Br. Fruits

3 mm long, lobes 8 mm long, oblong, obtuse, corona of numerous linear scales some inserted with the filaments and some on the corolla-lobes. Fruits are pair of two distinct pendulous green slender paired follicles, 25-50 cm by 6-8 mm cylindric slightly tapering to both ends, glabrous, striate, cohering at the tip only. Seeds 1.3-2 mm long, pointed at the apex, linear, glabrous, light yellowish-gray crowned with a deciduous coma or a tuft of white silky hairs of more than 3.8 cm long at the base by which they are disseminated in air. The hairy seeds are released as the fruit dehisces. The seeds resemble the seeds of Jau (Barley), this is the reason it is known as Indrajau. An outstanding characteristic feature that helps us to identify the tree is the organisation of its paired long follicles, joined at their tips. As the fruit dehisces along only one of its seams, long seeds with an attenuated apex and a cluster of air-filled hairs at their bases are released. Even so, they are not as well dispersed by air, as they should have been, because these hairs are deciduous, falling off rather early after release from the fruit (Kirtikar and Basu, 1975; Malvia, 1975; Mahadevan *et al.*, 1998; Reddy *et al.*, 1999).

W. tinctoria seed fibers are unicellular yellowish-buff in color, 1.2-1.4 cm long, 25-27 mm in diameter having pointed apex and large lumen with thin wall. The fibers are easily distinguishable from cotton and jute as evident from physical properties. *W. tinctoria* seed fibers shows presence of lignified tissues and very less quantity of cellulose, and absence of true cellulose and cuticle layer. Oxidizing agents disintegrates the lignified walls. *W. tinctoria* seed fibers are inherently wettable, solublize easily in acidic and basic medium, tensile strength $1.25´10^7$ N/M^2 which may ensure easy dispersibility in wounds (Bigoniya and Rana, 2006).

W. tinctoria is commonly used as adulterant of an important antidysentric drug *Holarrhena antidysentrica* another apocynaceae plant (Chopra *et al.*, 1956; Chopra *et al.*, 1958). The therapeutic properties of *W. tinctoria* are similar to that of *H. antidysentrica*, which contains several steroidal alkaloids and is an established antidiarrhoeal drug (Glasby, 1975; Khan, 1987). *W. tinctoria* plants as well as leafs are smaller in size than *H. antidysentrica*. The Holarrhena has longer and greener leaves while the leaves of Wrightia are not as large or as green as former. *W. tinctoria* has white flavored flowers and dark brown to black colored root which are less bitter than *H. antidysentrica*. *H. antidysentrica* seeds have their air-filled hairs at the apex, while in Wrightia the tuft of air filled hairs is at the base of the seed. A comparative study was carried out on both the seeds by Jolly and Mechery, (1996) which included pharmacognostical and physiochemical evaluation. *W. tinctoria* barks can be differentiated from *H. antidysentrica* as the former is less bitter or taste less, soothing and color is reddish-brown (Atal and Sethi, 1962).

Traditional and Ethnopharmacological Uses

Sweet Indrajao is called dhudi (Hindi) because of its preservative nature. Supposedly a few drops of its sap in milk prevent curdling and enhance its shelf life, without the need to refrigerate. The wood of Sweet Indrajao is extensively used for all classes of turnery. It is made into cups, plates, combs, pen holders, pencils and bed stead legs. It is commonly used for making Chennapatna toys.

Fresh leaves are acrid, pungent and are chewed for relief from toothache (Kirtikar and Basu, 1975; The Wealth of India, 1976). Bark and seeds are astringent, acrid, thermogenic, carminative, digestive, stomachic, antidysenteric, constipating, depurative, anthelmintic, aphrodisiac, febrifuge and diuretic. They are useful in vitiated conditions of pitta and kapha, dyspepsia, bilious affections, flatulence, colic stomach pain, diarrhoea, leprosy, psoriasis, haemorrhoids, helminthiasis, fever, burning sensation and dropsy. The plant is very useful as stomachic, in the treatment of abdominal pain, skin diseases, as antidiarrhoeal and antihaemorrhagic (Nadkarni, 1976; Joshi *et al.*, 1980; Singh *et al.*, 1980; Shah and Gopal, 1988).

The leaves are applied as a poultice for mumps and herpes and sometimes they are also munched to relieve toothache. Tribes in Tamil Nadu applies "Vetpalai" a paste of the leaves, mixed with neem (nimba: *Azadirachta indica* A.Juss.) oil for eczema (Anesan *et al.*, 2007).

In folk medicine, the dried and powdered roots of Wrightia along with *Phyllanthus amarus* (keezhanelli) and *Vitex negundo* (nochi) is mixed with milk and orally administered to women for improving fertility. The bark and seeds are effective against psoriasis and non-specific dermatitis. It has antiinflammatory and antidandruff properties and hence is used in hair oil preparations. Hill tribes use latex of the bark and unripe fruits for coagulating and solidifying milk. *W. tinctoria* produces thick and milky white latex. It is also said that Palakkad (Palghat), in Kerala got its name (pala = milky latex-bearing tree and kaadu = forest) due to the predominance of *W. tinctoria* trees in the drier forests (Ranjit Daniels *et al.*, 2007).

All parts of the plant yield a purple dye called pala-indigo. Bark powder is very useful when taken every day in small quantity for indigestion, acidity and stomach pain. It is also used in chronic lung diseases and asthma. Massage of *W. tinctoria* powder reduces bleeding gum and fowl smell in gum pyorrhea. A decoction of the leaves and bark is rubbed over the body in dropsy. The bark is used as tonic and mineral supplement. The seeds possess aphrodisiac and anthelmintic properties (Pandey, 1992; The Wealth of India, 1976).

Traditional healers of Chhattisgarh use Indrajau both internally and externally in the treatment of about 16 diseases. Aqueous paste of Indrajau root is given to the patients having intestinal worm problem. The traditional healers mix Indrajau bark to Giloi decoction mixture to make it more effective. Germinated seeds of Idrajau are being recommended for patients suffering from jaundice. The bark is used externally in skin troubles. The healers prepare paste by mixing Indrajau bark powder with cow urine and apply it to effected parts. Indrajau bark is given with cow milk in urinary troubles and with dahi (curd) in renal calculi. In treatment of fever, Indrajau is a main ingredient in popular herbal combinations. The use of Indrajau in treatment of jaundice, fever and worm problem is very popular among the traditional healers (Oudhia, 2003).

Phytochemistry

The very first approach towards the separation of alkaloidal constituents of *W. tinctoria* by TLC was approached by P. D. Sethi (1970). Dried bark powder of *W. tinctoria* was extracted with ethyl alcohol-chloroform (1:4) mixture for separation of total alkaloids. Different solvent systems were tried to separate individual alkaloids by TLC using Modified Dragendorff's spraying reagent. Maximum six spots have been revealed and best separation has been effected with benzene-chloroform-ethyl alcohol (4:2:1) on alkaline silica gel G layer.

Reddy *et al.* (1999) carried out pharmacognostical studies on *W. tinctoria* bark to establish standards for identification of the drug. Macroscopy, histology, microchemical and phytochemical tests along with ash and extractive values were reported. Successive cold extraction of dried *W. tinctoria* bark collected from Mothapalayam of Nilgiri hills, Tamil Nadu, India in the month of June showed presence of the following constituents in qualitative phytochemical tests - Petroleum ether extract: steroids; chloroform extract: steroids and triterpenoids; ethylacetate extract: steroids, triterpenoids, saponins, flavonoids, tannins and phenolics; acetone and methanol extract: glycosides, steroids, triterpenoids, saponins, carbohydrates and flavonoids, tannins and phenolics. All extracts gave negative tests for alkaloids, fixed oils, cumarins, gums and resins.

The stem bark of *W. tinctoria* contains β-amyrin, lupeol, β-sitosterol and a new triterpenoid as reported by Rangaswami and Rao, (1963). The powdered bark was exhausted by cold percolation with petroleum ether. The petroleum ether extract contained a lot of rubbery material elimination of which gives one triterpene compound obtained by direct fractional crystallization from ethyl alcohol, but that cannot be identified (m.p. 170-72°C). The mother liquors after suitable fractionation technique yield β-amyrin acetate (m.p. 238-40°C), lupeol benzoate (m.p. 266-70°C) and β-sitosterol (m.p. 132-34°C). The identity has been established by color reactions, elementary analysis, optical rotation and mixed melting point with authentic sample.

Triacontanol and tryptanthrin (m.p. 265-67°C) have been isolated from *W. tinctoria* leaves as reported by George *et al.* (1996). β-amyrin benzoate (m.p. 229-31°C) was isolated from the petroleum ether extract of powdered leaves.

The powdered pods (freed from seeds), were extracted with hexane followed by hot chloroform. The hexane extract gave a mixture of terpenoids. Ursolic acid (m.p. 280-82°C) was obtained from

Figure 3.4: Isolated Compound of *Wrightia tinctoria*

Bark

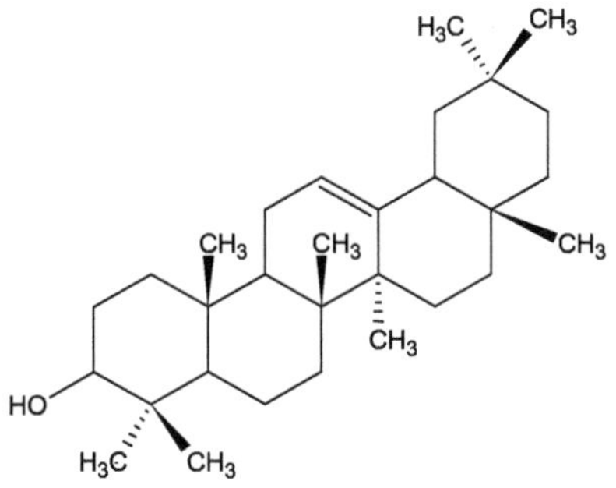

β-amyrin 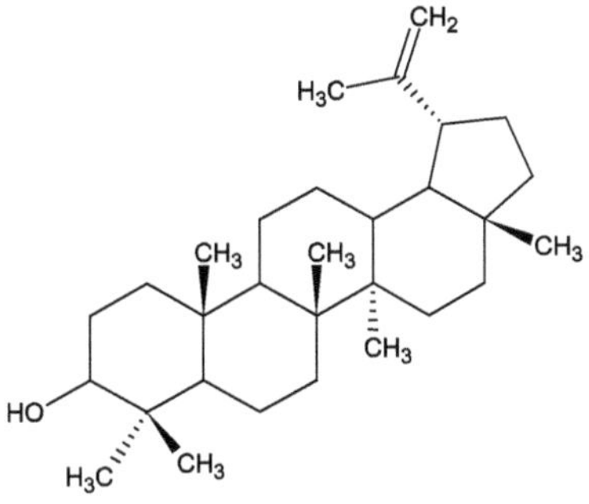 **Lupeol** 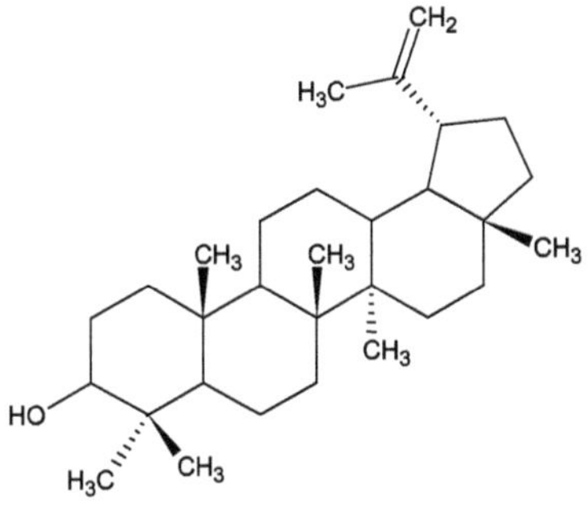 **β-Sitosterol**

Leaf

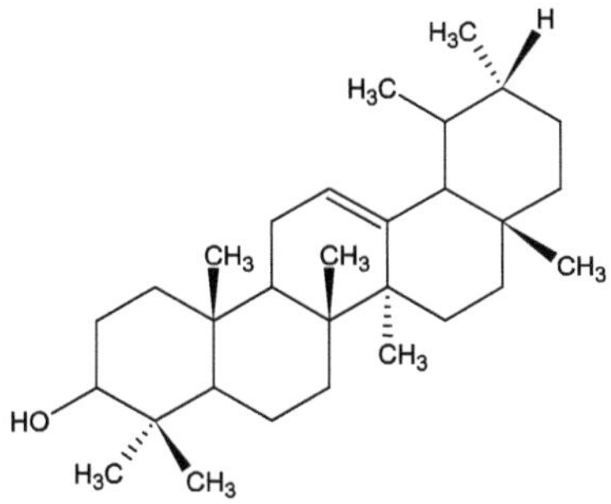

α-amyrin 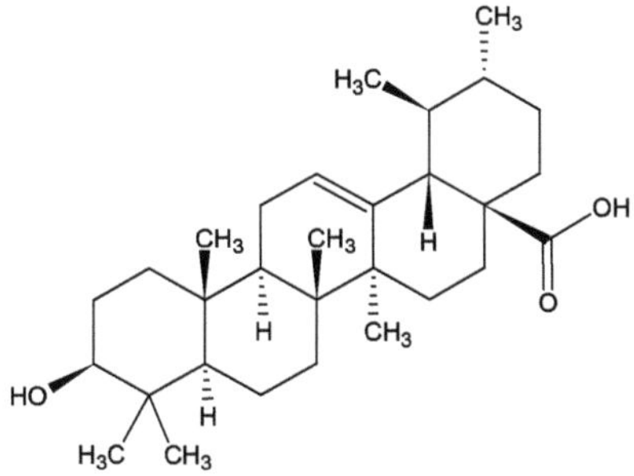 **Ursolic acid** 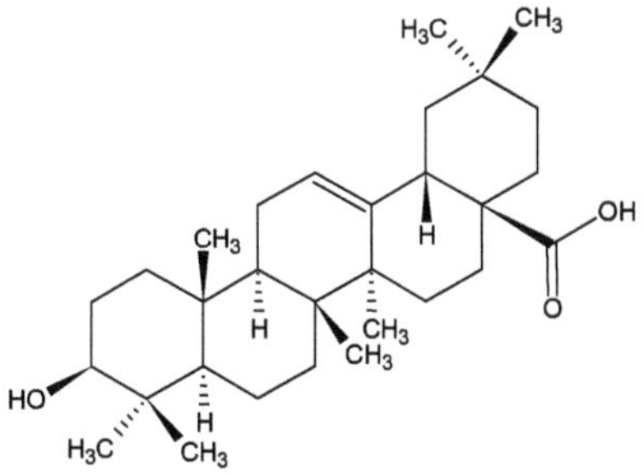 **Oleanolic acid**

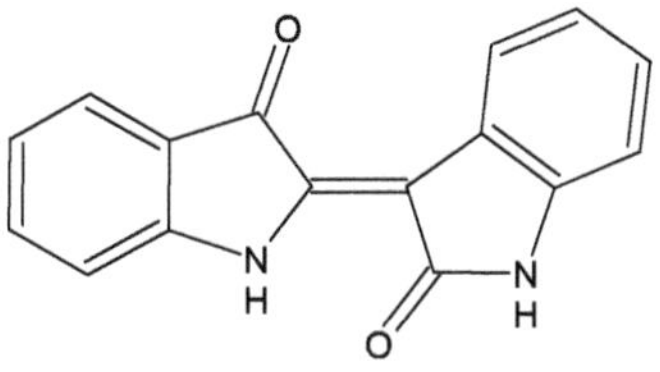

Indirubin 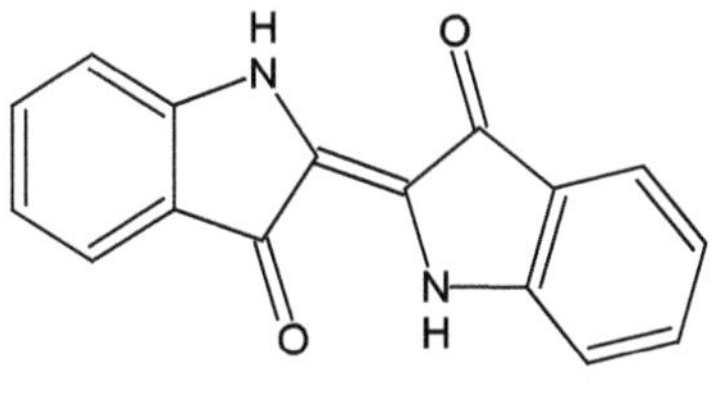 **Indigotin** 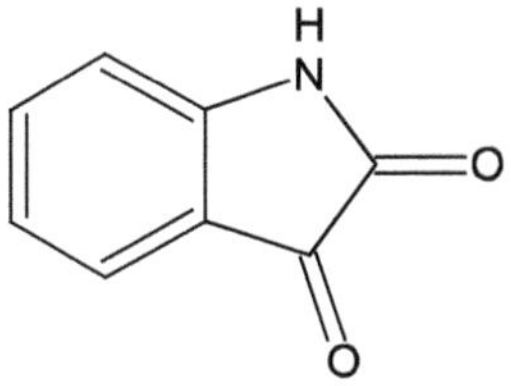 **Isatin**

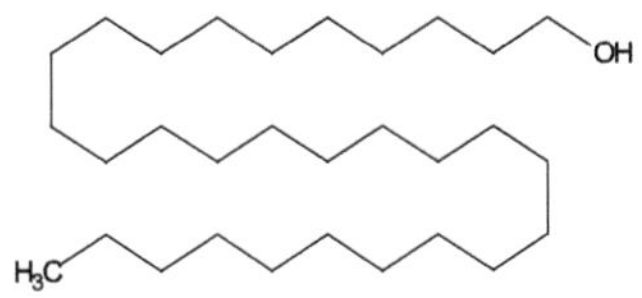

Triacontanol (Myricyl alcohol) 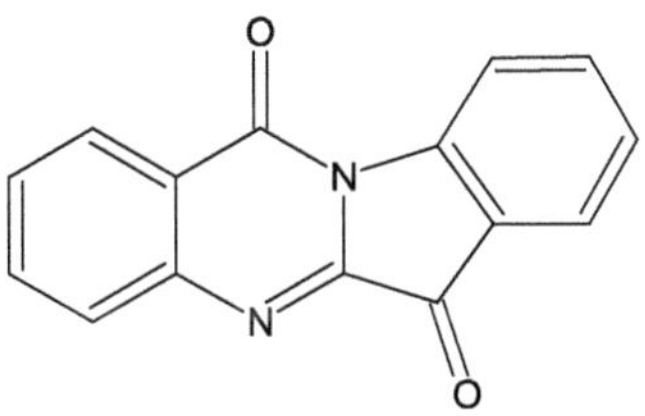 **Tryptanthrin** 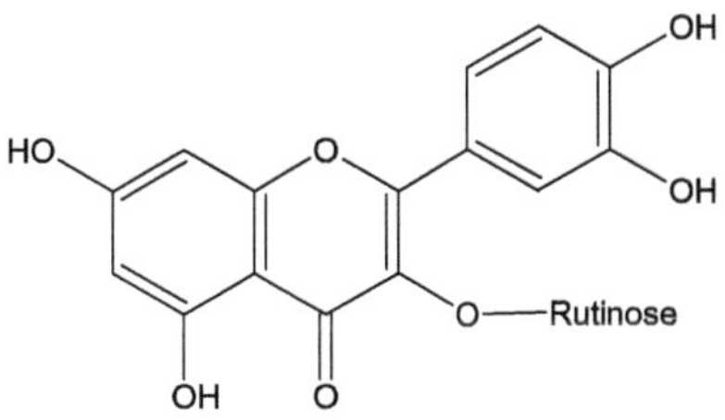 **Rutin**

Contd...

Figure 3.4–Contd...

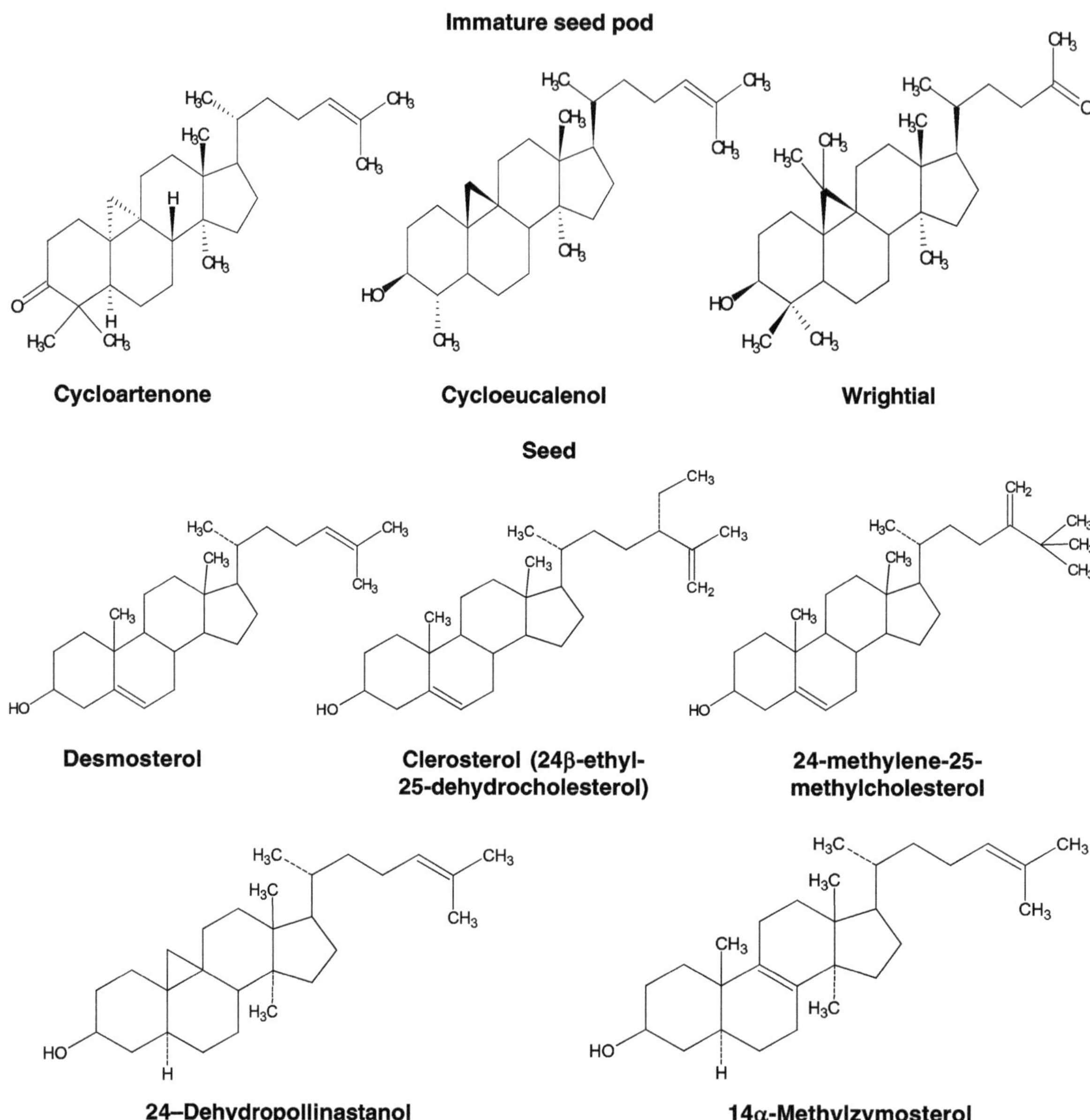

Seed Oil

CH_3-$(CH_2)_4$-CH=CH-$(CH_2)_2$-CH(OH)-$(CH_2)_7$-COOH
Isoricinoleic acid (Strophanthus acid)

chloroform extract of pods besides another triterpene acid (m.p. 130-31°C) from mother liquors which cannot be identified (Rao *et al.*, 1966). In continution to their studies Rao *et al.* (1968) reported isolation of α-amyrin (m.p. 182-84°C), β-sitosterol and ursolic acid from hexane extract of pods. oleanolic acid (m.p. 250-53°C) was reported to isolate from mother liquors of ursolic acid.

Column chromatography (petroleum ether, benzene and chloroform) of methanol extract of *W. tinctoria* immature dried seed pods gave five compounds. Four of these compounds were identified as cycloartenone, b-amyrin, cycloeucalenol and b-sitosterol and fifth one was identified as wrightial (m.p. 99°C), a new terpene. Petroleum ether–chloroform elute (1:1) gave a colourless compound identified as cycloartenone (m.p. 102-103°C) and a white solid which was identified as b-amyrin (m.p. 196°C). The chloroform elute gave colourless solid, wrightial (m.p. 99°C), cycloeucalenol (m.p. 140°C) and β-sitosterol (Ramchandra *et al.*, 1993).

Isolation and characterization of a new sterol 14α-methylzymosterol in addition to four rare plant sterols, desmosterol (m.p. 95-97°C), clerosterol (m.p. 122-24°C), 24-methylene-25-methylcholesterol (m.p. 145-48°C) and 24-dehydropollinastanol (m.p. 75-78°C) have been reported from *W. tinctoria* seeds. Air dried and powdered seeds were extracted with petrol in a soxhlet extractor. Preparative TLC of the unsaponifiable lipid (petrol extract) gave sterol fraction which was further separated by argentation TLC, final isolation of each component from individual fractions was performed by HPLC (Akihisa *et al.*, 1988).

W. tinctoria seeds contain 30 per cent of oil out of which 70 per cent is hydroxy acid. Oil is rich in isoricinoleic acid or 9-hydroxy-cis-12-octadecenoic acid (strophanthus acid) like some other plants of Apocynaceae family (Everett *et al.*, 1981). Ahmad and Lie Ken Jie, (2008) carried out derivatization of methyl 9-hydroxyoctadec-12-ynoate to obtain the industrially important fatty compounds. Methyl 9-hydroxyoctadec-12-ynoate was subjected to mesylation and demesylation reactions in which an unknown compound methyl 9-ethoxyoctadec-12-ynoate was furnished in good yield, in addition to an inseparable mixture of enynoic esters. In another set of reactions methyl 9-hydroxyoctadec-12-ynoate was oxidized with trimethyl chlorochromate wherein the resulting methyl 9-oxooctadec-12-ynoate was subjected to three condensation reactions–with 1,2-ethanedithiol, ethylene glycol and b-mercaptoethanol separately–to yield diethyl 9,9-ethylenedisulfide octadec-12-ynoate, 9,9-ethylenedioxyoctadec-12-ynoate and 9-oxathiolaneoctadec-12-ynoate respectively in excellent yields. Their structures have been established using infrared (IR) spectroscopy, ^{1}H nuclear magnetic resonance (NMR) spectroscopy, ^{13}C NMR spectroscopy and mass spectral studies.

Rajesh *et al.* (2007) compared the clot inducing and dissolving properties of *Calotropis gigantea* R. Br. (Asclepiadaceae), *Synadenium grantii* Hook. f. (Euphorbiaceae) and *Wrightia tinctoria* R. Br. (Apocynaceae) latex extracts. All the three latex extracts hydrolyzed casein, fibrinogen and crude fibrin dose-dependently. The proteolytic action on fibrinogen subunit was in the order of alpha > beta > gamma. All extracts exhibited procoagulant activity as assayed by re-calcification time. However thrombin like activity is restricted to *C. gigantea*. In addition the extracts dose-dependently hydrolyzed blood and plasma clots. Furthermore, the hydrolyzing pattern of fibrin in the plasma clot was substantiated by SDS-PAGE. The extracts hydrolyzed all the subunits (alpha polymer, alpha-chains, gamma-gamma dimer and beta-chain) of fibrin efficiently. Both fibrinogenolytic and fibrinolytic activity potency of the extracts were in the order of *C. gigantea* > *S. grantii* > *W. tinctoria*. *S. grantii* and *W. tinctoria* latex extracts were non-toxic and did not induce any hemorrhagic effect at the tested dose (> 200 microg). The proteolytic activities of *S. grantii* and *W. tinctoria* were inhibited by PMSF. Thus, this study provides the basis for the probable action of plant latex proteases to stop bleeding and effect wound healing as exploited in folk medicine.

A new protease named "wrightin" was purified from the latex of the plant *W. tinctoria* by cation-exchange chromatography. The enzyme is a monomer having a molecular mass of 57.9 kDa (MALDI-TOF), an isoelectric point of 6.0 and an extinction coefficient (1 per cent; 280) of 36. 4. Optimun activity is achieved at a pH of 7.5-10 and a temperature of 70°C. Wrightin hydrolyzes denatured natural substrates such as casein, azoalbumin, and hemoglobin with high specific activity; for example, the Km value is 50 mM for cadein as substrate. Wrightin showed weak amidolytic activity toward l-Ala-Ala–p-nitroanilide but completely failed to hydrolyze N-alpha-benzoyl–dl-arginine–p-nitroanilide (BAPNA), a preferred substrate for trypsin-like enzymes. Complete inhibition of enzyme activity by serine protease inhibitors such as PMSF and DFP indicates that the enzyme belongs to the serine protease class. The enzyme was not inhibited by SBTI and resists autodigestion. Wrightin is remarkably thermostable, retaining complete activity at 70°C after 60 min of incubation and 74 per cent of activity after 30 min of incubation at 80°. Besides, the enzyme is very stable over a broad range of pH from 5.0 to 11.5 and remains active in the presence of various denaturants, surfactants, organic solvents and metal ions. Thus wrightin might be a potential candidate for various applications in the food and biotechnological industries, especially in operations requiring high temperatures (Tomar *et al.*, 2008).

Pharmacology

W. tinctoria bark is effective in psoriasis and nonspecific dermatitis. The leaves are used in various skin disorders including herpes. Oil emulsion of *W. tinctoria* pods is used to treat psoriasis (Anonymous, 1987). Psoriasis is characterized by epidermal hyperplasia and a greatly accelerated rate of epidermal turnover. The lesions are characteristically dry, well demarcated, red, slightly raised and scaly. Gentle scraping of the lesion removes scales and produces many pinpoint bleeding sites, the so-called "Auspitz sign". The lesions are discrete or confluent erythromatous plaques and papules covered with white or silvery scales found on the extensor surfaces such as the elbows, knees, back and scalp.

Krishnamurthy *et al.* (1981) carried out clinical study of vetpalai (*Wrightia tinctoria* L.) oil in the treatment of kalanjagapadai (psoriasis). Alam *et al.* (1985) reported effect of insulation on "777 oil" used for psoriasis in Siddha system of medicine. According to Siddha system the fat soluble material of the leaves of *W. tinctoria* (Roxb.) R.Br. was extracted into the oil in sunlight, this method is called suryaputa. The fat soluble substances are claimed to have keratolytic action. Phytochemical studies carried out on the extract exposed to sunlight for four hours showed an increase in acid and iodine values. Process and product standardisation of "777 oil" used for psoriasis in Siddha medicine was reported by Alam *et al.* (1986). 777 oil was prepared from the leaves of *W. tinctoria* (Roxb.) R.Br. by insolation with coconut or gingelly oil as a base. In this study the drug prepared by insolation (exposure to sunlight) was compared with that prepared in darkness. The insolated drug had a higher iodine number, indicating the production of more unsaturated compounds.

A US patent has been issued by the title "Herbal medication for the treatment of psoriasis" on January 12, 1999. The invention includes a composition comprising a latex extracted from the leaves of the *W. tinctoria* R. Br. plant, water, urea, and polyethylene glycol for topical treatment of skin disorders, particularly psoriasis. The pharmaceutical preparation is a hydrophilic ointment that is capable of delivering the active drugs without being greasy or irritating to the skin (Herbal medication for the treatment of psoriasis, US). The antibacterial screening of the various extracts of the seeds of *H. antidyssenterica* and *W. tinctoria* were carried out and the chloroform and methanolic extracts of both the seeds were found to possess antibacterial activity (Jolly and Mechery, 1996).

Muruganandam *et al.* (1998a) reported effect of *W. tinctoria* leaf methanolic extract on anxiety patterns in rats. The effect of acute administration of *W. tinctoria* leaves methanolic extractives, constituting indigotin (HPTLC, relative abundance 21.97 per cent), indirubin (27.13 per cent), tryptanthrin (21 per cent), isatin (2.70 per cent) and rutin (14.24 per cent), was studied on the rat brain concentrations of monoamines and their metabolites in five different brain regions, *viz.* hypothalamus, hippocampus, striatum, pons medulla and frontal cortex. *W. tinctoria* extract was administered at the doses of 25 and 50 mg/kg, i.p. and the brain monoamines were assayed after 30 minutes of the treatment. *W. tinctoria* treatment significantly and dose dependently decreased the levels of serotonin (5-HT), its metabolite 5-hydroxy indole acetic acid (5-HIAA) and their turnover in all the brain regions assayed. On the other hand, extract treatment significantly and dose dependently augmented the levels of norepinephrine (NE), its metabolite methyl hydroxy phenyl glycol (MHPG) and also the turnover in all the brain regions studied. Similarly, the levels of dopamine (DA) was also significantly augmented in the hypothalamus, striatum and frontal cortex. Likewise, the levels of dihydroxy phenyl acetic acid (DOPAC), a metabolite of DA, was also increased in hypothalamus and frontal cortex. However, the treatment produced a significant decrease in the DOPAC in striatum. This differential modulation of the neurotransmitters and their metabolites can explain the behavioral effects of *W. tinctoria*, namely anxiolytic and antidepressant effect (Muruganandam *et al.*, 1998b).

An experimental histological evaluation of *W. tinctoria* was conducted on reversal of parakeratosis to orthokeratosis based on mouse tail test. *W. tinctoria* showed nearly 90 per cent reversal when compared with treatment using retinoids and betamethasone (Mitra *et al.*, 1998). *W. tinctoria* has antidandruff activity and is used in the treatment of various scalp and skin disorders. *W. tinctoria* have antipityrosporum activity in combination with *Hibiscus rosasinensis in vitro* against isolates of *Pityrosporum ovale* recovered from dandruff. The drug combination exhibited fungicidal activity at a concentration ranging between 500 to 1000 mg/ml (Krishnamoorthy and Ranganathan, 2000). Ethyl acetate, acetone and methanolic extracts of *W. tinctoria* bark showed significant antinociceptive activity in mice comparable with acetylsalicylic acid, studied by acetic acid induced writhing test (Reddy *et al.*, 2000). Ethanolic extract of *W. tinctoria* bark showed wound healing effect in rats may be due to its antimicrobial activity controlling microbial colonization and subsequent proliferation thus promoting the healing of wounds (Veerapur *et al.*, 2004). Chandrashekhar, *et al.* (2004) reported hepatoprotective activity of *W. tinctoria* in rats.

Wrightia tinctoria leaves possessed potent antimicrobial properties against dermatophytic microbes as reported by Kannan *et al.* (2006). In particular, methanol and ethanol extracts were active against bacteria and hexane extract was active against dermatophytic fungi, suggesting that the active principles may be useful in the topical treatment of superficial skin infections. Leaf hexane, methanol and ethanol extracts were screened *in vitro* against skin bacteria and dermatophytes. The extracts were tested using agar dilution method and broth micro dilution method. Methanol and ethanol extracts showed antibacterial activity. The MIC was 0.5 mg/ml for *Bacillus subtilis* and *Staphylococcus epidermidis* and 0.25 mg/ml for *Staphylococcus aureus*. The hexane extract showed antifungal activity against *Trichophyton rubrum* and *Trichophyton tonsurans* at 2 mg/ml. The MIC of 2 mg/ml was observed for methanol extract against *Trichophyton mentagrophytes* and IC_{50} (2 mg/ml) was determined for *Trichophyton rubrum* and *Epidermophyton floccosum*.

Mycotic infection of the skin by the dermatophytes may be categorized into superficial and deep fungal infections. *Malassezia furfur (Pityrosporum ovale)*, a lipophilic fungus, affects the hair and causes diseases called dandruff. Dandruff is a condition, which causes small white flakes of skin that separate and fall from the scalp. People who suffer from dandruff have over active sebaceous glands, which make their scalp oily. It has been investigated and reported that there was no complete cure for this disease. The influence of the plant extracts of 19 species on the growth of *M. furfur* has been investigated and reported. Vijayakumar *et al.* (2006) carried out investigation of nineteen plant extracts for the antimycotic activity against *M. furfur*. *Aloe vera, Eucalyptus globulus, Phyllanthus emblica and Wrightia tinctoria* leaf extracts and oil showed antifungal property as they progressively inhibited the growth of *M. furfur* on Sabouraud's destrose agar medium.

W. tinctoria bark ethanolic extract was shown to posses antiulcer activity against experimentally induced acute gastric ulcer model as the extract reduced both pyloric ligated and ethanol induced ulceration in rats in a dose dependent manner. The extract significantly reduced the ulcers index induced by both pyloric ligation and ethanol at 1000 mg/kg dose. Extract treatment significantly reduced the secretary parameters like volume and pH of gastric juice, free and total acidity. The extract has significant effect on gastric mucous substances by increasing total carbohydrate content and decreasing total protein content in pyloric ligated ulceration, all these effects are comparable to ranitidine (20 mg/kg). The results indicate that *W. tinctoria* bark extract protects gastric mucous membrane by improving microcirculation, increased capillary resistance or by precipitating microproteins (Bigoniya *et al.*, 2006).

Investigation of the pharmacological profile of hydro-alcoholic extract of *Wrightia tinctoria* bark hydro-alcoholic extract was carried out in mice and rats using various models. The effects of the extract were observed in three different dose levels 300, 500 and 1000 mg/kg as extract does not show any sign of toxicity up to 3000 mg/kg dose. Investigations were carried out against thermal, chemical and mechanical noxious stimuli to study antinociceptive activity, pentobarbitone induce hypnosis and diuretic activity. Carrageenan-induced paw edema and cotton pellet induced granuloma model were employed to test antiinflammatory activity. Study revealed moderate analgesic effect against thermal and chemical noxious stimuli and antiinflammatory activity at the 1000 mg/kg dose. Extract is devoid of any sedative activity. *W. tinctoria* extract considerably increases urine volume, acting as strong kaliuretic (Bigoniya *et al.*, In press; Asian Journal of Experimental Sciences).

Immunomodulatory activity of *W. tinctoria* bark alcoholic extract was evaluated on nonspecific and specific immune responses, studying the parameters like survival study, carbon clearance test, delayed type hypersensitivity and estimation of hemagglutinating antibody titer. *W. tinctoria* extract at 400 mg/kg b.w increased the survival rate of rats against *E. coli* induced abdominal sepsis upto 15 days post infection. Extract showed significant haemopoietic activity and also raised neutrophils count significantly which was further confirmed by increased phagocytic response against inert particles. *W. tinctoria* exhibited extremely significant inhibition of DTH response. Extract enhanced both primary and secondary humoral responses in rats sensitized with BSA. The results of the study substantiate *W. tinctoria* bark extract as moderate non-specific immunostimulant. The decreased DTH reaction may be due to simultaneous presence of high antibody titres, promoting the elimination of antigen (Bigoniya *et al.*, In press; Current Pharma Research Journal).

Marketed Products

W. tinctoria has been used as one of the ingredient in preparation of various polyherbal formulations for medicinal use. It has number of herbal preparation against psoriasis.

Antipsoriasis

Psorayur Ointment (Garry and Sun, USA)

Ayurveda recommends the local application of a herbal balm which is blended with vata and kapha balancing herbs. Psorayur is an ideal combination of such various time tested herbs, which act as a herbal balm processed with *Vata* and *Kapha* balancing herbs.

Each g of Psorayur Ointment contains:

- Oily extract of *Cocos nucifera* 666.66 mg processed with
- *Wrightia tinctoria* 140 mg
- *Cynadon dactylon* 35 mg
- *Melia azaderachta* 20 mg
- *Cinnamomum camphora* 20 mg
- *Hydnocarpus laurifolia* 0.03 ml
- Purified Honey in Beeswax base q.s.

Use

Use and application of Psorayur ointment is very simple like using any other herbal balm. Apply Psorayur ointment on the affected lesions, during the scaling stage of Psoriasis once or twice a day.

Side-effect and Contraindications

There is no known side-effect or contra indication that has been reported with the use of Psorayur ointment. However, in very rare cases, mild skin rashes over the lesions might be observed at the initial onset of application, it is not a matter to be worried as such mild rashes automatically disappear after few days of regular application.

Psorolin Ointment (Garry and Sun, USA)

Composition

- Oil extracts of *Wrightia tinctoria* (Swetha kutaja) : 33.3 per cent
- *Cynadon dactylon* (Duoorva) : 33.3 per cent and Base Q.S.

Dosage/Use

External application in combination with 777 Oil/separately at morning and or night over affected areas.

Contraindication

There is no known contraindication. In some cases, mild skin rashes may be seen over the lesions at the beginning of the therapy such lesions will disappear within few days after regular use.

Psorvate Ointment (Indian Herbal Store, New Delhi)

Content

Psorvate ointment is made from *Wrightia tinctoria* and beeswax. No added perfumes, dyes or other irritants.

Use

Wash afflicted area well with a natural soap before applying this ointment. Apply liberally and spread a thin film on affected areas twice daily or as directed. Relieves and helps prevent recurrence of itching, irritation, redness, flaking and scaling associated with psoriasis.

Psoria Oil–Double Strength of 777 Oil (Indian Herbal Store, New Delhi)

This is wonderful oil for psoriasis as well as other skin conditions similar to it. It is made from *Wrightia tinctoria* leaves.

Contents

Psoria contains *Wrightia tinctoria* and is the only ingredient with a coconut oil base, but in a more concentrated form, and in this way it is different and more effective than its competitive products (almost double the quantity of Wrightia). Psoria is prepared without any cooking process and hence it retains the original crude smell of the herb and coconut oil. Natural color and smell is retained, without adding any additives to it, so that no change is caused to its positive action on the skin.

Usage

Apply to afflicted areas 30 to 60 minutes before soaking in tub of warm water, without using any soap. It is ideal to apply Psoria early morning and to expose the affected skin areas to sun light or other warming. For better results 5ml of Psoria could be taken internally with 25ml hot water twice daily. Oil is food grade, 100 per cent pure.

777 Oil (Garry and Sun, USA)

777 oil is a single herbal formulation prepared by lipid extraction procedure. This drug is found to be effective in the management of Psoriasis. This formulation has already been clinically evaluated several thousand of patients benefited across India and many parts the world and has been proven to be very effective for long-term usage.

Composition

- *Oil extracts of Wrightia tinctoria (Swetha kutaja): 50 per cent W/V*
- *Oleum Cocus nucifera* (Narikela): 50 per cent W/V

External Use

Application after bath as a thin coating over affected surface. Expose to morning sun for 15 minutes after application. Use fingertips for application on scalp. Use natural cleaning agents like Shikakai powder for washing hair and body.

Indications

All types of psoriasis, dandruff, fissure foot, icthyosis, fungal dermatosis, ulcerative gingivitis, apthous ulcers of mouth and first-degree burns.

Contraindication

There is no known contraindication. Mild skin rashes in some cases are reported over the lesions at the beginning of the therapy. Such lesions will disappear within few days after regular use.

Psoroban Oil (GS Ayurveda Pharmaceuticals)

Psoraban is an effective preparation in an oil base to combat Psoriasis, chronic eczematous, fungal and related skin diseases. Its efficacy is undoubted in almost every skin ailment with key ingredients accepted the world over for efficacy in Psoriasis and other skin ailments.

Contents

Wrightia tinctoria (Stree Kutaja), *Psoralia corylifolia* (Bakuchi), *Azhadirachta indica* (Nimba), *Albizzia lebbeck* (Shireesh) and *Acacia catechu* (Khadeer). This is particularly efficacious in chronic skin ailments under prolonged steroid treatments.

Usage

To be applied liberally on the affected part and washed off after 30–45min. using a mild soap or herbal powder. Acute cases respond to Psoraban within 2-3 days of application. For chronic cases on prolonged medication, improvements can be appreciated by about 15 days of regular use. Complete cure can be expected by regular use for 1month–6 months.

Psorolin Soap (India Abundance; Indian Herbal Store, New Delhi)

Composition

- ✰ Oil extracts of *Wrightia tinctoria* (Swetha kutaja): 7.5 mg
- ✰ Oil extracts of Kumari (*Aloe vera*): 7.5 mg

Indications

Psorolin medicated bathing bar is indicated for treating skin conditions such as all types of psoriasis and other dry skin conditions. Psorolin medicated bathing bar contains oil of extracts of *Wrightia tinctoria* and aloe vera that have excellent therapeutic properties for management of psoriasis and in general for improving the overall skin condition and maintaining lusture.

Antidandruff

Herbal Antidandruff Hair Oil (Himalaya Herbal Health Care, India)

Massaging of hair and scalp with a proper nutrient hair oil gives additional nutrition to the scalp and prevents hair loss. Massaging also increases the blood circulation in the scalp and this keeps the hair roots strong. Dandruff hair oil prevents dandruff by eliminating microbial infections of the scalp.

Ingredients

Wrightia tinctoria (Sweet Indrajao, Hyamaraka); used to treat various scalp and skin disorders. *Rosmarinus officinalis* (Rosemary, Rusmari); useful in treating dandruff and other scalp infections. *Melaleuca leucodendron* (Tea Tree, Kayaputi); has antibacterial, antifungal, antiseptic and antidandruff properties. *Azadirachta indica* (Neem, Nimba); has an antidandruff action.

Use

Apply oil all over the scalp. Massage the scalp gently with fingers in a circular motion, so that the oil gets absorbed into the scalp, gradually. Leave for an hour or more before washing with an Ayurvedic Concepts' cleansing shampoo.

Control White Discharge

Lukol: Herbal to Control Women's White Discharge (Himalaya Herbal Health Care, India)

Lukol has a stimulatory action on the endometrium. Lukol's tonic property improves uterine circulation, and its antimicrobial and astringent actions on the mucous membrane of the genital system control leukorrhea. Lukol also improves general health and relieves the symptoms associated with leukorrhea. It controls white discharge. Lukol is useful when the following symptoms are displayed: 1. Non-specific leukorrhea 2. Malaise and backache associated with leukorrhea 3. Pelvic inflammatory disease.

Composition

60 tablets Extract of Dhataki (*Woodfordia fruticosa*) 40mg, Kokilaksha (*Hygrophila auriculata* Syn. *Asteracantha longifolia*) 40mg, Shatavari (*Asparagus racemosus*) 40mg, Sarpagandha (*Rauwolfia serpentina*) 20mg, Punarnava (*Boerhaavia diffusa*) 10mg, Vasaka (*Adhatoda zeylanica*) 10mg, Pdrs. Puga (*Areca catechu*) 20mg, Jatiphalam (*Myristica fragrans*) 16mg, Ela (*Elettaria cardamomum*) 11mg, Nagkesara (*Mesua ferrea*) 11mg, Jeeraka (*Cuminum cyminum*) 10mg, Chandana (*Santalum album*) 10mg, Bilva (*Aegle marmelos*) 5mg, Sunthi (*Zingiber officinale*) 5mg, Triphala 5mg, Maricha (*Piper nigrum*) 5mg, Hyamaraka (*Wrightia tinctoria*) 5mg, Guggulu (*Commiphora wightii*) 5mg, Palasa (*Butea frondosa* Syn. *B.monosperma*) 4mg, Shilajeet (Purified) 9mg, Praval bhasma 7mg, Loh bhasma 5mg, Trivang 5mg.

Dosage

Initially 2 tablets twice daily. Followed by one tablet twice daily or as directed by your physician.

Dano Antidandruff Herbal Hair Oil (Herbalcare, India)

Dano is considered as the best herbal solution to suppress and then cure the dandruff problem that is a nuisance in this world today. Dano equipped with the power of ayurveda had been a herbal answer to all kinds of dandruff problems. Dano is very effective in Dandruff Management. For most of the antidandruff products (shampoo etc.) the effect is fungi static *i.e.* the product removes the dead cell from the top but do not address the root cause. Hence there is further recurrence. Where as Dano has fungicidal effect. Being hair oil, it goes inside the hair root and there from it removes the problems and hence eliminates the chance of recurrence, provided proper hygiene is maintained. Dano is a powerful herbal stimultant that contains active herbals essential for getting rid of dandruff and infection that might occur on the scalp due to some negligence or unknown etiology.

Indications

Dandruff, hair fall, itching on scalp, Irritation and allergy on scalp.

The *in vivo* experiments suggest that Dano may be very effectively in killing the cells of *P. ovale*. Dano is very effective against *P. ovale in vitro*. It has been reported that the oil extracts of *W. tinctoria* possess antifungal activity especially against *P. ovale*. Similarly, the bitter fraction of neem is also known to possess antifungal activity (Krishnamoorthy and Ranganathan, 2000). The extracts of *W. tinctoria* are also known to have an effect on keratinocyte proliferation (cell line study, unpublished data). The antifungal activity coupled with keratinocyte proliferation inhibition activity of *W. tinctoria* in Dano makes the oil very effective in the management of dandruff. Further, the localized immune elicitation activity of bitter fraction of neem also offers better protection against relapse of dandruff for prolonged period of time (Krishnamoorthy *et al.*, 2006).

Antidiarrhoeal

Amaebsan Tablets (Clesstra Health Care Pvt. Ltd., India)

Diarrhoea and dysentery are results of indigestion of food and water borne microbial and worms infections. Patient suffers from loose motions with or without abdominal pain, mucous and blood. The electrolyte balance gets disturbed and the patient becomes dehydrated and weak.

Contents

Amaebsan is a combination of herbal antidiarrhoeals. It contains extracts of selected medicinal herbs that have been used from ancient times to provide relief in diarrhoea and dysentery. Kutaj alkaloids had strong antiamoebic and antiprotozoal action. Extract helps in clearing very chronic cases of amoebic dysentery; other ingredients are very useful to control diarrhoea and dysentery by their astringent action on the bowel.

Lip Balm

Protective Lip Salve/Himalaya Ayurvedic Lip Balm (Himalaya Herbal Health Care, India)

Lip Balm prevents chapping, drying and cracking of the lips. It contains a natural UV filter and Vit.E which nourishes, tones and softens the lips. It is an Ayurvedic propriety medicine, completely safe and nontoxic.

Ingredients

Eranda (*Ricinus communis*, Castor) oil is used externally to relieve various inflammatory conditions of the skin and mucus membrane. Narikela (*Cocos nucifera*, Coconut) oil extract is a good emollient and can be used externally for softening the lips. The oil extract is used in various cosmetics. Godhuma (*Triticum sativum*, Common Wheat) oil is a rich natural source of vitamin E, which nourishes and prevents loss of moisture from the skin. It is used to tone and soften the lips. It has a potent antioxidant activity. Hyamaraka (*Wrightia tinctoria*, Sweet Indrajao) leaves are used in various skin disorders including herpes. It has astringent and antiinflammatory activities and is used as an antibacteial in several skin disorders. Garijara (*Daucus carota*, Carrot) seed oil is used as a sunscreen and fragrance component in soaps, creams and lotions.

Indications

To be applied on the lips when dry or when necessary. Good for chapped, cracked or dry lips.

Rejuvenation of Joint Function

Move EZ 100 Tabs (Komal; AyurBest, India)

Move EZ is a proprietary formula combining numerous herbs which are used in Ayurvedic tradition to provide joint comfort and flexibility. Improper digestion and elimination may lead to toxic residue in the body. Certain types of residue may have a tendency to accumulate in the joints leading to joint discomfort. Promotes flexibility and comfortable movement of the joints, muscles and vertebral column. Helps relieve neck, upper back and lower back discomfort. Enhances the rejuvenation and strengthening of the skeletal and neuromuscular systems. Supports the elimination of toxins that impact healthy joint function. Supports the body's natural inflammation response.

Ingredients

Each Tablet of 240 mg Contains Blend of Trikatu (Dry Ginger, Black pepper, Long pepper), Chavak (*Chavica roxburghi*), Long pepper (*Piper longum*), Cummin seeds, Leadwort (*Plumbago zeylanica*), Asafoetida (*Ferula foetida*), White mustard seeds (*Brassica alba*), Chasteberry (*Vitex agnus castus*), Inderjav (*Wrightia tinctoria*), Vidang (*Embelia ribes*), Gajpimpali (*Scindapsus officinalis*), Kutki (*Picrrorrhiza kurroa*), Bharangmool (*Clerodendron serratum*), Vacha (*Acorus calamus*), Triphala, Gokshur (*Tribulus terrestris*), Jatamansi (*Nardostachys jatamansi*), Ashwagandha (*Withania somnifera*), Guggul (*Commiphora mukul*) and Gum Acacia. Triphala is an antioxidant and well known digestive that also assists in the elimination process. Guggul, Trikatu and Embelia are known for eliminating the toxins that can impact healthy joint function. Ashwagandha is an adaptogenic herb which is added to balance stress and support the immune system. *Brassica alba, Piper longum, Vitex agnus castus* along with the additional herbs present in the formula, work together to rejuvenate and strengthen the skeletal and neuromuscular systems. This powerful combination supports the body's natural inflammation response.

Usage

1-2 tablets 3 times a day, preferably 30 minutes after meals. Take daily over a period of at least 2-3 months. Noticeable changes may be observed in 2-3 months. Not recommended for children.

Discussion and Conclusion

In the present review we have congregated information pertaining to botanical, ethnopharmacological, phytochemical and pharmacological claims and published scientific studies on *Wrightia tinctoria*. This plant has immense potential and have broad spectrum of activity on several ailments. Fresh leaves are acrid, pungent and are chewed for relief from toothache. Bark and seeds are carminative, digestive, stomachic, antidysenteric, anthelmintic, aphrodisiac, bilious affections, leprosy, psoriasis, haemorrhoids, febrifuge and diuretic. The plant is reported to contain alkaloid, flavonoids, sterols and terpens. Literature search revels the isolation and identification of sterols, terpenes and some coloring pigments.

Review of literature also pin points that although number of diseases for which *W. tinctoria* finds its uses in traditional system is fairly large, though its therapeutic efficacy has been assessed in few plausible medicinal application. Very little pharmacological work has been done on medicinal application of the isolated compounds so imperative that more pharmacological and clinical studies should be conducted to investigate unexploited potential of this plant. Most of the isolated compounds of *W. tinctoria* lack the reported pharmacological activities which provide scope for further pharmacological studies. Exploration of chemical constituents and further pharmacological evaluation will give us basis for its therapeutic use in diarrhoea, pitta and kapha, bilious affections, liver disease, flatulence, colic stomach pain, haemorrhoids and helminthiasis. Very less information is available regarding the chemicals constituents of this plant like flavonoids and alkaloids. There is lack of phyto-pharmacological studies. Depending on the primary information available further studies can be carried out like phyto-pharmacological standardization of extracts, isolation and identification of active constituents, pharmacological studies on isolated compounds, mode of action, toxicity study. These studies may be followed by development of active molecules and clinical trial as s tool for modern drug development and serve the purpose of Ayurvedic formulation development.

The medicinal applications of this plant have countless possibilities for investigation in relatively new areas of its function to explore its therapeutic efficacy. The global changing scenario is showing a tendency towards use of nontoxic plant products having good traditional medicinal background. This review will definitely help the researcher and traditional healers in scientific standardization of this plant. *W. tinctoria* is easily available plant which grows in large quantity in the dry hilly areas of North and Central India. This plant can be used as a cheap source of active therapeutics. The present review showed the plant has potent antimicrobial properties against dermatophytic microbes, which is used extensively in superficial skin ailments like eczema, psoriasis, keratosis and dandruff. A number of poly herbal formulations containing *W. tinctoria* as one of the active phyto-pharmaceutical is available in market for psoriasis, diarrhoea and dysentery, dandruff and for rejuvenation of joint function, having reach in overseas markets also. This plant has proved effectiveness against commonly occurring ailments and can be used for long duration for alleviation of peptic ulcer, cut and wounds, immunosuppression, anxiety and depression and in arthritis and pain relief by the poor and under privileged people of central India region

Acknowledgements

The All India Council of Technical Education, New Delhi is highly acknowledged for awarding National Doctoral Fellowship grant to one of the authors (Dr. Papiya Bigoniya) to support this work.

References

Ahmad, I. and Lie Ken Jie, M.S.F. (2008). Oleochemicals from Isoricinoleic Acid (*Wrightia tinctoria* Seed Oil). *Indian Journal of Engineering and Chemical Research,* 47(6): 2091-2095

Akihisa, T., Ahmad, I., Singh, S., Tamura, T. and Matsumoto, T. (1988). 14α-methylzymosterol and other sterols from *Wrightia tinctoria* seeds. *Phytochemistry,* 27(10): 3231-3234.

Alam, M., Rukmani, B. and Anandan, T. (1985). Effect of insulation on "777 oil" used for psoriasis in Siddha system of medicine. *Ancient Science of Life,* 5(1): 17-20.

Alam, M., Rukmani, B., Joy, S., Anandan, T. and Veluchamy, G. (1986). Process and product standardisation of "777 oil" used for psoriasis in Siddha medicine. *Ancient Science of Life,* 6(1): 35-41.

Anesan, S.G., Amar, N.R., Andi, P. and Anumathy, N.B. (2007). Ethnomedicinal Survey of Alagarkoil Hills (Reserved forest), Tamil Nadu, India. *Electronic Journal of Indian Medicine,* 1: 1–19.

Anonymous. (1987). Clinical and Experimental Studies on the Efficacy of 777 oil, A Siddha Preparation in the Treatment of Kalanjagapadai (Psoriasis). A Monograph Published by Central Council of Research in Ayurveda and Siddha, Ministry of Health and Family Welfare, Govt. of India, New Delhi.

Anonymous; Scientific Correspondence. (2005). Floral device for obligate selfing by remote insect activity and anemochory in *Wrightia tinctoria* (Roxb.) R.Br. (Apocynaceae). *Current Science,* 88(9): 1378-79.

Atal, C.K. and Sethi, P.D. (1962). *Wrightia tinctoria* bark, an adulterant of Kurchi. *Journal of Pharmacy and Pharmacology,* 14: 41-45.

Bigoniya, P. and Rana, A.C. (2006). Comparative macroscopic, microscopic and Physico-chemical studies and quantitative physical evaluation of *Wrightia tinctoria* seed fibres with cotton and jute. *Planta Indica,* 2(1): 44-50.

Bigoniya, P., Rana, A. C. and Lariya, S. Immunomodulatory activity of *Wrightia tinctoria* bark alcoholic extract on rats. *Current Pharma Research Journal,* (In press).

Bigoniya, P., Rana, A.C. and Agrawal, G.P. (2006). Evaluation of the antiulcer activity of hydro-alcoholic extract of *Wrightia tinctoria* bark in experimentally induced acute gastric ulcers on rat. *Nigerian Journal of Natural Product and Medicine,* 10: 36-40.

Bigoniya, P., Shukla, A., Agrawal, G.P. and Rana, A. C. Pharmacological screening of *Wrightia tinctoria* bark hydro-alcoholic extract. *Asian Journal of Experimental Sciences,* (In press)

Chandrashekhar, V.M., Abdul Haseeb, T.S., Habbu, P.V. and Nagappa, A.N. (2004). Hepatoprotective activity of *Wrightia tinctoria* (Roxb) in rats. *Indian Drugs,* 41: 366-70.

Chary, S.T.R. (1980). Floristic Study of Achampet Taluk Mahabubnagar of Andhra Pradesh, India, Ph.D. Thesis. Osmania University, Hyderabad, India, pp. 285.

Chopra, R.N., Chopra, I.C., Handa, K.L. and Kapur, L.D. (1958). Indigenous Drugs of India. 2nd Ed., MN Dhar and Sons, Calcutta, India, pp. 56-7,187-89, 342-51,181-83, 342, 426-28, 431-33, 530.

Chopra, R.N., Nayar, S.L. and Chopra, I.C. (1956). Glossary of Indian Medicinal Plants, Council of Science and Industrial Research, New Delhi, India.

Everett, H., Pryde, L., Princen, L. and Kumar, D. (1981). New Sources of Fats and Oils. The American Oil Chemists Society, New York, pp.114-117.

George, V., Koshy, A.S., Singh, O.V., Nayar, M.N.S. and Pushpangadan, P. (1996). Tryptanthrin from *Wrightia tinctoria*. *Fitoterapia,* LXVII(6): 553-554.

Glasby, J. S. (1975). Encyclopedia of the Alkaloids. Plenum Press, New York.

Herbal medication for the treatment of psoriasis. US Patent Issued on Jan 12, 1999, Application No. 928959. Filed on 1997-09-12. Document Type and Number: United States Patent 5858372. Available at: http://www.freepatentsonline.com/585872.html

Jolly, C.I. and Mechery, N.R. (1996). Comparative pharmacognostical, physico-chemical and antibacterial studies on seeds of *Holarrhena antidysenterica* wall and *Wrightia tinctoria* R.Br. *Indian Journal of Pharmaceutical Sciences,* 58(2): 51-54.

Joshi, M.C., Patel, M.B. and Mehta, P..J. (1980). Some folk medicines of Dangs, Gujarat State. *Bulletin of Medicinal and Ethnobotanical Research,* 1: 8-24.

Kannan, P., Shanmugavadivu, B., Petchiammal, C. and Hopper, W. (2006). *In vitro* antimicrobial activity of *Wrightia tinctoria* leaf extracts against skin microorganisms. *Acta Botanica Hungarica,* 48(3-4): 323-329.

Khan, P.S.H. (1987). Comparative seed structure of medicinally important *Holarrhena antidysenterica* (Roth.) A.D.C. and its adulterant, *Wrightia tinctoria* R.Br. (Apocynaceae). *International Journal of Crude Drug Research,* 25(2): 81-86.

Kirtikar, K.R. and Basu, B.D. (1975). Indian Medicinal Plants. Vol. 11, 2nd and reprint Ed., Jayyed Press, Delhi, pp. 1581.

Krishnamoorthy, J.R. and Ranganathan, S. (2000). Antipityrosporum ovale activity of a herbal drug combination of *Wrightia tinctoria* and *Hisbiscus rosasinensis*. *Indian journal of Dermatology,* 45(3): 125-126.

Krishnamoorthy, J.R., Ranganathan, S., Gokul Shankar, S. and Ranjith, M.S. (2006). Dano: A herbal solution for dandruff. *African Journal of Biotechnology Academic Journals,* 5(10): 960-962.

Krishnamurthy, J.R., Kalaimani, S. and Veluchamy, G. (1981). Clinical study of vetpalai (*Wrightia tinctoria* L.) oil in the treatment of kalanjagapadai (psoriasis). *Journal of Research in Ayurveda and Siddha,* 2(1): 58-66.

Mahadevan, N., Moorthy, K.., Perumal, P. and Varadha Raju, S. (1998). Pharmacognosy of leaves of *Wrightia tinctoria* R.Br. *Ancient Science of Life,* 18(1): 78-83.

Malvia, P. (1975). Pharmacognostical investigation of seeds of *Wrightia tinctoria* and *Holarrhena antidysenterica* Wall. *Indian Journal of Pharmaceutical Education,* 9(1): 25.

Mitra, S.K., Seshadri, S.J., Venkataranganna, M.V. and Gopumadhvan, S. (1998). Reversal of parakeratosis, a feature of psoriasis by *Wrightia tinctoria* (in emulsion) histological evaluation based on mouse tail. *Indian journal of Dermatology*, 43(3): 102-104.

Muruganandam, A.V., Jaiswal, A.K., Bhattacharya, S.K. and Ghosal, S. (1998a). Effect of *Wrightia tinctoria* on anxiety patterns in rats. *Indian Journal of Pharmacology*, 30(2): 124 (abstract No. 56).

Muruganandam, A.V., Jaiswal, A.K., Ghosal, S. and Bhattacharya, S.K. (1998b). Effect of *Wrightia tinctoria* on the brain monoamines and metabolites in rats. *Biogenic Amines*, 14: 655-665.

Nadkarni, K.M. (1976). Indian Materia Medica, Vol. 1, Popular Prakashan, Bombay, India, pp. 1296.

Ngan P.T. (1965). A revision of the genus Wrightia (Apocynaceae). Annals of the Missouri Botanical Garden, 52(2): 114-175.

Oudhia, P. (2003). Medicinal herbs of Chhattisgarh. India having less known traditional uses, II. Indrajau (*Wrightia tinctoria*, family: Apocynaceae), Research note, [on line], Botanical.com, cited 4th May 2007. Available at: http://www.botanical.com/site/column_poudhia/155_indrajau.html

Pandey, G.S. (1992). Bhavaprakasa Nighantu. *In:* Indian Materia Medica, Ed. By Mishra, B., Chaukhambha Bharti Academy, Varanashi, pp. 308 and 76-77.

Rajesh, R., Shivprasad, H.V., Gowda, C.D., Nataraju, A., Dhananjaya, B.L. and Vishwanath, B.S. (2007). Comparative study on plant latex proteases and their involvement in hemostasis: a special emphasis on clot inducing and dissolving properties. *Planta Medica*, 73(10): 1061-67.

Ramchandra, P., Basheermiya, M., Krupadanam, G.L.D. and Srimannarayana, G. (1993). Wrightial, a new terpene from *Wrightia tinctoria*. *Journal of Natural Products*, 56(10): 1811-1812.

Rangaswami, S. and Rao, M.N. (1963). Crystalline chemical components of the bark of *Wrightia tinctoria*, BR. *Proceedings of the Indian academy of Sciences*, 57(A): 115-120.

Ranjit Daniels, R.J., Ramachandran, V.S., Vencatesan, J., Ramakantha, V. and Puyravaud, J.P. (2007). Dispelling the myth of tropical dry evergreen forests of India. *Current Science*, 92(5): 586-87.

Rao, M.N., Rao, E.V. and Rao, V.S. (1966). Triterpenoid components of the leaves and pods of *Wrightia tinctoria*. *Current Science*, 35: 518-519.

Rao, M.N., Rao, E.V. and Rao, V.S. (1968). Occurrence of oleanolic acid in the pods of *Wrightia tinctoria* Br. *Current Science*, 22(20): 645.

Reddy, Y.S.R., Venkatesh, S., Ravichandran, T., Murugan, V. and Suresh, B. (2000). Antinociceptive activity of *Wrightia tinctoria* bark. *Fitoterapia*, 73: 421-423.

Reddy, Y.S.R., Venkatesh, S., Ravichandran, T., Subburaju T. and Suresh, B. (1999). Pharmacognostical studies on *Wrightia tinctoria* bark. *Pharmaceutical Biology*, 37(4): 291-295.

Sethi, P.D. (1970). Separation of alkaloidal constituents of *Wrightia tinctoria* by TLC. *Planta Medica*, 18(1): 26-9.

Shah, G.L. and Gopal, G.V. (1988). Ethnomedical notes from the tribal inhabitats of the north Gujarat (India). *Journal of Ecotoxicology and Botany*, 6: 193-221.

Singh, V.P., Sharma, S.K. and Kare, V.S. (1980). Medicinal plants from Ujjain District, Madhya Pradesh; Part 2. *Indian Drugs*, 17: 7-12.

The Wealth of India: Raw Materials. (1976). Vol. 10, Council of Scientific and Industrial Research, New Delhi, India, pp. 588-590.

Tomar, R., Kumar, R. and Jagannadham, M.V. (2008). A Stable Serine Protease, Wrightin, from the Latex of the Plant *Wrightia tinctoria* (Roxb.) R. Br.: Purification and Biochemical Properties. *Journal of Agriculture and. Food Chemistry*, 56(4): 1479–1487

Veerapur, V.P., Palkar, M.B., Srinivasa, H., Kumar, M.S., Patra, S., Rao, P.G.M. and Srinivasan, K.K. (2004). The effect of ethanol extract of *Wrightia tinctoria* bark on wound healing in rats. *Journal of Natural Remedies*, 4(2): 155-159.

Vijayakumar, R., Muthukumar, C., Kumar, T. and Saravanamuthu, R. (2006). Characterization of *Malassezia Furfur* and its control by using plant extracts. *Indian Journal of Dermatology*, 51(2): 145-148.Table, Figures and photograph citation details.

Medicinal Plants: Phytochemistry, Pharmacology and Therapeutics, Vol. 1 *Pages 75–97*
Editors: **V.K. Gupta, G.D. Singh, Surjeet Singh and A. Kaul**
Published by: **DAYA PUBLISHING HOUSE, NEW DELHI**

Chapter 4

Genotoxicity: Its Methods of Evaluation and the Significance–A Review

S. Singh*, R. Sharma, G.D. Singh, A. Kaul,
A. Khajuria, P. Koul and V.K. Gupta
Indian Institute of Integrative Medicine (CSIR),
Canal Road, Jammu - 180 001, J&K State, India

ABSTRACT

There is a little information available on the possible risks that natural products may pose to health. Although general toxicity of the natural products which are commonly used as medicines has been carried out in most of the cases but not the genotoxicity. Many plant products contain compounds known to cause various diseases or even death in animals and humans. Recently, various lines of evidence have suggested that plant-derived constituents may play an important role in determining spontaneous rate of genetic damage and tumor incidence. Genotoxicity is the requirement of the OECD now a day. Genotoxicity studies of both naturally occurring and synthetic substances are of great interest because of the widespread and often chronic use of specific herbal as well as modern medicinal products, of food ingredients and other household and environmental chemicals. The present review gives the details of the genotoxicity. Mutagenicity is defined as a permanent change in the content or structure of the genetic material of an organism. A mutagenic hazard can be manifested as a heritable change resulting from germ line mutations and/or somatic mutations leading to cancer or other chronic degenerative processes such as aging. Germ cell mutagens/genotoxins are substances that cause heritable (passed on to progeny) changes in the genetic material in germ cells, namely spermatocytes or oocytes. The term *mutagen* refers to a substance that induces transmissible changes in DNA

* Corresponding Author: E-mail: surjeet58@yahoo.com.

structure involving a single gene or a group of genes. Genotoxins are a broader category of substances that induce changes to the structure or number of genes via chemical interaction with DNA and/or non-DNA targets. The term *genotoxicity* is generally used unless a specific assay for mutations is being discussed. Currently, millions of people all over the world are exposed unknowingly to the ubiquitous element in exposure levels leading to long-term toxicity, in particular cancer. The marketed pharmaceuticals which are used for the treatment of different types of the ailments are not devoid of such effects. As a matter of fact they are not been checked for such effects *i.e.*, genotoxicity. A data survey of 467 marketed drugs on genotoxicity revealed that 115 drugs had no published genotoxicity data. Most regulatory agencies and international authorities recommend a test scheme consisting of *in vitro* and *in vivo* methods to identify genotoxic/mutagenic substances. This review is going to give some exposure to the readers regarding the genotoxicity its significance and evaluation.

Keywords: *Genotoxicity, DNA damage, Micronuclei, Chromosome aberration, OECD.*

Introduction

Toxicology is the study of the adverse effects of chemicals on living organisms, whether they be human, animal, plant or microbes. 'Adverse effect' can range from a life threatening injury to something that might be considered a minor annoyance. Toxicology (derived from the greek words *toxicos* and *logos*) is the study of symptoms, mechanisms, treatments and detection of poisoning, especially the poisoning of people.

The term toxicity is used to describe the ability of a substance to cause a harmful effect. It is used in two contrasting senses *i.e.*, to denote the capacity to cause harm to a living organism and to indicate the adverse effects caused by a chemical. In other words it is the degree to which a substance is able to damage an exposed organism, such as an animal, plant or bacterium, as well as the effect on substructure of the organism, such as cell (cytotoxicity) or an organ (organotoxicity), such as the liver (hepatotoxicity). By extension, the word may be metaphorically used to describe toxic effects on larger and more complex groups, such as the family unit or society at large. A central concept of toxicology is that, the effects are dose dependent; even water can lead to water intoxication when taken in large enough doses, whereas for even a very toxic substance such as snake venom there is a dose below which there is no detectable toxic effects. Dose is the amount of something you are exposed to, or come in contact with. The less the toxicity, the greater the dose you can tolerate without ill effects. The greater the toxicity, the less dose you can tolerate without becoming sick.

There is a little information available on the possible risks that natural products may pose to health (Dias *et al.*, 1994). Although general toxicity of the natural products which are commonly used as medicines has been carried out in most of the cases but not the genotoxicity. Genotoxicity studies of both naturally occurring and synthetic substances are of great interest because of the widespread and often chronic use of specific herbal medicines, of modern medicinal products, of food ingredients as well as other household and environmental chemicals (Umar-Tsafe *et al.*, 2004). Many plant products contain compounds known to cause various diseases or even death in animals and humans (Dearfield *et al.*, 2002). Moreover plant foods contain natural or processing-induced constituents with biological activity in mammals. Among these are glycoalkaloids, amines, glucosinolates, cyanogenic glycosides, protease inhibitors, oxalates, coumarins, polyphenols, cyclopropenoid fatty acids, phytates, xanthines and essential oils are predominant. Recently, various lines of evidence have suggested that plant-derived constituents may play an important role in determining spontaneous rates of genetic damage and tumor incidence. Genotoxic constituents such as certain flavones, anthraquinones, browning products, benzoxazinones, and acetals have been identified in plant-derived foods, and unsaturated oilseed lipids have been found to increase cancers of certain sites, particularly intestine and breast, in laboratory animals (MacGregor,1986). Henceforth it is necessary to evaluate genotoxicity potential of natural plant products before their human use.

Any substance capable of causing damage to cellular DNA and thus producing mutations or cancer is called genotoxicant and the effect is called genotoxicity. Toxic substances that are genotoxic may bind directly to DNA or act indirectly leading to DNA damage by affecting enzymes involved in DNA replication, thereby causing mutations which may or may not lead to cancer or birth defects (inheritable damage). Genotoxic substances are not necessarily carcinogenic.

Although most of the cancer chemotherapeutic agents are mutagenic and carcinogenic yet they are extensively used for the treatment of various types of cancers, as at times they cure the disease or at least increase the life expectancy of cancer patients. However, as these chemicals are not target specific and mostly S-phase dependent, numerous non-cancerous cells are also affected during chemotherapy, particularly the proliferative ones. One outcome of it is the occurrence of secondary tumors and mostly leukemia's in cancer patients who survive for a longer period after chemotherapy. This serious concern has warranted the detailed genotoxicity testing of various cancer chemotherapeutics. On the other hand, efforts are also being made to make them target specific.

Every new chemical entity (NCE) has to pass through genotoxicology tests in order to get regulatory approval. A 'negative' on this crucial test takes the sample drug one step closer to the market. Drug discovery has remained one of the most challenging aspects for pharmaceutical companies. It is the process of taking new chemical leads, the output of which is the emergence of NCEs. Though NCEs are the precursors for any drug discovery, their actions on biological targets and subsequent genetic changes still baffle researchers and the medical fraternity.

Few decades ago, 'chemical mutagenicity' was central to drug discovery and the term 'genotoxicology' was struggling to find a place in medical textbooks. However, intervening period saw chemical mutagenicity getting replaced by genotoxicology. Today, there are many organizations and journals that are completely dedicated to genotoxicology. Indeed, geno-toxicology has left a strong impression on many organizations concerned with detrimental health effects of toxic chemicals. It is a general belief that the field of genotoxicology was discovered by H J Muller and C Auerbach, who had narrated the first chemical and physical mutagens by using sub-mammalian species.

Genotoxicity testing of new chemical entities is generally used for hazard identification with respect to DNA damage and its fixation (Madle *et al.*, 1987). These damages can be manifested in the form of gene mutation, structural chromosomal aberration, recombination and numerical changes. These changes are responsible for heritable effects on germ cells and impose risks to future generations (Wassom *et al.*, 1992). Somatic mutations can also play an important role in malignancy (Tennant *et al.*, 1987). These tests have been used mainly for the prediction of carcinogenicity and genotoxicity because compounds, which are positive in these tests, have the potential to be human carcinogens and/or mutagens.

The discovery of new drugs needs a thorough investigation for its safety and efficacy before their release into the market (Purves *et al.*, 1995). The primary objective of drug safety evaluation is to obtain biological information indicative of toxicity, which can be interpreted and/or extended to the assessment of health risk to the humans (Nath and Krishna, 1998). Most of the countries are having the specific guidelines for testing of pharmaceuticals for genotoxicity. In India, schedule 'Y' of Drugs and Cosmetic Rules 1988, Central Drugs Standard Control Organizations (CDSCO), Directorate General of Health Services (DGHS), New Drugs Division issued by Ministry of Health and Family Welfare, Government of India, deals with the prerequisites to carry out the clinical trials of the new drugs before its marketing, depending upon the status of the drugs in other countries. As per the regulatory requirements, the mutagenicity and carcinogenicity testing are required, when the compound or its metabolite is structurally related to a known carcinogen or when the nature and the action of the drugs suggest a mutagenic/carcinogenic potential (Malik, 1999). In U.S., the FDAs (Food and Drug Administration) Centre for Drugs and Biologics Evaluation and Research (CDER and CBER) recommend genotoxicity testing for all new drugs (Hutt, 1991). In Japan, the Ministry of Health and Welfare (MHW) adopted mutagenicity tests in 1984 as one of the several toxicity studies required for the approval to manufacture or import of new drugs.

The Organization for Economic Cooperation and Development (OECD) guidelines are specifically important because by complying the same one can ensure the acceptance of toxicity data in each of the thirty member countries of the OECD (OECD, 1996). The International Conference on Harmonization (ICH) brings together the regulatory authorities of Japan, Europe and U.S.A. Most of the guidelines recommended by various regulatory authorities are represented in the four–test battery. These tests include

- ✰ A gene mutation in bacteria,
- ✰ A test for chromosome aberration in mammalian cells *in vitro,*
- ✰ A test for gene mutation in eukaryotic cells *in vitro*
- ✰ *In vivo* test for genetic damage.

The compound under study complies genotoxicity testing, when the result of the entire test in the four-test battery are uniformly negative. Further experiments are suggested when the test results are not uniform in the four-test battery. The development of genetic toxicology began in the 1960s in the midst of increasing awareness of human exposure to toxic chemicals in the environment. Early genetic toxicology studies were designed to detect reproductive toxicants. It was not until the 1970s that most of the current routine genetic toxicology tests were developed and test results were used for identification of carcinogens and risk characterization for cancer risk assessment (Brusick, 1987a).

The distinct advantage in applying these tests is that it opens the door to the possibility of detecting future health problems before they arise as major issues for an industry or company. "Early detection" is rationale for applying these tests. On the other hand, products that lower one's risk of genetic damage could be used to positive advantage for the human welfare and exploited accordingly.

Toxicology

The term toxicity is used to describe the ability of a substance to cause a harmful effect. It is used in two contrasting senses *i.e.*, to denote the capacity to cause harm to a living organism, and to indicate the adverse effects caused by a chemical. Toxicity is often subdivided into acute, sub-acute and chronic toxicity.

Acute Toxicity

Adverse effects are observed within a short time of exposure to the chemical. This exposure may be a single dose, or a short continuous exposure, or multiple doses administered over 24 hours or less. Acute toxicity looks at lethal effects following oral, dermal or inhalation exposure. It is classified in to five categories of severity (GHS categories) where category 1 requires the least amount of exposure to be lethal and category 5 requires the most exposure to be lethal (Table 4.1).

Table 4.1: Five Categories of the Severity of the Dosage

Mode of Exposure	*Category*	*Dose (according to body weight)*
Oral	Category 1	LD 50 ≤ 5 mg/kg
	Category 2	LD 50 ≤ 50 mg/kg
	Category 3	LD 50 ≤ 300 mg/kg
	Category 4	LD 50 ≤ 2000 mg/kg
	Category 5	LD 50 ≤ 5000 mg/kg
Dermal	Category 1	LD 50 ≤ 50 mg/kg
	Category 2	LD 50 ≤ 200 mg/kg
	Category 3	LD 50 ≤ 1000 mg/kg
	Category 4	LD 50 ≤ 2000 mg/kg
	Category 5	LD 50 ≤ 5000 mg/kg
Inhalation–gases	Category 1	LC 50 ≤ 100 ppmV
	Category 2	LC 50 ≤ 500 ppmV
	Category 3	LC 50 ≤ 2500 ppmV
	Category 4	LC 50 ≤ 20000 ppmV
	unclassified	LC 50 ≤ 5000 mg/kg
Inhalation–Vapour	Category 1	LC 50 ≤ 100 ppmV
	Category 2	LC 50 ≤ 0.5 mg/l
	Category 3	LC 50 ≤ 2.0 mg/l
	Category 4	LC 50 ≤ 10 mg/l
	unclassified	LC 50 ≤ 10 mg/l
Inhalation–Dust and Mist	Category 1	LC 50 ≤ 0.05 mg/l
	Category 2	LC 50 ≤ 0.5 mg/l
	Category 3	LC 50 ≤ 1.0 mg/l
	Category 4	LC 50 ≤ 5.0 mg/l
	unclassified	LC 50 ≤ 5.0 mg/l

Sub Acute (Sub chronic) Toxicity

Adverse effects are observed following repeated daily exposure to a chemical, or exposure for a significant part of an organism's lifespan (usually not exceeding 10 per cent). With experimental animals, the period of exposure may range from a few days (28) to 3 months.

Chronic Toxicity

Adverse effects are observed following repeated exposure to a chemical during a substantial fraction of an organism's lifespan (usually more than 50 per cent) or some time up to the full span of the animal. For humans, chronic exposure typically means several decades; for experimental animals, it is typically more than 3 months and up to 2 years. Chronic exposure to chemicals over a period of 2 years using rats or mice may be used to assess the carcinogenic potential of chemicals. Apart from the general toxicity, genotoxicity is one of the most important parts of the toxicity study. Moreover it is the requirement of the OECD for all the new drug molecules to be taken for the clinical trial study.

Genotoxicity

Genotoxicity describes a deleterious action on a cell genetic material affecting its integrity. Genotoxic substances are known to be potentially mutagenic or carcinogenic, especially those capable of causing genetic mutations and of contributing to the development of tumors. This includes both certain chemical compounds and certain types of radiations. Typical genotoxins like aromatic amines are believed to cause mutations because they are nucleophilic and form strong covalent bonds with DNA resulting with the formation of aromatic amine-DNA adducts, preventing accurate replication. Genotoxins affecting sperms and eggs can pass genetic changes down to descendants who have never been exposed to the genotoxin (Smith M.T., 1996). From these observations this can be predicted that the DNA part is the main functioning unit for the genotoxicity. This becomes essential to look into the DNA in depth. Other than DNA, micronuclei formation, chromosomal aberrations and sperm abnormalities are the major parameters of concern.

Principle of Genotoxicity Testing

Most human carcinogens are genotoxic in nature. The science of genotoxicity mainly concerns that chemicals, which induce mutations in various experimental models, may conceivably affect the incidence of heritable mutations in man (Davidson *et al.*, 1986 and Douglasss *et al.*, 1988). Genotoxicity test can be defined by *in vitro* or *in vivo* tests designed to detect drugs, which can induce genetic damage directly or indirectly by various mechanisms of action. Genotoxicity test enable hazard identification with respect to DNA damage and fixation in the form of gene mutations, large scale chromosomal damage, recombination and numerical chromosomal changes. Drugs that are positive in these tests that detect such kind of damage have the potential to be human carcinogen and/or mutagens *i.e.*, may induce cancer and/or heritable defects. To detect these tests during the last two decades, several test systems with different end points have been introduced successfully in routine genotoxicity testing (Tweats, 1984). Three levels (gene, chromosome and genome) of information are required to give the comprehensive coverage of the mutagenic potential of a new drug substance (Shelby, 1988) to minimize the risk factors a new chemical entity (NCE) has to be subjected to a battery of genotoxicity tests and a judicious test selection is essential to determine the risk potential of NCE completely.

Selection of Test Battery

For setting up of a test battery in genotoxicity testing, it has always been observed that *in vitro* tests play a major role due to their high sensitivity and rapidity. Preliminary tests are designed in such a way that it can detect majority of the genotoxic carcinogens (Mac Gregor *et al.*, 1995). One of the most important criteria considered for *in vitro* test evaluation is the relative sensitivity of different cell lines and their genetic diversity (Kirkland, 1998). The *in vivo* tests models are generally designed to see the chemical effects on the route of exposure, duration of treatment, metabolism and target organ exposure therapeutically relevant to humans. On the basis of the requirement different types of experimental protocol design and guidelines have been developed to conduct genotoxic evaluations (Kirkland, 1990; Maron *et al.*, 1983).

Significance of Genotoxicity Study

Genotoxicity study can be defined as *in vitro* and *in vivo* tests designed to detect compounds that induce genetic damage directly or indirectly by various mechanisms. These tests should enable hazard identification with respect to damage to DNA and its fixation. Fixation of damage to DNA in the form of gene mutations, large scale chromosomal damage, recombination and numerical chromosome changes is generally considered to be essential for heritable effects and in the multistep process of malignancy, a complex process in which genetic changes may play only a part. Compounds which are positive in tests that detect such kinds of damage have the potential to be human carcinogens and/or mutagens, *i.e.*, may induce cancer and/or heritable defects. Because the relationship between exposure to particular chemicals and carcinogenesis is established for man, while a similar relationship has been difficult to prove for heritable diseases. Genotoxicity tests have been used mainly for the prediction of carcinogenicity. Nevertheless, because germ line mutations are clearly associated with human disease, the suspicion that a compound may induce heritable effects is considered to be just as serious as the suspicion that a compound may induce cancer. In addition, the outcome of such tests may be valuable for the interpretation of carcinogenicity studies. To study all these effects DNA is the main cellular target which should be looked in detail for the evaluation of the genotoxicity.

DNA

Deoxyribonucleic acid (DNA) is a nucleic acid that contains the genetic instructions used in the development and functioning of all known living organisms and some viruses. The main role of DNA molecules is the long-term storage of information. DNA is often compared to a set of blueprints, since it contains the instructions needed to construct other components of cells, such as proteins and RNA molecules. The DNA segments that carry this genetic information are called genes, but other DNA sequences have structural purposes, or are involved in regulating the use of this genetic information.

DNA Damage

DNA damage, due to environmental factors and normal metabolic processes inside the cell, occurs at a rate of 1,000 to 1,000,000 molecular lesions per cell per day (Lodish *et al.*, 2004) while this constitutes only 0.000165 per cent of the human genome's approximately 6 billion bases (3 billion base pairs), unrepaired lesions in critical genes (such as tumor suppressor genes) can impede a cell's ability to carry out its function and appreciably increase the likelihood of tumor formation.

The vast majority of DNA damage affects the primary structure of the double helix; that is, the bases themselves are chemically modified. These modifications can in turn disrupt the molecules' regular helical structure by introducing non-native chemical bonds or bulky adducts that do not fit in the standard double helix. Unlike proteins and RNA, DNA usually lacks tertiary structure and therefore damage or disturbance does not occur at that level. DNA is, however, super coiled and wrapped around "packaging" proteins called histones (in eukaryotes), and both superstructures are vulnerable to the effects of DNA damage.

Sources of Damage

DNA damage can be subdivided into two main types:

1. *Endogenous damage* such as attack by reactive oxygen species produced from normal metabolic byproducts (spontaneous mutation), especially the process of oxidative deamination
2. *Exogenous damage* caused by external agents such as:
   - ✰ Ultraviolet [UV 200-300nm] radiation from the sun

- Other radiation frequencies, including x-rays and gamma rays
- Hydrolysis or thermal disruption
- Certain plant toxins
- Human-made mutagenic chemicals, especially aromatic compounds that act as DNA intercalating agents
- Cancer chemotherapy and radiotherapy

The replication of damaged DNA before cell division can lead to the incorporation of wrong bases opposite damaged ones. Daughter cells that inherit these wrong bases carry mutations from which the original DNA sequence is unrecoverable (except in the rare case of a back mutation, for example, through gene conversion).

Types of DNA Damage

1. All four of the bases in DNA (A, T, C, and G) can be covalently modified at various positions. *Hydrolysis* of bases, such as deamination, depurination and depyrimidination. One of the most frequent is the loss of an amino group ("deamination")–resulting, for example, in a C being converted to a U.
2. *Mismatches* of the normal bases because of a failure of proofreading during DNA replication. Common example: incorporation of the pyrimidine U (normally found only in RNA) instead of T.
   - *Breaks* in the backbone can be limited to one of the two strands (a single-stranded break, *SSB*) or on both strands (a double-stranded break, DSB). Ionizing radiation is a frequent cause, but some chemicals produce breaks as well.
   - *Cross links* Covalent linkages can be formed between bases on the same DNA strand ("intrastrand") or on the opposite strand ("interstrand").
3. Several chemotherapeutic drugs used against cancers crosslink DNA.
4. Oxidation of bases [*e.g.* 8-oxo-7,8-dihydroguanine (8-oxoG)] and generation of DNA strand interruptions from reactive oxygen species,
5. alkylation of bases (usually methylation), such as formation of 7-methyl guanine, 1-methyladenine, O6 methyl guanine

Damage caused by exogenous agents comes in many forms. Some examples are:

- *UV-B light* causes cross linking between adjacent cytosine and thymine bases creating *pyrimidine dimers*. This is called direct DNA damage.
- *UV-A light* creates mostly free radicals–especially if sunlight penetrated into the skin.
- The damage caused by free radicals is called indirect DNA damage.
- *Ionizing radiation* such as that created by radioactive decay or in *cosmic rays* causes breaks in DNA strands.
- *Thermal disruption* at elevated temperature increases the rate of depurination (loss of purine bases from the DNA backbone) and single strand breaks *e.g.*, hydrolytic depurination is seen in the thermophilic bacteria, which grow in hot springs at 85–250 °C

The rate of depurination (300 purine residues per genome per generation) is too high in these species to be repaired by normal repair machinery; hence a possibility of an adaptive response cannot be ruled out.

Mutation

In biology, mutations are changes to the nucleotide sequence of the genetic material of an organism. Mutations can be caused by copying errors in the genetic material during cell division, by exposure to UV or ionizing radiations, chemical mutagens, or viruses, or can be induced by the organism, itself, by cellular processes such as hypermutation.

DNA Damage and Mutation

It is important to distinguish between DNA damage and mutation, the two major types of error in DNA. DNA damage and mutation are fundamentally different. Damages are physical abnormalities in the DNA, such as single and double strand breaks, 8-hydroxydeoxyguanosine residues and polycyclic aromatic hydrocarbon adducts. DNA damages can be recognized by enzymes, and thus they can be correctly repaired if redundant information, such as the undamaged sequence in the complementary DNA strand or in a homologous chromosome, is available for copying. If a cell retains DNA damage, transcription of a gene can be prevented and thus translation into a protein will also be blocked. Replication may also be blocked and/or the cell may die.

In contrast to DNA damage, a mutation is a change in the base sequence of the DNA. A mutation cannot be recognized by enzymes once the base change is present in both DNA strands, and thus a mutation cannot be repaired. At the cellular level, mutations can cause alterations in protein function and regulation. Mutations are replicated when the cell replicates. In a population of cells, mutant cells will increase or decrease in frequency according to the effects of the mutation on the ability of the cell to survive and reproduce. Although distinctly different from each other, DNA damages and mutations are related because DNA damages often cause errors of DNA synthesis during replication or repair and these errors are a major source of mutation.

Given these properties of DNA damage and mutation, it can be seen that DNA damages are a special problem in non-dividing or slowly dividing cells, where unrepaired damages will tend to accumulate over time. On the other hand, in rapidly dividing cells, unrepaired DNA damages that do not kill the cell by blocking replication will tend to cause replication errors and thus mutation. The

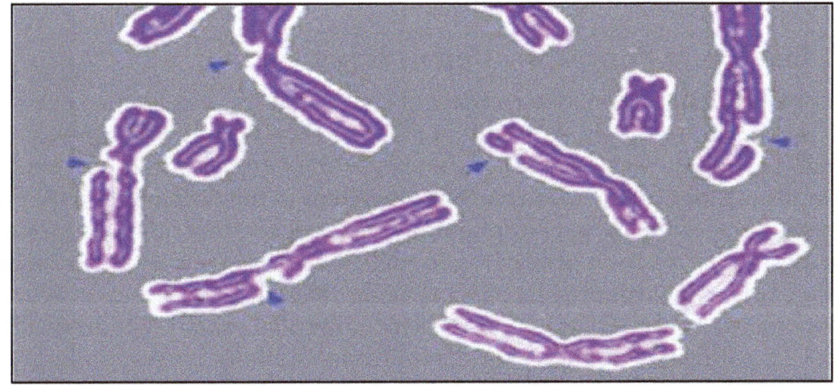

Figure 4.1: DNA Damage Resulting in Multiple Broken Chromosomes

great majority of mutations that are not neutral in their effect are deleterious to a cell's survival. Thus, in a population of cells comprising a tissue with replicating cells, mutant cells will tend to be lost. However infrequent mutations that provide a survival advantage will tend to clonally expand at the expense of neighboring cells in the tissue. This advantage to the cell is disadvantageous to the whole organism, because such mutant cells can give rise to cancer. Thus DNA damages in frequently dividing cells, because they give rise to mutations, are a prominent cause of cancer. In contrast, DNA damages in infrequently dividing cells are likely a prominent cause of aging.

Mutagens

A mutagen (Latin, literally *Origin of change*) is a physical or chemical agent that changes the genetic information (usually DNA) of an organism and thus increases the frequency of mutations above the natural background. As many mutations cause cancer, mutagens are typically also carcinogens but sometimes mutations occur spontaneously due to DNA replication, repair and recombination.

Agents that Damage DNA

1. Certain wavelengths of *radiation*
   - ✰ Ionizing radiation such as gamma rays and x-rays
   - ✰ *Ultraviolet rays*, especially the UV-C rays (~260 nm) that are absorbed strongly by DNA but also the longer-wavelength UV-B that penetrates the ozone shield
2. Highly-reactive *oxygen radicals* produced during normal cellular respiration as well as by other biochemical pathways.
3. Chemicals in the *environment*
   - ✰ Many hydrocarbons, including some found in cigarette smoke
   - ✰ Some plant and microbial products, *e.g.* the aflatoxins produced in moldy peanuts
4. Chemicals used in *chemotherapy*, especially chemotherapy of cancers

Consequences of Damaged DNA

The biological consequences of individual damaged bases have been deduced by a combination of experimental approaches (Wallace, 2002). The possible consequences of fertilization with sperm possessing abnormal DNA are shown in Figure 4.2.

Pathological Effeccts of Poor DNA Repair (Figure 4.3)

DNA repair rate is an important determinant of cell pathology. In a healthy cell the rate of DNA damage is equal to the rate of repair. Any shift of their balance leads to pathological effects of DNA repair. Experimental animals with genetic deficiencies in DNA repair often show decreased lifespan and increased cancer incidence. For example, mice deficient in the dominant NHEJ pathway and in telomere maintenance mechanisms get lymphoma and infections more often, and consequently have shorter lifespan than wild-type mice similarly, mice deficient in a key repair and transcription protein that unwinds DNA helices have premature onset of aging-related diseases and consequent shortening of lifespan. However, not every DNA repair deficiency creates exactly the predicted effects; mice deficient in the NER pathway exhibited shortened lifespan without correspondingly higher rate of mutation.

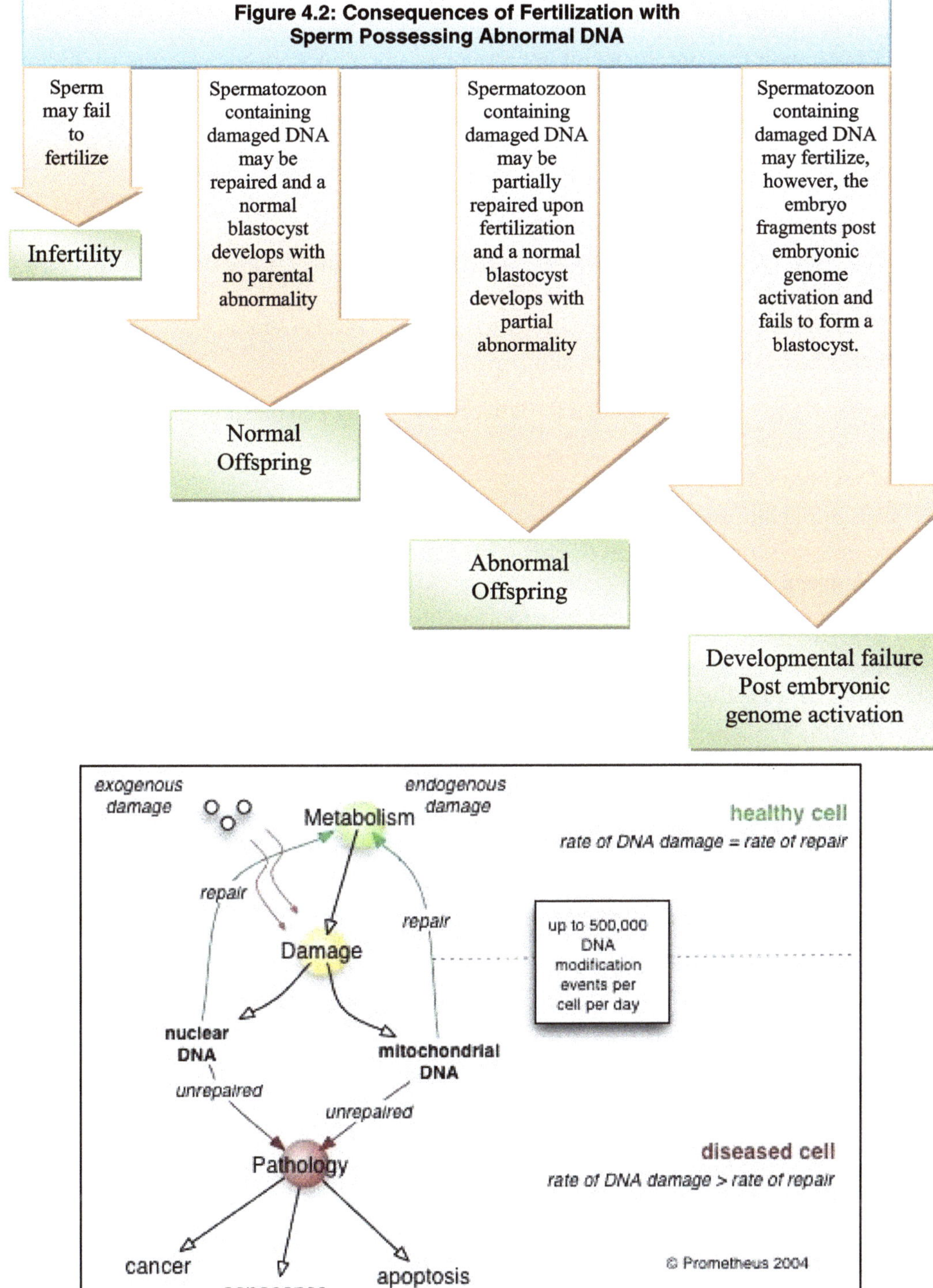

Figure 4.2: Consequences of Fertilization with Sperm Possessing Abnormal DNA

Figure 4.3: Pathological Effeccts of Poor DNA Repair

If the rate of DNA damage exceeds the capacity of the cell to repair it, the accumulation of errors can overwhelm the cell and result in early senescence, apoptosis or cancer. Inherited diseases associated with faulty DNA repair functioning result in premature aging, increased sensitivity to carcinogens, and correspondingly increased cancer risk. On the other hand, organisms with enhanced DNA repair systems, such as *Deinococcus radiodurans*, the most radiation-resistant known organism, exhibit remarkable resistance to the double strand break-inducing effects of radioactivity, likely due to enhanced efficiency of DNA repair and especially NHEJ.

Hereditary Consequences of Damaged DNA

1. Xeroderma pigmentosum: hypersensitivity to sunlight/UV, resulting in increased skin cancer incidence and premature aging
2. Cockayne syndrome: hypersensitivity to UV and chemical agents
3. Trichothiodystrophy: sensitive skin, brittle hair and nails

Mental retardation often accompanies the latter two disorders, suggesting increased vulnerability of developmental neurons.

Other DNA repair disorders include:

1. Werner's syndrome: premature aging and retarded growth
2. Bloom's syndrome: sunlight hypersensitivity, high incidence of malignancies (especially leukemias).
3. Ataxia telangiectasia: sensitivity to ionizing radiation and some chemical agents

All of the above diseases are often called "segmental progerias" ("accelerated aging diseases") (Wei *et al.*, 2007) because their victims appear elderly and suffer from aging-related diseases at an abnormally young age.

Other diseases associated with reduced DNA repair function include Fanconi's anemia, hereditary breast cancer and hereditary colon cancer.

Repairing Damaged Bases (Figure 4.4)

Thankfully, cells have evolved many complex mechanisms to detect and repair DNA damage, and most of the time a cell repairs its damaged DNA without a problem. But, just like the machinery that copies DNA, a cell's repair machinery is not 100 per cent efficient and not every single error is corrected. Maintenance of genome integrity is essential to minimize heritable mutations and to promote healthy survival of organisms. The DNA damage response (DDR) has evolved to optimize cell survival following DNA damage. It involves the actions of DNA repair proteins together with the "checkpoint" events that slow down or arrest cell-cycle progression while the damage is being removed. The inability to properly face a genotoxic threat leads to genomic instability, and eventually to tumoral transformation.

DNA damage is caused by a variety of sources. The cellular response to damage may involve activation of a cell cycle checkpoint, commencement of transcriptional programs, execution of DNA repair, or when the damage is severe, initiation of apoptosis.

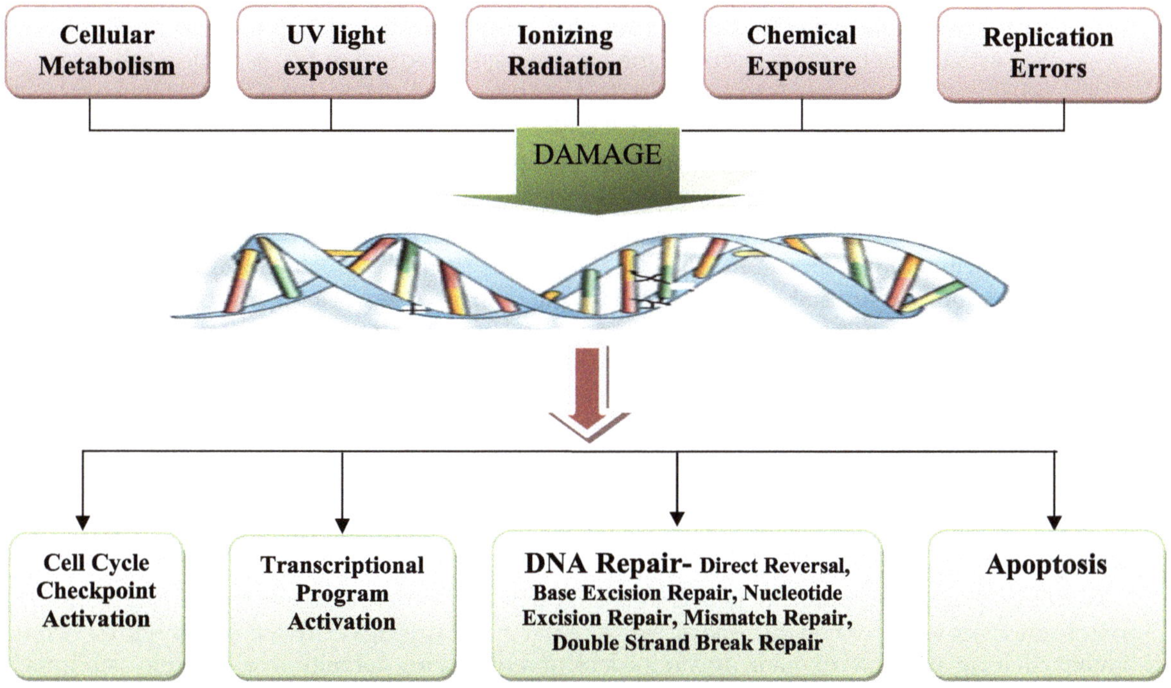

Figure 4.4: DNA Damage Response

The DNA damage response or inappropriate bases can be repaired by several mechanisms such as

1. Direct chemical reversal of the damage
2. Excision Repair, in which the damaged base or bases are removed and then replaced with the correct ones in a localized burst of DNA synthesis. There are three modes of excision repair, each of which employs specialized sets of enzymes.
   - Base Excision Repair (BER)
   - Nucleotide Excision Repair (NER)
   - Mismatch Repair (MMR)

The genotoxicity of the drug like molecule can be tested on the basis of the observations of the different parameters in the experimental animals *viz.*, micronuclei, chromosomal aberrations and sperm aberrations.

Detection of Damaged DNA

Various methods have been developed to detect damaged DNA.

1. *UDS*: UDS (unscheduled DNA synthesis) most common complementary assay and can be detected *e.g.* by an elevated incorporation of [3H]–thymidine in to the DNA of cultured mammalian cells during the repair of damage. This can be detected by autoradiography or liquid scintillation counting.

The UDS assay measures repairable DNA damage induced by test article. The UDS assay is customarily conducted in hepatocytes, both *in vitro* and *in vivo*. Metabolic activation of the test article is believed to occur in the hepatocytes proximal to DNA, which enhances the sensitivity of mutagen detection. This test has been proposed by the ICH guidelines to be an additional assay for the clarification of equivocal *in vitro* test.

Both *in vitro* and *in vivo* UDS assays are most useful in detecting liver carcinogens and less reliable in detecting carcinogens of other organs.

2. *Comet Assay*: the comet assay is a relatively simple, but sensitive and well validated tool for measuring strand breaks in DNA in single cells (Wong *et al.*, 2005). In the comet assay, nucleated cells are embedded in low melting point agarose on a microscopic slide, and the membranes and histones are removed by high salt solutions (singh *et al.*, 1988). DNA is unwinds and spills out as a 'halo' surrounding the nucleoid (Cook *et al.*, 1976). Electrophoresis at neutral, mildly alkaline or strongly alkaline conditions follows the unwinding step (Tice and Strauss, 1995). The comet is visualized by a DNA staining fluorescent dye (Tice *et al.*, 2000) and DNA damage is then scored using either visual or computerized image analysis.

Micronuclei

Micronucleus is the small nucleus that forms whenever a chromosome or a fragment of a chromosome is not incorporated into one of the daughter nuclei during cell division or by chromosome fragments that lag at the cell division due to the lack of centromere, damage, or a defect in cytokinesis (Heddle *et al.*, 1991). In newly formed red blood cells in humans, these are known as Howell-Jolly bodies. In normal people and many other mammals, which do not have nuclei in their red blood cells,

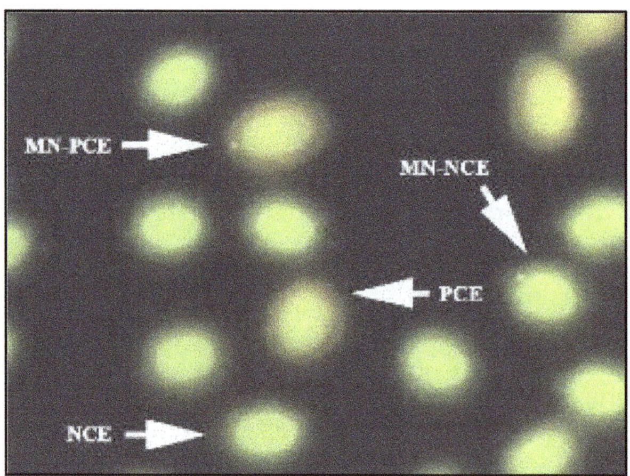

Figure 4.5: Acridine Orange Stained Peripheral Blood Erythrocytes of *C. auratus*

Arrows; NCE: Normochromatic (mature) erythrocyte; MN-NCE: Micronucleated normochromatic erythrocyte; PCE: Polychromatic (young) erythrocyte with RNA-containing cytoplasm; MN-PCE: Micronucleated polychromatic erythrocyte (Cavas, 2008).

the micronuclei are removed rapidly by the spleen. Hence high frequencies of micronuclei in human peripheral blood indicate a ruptured or absent spleen. In mice, these are not removed, which is the basis for the *in vivo* Micronucleus test.

A "micronucleus" is literally a small nucleus. In the micronucleus test, animals are treated with a chemical and then the frequency of micro nucleated cells is determined at some specified time after treatment. If a treated group of animals shows significantly higher frequencies of micro nucleated cells than do the untreated control animals, the chemical is considered to be capable of inducing structural and/or numerical chromosomal damage.

The micronucleus test is performed in a variety of ways, depending upon the questions the investigator is attempting to answer, the test organism, the cell type that is assayed, and the mode of action of the chemical. The tissues most often assessed for frequency of micronuclei are bone marrow and peripheral blood. Erythrocytes (red blood cells) are the cells that are scored in the bone marrow or the blood for presence of micronuclei. Micronucleus tests must be performed on cells that are dividing. Erythrocytes arise from "stem cells" in the bone marrow and are produced by a series of divisions in a precursor cell population. The constant, rapid turn over of precursor cells make erythrocytes an ideal cell type for a micronucleus test. Another unique feature of the erythrocyte is that in the cell division immediately prior to formation of the fully differentiated erythrocyte, the nucleus is pushed out of the cell, erythrocytes are the only mammalian cell type that does not contain a nucleus, and therefore, the differentiated erythrocyte cannot further divide. Thus the bone marrow stem cells are continuously producing new erythrocytes to replace the ones that eventually die. If a chemical damages a stem cell and a micronucleus is formed as a consequence of this damage, the micronucleus remains in the cell after the main nucleus has been pushed out and is very easy to observe microscopically. Micronuclei are chromatin containing structures in the cytoplasm surrounded by a membrane without any detectable link to the cell nucleus. They are formed by exclusion of whole chromosomes or chromatin fragments during cell division. Micronuclei can be detected using different DNA dyes and their frequency can be quantified microscopically or with flow cytometry. It can be determined with immunofluorescence staining whether micronuclei contain kinetochores and thus the centromeric region of the chromosomes. This region can be present in the micronuclei if a whole chromatid/ chromosome or if the centromeric region is included. If a high frequency (in the order of 7-100 per cent) of micronuclei contains a kinetochore, the compound is generally considered aneugenic, since non random breakage of centromeric chromosome fragments at such high frequencies is considered unlikely. Since induction of aneuploidy is the cause of hereditary disease in the new born child and could be associated with the formation of cancer, detection of aneugene is an important end point in the genotoxicity testing. A micronucleus is without kinetochore if it contains an eccentric's fragment or if the kinetochore is lost from the centromere. This loss of kinetochore protein can be investigated by fluorescence in situ hybridization with DNA probes that bind to centromeric DNA sequences. If the frequency of kinetochore containing micronuclei is low (in the order of 0-30 per cent),the compound is generally considered clastogenic because it is considered that kinetochore loss at such a high percentage is unlikely and thus chromosome breakage must have occurred. Knowledge of the contents of micronuclei is the crucial step in understanding of their formation. Schiffmann and DoBoni showed the high ultra structural similarity of micronuclei with cell nuclei. The amount of DNA in micronuclei is dependent on chromosomal distribution, cell cycle phase at micronucleus detection and the occurrence of whole chromosomes/fragments in them. One approach to determine this is to measure the micronucleus sizes relative to the cell nucleus sizes.

Detection of Micronuclei

The origination of the micronuclei, whether by chromosome breaks or non disjunction, can be distinguished immunochemically for the presence of the kinetochore protein in the micronuclei (Gudi *et al.*, 1990), or by in situ DNA hybridization of the centromeric sequence in the micronuclei (Hayashi *et al.*, 1994). The presence of kinetochore protein or the centromeric DNA sequences indicates that the micronuclei were derived from whole chromosome as a result of aneuploidy induction.

The procedure of the micronuclei test can vary slightly, depending upon the type of data desired for the study (Tinwell, 1990). For a typical rodent bone marrow micronucleus assay, there are at least three acceptable dosing and bone marrow harvest schedules. Bone marrow suppression is monitored by a decrease in ratio of PCE to NCE, or PCE to total erythrocytes (RBC, PCE+ NCE) which are commonly referred to as PCE/NCE or PCE/RBC ratio. Bone marrow smears are prepared on microscopic slides, stained with giemsa (Schmid, 1976) or nucleic acid specific fluorescent dye (like Acridine Orange, A.O.) (Hayashi *et al.*, 1983) and scored for micronucleated PCEs. An increase of the micronucleated PCE indicates clastogenecity of test article. Commonly used statistical methods are acceptable for data analysis. Micronuclei can also be scored in the PCE in mouse peripheral blood (MacGregor *et al.*, 1983; 1986).

Chromosomal Aberration

Chromosomes are organized structures of DNA and proteins that are found in cells. A chromosome is a continuous piece of DNA, which contains many genes, regulatory elements and other nucleotide sequences. Chromosomes also contain DNA-bound proteins, which serve to package the DNA and control its functions.

Chromosomal aberrations are disruptions in the normal chromosomal content of a cell, and are a major cause of genetic diseases in humans, such as Down syndrome. Some chromosome abnormalities do not cause disease in carriers, such as translocations, or chromosome inversions, although they may lead to a higher chance of birthing a progency with a chromosome disorder. Abnormal numbers of chromosomes or chromosome sets, aneuploidy, may be lethal or give rise to genetic disorders. Genetic counseling is offered for families that may carry a chromosome rearrangement.

The gain or loss of chromosome material can lead to a variety of genetic disorders. Human examples include.

- ✫ *Cri du chat*, which is caused by the deletion of part of the short arm of chromosome 5. "Cri du chat" means "cry of the cat" in French, and the condition was so-named because affected babies make high-pitched cries that sound like those of a cat. Affected individuals have wide-set eyes, a small head and jaw, and are moderately to severely mentally retarded and very short.
- ✫ *Wolf–Hirschhorn syndrome*, which is caused by partial deletion of the short arm of chromosome 4. It is characterized by severe growth retardation and severe to profound mental retardation.
- ✫ *Down's syndrome*, usually is caused by an extra copy of chromosome 21 (trisomy 21 it is an example of trisomics.). Characteristics include decreased muscle tone, stockier build, asymmetrical skull, slanting eyes and mild to moderate mental retardation (Miller 2000).
- ✫ *Edward syndrome*, which is the second-most-common trisomy; Down syndrome is the most common. It is a trisomy of chromosome 18. Symptoms include mental and motor retardation and numerous congenital anomalies causing serious health problems. Ninety percent die

in infancy; however, those that live past their first birthday usually are quite healthy thereafter. They have a characteristic clenched hands and overlapping fingers.

- *Patau syndrome* also called D-Syndrome or trisomy-13. Symptoms are somewhat similar to those of trisomy-18, but they do not have the characteristic hand shape.
- *Idic 15*, abbreviation for Isodicentric 15 on chromosome 15; also called the following names due to various researches, but they all mean the same; IDIC(15), Inverted duplication 15, extra Marker, Inv dup 15, partial tetrasomy 15
- *Jacobsen syndrome* also called the terminal 11q deletion disorder (European Chromosome 11 network). This is a very rare disorder. Those affected have normal intelligence or mild mental retardation, with poor expressive language skills. Most have a bleeding disorder called Paris–Trousseau syndrome.
- *Klinefelter's syndrome (XXY)*. Men with Klinefelter syndrome are usually sterile, and tend to have longer arms and legs and to be taller than their peers. Boys with the syndrome are often shy and quiet, and have a higher incidence of speech delay and dyslexia. During puberty, without testosterone treatment, some of them may develop gynecomastia.
- *Turner syndrome (X instead of XX or XY)*. In Turner syndrome, female sexual characteristics are present but underdeveloped. People with Turner syndrome often have a short stature, low hairline, abnormal eye features and bone development and a "caved-in" appearance to the chest.
- *XXY syndrome*. XYY boys are usually taller than their siblings. Like XXY boys and XXX girls, they are somewhat more likely to have learning difficulties.
- *Triple-X syndrome (XXX)*. XXX girls tend to be tall and thin. They have a higher incidence of dyslexia.
- *Small supernumerary marker chromosome*. This means there is an extra, abnormal chromosome. Features depend on the origin of the extra genetic material. Cat–eye syndrome and isodicentric chromosome 15 syndrome (or Idic15) are both caused by a supernumerary marker chromosome, as is pallister–Killian syndrome.

Chromosomal mutations produce changes in whole chromosomes (more than one gene) or in the number of chromosomes present.

- Deletion–loss of part of a chromosome
- Duplication–extra copies of a part of a chromosome
- Inversion–reverse the direction of a part of a chromosome
- Translocation–part of a chromosome breaks off and attaches to another chromosome

Most mutations are neutral–have little or no effect. All mutagenic agents induce lesions in the cellular DNA and they are repaired efficiently by different repair mechanisms. Un-repaired and mis-repaired lesions lead to chromosomal aberrations (CAs) (Natarajan and Palitti, 2008).

Karyotype

In general, the karyotype is the characteristic chromosome complement of a eukaryote species (White, 1973). The preparation and study of karyotypes is part of cytogenetics. There may be variation between species in chromosome number and in detailed organization. In some cases, there is significant variation within species. Often there is 1) variation between the two sexes; 2) variation between the germ-line and soma (between gametes and the rest of the body); 3) variation between members of a population, due to balanced genetic morphism; 4) Geographical variation between races; 5) mosaics or otherwise abnormal individuals. Also, variation in karyotype may occur during development from the fertilized egg.

The technique of determining the karyotype is usually called *karyotyping*. Cells can be locked part-way through division (in metaphase) *in vitro* (in a reaction vial) with colchicine. These cells are then stained, photographed, and arranged into a *karyogram*, with the set of chromosomes arranged, autosomes in order of length, and sex chromosomes.

Standard karyotyping, successfully used for the last 50 years in investigating the chromosome etiology in patients with infertility, fetal abnormalities and congenital disorders, is constrained by the limits of microscopic resolution and is not suited for the detection of subtle chromosome abnormalities. The ability to detect submicroscopic chromosomal rearrangements that lead to copy-number changes has escalated progressively in recent years with the advent of molecular cytogenetic techniques. The procedure for the chromosome aberration assay varies slightly with different cell types (Ishidate *et al.*, 1998). Recently Gouas *et al.* (2008) reviewed some gene dosage methods, such as FISH, PCR-based approaches (MLPA, QF-PCR, QMPSF and real time PCR), CGH and array-CGH, that can be used for the identification and delineation of copy-number changes for diagnostic purposes.

Sperm Abnormalities

Sperms are a highly specialized cell type derived to deliver the paternal haploid genome to the oocyte. The epigenetic, or gene regulatory, properties and mechanisms of the sperm assist in preparation of the paternal genome to contribute to embryogenesis and the genome of the zygote. Many recent studies have addressed the issue of altered epigenetic processes in the sperm. Benjamin and Douglas (2006) evaluated the current understanding of DNA damage, chromosome aneuploidy, reduced telomere length, malformations of the centrosome, genomic imprinting errors, altered mRNA profiles, and abnormal nuclear packaging in the sperm prior to fertilization and the observed effects on embryogenesis.

Spermatogenesis is a highly regulated process that takes place in the seminiferous tubules, where morphological alterations lead to the formation of differentiated sperm (Russell *et al.*, 1990a). Spermatogenesis can be subdivided into three main phases: spermatogonial proliferation, meiosis of spermatocytes and spermiogenesis of haploid spermatids (Russell *et al.*, 1990b). During spermiogenesis, the round haploid spermatids undergo an elongation phase and transformation of the germ cell in which the majority of the somatic histones are replaced, first by transition proteins and then protamines, packing the DNA into the sperm cell nucleus (Sassone-Corsi, 2002). A proportion of the spermatozoa produced by males of many mammalian species are morphologically abnormal. A high incidence of abnormal sperm may cause lower fertility or abnormal embryos, since a high incidence of abnormal karyotypes were found in embryos that had been inseminated with morphologically abnormal sperm (Kishikawa *et al.*, 1999). Therefore, it was suggested that morphologically abnormal sperm have some abnormalities in terms of producing progeny. A mouse would be useful model for analyzing the correlation between sperm morphology and fertilization or development. In the mouse, spermatogenesis begins after birth; approximately 35 days are required for the development of mature sperm. This initial spermatogenesis after birth is referred to as the first wave of spermatogenesis (Hiroshi *et al.*, 2009).

While evaluating the effects of any agent in an organism it is highly relevant to study the genotoxic effects on the germinal cells also, because it provides information on transmissible genetic damage from one generation to other (Au and Hsu, 1980). Chemicals that showed positive responses in the sperm abnormality test are also proved to be carcinogenic (Wyrobek *et al.*, 1983). The change in the sperm parameters probably arise from inference by the test substance with the genetically controlled differentiation of the sperm cells, and therefore, these assays are intrinsically relevant to safety evaluation and assessment of potential and possible reproductive outcomes. Sperm shape test provides a direct measure of the quality of sperm production during chemically treatment conditions.

Many different types of sperm abnormalities occur. A common classification scheme is based on the location of the abnormalities. Those that are located in the sperm head are classified as primary. Abnormalities associated with neck, mid-piece or tails are classified as secondary abnormalities. Included in the secondary abnormalities is the presence of cytoplasmic droplets. Normal and abnormal sperm are shown below within a species (Figure 4.6).

Detection of Sperm Abnormalities

Various assays have been developed to get informations regarding sperm abnormalities, most common are sperm morphology assay, sperm count assay and reactive oxygen evaluations of sperms. For the sperm morphological evaluations sperm samples collection from cauda epididymis followed by mincing and smear preparation on microscopic slides for examination. Sperm count by the counting chamber which provides functional spermatozoa count.

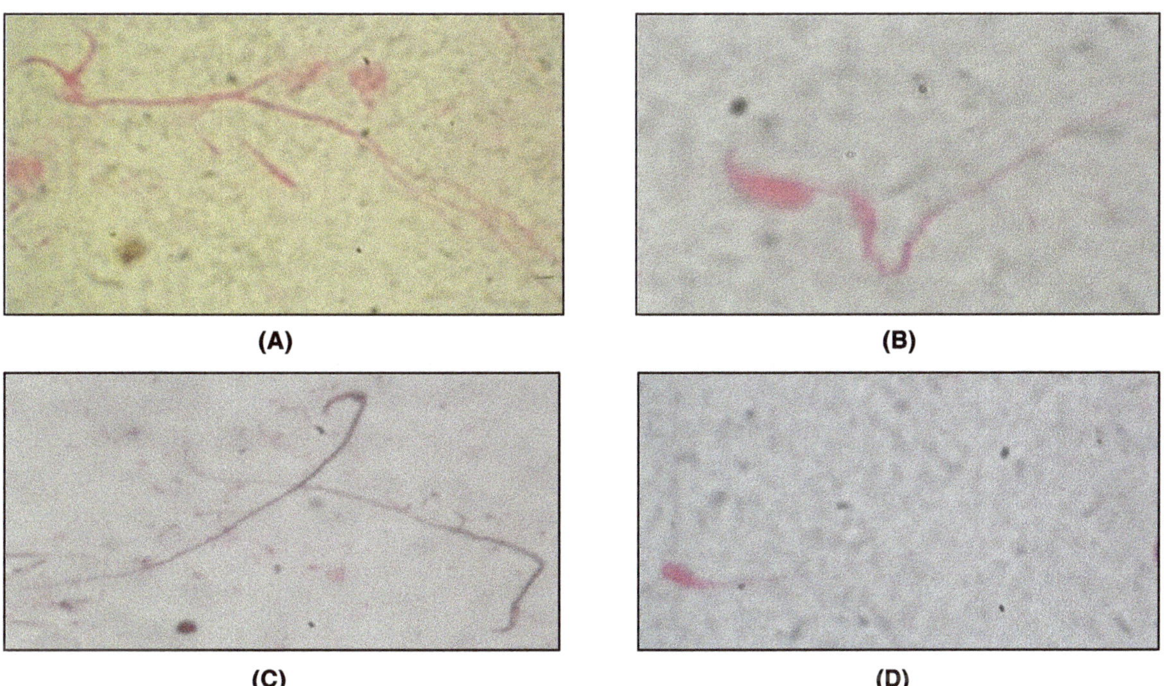

(A) (B)

(C) (D)

Figure 4.6: Abnormal Sperms

A: Double head and double tail; B: Bend filament;
C: Bending at cephalocaudal region; D: Amorphous head

Generial Purpose of Genotoxicity Testing

Genotoxicity tests can be defined as *in vitro* and *in vivo* tests designed to detect compounds that induce genetic damage directly or indirectly by various mechanisms. These tests should enable hazard identification with respect to damage to DNA and its fixation. Fixation of damage to DNA in the form of gene mutations, larger scale chromosomal damage, recombination and numerical chromosome changes is generally considered to be essential for heritable effects and in the multistep process of malignancy, a complex process in which genetic changes may play only a part. Compounds which are positive in tests that detect such kinds of damage have the potential to be human carcinogens and/or mutagens, *i.e.*, may induce cancer and/or heritable defects. Because the relationship between exposure to particular chemicals and carcinogenesis is established for man, while a similar relationship has been difficult to prove for heritable diseases, Genotoxicity tests have been used mainly for the prediction of carcinogenicity. Nevertheless, because germ line mutations are clearly associated with human disease, the suspicion that a compound may induce heritable effects is considered to be just as serious as the suspicion that a compound may induce cancer. In addition, the outcome of such tests may be valuable for the interpretation of carcinogenicity studies.

Limitations of the Present Regulatory System to Test Genotoxicity

- ✰ Guidelines followed for the study of preclinical safety of a drug are very time consuming, resource intensive process and need a large number of animals for experimentation.
- ✰ The *in vitro* and *in vivo* protocols measured in the guidelines are not validated for detection of genome mutations (aneuploidy) and somatic point mutations.
- ✰ There are no details regarding the choice of specific test system and test protocols for certain categories of pharmaceuticals, which need critical experimental evaluation.
- ✰ Most guidelines are devoid of recommendations for compounds, which are genotoxic, but seem to act by non-DNA targets (Tenant *et al.*, 1987).
- ✰ There are also no specific recommendations on the threshold of different genotoxic and tumorigenic compounds and their organ–specific effects when they are intended to use therapeutically (Scott *et al.*, 1991).

References

Au, W.W. and Hsu, T.C. (1980). The genotoxic effects of adriamycin in somatic and germinal cells of mouse. *Mutat Res.*, 79: 351–361.

Benjamin, R., Douglas, E. and Carrell, T. (2006). The effect of epigenetic sperm abnormalities on early embryo-genesis. *Asian J Androl.*, 8 (2): 131–142.

Brusick, D.J. (1987a). Implications of treatment–condition–induced Genotoxicity for chemical screening and data interpretation. *Mutat. Res.*, 189(1): 1-6.

Cavas, T. (2008). *In vivo* genotoxicity of mercury chloride and lead acetate: Micronucleus test on acridine orange stained fish cells. *Food and Chemical Toxicology*, 46 (1): 352-358.

Cook, P.R., Brazell, I.A. and Jost, E. (1976). Characterization of nuclear structures containing superhelical DNA. *Journal of Cell Science*, 22: 303-24.

Davidson, I.W.F., Parker, J.C. and Beliles, R.P. (1988). Biological basis for extrapolation across mammalian species. *Regul Toxicol Pharmacol.*, 6: 211–37.

Dearfield, K.L., Cimino, M.C., McCarroll, N.E., Mauer, I. and Valcovic, L.R. (2002). Genotoxicity risk assessment: a proposed classification strategy. *Mutat. Res.*, 521: 121–135.

Dias, F.D.L. and Takahashi, C.S. (1994). Cytogenetic evaluation of aqueous extracts of the medicinal plants *Alpinia nutans* Rose (Zingerberaceae) and *Pogostemum hyneanus* benth (Labitae) on Wistar rats and *Allium cepa* Linn (Liliaceae) root tip cells. *Rev. Brasil Genet.*, 17: 175–180.

Douglass, G.R., Blakey, D.H. and Clayson, D.B. (1988). Genotoxicity tests as predictors of carcinogens: an analysis, ICPEMC working paper no. 5. *Mutat Res.*, 196: 83–93.

European Chromosome 11 network: www.11q.org.

Genomics.energy.gov: Gene Gate Way–Genes and Genetic disorders *in* Human Genome Project information.

Gouas, L., Goumy, C., Véronèse, L., Tchirkov, A. and Vago, P. (2008). Gene dosage methods as diagnostic tools for the identification of chromosome abnormalities. *Pathologique Biologique.*, 56: 345-353.

Gudi, R., Sandhu, S.S. and Athwal, R.S. (1990). Kinetochore identification in micronuclei in mouse bone marrow erythrocytes. An assay for the detection of aneuploidy inducing agents. *Mutat Res.*, 234: 263-268.

Hayashi, M., Marki-paakkanem, J., Tanabe, H., Houma, M., Suzuki, T., Matsmoka, A., Mizusawa, H. and Sofuni, T. (1994). Isolation of micronuclei from mouse blood and fluoresce in situ hybridization with a mouse centromeric DNA probe. *Mutat Res.*, 307: 245–251.

Hayashi, M., Sofuni, T. and Ishidate, M., Jr. (1983). An application of acridine orange fluorescent staining to the micronucleus test. *Mutat Res.*, 120: 241-247.

Heddle, J.A., Cimino, M.C., Hayashi, M. *et al.* (1991). Micronuclei as an index of cytogenetic damage: past, present and future. *Environ Mol Mutagen.*, 18: 277-291.

Hiroshi, Ohta, Yuko, Sakaide and Teruhiko, Wakayama. (2009). Age–and substrain–dependent sperm abnormalities in BALB/c mice and functional assessment of abnormal sperm by ICSI. *Human Reproduction*, 1(1): 1–7.

Hutt, P.B. and Merril, R. (1991). Food and Drug Law: Cases and Materials. Mineola, New York: Foundation Press.

Ishidate, M., Miura, Dr, k.F. and Sofuni, T. (1998) Chromosome aberration assays in genetic testing *in vitro*. *Mutat Res.*, 404: 167-172.

Kirkland, D.J. (1998). Chromosome aberration testing in genetic toxicology–past, present and future. *Mutat res.*, 404: 173–85.

Kirkland, J. (1990). Report of the UKEMS sub–committee Guidelines for Mutagenesity Testing. Part-I: Basic test battery–Revised. Cambridge University Press.

Kishikawa, H., Tateno, H. and Yanagimachi, R. (1999). Chromosome analysis of BALB/c mouse spermatozoa with normal and abnormal head morphology. *Biol Reprod.*, 61:809–812.

Lodish, H. *et al.* (2004). Molecular Biology, 5th ed. WH Freeman and Company. New York.

Macgregor, J.T. (1986). Naturally-occurring toxicants in horticultural food crops. ISHS Acta Horticulturae 207:

Mac Gregor, J.T., Farr, S., Tucker, J.D., Heddle, J.A., Tice, R.R. and Turtletaub, K.W. (1995). New molecular end points and methods for routine toxicity testing. *Food Apple Toxicol.*, 26: 156-73.

Mac Gregor, J.T., Schelegel, R., Choy, W.M. and Wehr, C.M. (1983) Micronuclei in circulating erythrocytes: A rapid screen for chromosomal damage during routine toxicity testing in mice. In: Development in the science and practice of toxicology. Amsterdam: Elsevier, Pp 555–558.

Madle, S., Korte, A. and Ball, R. (1987). Experience with mutagenicity testing of new drugs: view point of a regulatory agency. *Mutate Res.*, 182: 187-92.

Malik V. (1999). Requirement and guidelines on clinical trials for import and manufacture of new drugs. In: Drugs and Cosmetic Act, 1940, 12th ed. Luckhnow: Eastern Book Company; P. 394–404.

Maron, D.M. and Ames, M.N. (1983). Revised methods for the Salmonella mutagenesity test. *Mutat Res.*, 111: 173–215.

Miller, Kenneth, R. (2000). "9-3". *Biology* (5 ed.). Upper Saddle River, New Jersey: Prentice Hall. pp. 194–195. ISBN 0-13-436265–9.

Natarajan, Adayapalam, T. and Palitti Fabrizio (2008). DNA repair and chromosome alterations. *Mutat Res.*, 657: 3-7.

Nath, J. and Krishna, G. (1988). Safety screening of drugs in cancer therapy. *Acta Haematol.*, 99: 138-47.

OECD (1996). (Organization of Economic Cooperation and Development) guidelines for the testing of chemicals, updated guideline 473, Genetic Toxicology: *in vitro* mammalian chromosome aberration test. Paris: Organization of Economic Cooperation and Development.

Purves, D., Harvey, C., Tweats, D. and Lumley, C.E. (1995). Genotoxicity testing: current practices and strategies used by the pharmaceutical industry. *Mutagenesis*, 10: 297–312.

Russell, L.D., Ettlin, R.A., SinhaHikim, A.P. and Clegg, E.D. (1990a). Mammalian Spermatogenesis in Histological and Histopathological Evaluation of the Testis. St. Louis: Cache River Press, 1–40.

Russell, L.D., Ettlin, R.A., SinhaHikim, A.P. and Clegg, E.D. (1990b). Mammalian Spermatogenesis in Histological and Histopathological Evaluation of the Testis. St. Louis: Cache River Press, 41–58.

Sassone-Corsi, P. (2002). Unique chromatin remodeling and transcriptional regulation in spermatogenesis. *Science*, 296: 2176–2178.

Schmid, W. (1976). The micronucleus test for cytogenetic analysis. In: Hollander, ed. Chemical mutagens: Principles and Methods for their detection. Vol 4, New York: Plenum Press, pp 31–53.

Scott, D., Galloway, S.M., Marshall, R.R., Ishidate, Jr. M, Brisick, D., Ashby. J, *et al.* (1991).Genotoxicity under extreme culture conditions. A report from ICPEMC Task Group 9. *Mutat Res.*, 257: 147–204.

Shellby, M. (1988). The genetic toxicity of human carcinogens and its implications. *Mutat Res.*, 204: 3-15.

Singh, N.P., McCoy, M.T., Tice, R.R. and Schneider, E.L. (1988). A simple technique for quantization of low levels of DNA damage in individual cells. *Experimental cell research*, 175: 184–191.

Smith, M. T. (1996). The Mechanism of Benzene-induced Leukemia: A Hypothesis and Speculations on the Causes of Leukemia. *Environment Health Perspect*,104 (6): 1219–1225.

Tennat, R., Margolin, B., Shelby, M., Zeiger, E., Haseman, J. and Spalding, J. (1987). Prediction of chemical carcinogenicity in rodents from *in vivo* genotoxicity assays. *Science*, 236: 933-41.

Tice, R.R., Agurell, E., Anderson, D., Burlinson, B., Hartmann, A., Kobayashi, H., Miyamae, Y., Rojas, E., Ryu, J.C. and Sasaki, Y.F. (2000). Single cell gel/comet assay: guidelines for *in vitro* and *in vivo* genetic toxicology testing. *Environmental and Molecular Mutagenesis*, 35: 206-221

Tice, R.R., and Strauss, G.H. (1995). The single cell gel electrophoresis/comet assay: a potential tool for detecting radiation induced DNA damage in humans. *Stem Cells,* 13: S207–S214.

Tinwell, H. (1990). Serial versus single dosing protocol for the rodent bone marrow micronucleus assay. *Mutat Res.,* 234: 111-261.

Tweats, D. (1984). The predictive value of batteries of short term tests for carcinogens. *Food Add. Contam.,* 1: 189–197.

Umar-Tsafe, Nasir, Mohamed-Said, Mohamed Saifulaman, Rosli, R., Din, L. B. and Lai, L. C. (2004). Genotoxicity of goniothalamin in CHO cell line. *Mutat. Res.,* 562: 91–102.

Wallace, Susane S. (2002). Biological consequences of free radical–damaged DNA bases. *Free Radical Biology and Medicine,* 33(1): 1–14.

Wassom, J. (1992). Origins of genetic toxicology and the Environmental Mutagen Society. *Environ Mol Mutagenesis,* 14: 1-6.

Wei, Qingyi and Lei Li, David Chen, (2007). *DNA Repair, Genetic Instability, and Cancer.* World Scientific.ISBN 9812700145.

White, M.J.D. (1973). *The chromosomes.* 6th ed, Chapman and Hall, London. p28.

Wong, Vincy W.C., Szeto, Y.T., Collins, A.R. and Benzie, I.F.F. (2005). The Comet Assay: a biomonitoring tool for nutraceutical research. *Current Topics in Nutraceutical Research,* 3: 1-14.

Wyrobek, A.J., Gordon, L.A., Burkhart, J.G., Francis, M.W., Kapp, R. W., Letz, G., Malling, H. V., Topham, J.C. and Whorton, M.D. (1983). An evaluation of human sperm as indicators of chemically induced alterations of spermatogenic functions, *Mutat Res.,* 115: 73-148.

Medicinal Plants: Phytochemistry, Pharmacology and Therapeutics, Vol. 1 *Pages* ***98–130***
Editors: **V.K. Gupta, G.D. Singh, Surjeet Singh and A. Kaul**
Published by: **DAYA PUBLISHING HOUSE, NEW DELHI**

Chapter 5

Vasodilatory Activity Induced by Natural Products

Gisele Zapata-Sudo*, Juliana Montani Raimundo and Roberto Takashi Sudo
Departamento de Farmacologia Básica e Clínica, Instituto de Ciências Biomédicas, Universidade Federal do Rio de Janeiro, Rio de Janeiro, Brazil

ABSTRACT

Medicinal plants have been used to treat diseases since the time of ancient civilizations, and there is currently growing interest in the therapeutic use of natural products. Although modern medicine is well-developed in most of the world, medicinal plants are still used for primary health care in developing countries. Furthermore, medicinal plants are gaining the interest of researchers seeking to discover and develop new bioactive components. At present, 25 per cent of modern medicines are developed from plants that were first used traditionally: many synthetic drugs have also been obtained from natural precursors. Despite this, the phytochemical and pharmacological characteristics of only a small percentage of plant species have been studied. The development of new medicines from plants implies the screening of extracts for their biological activities and further isolation of bioactive compounds. This review examines plant extracts that affect the cardiovascular system, focusing on vasodilatory activity. Vasodilation is particularly important in arterial hypertension, which contributes to at least 50 per cent of cardiovascular disease and is a significant cause of premature death worldwide. We describe recent pharmacological studies on vascular reactivity induced by plants extracts in isolated arteries (*e.g.*, aorta and mesenteric arteries) and the effects of these extracts on blood pressure.

* Corresponding Author: E-mail: gsudo@farmaco.ufrj.br.

The plant species and active compounds isolated from them are described according to their mechanism of action. Plant extracts that promoted relaxation of vascular smooth muscle *in vitro* were found to be effective in reducing arterial blood pressure *in vivo*, and may be useful in treatment of cardiovascular diseases such as arterial hypertension.

Keywords: *Arterial hypertension, Blood pressure, Extract, Natural products, Plants, Smooth muscle, Vascular, Vasodilatory activity.*

Introduction

Medicinal plants are important both to the development of pharmaceuticals and to address the growing interest in the therapeutic use of natural products. Clinical, pharmacological and chemical studies of the traditional plant-based medicines, allowed the development of most early medicines, such as digitoxin from *Digitalis purpurea*, aspirin from *Salix alba* and ephedrine from *Ephedra sinica* (Butler, 2004; Mashour *et al.*, 1998). The molecular diversity and beneficial biological properties of medicinal plants have made them central to pharmacological discovery of new bioactive components (Koehn and Carter, 2005). Currently, 25 per cent of modern medicines are made from plants first used traditionally (WHO, 2003) and a large number of synthetic drugs have also been obtained from natural precursors. Natural products are still a significant source of new drugs, especially in anticancer and antihypertensive therapy (Newman *et al.*, 2003). Despite this importance, only a small percentage of plant species has been phytochemically and pharmacologically studied (Calixto, 2005).

Since the development of new medicines from plants implies the screening of extracts for their biological activities and further isolation of the bioactive compounds, this review examines plant extracts that affect the cardiovascular system, focusing especially on vasodilatory activity. Vasodilation is particularly important in the treatment of arterial hypertension, which contributes to at least 50 per cent of cardiovascular disease and is one of the most important causes of premature death worldwide. Approximately 600 million people worldwide are affected by hypertension and 17 million die each year (Tenorio *et al.*, 2005; WHO, International Society of Hypertension Writing Group, 2003). Although modern medicine is responsible for the effective lowering of blood pressure in most of the world, medicinal plants and herbal medicines are still largely used for primary health care in many regions. One of the first drugs clinically used for the treatment of high blood pressure is reserpine, from the herb *Rauwolfia serpentina*, which was described many centuries ago in Indian Ayurvedic monographs (Engel and Straus, 2002). Herbal treatments have been used for the treatment of many cardiovascular diseases, including congestive heart failure, systolic hypertension, angina pectoris, atherosclerosis, cerebral insufficiency, venous insufficiency, and arrhythmia (Mashour *et al.*, 1998).

The present review describes recent pharmacological studies of vascular reactivity induced by plant extracts of in isolated arteries (*e.g.* aorta and mesenteric arteries) and their effects on blood pressure. The species and the active compounds isolated from them are described according to their mechanism of action. Many plant extracts that promoted relaxation of vascular smooth muscle *in vitro* were also effective in reducing arterial blood pressure *in vivo*, revealing good potential for treatment of cardiovascular diseases such as hypertension.

Data Collection

The data for this review were collected using the PubMed literature system of the National Library of Medicine (NLM) and were gathered from articles published during the 2000-2008 time period.

Abstracts containing adequate information were also included. Species were selected and classified according to their mechanism of vasodilation. The scientific name, part used, extract, active constituent, animal model, mechanism of action and references are listed in Tables 5.1–5.3.

Pharmacological Evaluation

Rat aorta was the most frequently used animal model for assessment of vasorelaxant activity followed by rat mesenteric artery, dog carotid artery, porcine coronary artery, and guinea pig aorta. Vasodilatory activity of a substance can be investigated by measuring resting tension of the vessel or by using pre-contracted vessels. Vascular smooth muscle cells contract when there is a sufficient increase in intracellular concentration of calcium (Ca^{2+}). This increase may be due to a change in membrane potential or to the binding of a contractile agonist to a specific receptor. Membrane despolarization leads to activation of a voltage-operated Ca^{2+} channel, thus augmenting Ca^{2+} cytosolic levels. On the other hand, receptor binding of a contractile agonist provokes an increase in Ca^{2+} levels through the generation of second messengers, without a prior change in membrane potential (Orallo, 1996). In most studies, contractures of vascular smooth muscle were induced through exposure to an adrenoceptor agonist, such as phenylephrine and noradrenaline, or to KCl (potassim chloride). The high potassium (K^+)-induced contraction of smooth muscle is mediated by an increase in Ca^{2+} influx through voltage-operated Ca^{2+} channels.

Endothelium-dependent Vasodilation

Vascular tone is an essential component of blood pressure regulation. The contractile state of arteries is a major determinant of the peripheral resistance, which is elevated in sustained arterial hypertension. The endothelium cells play an important role in the blood flow regulation and vascular tone through the production and release of modulatory factors that contract or relax vascular smooth muscle (Orallo, 1996). Nitric oxide (NO) and prostacyclin (PGI_2) are the major vasodilators released by the endothelium. Endothelium-derived hyperpolarizing factor (EDHF) may also participate in vasodilation, especially in small arteries when NO and PGI_2 production is inhibited (Achike and Kwan, 2003). The release of these substances produces endothelium-dependent vasorelaxation of different vascular beds in animal models, including rat aorta (Andriambeloson *et al.*, 1998).

After stimulation of endothelial receptors, endothelial NO synthase can be activated to synthesize NO from L-arginine. NO diffuses from the endothelium to the vascular smooth muscle, where it stimulates soluble guanylyl cyclase to generate cyclic guanosine monophosphate (cGMP), leading to relaxation (Bryan *et al.*, 2005). Similarly, cyclooxigenase can synthesize PGI_2, which causes vasodilation predominantly via the generation of cyclic adenosine monophosphate (cAMP) (Parkington *et al.*, 2004). EDHF produces vasodilation by hyperpolarizing the vascular smooth muscle through potassium channel activation. The smooth muscle hyperpolarization elicits relaxation by decreasing the concentration of cytoplasmatic Ca^{2+} through the closure of voltage-operated Ca^{2+} channels in the membrane (Bryan *et al.*, 2005).

Many plants and the compounds isolated from them (Table 5.1) have been shown to have effects on the NO signaling pathway and to promote *in vitro* endothelium-dependent vasorelaxation (Achike and Kwan, 2003; Andriambeloson *et al.*, 1998). Endothelial involvement in the vasorelaxant activity of a substance can be investigated in endothelium-intact and endothelium-denuded preparations. Most studies have investigated the particular mediators involved in endothelium-dependent vasodilation through the pretreatment of tissues with inhibitors such as: N^G-nitro-l-arginine methyl ester (L-NAME), an NO synthase inhibitor; methylene blue, a guanylyl cyclase inhibitor; and indomethacin, a

Table 5.1: Plant Extracts and Isolated Compounds that Show Significant Vasodilatory Activity in Animal Models through Endothelium-Dependent Mechanisms

Scientific Name	Part Used	Extract	Possible Active Components	Animal and Model	Mechanism of Action	Reference
Aconitum japonicum			Mesaconitine	Rat aorta	NO	Mitamura *et al.*, 2002
Anacardium occidentale	Leaf	Methanol		Rat aorta	NO	Runnie *et al.*, 2004
Angelica keiskei	Root	Ethyl alcohol;	Xanthoangelol;	Rat aorta	NO; EDHF	Matsuura *et al.*, 2001
		ethylacetate fraction	4-hydroxyderricin; xanthoangelols E and F			
Apocynum venetum	Leaf	Aqueous; ethanol fraction		Rat aorta; rat mesenteric artery	NO, K^+ channel activation	Kwan *et al.*, 2005
Arbutus unedo L.	Root	Aqueous		Rat aorta	NO	Ziyyat *et al.*, 2002
	Leaf	Aqueous	Tannins; catechin gallate	Rat aorta	NO	Legssyer *et al.*, 2004
Caesalpinia sappan L.	Heartwood	Methanol	Brazilin; hematoxylin	Rat aorta	NO/cGMP	Xie *et al.*, 2000
			Brazilin	Rat aorta	NO/cGMP	Hu *et al.*, 2003
Carica papaya	Leaf	Methanol		Rat aorta	NO	Runnie *et al.*, 2004
Cecropia lyratiloba Miquel.	Leaf	Methanol, flavonoid fraction		Rat aorta	NO	Almeida *et al.*, 2006
Crataegus			Procyanidins		NO/cGMP; K^+ channel activation	Kim *et al.*, 2000
Crotalaria sessiliflora L.	Aerial parts	Aqueous		Rat aorta	NO/cGMP; muscarinic receptor activation	Hoh *et al.*, 2007
Cymbopogon citratus	Stalk	Methanol		Rat aorta; rat perfused mesenteric artery	NO; EDHF; prostanoids	Runnie *et al.*, 2004
Diospyros kaki Thumb.	Leaf	Hexane; n-butanol		Rat aorta	NO	Yin *et al.*, 2005
Echinodorus grandiflorus	Leaf	Aqueous		Rabbit aorta	NO/cGMP; PAF receptor activation	Tibiricá *et al.*, 2007
Elaeis guineensis	Oil	Methanol		Rat aorta; rat mesenteric vascular bed	NO	Abeywardena *et al.*, 2002

Contd...

Table 5.1–Contd...

Scientific Name	*Part Used*	*Extract*	*Possible Active Components*	*Animal and Model*	*Mechanism of Action*	*Reference*
Eleutherococcus senticosus Maxim.	Root	Aqueous		Rat aorta; rat mesenteric artery; dog carotid artery	NO; EDHF; K^+ channel and muscarinic receptor activation	Kwan *et al.*, 2004c
Eucommia ulmoides Oliv.	Leaf; bark	Aqueous; methanol		Rat aorta; dog carotid artery	NO, K^+ channel activation	Kwan *et al.*, 2004a
	Bark	Aqueous		Rat aorta; rat mesenteric artery	NO; EDHF	Kwan *et al.*, 2004b
Euterpe oleracea Mart.	Stone	Hydro-alcoholic		Rat mesenteric vascular bed	NO/cGMP, EDHF	Rocha *et al.*, 2007
Fritillaria ussuriensis maxim.	Bulb	Aqueous; ethyla-cetate; butanol; hexane		Rat aorta	NO/cGMP	Kang *et al.*, 2002
Ginkgo biloba	Leaf	GBE	quercetin	Rat aorta	NO	Kubota *et al.*, 2001
	Leaf	GBE	bilobalide	Rat aorta	NO; Ca^{2+} channel blocking; K^+ channel activation	Nishida and Satoh, 2003
Gynandropsis gynandra	Leaf	Methanol		Rat aorta	NO	Runnie *et al.*, 2004
Hancornia speciosa	Leaf	Ethanol		Rat superior mesenteric artery	NO, EDHF, K^+ channel activation	Ferreira *et al.*, 2007a
	Leaf	Ethanol		Rat aorta	NO, PI3K	Ferreira *et al.*, 2007b
Ipomoea batatas	Leaf	Methanol		Rat aorta	NO	Runnie *et al.*, 2004
Lepechenia caulescens		Methanol	ursolic acid	Rat aorta	NO/cGMP	Aguirre-Crespo *et al.*, 2006
Ligustici wallichii		Chloroform		Rat aorta	NO	Rhyu *et al.*, 2004
Magnolia liliflora Desr.	Flower	Hexane; ethyl-acetate; n-butanol		Rat aorta	NO	Yin *et al.*, 2005
Mentha arvensis	Leaf	Methanol		Rat aorta	NO	Runnie *et al.*, 2004
Mitragyna inermis (Wild) O. Kuntze	Bark of the trunk	Aqueous		Porcine coronary artery	NO	Quédraogo *et al.*, 2004

Contd...

Table 5.1–Contd...

Scientific Name	*Part Used*	*Extract*	*Possible Active Components*	*Animal and Model*	*Mechanism of Action*	*Reference*
Morus bombycis Koidzumi	Root bark	100 per cent ethanol		Rat aorta	NO	Oh *et al.*, 2007
Musanga cecropioides R. Brown	Leaf	Aqueous		Rat aorta	NO	Dongmo *et al.*, 2002
Ouratea semiserrata	Stem	Hydroethanol; ethylacetate fraction		Rat aorta	NO	Côrtes *et al.*, 2002
Persea americana Mill.	Leaf	Aqueous		Rat portal vein; rat aorta	NO	Ojewole *et al.*, 2007
	Leaf	Aqueous		Rat aorta	NO/cGMP; prostanoids; Ca^{2+} channel blocking	Owolabi *et al.*, 2005
Piper betle	Leaf	Methanol		Rat aorta; rat perfused mesenteric artery	NO; EDHF; prostanoids	Runnie *et al.*, 2004
Polygonun aviculare L.	Whole plant	Hexane; n-butanol		Rat aorta	NO	Yin *et al.*, 2005
Psittacanthus calyculatus	Leaf	Ethanol		Rat aorta	NO	Rodríguez-Cruz *et al.*, 2003
Raphanus sativus	Seed	Aqueous			NO; muscarinic receptor activation	Ghayur and Gilani, 2006
Rheum undulatum L	Rhizome	Aqueous		Rat aorta	NO/cGMP	Moon *et al.*, 2006
Sclerocarya birrea Hochst	Stem bark	Aqueous		Rat aorta	NO	Ojewole, 2006
Selaginella tamariscina Spr.	Whole plant	Ethylacetate; n-butanol		Rat aorta	NO	Yin *et al.*, 2005
			Amentoflavone	Rat aorta	NO/cGMP; K^+ channel activation	Kang *et al.*, 2004

Contd...

Table 5.1–Contd...

Scientific Name	*Part Used*	*Extract*	*Possible Active Components*	*Animal and Model*	*Mechanism of Action*	*Reference*
Sorbus commixta Hedl	Stem bark	n-butanol		Rat aorta	NO	Yin *et al.*, 2005
	Cortex	Methanol		Rat aorta	NO/cGMP	Kang *et al.*, 2005
Tribulus terrestris L.	Whole plant	Methanol; aqueous		Rat mesenteric vascular bed	NO; EDHF	Phillips *et al.*, 2006
Urtica dioica L.	Root	Aqueous; methanol; purified fractions		Rat aorta	NO, K^+ channel activation	Testai *et al.*, 2002
Vitis			Vitisin C	Rabbit aorta	NO	Seya *et al.*, 2003
Vitis labrusca	Skin	Alcohol-free grape		Rat mesenteric vascular bed	NO	Soares de Moura *et al.*, 2002
	Skin	Alcohol-free grape		Rat mesenteric vascular bed	NO; EDHF	Madeira *et al.*, 2005

Table 5.2: Plant Extracts and Isolated Compounds which Show Vasodilatory Activity that in Animal Models through Endothelium-Dependent and Independent Mechanisms

Scientific Name	*Part Used*	*Extract*	*Possible Active Components*	*Animal and Model*	*Mechanism of Action*	*Reference*
Albizia inopinata G. P. Lewis	Leaf	Ethanolic; aqueous fraction		Rat aorta	NO	Pires *et al.*, 2000
	Leaf	Ethanolic; aqueous fraction		Rat aorta	Ca^{2+} channe blocking; inhibition of intracellular Ca^{2+} mobilization	Maciel *et al.*, 2004l
Alpinia henryi K. Schum.			Cardamonin; alpinetin	Rat mesenteric artery	NO; Ca^{2+} channel blocking; inhibition of intracellular Ca^{2+} release	Wang *et al.*, 2001
Alpinia officinarum			Galangin	Rat aorta	NO; Ca^{2+} channel blocking	Morello *et al.*, 2006
Coscinium fenestratum (Gaertn.) Colebr.	Stem	Aqueous		Rat aorta	NO	Wongcome *et al.*, 2007
Cuphea carthagenesis	Aerial parts	Hydroalcoholic; butanolic fraction		Rat aorta	NO/cGMP	Schuldt *et al.*, 2000
Glycine max			Genistein; daidzein	Rat aorta; rat pulmonary artery	NO	Mishra *et al.*, 2000
	Leaf	Butanol		Rat carotid artery	Prostaglandin antagonism	Ho *et al.*, 2002
Hibiscus sabdariffa Linn.	Calyce	Methanolic		SHR aorta	NO/cGMP; Ca^{2+} channel blocking	Ajay *et al.*, 2007
Melaleuca quinquenervia	Leaf	Methanolic	Glycosides	Rat aorta	NO	Lee *et al.*, 2002
Mentha x villosa	Aerial parts	Essential oil		Rat aorta	NO, PGI_2, Ca^{2+} channel blocking	Guedes *et al.*, 2004
	Aerial parts	Essential oil		Rat aorta	NO	Lahlou *et al.*, 2002a
	Aerial parts	Essential oil	Rotundifolone	Rat aorta	NO, PGI_2, muscarinic receptor activation	Guedes *et al.*, 2002

Contd...

Table 5.2–Contd...

Scientific Name	*Part Used*	*Extract*	*Possible Active Components*	*Animal and Model*	*Mechanism of Action*	*Reference*
Mitragyna ciliata	Stem bark	Methanol		Rat and guinea pig aorta	Ca^{2+} channel blocking	Dongmo *et al.*, 2004
Morinda lucida	Leaf	Aqueous		Rat aorta	NO/cGMP	Ettarh and Emeka, 2004
Ocotea duckei Vattimo	Stem		Reticuline	Rat aorta	NO; muscarinic receptor activation; Ca^{2+} channel blocking; inhibition of intracellular Ca^{2+} release	Dias *et al.*, 2004
Panax ginseng			Ginsenosides	Rat aorta	NO/cGMP; Ca^{2+} activated K^+ channel	Li *et al.*, 2001b
Peucedanum japonicum Thunb.	Root	Methanol; $CHCl_3$ soluble fraction	Pyranocoumarin	Rat aorta	NO/cGMP; Ca^{2+} channel blocking	Lee *et al.*, 2002
Uncarie ramulus et Uncus	Hook	Methanolic	Geissoschizine methyl ether	Rat aorta	NO; Ca^{2+} channel blocking	Yuzurihara *et al.*, 2002
Viguiera robusta	Root		Kaurenoic acid	Rat carotid artery		Tirapelli *et al.*, 2002
	Root		Kaurenoic acid	Rat aorta	NO/cGMP; K^+ channel activation	Tirapelli *et al.*, 2004

Table 5.3: Plant Extracts and Isolated Compounds that Show Vasodilatory Activity in Animal Models through Endothelium-Independent Mechanisms

Scientific Name	*Part Used*	*Extract*	*Possible Active Components*	*Animal and Model*	*Mechanism of Action*	*Reference*
Allium sativum	Raw and frozen cloves	Methanol		Rat aorta; rat mesenteric artery	Ca^{2+} channel blocking; inhibition of intracellular Ca^{2+} mobilization	Ganado *et al.*, 2004
Alseis yucatanensis	Bark	Aqueous		Rat aorta	Ca^{2+} channel blocking; inhibition of intracellular Ca^{2+} mobilization; K^+ channel activation	Slish *et al.*, 2004
Bidens pilosa	Leaf	Neutral		Rat aorta	Ca^{2+} channel blocking	Nguelefack *et al.*, 2005
Brillantasia nitens Lindau	Leaf	Aqueous; methylene chloride; methanol; methylene choride/ methanol		Rat aorta	Ca^{2+} channel blocking; ATP-sensitive K^+ channel activation	Dimo *et al.*, 2007
Bupleurum fruticosum L.	Root	chloroformic		Rat aorta	Ryanodine-sensitive Ca^{2+} channel blocking	Testai *et al.*, 2005
Chinese motherwort			Leonurine	Rat aorta	Ca^{2+} channel blocking; inhibition of intracellular Ca^{2+} mobilization	Chen *et al.*, 2001
Chondrodendron platyphyllum A.St. Hil			Curine	Rat mesenteric artery	Ca^{2+} channel blocking; inhibition of intracellular Ca^{2+} mobilization	Dias *et al.*, 2002
			12-O-methylcurine	Rat aorta	Ca^{2+} channel blocking	Guedes *et al.*, 2002b
Dioclea grandiflora			Dioclein	Rat aorta	Ca^{2+} channel blocking; inhibition of intracellular Ca^{2+} mobilization	Trigueiro *et al.*, 2000
			Dioclein	Rat mesenteric artery	K^+ channel activation	Côrtes *et al.*, 2001
			Floranol	Rat aorta		Lemos *et al.*, 2006

Contd...

Table 5.3–Contd...

Scientific Name	*Part Used*	*Extract*	*Possible Active Components*	*Animal and Model*	*Mechanism of Action*	*Reference*
Gentiana kochiana Perr. Et Song.	Root	Methanol		Rat aorta		Uncini Manganelli *et al.*, 2000
	Root	Methanol		Rat aorta	Ryanodine-sensitive Ca^{2+} channel blocking	Baragatti *et al.*, 2002
			Genticaulein; gentiakochianin	Rat aorta		Chericoni *et al.*, 2003
Iostephane heterophylla			Xanthorrhizol	Rat aorta	Ca^{2+} channel blocking	Campos *et al.*, 2000
Jacaranda mimosaefolia D.Don	Leaf	Methanol		Rat aorta	Adrenergic receptor blocking	Nicasio *et al.*, 2005
Marrubium vulgare	Aerial parts	Aqueous		Rat aorta		El Bradai *et al.*, 2001
			Marrubenol	Rat aorta		El Bradai *et al.*, 2003a
			Marrubenol	Rat aorta	Ca^{2+} channel blocking	El Bradai *et al.*, 2003b
Michelia figo Spreng.	Leaf	Methanol; Fraction S4		Rat aorta	Ryanodine-sensitive Ca^{2+} channel blocking	Chericoni *et al.*, 2004
Peganum harmala L.	Seed	Methanol		Rat aorta	cAMP phosphodiesterase inhibition	Berrougui *et al.*, 2002
			Harmine	Rat aorta	Ca^{2+} channel blocking; phosphodiesterase inhibition	Berrougui *et al.*, 2006
			Harmaline	Rat aorta	Ca^{2+} channel blocking; phosphodiesterase inhibition; NO; PGI_2	Berrougui *et al.*, 2006
Piper methysticum Forst.			Kavain	Rat aorta	Ca^{2+} channel blocking	Martin *et al.*, 2002
Piper truncatum Vell.	Leaf; stem	Hexane		Rat aorta		Raimundo *et al.*, 2004

Contd...

Table 5.3–Contd...

Scientific Name	*Part Used*	*Extract*	*Possible Active Components*	*Animal and Model*	*Mechanism of Action*	*Reference*
Platycapnos spicata Bernh.			(+)-natenine	Rat aorta	Ca^{2+} channel blocking	Orallo *et al.*, 2001
Salvia miltiorrhiza	Whole plant	Aqueous	Salvianolic acid B	Rat coronay artery	Ca^{2+} channel blocking	Lam *et al.*, 2006
	Whole plant	Aqueous	danshensu	Rat coronay artery	Ca^{2+} channel blocking	Lam *et al.*, 2007
	Whole plant	Ethanol	Cryptotanshinone	Rat coronay artery	Ca^{2+} channel blocking	Lam *et al.*, 2008
			3-(3, 4-dihydroxyphenyl)-2-hydroxypropanoate	Rat mesenteric artery	Ca^{2+} channel blocking; inhibition of intracellular Ca^{2+} mobilization; K^+ channel activation	Wang *et al.*, 2008
Stevia reubadiana Bertoni			Stevioside	SHR aorta	Ca^{2+} channel blocking	Lee *et al.*, 2001
			Stevioside	Rat aorta	Ca^{2+} channel blocking; NO/cGMP	Bornia *et al.*, 2008
			Isosteviol	Rat aorta	K^+ channel activation	Wong *et al.*, 2004

cyclooxigenase inhibitor. Receptor involvement can be evaluated using antagonists, such as atropine (muscarinic-receptor antagonist), propranolol (β-adrenoceptor antagonist) and tripolidine (hitamine H_1 receptor antagonist).

There are several traditional medicinal herbs that are typically used to treat arterial hypertension or to remove blood clots and produce vascular relaxation (Kwan, 1995); many of these act via an endothelium-dependent mechanism mediated by NO (Achike and Kwan, 2003). The characteristics and application of predominant traditional herbs that have been so used are summarized below.

Leaves of *Apocynum venetum*, known as Luobuma in China, are traditionally used to treat hypertension. In addition to its known diuretic effect, this plant has been shown to relax aortas and superior mesenteric arteries with intact endothelium from rats. In the aorta, the relaxation evoked by the leaf extract (AVLE) was totally reversed by pre-incubation with L-NAME, indicating that the effect was mediated by the release of NO. In the mesenteric artery, relaxation was mediated by the release of NO and EDHF, as commonly occurs in small arteries (Vanhoutte, 2004). The vasodilatory activity induced by AVLE was associated with the activation of K^+ channels, but not with the activation of muscarinic or β-adrenergic receptors (Kwan *et al.*, 2005). When administrated *in vivo*, AVLE significantly decreased systolic blood pressure in animal models of hypertension, such as spontaneously hypertensive rats (SHR), renal hypertensive rats and NaCl-induced hypertensive rats, supporting its traditional use as antihypertensive (Kim *et al.*, 2000).

Interestingly, similar effects have been observed with *Eucommia ulmoides* Oliv. (known in China as Du-Zhong) and *Eleutherococcus senticosus* (Siberian ginseng), widely used for the treatment of hypertension and improvement of well-being, respectively. Both herbs also elicit NO-mediated vasorelaxation, with the involvement of EDHF in the mesenteric artery. Aqueous extracts from the leaf and bark of *Eucommia* produced a concentration-dependent relaxation in isolated rat aorta and dog carotid artery, but the methanol extract of the leaf had no effect. As observed with AVLE, the relaxant effect was not mediated by mucarinic receptors and may involve the activation of K^+ channels (Kwan *et al.*, 2004a). *E. ulmoides* bark extract was also found to relax rat mesenteric artery (Kwan *et al.*, 2004b). Recently, Lang *et al.* (2005) reported that crude extract from *E. ulmoides* is non-toxic and effective in reducing systolic blood pressure in SHR. Many chemical constituents have been identified and isolated from aqueous *E. ulmoides* extracts, including glycosides and polyphenols, which are compouds with known vascular effects (Ajay *et al.*, 2003; Deyama *et al.*, 2001).

The aqueous root extract from *Eleutherococcus senticosus* showed a vasorelaxant effect on dog carotid artery, rat aorta and rat mesenteric artery. K^+ channels and muscarinic receptors may be involved in this response (Kwan *et al.*, 2004c). Siberian ginseng root contains a large quantity of lignans (Deyama *et al.*, 2001), a class of plant polyphenols reported to induce endothelium-dependent vasorelaxation (Achike and Kwan, 2003). Kwan (2004c) reports, however, that the active component in Siberian ginseng extract seems not to be of lignan origin.

Ligustici wallichii and *Fritillaria ussuriensis* maxim., which have been used to treat hypertension in traditional Chinese medicine, have been shown to dilate rat aortas with intact endothelium (Rhyu *et al.*, 2004; Kang *et al.*, 2002). The relaxant effect of *L. wallichii* chloroform extracts was abolished by pretreatment with NO synthase inhibitors, but was not altered by a muscarinic receptor antagonist and a cyclooxygenase inhibitor. The alkaloid tetramethylpyrazine, isolated from the extract, could be responsible for the vasodilatory activity; however, it induced an intense endothelium-independent vasodilation, and thus might not participate in the relaxation induced by *L. wallichi* (Rhyu *et al.*, 2004). The ethylacetate and butanol extracts of *F. ussuriensis* bulbs were shown to attenuate the angiotensin

I-induced contraction of endothelium-intact rat aorta and to significantly inhibit angiotensin I-converting enzime (ACE) activities. Hexanic, butanolic and aqueous extracts increased NO and cGMP productions in intact aorta. Moreover, intravenous injection of aqueous extract decreased mean arterial pressure of anesthetized rats in a dose-dependent manner (Kang *et al.*, 2002). Various alkaloids such as imperialine are present in *F. ussuriensis* bulb extract (Song-Lin *et al.*, 2000), but the constituents responsible for the hypotensive effect have not yet been identified.

Crataegus oxyacantha (hawthorn) and *Crataegus monogyna* Jacq. extracts are used to treat heart failure, angina pectoris and arterial hypertension. The extract, a mixture of flavonoids and procyanidins, has been shown to promote endothelium-dependent vasorelaxation. The flavonoids in *Crataegus* extract did not elicit endothelium-dependent vasodilation; rather, the procyanidins are likely responsible for the vasorelaxation, since they induce NO and cGMP production and may activate K^+ channels (Kim *et al.*, 2000).

Other extracts from medicinal plants used in traditional Oriental medicine to treat cardiovascular diseases also showed an endothelium-dependent vasorelaxant activity via the NO pathway. These include *Diospyros kaki* (leaf), *Polygonun aviculare* (whole plant), *Magnolia liliflora* (flower), *Sorbus commixta* (stem bark) and *Selaginella tamariscina* (whole plant) (Yin *et al.*, 2005). The methanolic extract of *Sorbus commixta* cortex induced NO-dependent relaxation of rat aorta (Kang *et al.*, 2005). Purifications of the ethyl acetate-soluble extract of *Selaginella tamariscina* resulted on the identification of the active bioflavonoid amentoflavone, which showed an NO/cGMP-dependent relaxation of the aorta with possible involvement of K^+ and Ca^{2+} channels (Kang *et al.*, 2004).

The heartwood of *Caesalpinia sappan* L. is a traditional Chinese medicine that has been reported to have several pharmacological activities. Xie *et al.* (2000) showed that its methanolic extract relaxes rat aorta and that two purified compounds, brazilin and hematoxylin, also had similar effects, suggesting that they may be responsible for the vascular effect of *C. sappan*. Similarly, Hu *et al.* (2003) showed that brazilin induces an NO-dependent vasodilation on aortas and an increase in NO formation in human umbilical vein endothelial cells.

Rheum undulatum (rhubarb) originated in Asia and has been used for centuries in traditional Chinese medicine. The aqueous extract of *R. undulatum* rhizomes was found to induce vasorelaxant activity via endothelium-dependent NO/GMPc signaling (Moon *et al.*, 2006). Similar results were obtained with the 100 per cent ethanol extract of *Morus bombycis* Koidzumi, widely used in traditional medicine in Asia (Oh *et al.*, 2007).

Aconiti tuber, *Aconitum japonicum* roots, has been used for centuries in the herbal medicines of Japan and China. Pharmacological evaluation of mesaconitine, an alkaloid isolated from Aconiti tuber, showed that it produces endothelium-dependent relaxation of rat aorta, due to the activation of endothelial NO production through the increase of intracellular concentration of Ca^{2+} (Mitamura *et al.*, 2002).

The medicinal use of *Ginkgo biloba* can be traced to the origins of traditional Chinese medicine. Its seeds and leaves were used for the treatment of many diseases, including those of the heart and lung. At present, *Ginkgo biloba* leaf extract (GBE), is widely used in Europe (designated Egb 761) for the treatment of peripheral vascular disease and cerebrovascular insufficiency (Mahady, 2002). GBE has been shown to produce relaxation of rat aorta due to the activation of NO synthesis and release by increasing the intracellular calcium level in vascular endothelial cells (Kubota *et al.*, 2001). In addition, GBE was found to be a potent stimulator of NO synthase activity in endothelial cells via Ca^{2+}-sensitive K^+ channels activation (Li *et al.*, 2001a). GBE is composed mainly of flavonoids such as quercetin and rutin, and terpenoids such as bilobalide and ginkgolides A, B and C. Recently, through high performance liquid chromatography (HPLC) analysis, GBE quality has been standardized to contain 22-27 per cent w/w flavonoid glycosides and 6 per cent w/w terpenoids (Kressmann *et al.*, 2002). A comparative study of the vasodilatory activity of GBE constituents demonstrated that all of them had a concentration-dependent vasorelaxant effect. The actions of bilobalide and ginkgolides A, B and C were weaker than GBE (Nishida and Satoh, 2004). Quecertin has been reported to produce vasodilation comparable to GBE in a NO-mediated manner, indicating its importance in the extract activity (Kubota *et al.*, 2001). However, the vascular effects of bilobalide seem to involve the activation of NO release and the inhibition of Ca^{2+} influx through Ca^{2+} channels (Nishida and Satoh, 2003). The antihypertensive effect of GBE has been detected in deoxycorticosterone acetate-salt (DOCA) hypertensive rats (Umegaki *et al.*, 2000) and SHR (Kubota *et al.*, 2006), but not in normotensive rats.

A study of common edible tropical plant extracts from Malasia showed that 6 of the 9 extracts tested produced vasodilation on aortic rings and isolated mesenteric artery preparations. *Ipomoea batatas, Piper betle, Anacardium occidentale, Gynandropsis gynandra, Carica papaya* and *Mentha arvensis* leaf extracts exhibited vasodilatory activity greater than 50 per cent on aortas, mediated by NO formation. Only *Piper betle* and *Cymbopogon citratus* showed comparable vasorelaxation on isolated perfused mesenteric artery preparations as a result of NO, prostanoids and EDHF release (Runnie *et al.*, 2004).

Angelica keiskei Koidzumi is used as a diuretic and laxative in Japan, and is also thought to have preventive effects on coronary disease and arterial hypertension. An ethyl acetate (EtOAc)-soluble fraction from a 50 per cent ethyl alcohol (EtOH) extract of *A. keiskei* roots produced relaxation of rat aorta, as did five active substances isolated from this fraction. Xanthoangelol, 4-hydroxyderricin and xanthoangelols E and F promoted vasodilation in an endothelium-dependent manner, with involvement of NO and EDHF. In contrast, the relaxant effect of xanthoangelol B was endothelium-independent although it was the more potent (Matsuura *et al.*, 2001).

Arbutus unedo L. is one of the most commonly used plants in Morocco to treat hypertension. The antihypertensive effects of the root aqueous extract have been demonstrated in many studies, including vascular effects on SHR and endothelium-dependent vasorelaxation on rat aorta (Ziyyat *et al.*, 2002). Recently, Legssyer *et al.* (2004) showed that the aqueous leaf extract of the plant also produces vasodilation comparable, in potency and efficacy, to that of the root extract. This effect is likely to be due to polyphenol compounds such as tannins and catechin gallate.

Similar results were observed with *Urtica dioica* L., also used in the traditional medicine of Morocco as an antihypertensive. Acute diuretic and hypotensive effects of the aqueous extract of aerial parts of *U. dioica* have been reported (Tahri *et al.*, 2000). The crude aqueous and methanolic extracts of the plant roots, as well as purified fractions, elicited a vasodilatory action in rat aorta mediated by the release of NO and opening of K^+ channels. The purified fraction F1W also produced a transient hypotensive effect on the blood pressure of anaesthetized rats, and seems to be the fraction containing active compounds in *U. dioica* roots (Testai *et al.*, 2002).

Raphanus sativus (radish) is traditionally used in the treatment of several diseases, including hypertension. Pharmacological studies have shown that radish has many biological effects, such as antioxidant activity (Salah-Abbès *et al.*, 2008). Its vasodilatory and hypotensive activities had been shown by Ghayur and Gilani (2006). Both effects were mediated through the activation of muscarinic receptors.

Crotalaria sessiliflora L., used in Asian folk medicine as a diuretic and cardiotonic, also produced a NO/cGMP-dependent relaxation of rat aorta. Intravenous injection induced an increase in plasma NO production, accompanied by a decrease in blood pressure. As with *R. sativus*, these effects were probably due to the activation of muscarinic receptors (Koh *et al.*, 2007).

Tribulus terrestris L. is widely distributed in Africa, western Asia, China, Japan, Korea and Europe, where it has been used to treat hypertension and coronary heart disease. Aqueous and methanolic *T. terrestris* extract produced vasodilation of the mesenteric vascular bed, which involved both NO production and membrane hyperpolarization. In addition, intravenous administration of the crude aqueous and methanolic extract produced dose-dependent reduction in blood pressure of SHR (Phillips *et al.*, 2006). Similar results were observed with the aqueous extract of *T. terrestris* fruits after chronic administration in 2-kidney 1-clip hypertensive rats (Sharifi *et al.*, 2003).

In Africa, aqueous extract from *Mitragyna inermis* (Wild) O. Kuntze is traditionally used for the treatment of many diseases, particularly hepatic illness, malaria and hypertension. This extract has been demonstrated to increase coronary flow in isolated hearts and produce relaxation in porcine coronary arteries in an endothelium-dependent manner, due to the release of NO and EDHF. Interestingly, in rat tail arteries, the relaxation induced by the extract is not dependent on the presence of endothelium (Ouédraogo *et al.*, 2004).

Musanga cecropioides R. Brown, known as the umbrella tree in Africa, is used to treat bronchopulmonary infections, hypertension and epileptic seizures. The aqueous leaf extract has been reported to produce endothelium-dependent vasodilation (Kamanyi *et al.*, 1991). Further investigations demonstrated that the vasorelaxant effect is due to the release of NO and that the extract also inhibits ACE activity. The aqueous leaf extract produced a dose-dependent fall in blood pressure in anaesthetized normotensive and hypertensive rats. The presence of procyanidins, flavonoids and saponins in the *M. cecropioides* extract may be responsible for these effects (Dongmo *et al.*, 2002).

Persea americana (avocado) is widely used in traditional African medicine; the extract of it leaves is taken as a diuretic and antihypertensive, and other products of the plant have been used for the treatment of many diseases. Some of these traditional uses have been pharmacologically studied. The aqueous leaf extract reduced the spontaneous myogenic contractions of portal veins and produced an NO-dependent relaxation of pre-contracted rat aorta (Ojewole *et al.*, 2007). However, a previous study showed that the vascular effect of *P. americana* on rat aorta was partially dependent on endothelium, with the involvement of NO, PGI_2 and Ca^{2+} channels (Owolabi *et al.*, 2005). Its hypotensive effect was demonstrated in both normotensive and hypertensive rats, indicating that the extract is effective in reducing blood pressure (Ojewole *et al.*, 2007).

Another species popularly used in Africa is *Sclerocarya birrea*, called "marula" or "maroela". The stem bark, roots and leaves of *S. birrea* are traditionally used for the treatment of many conditions, including malaria, dysentery, headaches and circulatory disorders. Pharmacological study of *S. birrea* showed that it produces NO-dependent relaxation of rat aorta and also induces, after bolus intravenous administration, reduction of blood pressure in anesthetized normotensive and hypertensive Dahl-sensitive rats (Ojewole, 2006).

Psittacanthus calyculatus and *Lepechinia caulescens* are used in Mexican traditional medicine for the treatment of hypertension. *P. calyculatus* ethanolic leaf extract has been reported to induce a small tension development in rat aorta at low concentrations, and relaxation at higher concentrations. The predominant effect of relaxation seems to be mediated by the release of NO, without the participation of PGI_2 (Rodríguez-Cruz *et al.*, 2003). The methanolic extract of *L. caulescens* has been shown to produce a significant NO/cGMP-dependent vasodilation. Ursolic acid had the same activity and seems to be the active component of the methanolic extract (Aguirre-Crespo *et al.*, 2006).

Evidence of the protective cardiovascular effects of the moderate consumption of red wine, which is rich in polyphenols, have stimulated the pharmacological study of species used for wine production. An alcohol-free grape-skin extract obtained from *Vitis labrusca*, largely used in Brazilian red wine production, has been shown to induce a significant reduction of blood pressure and an endothelium-dependent relaxation in rat mesenteric vascular beds (Soares de Moura *et al.*, 2002). This vasodilatory activity is mediated by the release of NO and EDHF (Madeira *et al.*, 2005). In addition, Seya *et al.* (2003) have shown that vitisin C, an oligostilbene from *Vitis* plants, produces vasorelaxation by enhancing NO release. The health benefits of plant-based polyphenols have also been studied. The extract of oil palm frond (*Elaeis guineensis*) has shown an important vasodilatory effect in rat aorta and isolated perfused mesenteric vascular bed, which was totally reversed in the presence of an NO synthase inhibitor (Abeywardena *et al.*, 2002).

Ouratea semiserrata was found to be the most potent among several Brazilian plants for *in vitro* inhibition of ACE, although it is not popularly used for the treatment of cardiovascular diseases. In addition, the stem hydroethanolic extract and its ethyl acetate fraction demonstrated an endothelium-dependent vasorelaxing activity in rat aorta, more potent with the fraction. A muscarinic antagonist and a cyclooxygenase inhibitor did not alter this response. The high content of proanthocyanidins in the fraction suggests that compounds of this class may play a role in vascular activity (Côrtes *et al.*, 2002).

Harconia speciosa Gomes, commonly known as mangaba, is used to treat many diseases in Brazil, including hypertension and diabetes. The vasodilatory action of the ethanolic extract of *H. speciosa* leaves was demonstrated in mesenteric artery rings with endothelium. This effect was mediated by the release of NO and EDHF and the activation of K^+ channels (Ferreira *et al.*, 2007a). Similar effects were observed in rat aortic rings, by a mechanism dependent on the activation of phosphatidyl-inositol 3-kinase (Ferreira *et al.*, 2007b).

Echinodorus grandiflorus is another plant widely distributed in Brazil and used in folk medicine. The crude aqueous extract of *E. grandiflorus* was shown to relax rabbit aorta in an NO-dependent manner, without the participation of prostaglandins or the activation of K^+ channels. This effect was dependent on the activation of platelet-activating factor (PAF) receptor (TibiriCá *et al.*, 2007). Rocha *et al.* (2007) investigated the vascular effects of the hydro-alcoholic extract obtained from stones of *Euterpe oleracea* Mart., a plant known as aCaí that is commonly consumed in Brazil. The study demonstrated that the extract's effect depends on the NO/cGMP pathway and EDHF release. The vasodilation induced by *E. oleracea* may be due to polyphenols.

We have reported for the first time that *Cecropia lyratiloba* produces vasodilation of precontracted rat aorta (Almeida *et al.*, 2006). Many species of *Cecropia* genus are traditionally used for the treatment of hypertension in Brazil. The methanolic extract and flavonoid fraction of *C. lyratiloba* produced an endothelium-dependent relaxation of rat aorta through stimulation of NO release. Muscarinic receptors and PGI_2 were not involved in this response. The flavonoids isolated from the flavonoid fraction, isoorientin and the mixture of orientin and isovitexin, do not seem to be responsible for its vasorelaxant activity (Almeida *et al.*, 2006).

Endothelium-dependent and Independent Vasodilation

The cytoplasmatic concentration of free Ca^{2+} is a major determinant of the contractile state of smooth muscle. In general, increases in Ca^{2+} concentration produce contractions, whereas decreases in Ca^{2+} relax the smooth muscle cell (Bryan *et al.*, 2005). The increase in cytosolic free Ca^{2+} occurs by raising the influx of the ion through voltage–and receptor-operated Ca^{2+} channels and releasing intracellular stored Ca^{2+} in the sarcoplasmatic reticulum (SR). In most vascular smooth muscle cells, L-type channels are the most numerous voltage-operated calcium channels and probably the most important route of the activator calcium influx. L-type Ca^{2+} channels are highly sensitive to dihydropyridines and other organic and inorganic calcium antagonists, which cause a decrease in cytosolic Ca^{2+} concentration, leading to relaxation of vascular smooth muscle. The accumulation of Ca^{2+} in the intracellular stores of the SR is accomplished by a Ca^{2+}-ATPase that is specifically inhibited by thapsigargin and cyclopiazonic acid. Two types of Ca^{2+} channels are thought to be involved in Ca^{2+} release from the SR: channels sensitive to inositol triphosphate (IP_3), and channels sensitive to the plant alkaloids ryanodine (from *Ryania speciosa*) and caffeine (from *Coffea arabica*) (Bolton *et al.*, 1999; Orallo, 1996).

Herbs can activate endothelium release of vasodilator agents such as NO, PGI_2 and EDHF, and can also act directly on the smooth muscle to cause vasodilation. Plant extracts may produce vasodilation by endothelium-dependent and–independent mechanisms. In this case, most of the reviewed plants exhibit mechanisms that involve the release of NO and blocking of Ca^{2+} channels, as described below (Table 5.2).

Peucedanum japonicum Thunb. is widely distributed in Korea, Japan and China, where the roots of the plant are used in the treatment of cold, cough and headache. Several coumarins have been isolated from the roots of this plant. Lee *et al.* (2002) reported that the trichloromethane ($CHCl_3$)-soluble fraction from the methanol extract of *P. japonicum* relaxed rat aorta. A pyranocoumarin was isolated and identified as one of the bioactive compounds of the fraction. This compound acts through NO release and L-type Ca^{2+} channel blockade.

Uncariae Ramulus et Uncus is traditionally used in China to relieve symptoms associated with hypertension. Several alkaloids isolated from the plant, such as rhynchophylline, corynoxeine and hirsutine, have been shown to relax vascular smooth muscle by blocking Ca^{2+} channels. The indole alkaloid geissoschizine methyl ether isolated from the hook of the plant also showed vasorelaxant activity, which was more potent than that of the other alkaloids. However, its effect was mediated both by NO and by Ca^{2+} channel blocking (Yuzurihara *et al.*, 2002).

Hibiscus sabdariffa Linn. has traditionally been used to treat hypertension. Its hypotensive effect has been confirmed after chronic administration in a 2-kidney 1-clip rat model of hypertension (Odigie *et al.*, 2003). Recently, Ajay *et al.* (2007) demonstrated that the crude methanolic extract of *H. sabdariffa* calyces induced relaxation of aorta from SHR, probably mediated through both the release of NO and the inhibition of Ca^{2+} influx.

Melaleuca quinquenervia leaves are used as a sedative and pain-reliever in Taiwan. Chemical studies revealed the presence of triterpenoids, flavones, polyphenols and glycosides in the leaves of the plant. Interestingly, two new glycosides, 4-benzoyl-2-C-b-glucopyranosyl-3-5-dihydroxy-6-methylphenyl b-D-glucopyranoside and roseoside, isolated from the methanolic extract of *M. quinquenervia* leaves exhibited a partially endothelium-dependent relaxation of rat aorta, with the involvement of NO. Conversely, four other known glycosides isolated from the extract induced endothelium-independent vasodilation (Lee *et al.*, 2002).

The stem bark of *Mitragyna ciliata* is used in African traditional medicine to treat fever, hypertension and bronchopulmonary diseases. *M. ciliata* stem bark extract has vasodilating properties, which are greater in aorta with intact endothelium than in aorta without endothelium. The magnitude of the effect was five times greater in KCl-contracted guinea pig aorta than in noradrenaline-contracted aorta, suggesting blockade of voltage-operated Ca^{2+} channels. Phytochemical studies indicate that the vasodilating effect of *M. ciliata* might be due to the presence of alkaloids and flavonoids (Dongmo *et al.*, 2004).

Morinda lucida Benth. is widely used in the treatment of malaria and diabetes in Africa and has also been reported to have a hypotensive effect in animal experiments. The aqueous extract of *M. lucinda* leaves was found to relax rat aorta via endothelium-dependent and–independent mechanisms. The endothelium-dependent component involves the NO/cGMP pathway (Ettarh and Emeka, 2004).

The aqueous fraction of the ethanolic extract of *Albizia inopinata* G. P. Lewis leaves has been reported to relax rat aorta precontracted with phenylephrine or KCl, in a partially endothelium-dependent manner. The fraction also produced a significant dose-dependent hypotension in conscious rats that was attenuated after NO synthase blockade with L-NAME (Pires et al, 2000). A second study suggested that the remaining vasodilatory effect was due to the inhibition of Ca^{2+} influx and/or inhibition of intracellular Ca^{2+} mobilization (Maciel *et al.*, 2004).

Alpinia officinarum and *Coscinium fenestratum* (Gaertn.) Colebr. are widely used as herbal medicines in Asia. Galangin, present in high concentrations in *A. officinarum,* was found to produce vasodilation of rat aorta through a dual mechanism. At low concentrations the effect of the flavonoid was partially dependent on the release of NO, and at high concentrations it was due to inhibition of Ca^{2+} entry and release from intracellular stores (Morello *et al.*, 2006). *C. fenestratum* also showed an endothelium-dependent and–independent vasodilatory effect in rat aorta, with the involvement of NO (Wongcome *et al.*, 2007). This activity could support the use of the hot-water extract of *C. fenestratum* stems as an antihipetensive in Thailand.

Kaurenoic acid, isolated from *Viguiera robusta*, has been shown to exert antispasmodic and relaxant actions on smooth muscle. Moreover, it was shown to relax both rat carotid artery (Tirapelli *et al.*, 2002) and aorta pre-contracted with either phenylephrine or KCl. This effect was mediated by the release of NO, opening of K^+ channels and inhibition of extracellular Ca^{2+} influx (Tirapelli *et al.*, 2004). Reticuline, isolated from the stem of *Ocotea duckei* Vattimo, also induced relaxation of rat aorta through multiple mechanisms. Its vasodilatory activity involves the activation of muscarinic receptors and consequent activation of NO production, blockade of voltage-operated Ca^{2+} channels and, possibly, inhibition of Ca^{2+} release from noradrenaline-sensitive intracellular stores. Moreover, it was shown to produce an intense hypotension in rats after intravenous injection, which was attenuated after NO synthase and muscarinic receptor blockade (Dias *et al.*, 2004).

Panax ginseng is an important Asian traditional medicine with diverse cardiovascular actions. Many substances have been isolated from *P. ginseng* and ginsenosides are considered to be the major biologically active component of the specie (Persson *et al.*, 2006). Ginsenosides induced vascular relaxation through both release of NO and activation of Ca^{2+}-activated K^+ channels (Li *et al.*, 2001b). *Alpinia henryi* K. Schum. is also used in Chinese traditional medicine. Among its active components are cardamonin and alpinetin, which are widely distributed in many medicinal plants. Wang and co-workers (2001) have shown that their vascular relaxant effect in rat mesenteric artery is partially dependent on endothelium and is mediated by multiple mechanisms, including the NO/cGMP pathway and inhibition of extracellular Ca^{2+} influx and intracellular Ca^{2+} release. Cardamonin and alpinetin may also inhibit the protein kinase C-dependent contractile mechanism.

Dietary soy products have been demonstrated to be useful in the prevention of cardiovascular diseases. Genistein and daidzein, isoflavones present in soybean (*Glycine max*), have been shown to induce partially NO-dependent vasorelaxation in rat aorta and pulmonary arteries (Mishra *et al.*, 2000). Butanol extract from soy leaves (*Glycine max*) also relaxed rat carotid arteries, but in an endothelium-independent manner. The extract was much more effective in relaxing vessels pre-contracted by a tromboxane A_2 agonist (U46619) and prostaglandin F_{2a} than phenylephrine, suggesting a prostaglandin antagonist action. Six kaempferol glycosides isolated from the leaf extracts and genistin were devoid of vasorelaxant activity, indicating that they are not responsible for the extract-induced vasodilation (Ho *et al.*, 2002).

Cuphea carthagenensis is widely distributed in Brazil and South America, where it is used in folk medicine to treat hypertension. Its hypotensive effect may be due to its vasodilatory activity (Schuldt *et al.*, 2000). The butanolic fraction of crude hydroalcoholic extract of *C. carthagenensis* induced relaxation of rat aorta through both endothelium-dependent and–independent mechanisms, with involvement of the NO/cGMP pathway.

Mentha x villosa Hudson is used in folk medicine in Brazil and is popularly known as "hortelã da folha miúda". Its cardiovascular effects have been extensively studied. The hypotensive activity of *Mentha x villosa* essential oil has been shown in normotensive (Lahlou *et al.*, 2001; 2002a) and DOCA-salt-hypertensive rats (Lahlou *et al.*, 2002b), and it may be due to a direct vascular effect. Guedes *et al.* (2004) showed that *Mentha x villosa* induced a vasorelaxant effect that was mediated by NO, PGI_2 and possibly by Ca^{2+} channel blockade. In the same way, rotundifolone, the major constituent of *Mentha x villosa* essential oil, induced hypotension in normotensive rats and relaxation of rat aorta, probably due to muscarinic receptor stimulation (Guedes *et al.*, 2002a).

Endothelium-independent Vasodilation

Several plant extracts produce vasodilation in an endothelium-independent manner through the mechanism of Ca^{2+} channel blocking. Interestingly, many isolated constituents that have already been tested exhibited this mechanism. Most of these extracts also inhibit the mobilization of intracellular Ca^{2+}.

Bidens pilosa Linn. is widely used in African traditional medicine to treat many diseases, including anemia and cardiovascular disturbances. Phytochemical studies of the plant revealed the presence of alkaloids, saponins, flavonoids, polyacetylenes, triterpenes, linoleic acid and linolic acid. The antihypertensive activity of the methanol extract of *B. pilosa* leaf has been demonstrated in rats fed a high-fructose diet (Dimo *et al.*, 2002). Similarly, the leaf neutral extract (a stage of bioguided fractionation) exhibited antihypertensive effects in normotensive rats and SHR (Dimo *et al.*, 2003). This extract also showed vasodilatory activity, which seemed to act by blocking Ca^{2+} channels (Nguelefack *et al.*, 2005). *Brillantaisia nitens* Lindau is another species widely used in African traditional medicine. The methylene chloride/methanol extract of *B. nitens* was shown to produce relaxation of rat aorta, which was mediated by the activation of ATP-sensitive K^+ channels and the inhibition of Ca^{2+} influx (Dimo *et al.*, 2007)

In Moroccan traditional medicine, *Marrubium vulgare* is used in association with *Foeniculum vulgare* to treat hypertension. Water extracts of both plants, administered orally, were shown to lower the systolic blood pressure of SHR but not of normotensive rats. *F. vulgare* and *M. vulgare* also produced vasodilation of rat aorta, with *M. vulgare* being more potent (El Bardai *et al.*, 2001). A diterpenoid characterized as marrubenol was isolated from the water extract of aerial parts of *M. vulgare* and also demonstrated a vasorelaxant activity (El Bardai *et al.*, 2003a). Marrubenol produced a more potent vasodilation in rat aorta pre-contracted with KCl than with noradrenaline. In addition, it decreased the cytosolic Ca^{2+} concentration in fura-2-loaded aorta in a concentration-dependent manner, and inhibited Ba^{2+} inward current in aortic smooth muscle cells (A7r5) in a voltage-dependent manner. Thus, marrubenol inhibits smooth muscle contraction by blocking L-type Ca^{2+} channels (El Bardai *et al.*, 2003b). El Bardai *et al.* (2004) have also demonstrated that interaction with the phenylalkylamine binding site seems to account for the inhibition of L-type Ca^{2+} channels by marrubenol.

Xanthorrhizol is a bisabolene isolated from *Iostephane heterophylla*, which is found in Mexico and is used in the treatment of rheumatism, diabetes, gastrointestinal complaints and liver ailments. Xanthorrhizol has been shown to inhibit contractions induced by different agonists in rat uterus, probably due to the blockade of voltage-operated Ca^{2+} channels (Ponce *et al.*, 1999). In a similar manner, the compound produced relaxation of pre-contracted rat aorta, with a greater effect on KCl–and $CaCl_2$-induced contractions. The vasorelaxant effect of xanthorrhizol was mediated by blocking of both voltage–and receptor-operated Ca^{2+} channels (Campos *et al.*, 2000).

(+)-Nantenine is an alkaloid found in several plant species, including *Platycapnos spicata* Bernh. In rat aorta, (+)-nantenine showed an endothelium-independent vasorelaxant effect and inhibited the uptake of $^{45}Ca^{2+}$ induced by noradrenaline and extracellular high K^+. These effects were mediated, in part, by blocking voltage–and receptor-operated Ca^{2+} channels (Orallo *et al.*, 2001). In anaesthetized normotensive rats, intravenous administration of (+)-nantenine produced reduction of arterial pressure, which seemed to be due, in part, to a combined α_1-adrenergic and 5-HT receptor blockade (Orallo, 2004)

The roots of *Piper methysticum* Forst. (kava) are widely used as anxiolytic, antiarthritic and antiasthmatic. The most prevalent compound among the active ingredients in the root is kavain, followed by demethoxyyangonin, methysticin and dihydromethysticin. Kavain has been reported to inhibit airway smooth muscle contraction (Martin *et al.*, 2000). Moreover, it induced relaxation of rat aorta through the inhibition of L-type Ca^{2+} channels, since its vasorelaxant effect was more effective in aorta contracted with a selective L-type channel activator and inhibited by nifedipine (Martin *et al.*, 2002). Our laboratory has demonstrated that *Piper truncatum* Vell. possesses similar smooth muscle relaxant activity. Both hexanic extracts of leaves and stems from *P. truncatum* produced comparable inhibition of aorta contraction in an endothelium-independent manner, and relaxation of pre-contracted trachea. The similarity in the results obtained with the two extracts indicates that the compounds responsible for these effects may be present in both leaf and stem extracts. However, the active constituents and the mechanisms of action of the extracts have not yet been identified (Raimundo *et al.*, 2004).

The dried root of *Salvia miltiorrhiza* (danshen) is an herbal medicine used in China for the treatment of cardiovascular diseases, such as angina pectoris, myocardial infarction and stroke. *S. miltiorrhiza* can be separated into lipophilic and hydrophilic fractions containing a number of active substances. The aqueous extract of danshen and two aqueous components, salvianolic acid B and danshensu, have shown vasodilatory properties in coronary artery rings, which were mediated by the inhibition of extracellular Ca^{2+} influx (Lam *et al.*, 2006; 2007). Similar results were found with danshen ethanol extract and with a lipophilic component, cryptotanshinone (Lam *et al.*, 2008). Pharmacological studies have examined the bioactive metabolites of danshen. Isopropyl 3-(3, 4-dihydroxyphenyl)-2-hydroxypropanoate, was identified as one of the main bioactive metabolites of danshen when administered orally. This substance has been reported to relax rat mesenteric arteries through the inhibition of Ca^{2+} release from intracellular stores and Ca^{2+} influx through voltage and receptor-operated Ca^{2+} channels and the activation of K^+ channels (Wang *et al.*, 2008).

Stevioside is a sweet glycoside isolated from *Stevia rebaudiana* Bertoni, which is traditionally used as a sugar substitute in Japan and Brazil. It has been shown to lower blood pressure in SHR when administered intravenously (Chan *et al.*, 1998). The intraperitoneal injection of stevioside also had an antihypertensive effect, and stevioside relaxed rat aorta contracted with vasopressin. Furthermore, it was effective in inhibiting Ca^{2+} influx stimulated by vasopressin in A7r5 cells. Thus, the vasorelaxation effect of stevioside was mainly through Ca^{2+} channel inhibition (Lee *et al.*, 2001). Bornia *et al.* (2008) recently showed that the NO/cGMP pathway is also involved in stevioside-induced vascular relaxation. Isosteviol, a derivative of stevioside, was also shown to induce relaxation of vasopressin-induced aortic contraction, with or without endothelium. Meanwhile, isosteviol-induced vasodilation was found to be related to the opening of K^+ channels (ATP-sensitive and small conductance Ca^{2+}-activated) (Wong *et al.*, 2004).

The roots and stems of *Blupeurum fruticosum* L. are used in the Mediterranean region as an antirheumatic remedy. The essential oil of this plant has been demonstrated to have antispasmodic and antiinflammatory activities. The chloroformic crude extract of *B. fruiticosum* roots was recently shown to produce an endothelium-independent vasorelaxant response. This effect was not altered by the treatment with nifedipine, an L-type Ca^{2+} channel blocker, or cyclopiazonic acid, a blocker of Ca^{2+}-ATPase of the SR. However, the extract produced a reduction of the contraction induced by caffeine (an opener of the ryanodine-sensitive Ca^{2+} channels), suggesting that the vasodilatory effect is due to the blockade of ryanodine-sensitive Ca^{2+} channels of the SR (Testai *et al.*, 2005).

Peganum harmala L. is found in the Mediterranean region and has been reported to have hypotensive effects. The methanolic extract from *P. harmala* seeds exhibited a relaxant activity in rat aorta, which was related to the inhibition of cAMP phosphodiesterase (Berrougui *et al.*, 2002). The alkaloids harmine and harmaline showed similar activity, acting through inhibition of voltage-operated Ca^{2+} channels and as inhibitors of phosphodiesterase; however, NO and PGI_2 also mediated the effect of harmaline (Berrougui *et al.*, 2006).

The same mechanism of action seems to be involved in the vasodilatory action of other species, such as *Gentiana kokiana* Perr. et Song. and *Michelia figo* Spreng.. In the traditional medicine of Tuscany, the roots of *G. kokiana* are employed in decoction form as antipyretic, spasmolytic and antihypertensive agents. The dried methanolic extract of the roots has been reported to have an endothelium-independent vasodilatory effect (Uncini Manganelli *et al.*, 2000), which was further described to involve the ryanodine-sensitive Ca^{2+} channels (Baragatti *et al.*, 2002). The xanthones gentiacaulein and gentiakochianin seemed to be the active principles responsible for this vasodilatory activity, while swertiaperennin did not show any vasodilatory effect (Chericoni *et al.*, 2003).

M. figo Spreng., commonly called banana shrub, is used to obtain essences and as an ornamental plant. The plant is also used in Indian folk medicine as an antihypertensive remedy. The methanolic extract and purified fractions of *M. figo* leaves showed a vasorelaxing effect on rat aorta. Investigation of the mechanism of action of the S4 fraction, that having the best vasodilator effect, indicated that it may block the ryanodine-sensitive Ca^{2+} channels (Chericoni *et al.*, 2004).

Allium sativum (garlic) has long been employed in traditional medicine. Many authors have described its effect on vascular smooth muscle, but its mechanism of action remains unclear (Ganado *et al.*, 2004). It has been proposed to have both endothelium–dependent and–independent mechanisms (Fallon *et al.*, 1998). A recent study investigated the effects of raw (RG) and frozen (FG) garlic extracts and fractions on rat aortas and mesenteric arteries. The contractions induced by noradrenaline and KCl were relaxed by all extracts and fractions of garlic. However, as the effect was higher with the fraction RG 20-100 and raw garlic is the more frequently consumed form, the mechanism of action of this fraction was further investigated. The vasorelaxant effect of RG 20-100 was found to be endothelium-independent and mediated by inhibition of the extracellular Ca^{2+} entry and mobilization of intracellular Ca^{2+} (Ganado *et al.*, 2004). The benefits of garlic in lowering blood pressure have been demonstrated in animal models of hypertension, as in the 2-kidney 1-clip rat model (Al-Qattan *et al.*, 2006) and SHR (Harauma and Moriguchi, 2006).

Chinese motherwort, *Leonurus artemisia* and *Leonurus heterophyllus*, has been widely used in China to treat gynecological disorders as well as myocardial ischemia and blood hyperviscosity. Leonurine, a plant alkaloid present in Chinese motherwort, has been reported to have uterotonic and antiplatelet aggregation actions. In addition, Chen and Kwan (2001) showed that the alkaloid produces endothelium-independent vasorelaxation of phenylephrine, KCl and prostaglandin F_{2a} pre-contracted rat aorta, probably acting by inhibiting Ca^{2+} influx and release of intracellular Ca^{2+}.

Chondrodendron platyphyllum A. St. Hil is used in Brazil for the treatment of fever, malaria and as an antispasmodic. Curine, a bisbenzyl isoquinoline alkaloid isolated from the root bark of the plant, has a non-depolarizing neuromuscular blocking action. Curine has also been reported to have a vasodilatory effect on rat mesenteric arteries blocking Ca^{2+} channels and the mobilization of intracellular Ca^{2+} from noradrenaline-sensitive stores (Dias *et al.*, 2002). 12-O-methylcurine, also isolated from *C. platyphyllum*, showed similar activities to curine, which were mediated by blocking Ca^{2+} influx through voltage–and receptor-operated Ca^{2+} channels (Guedes *et al.*, 2002b).

The roots of *Dioclea grandiflora*, known in Brazil as "olho de boi", are used in folk medicine. Phytochemical investigations have reported the presence of flavonoids in this plant and have led to the isolation of dioclein and floranol. Both compounds induced an endothelium-independent vasodilation in rat aorta (Trigueiro *et al.*, 2000; Lemos *et al.*, 2006). The vasorelaxant effect of dioclein involved the inhibition of extracellular Ca^{2+} influx and of intracellular Ca^{2+} release, as well as processes dependent on activation of protein kinase C (Trigueiro *et al.*, 2000). Dioclein showed a similar effect in rat mesenteric arteries, but its relaxant activity seemed to be mediated by the opening of K^+ channels and subsequent membrane hyperpolarization (Côrtes *et al.*, 2001). Studies have also demonstrated the hypotensive effect of dioclein after bolus administration in rats (Côrtes *et al.*, 2001).

Alseis yucatanensis Standley is found in Guatemala, Belize and Mexico. The aqueous extract of *A. yucatanensis* leaves or bark was shown to relax endothelium-denuded rat aorta (Slish *et al.*, 1999) by blocking both Ca^{2+} release from SR and voltage-operated Ca^{2+} channels. A long-term relaxation was observed at low doses, apparently due to the opening of K^+ channels (Slish *et al.*, 2004).

The leaves, flowers and seeds of *Jacaranda mimosaefolia* D. Don are used in Mexico to treat high blood pressure and amoebic infections. The hydroalcoholic extract from *J. mimosaefolia* leaves induced relaxation of noradrenaline pre-contracted aorta and also produced a rightward displacement of the concentration-response curve to noradrenaline, suggesting the blockade of α-adrenoceptors. The extract also showed a hypotensive effect in anesthetized rats (Nicasio *et al.*, 2005).

Conclusions

The benefits of lowering blood pressure are well-known. In clinical trials, antihypertensive therapy has been associated with 35 to 40 per cent mean reductions in stroke incidence and 20 to 25 per cent reduction in myocardial infarction incidence. Several classes of drugs are currently used in the treatment of hypertension, including angiotensin-converting enzyme inhibitors, angiotensin-receptor blockers, b-blockers, vasodilators, calcium channel blockers and diuretics. However, these drugs can have potentially unfavorable secondary effects and should be used with caution. Hence, demand for new antihypertensive drugs with less or no counter-indications persists. This review describes a large number of plant extracts and compounds that have been demonstrated to have vasodilatory activity and hypotensive effects in animal models. Consideration of these characteristics may be useful in the search for novel pharmacotherapies for cardiovascular diseases, especially hypertension.

References

2003 World Health Organization (WHO)/International Society of Hypertension (ISH) Statement on Management of Hypertension. (2003). *Journal of Hypertension*, 21: 1983-1992.

Abeywardena, M., Runnie, I., Nizar, M., Suhaila, M., Head, R., Suhaila, M. (2002). Polyphenol-enriched extract of oil palm fronds (*Elaeis guineensis*) promotes vascular relaxation via endothelium-dependent mechanisms. *Asia Pacific Journal of Clinical Nutrition*, 11: S467-S472.

Achike, F.I., Kwan, C.Y. (2003). Nitric oxide, human diseases and the herbal products that affect the nitric oxide signalling pathway. *Clinical and Experimental Pharmacology and Physiology*, 30: 605-615.

Aguirre-Crespo, F., Vergara-Galicia, J., Villalobos-Molina, R., Lópes-Guerrero, J.J., Navarrete-Vásquez, Estrada-Soto. (2006). Ursolic acid mediates the vasorelaxant activity of *Lepechinia caulescens* via NO release in isolated rat thoracic aorta. *Life Sciences*, 79: 1062-1068.

Ajay, M., Gilanib, A.H., Mustafa, M.R. (2003). Effects of flavonoids on vascular smooth muscle of the isolated rat thoracic aorta. *Life Sciences*, 74: 603-612.

Ajay, M., Chai, H.J., Mustafa, A.M., Gilani, A.H., Mustafa, M.R. (2007). Mechanisms of the antihypertensive effect of *Hibiscus sabdariffa* L. calyces. *Journal of Ethnopharmacology*, 109: 388-393.

Almeida, R.R., Raimundo, J.M., Oliveira, R.R., Kaplan, M.A.C., Gattass, C.R., Sudo, R.T., Zapata-Sudo, G. (2006). Activity of *Cecropia Lyratiloba* extract on contractility of cardiac and smooth muscles in Wistar rats. *Clinical and Experimental Pharmacology and Physiology*, 33: 109-113.

Al-Qattan, K.K., Thomson, M., Al-Mutawa'a, S., Al-Hajeri, D., Drobiova, H., Ali, M. (2006). Nitric oxide mediates the blood-pressure lowering effect of garlic in the rat two-kidney, one-clip model of hypertension. *The Journal of Nutrition*, 136: 774S-776S.

Andriambeloson, E., Magnier, C., Haan-Archipoff, G., Lobstein, A., Anton, R., Beretz, A., Stoclet, J.C., Andriantsitohaina, R. (1998). Natural dietary polyphenolic compounds cause endothelium-dependent vasorelaxation in rat thoracic aorta. *The Journal of Nutrition*, 128: 2324-2333.

Baragatti, B., Calderone, V., Testai, L., Martinotti, E., Chericoni, S., Morelli, I. (2002). Vasodilator activity of crude methanolic extract of *Gentiana kokiana* Perr. et Song. (Gentianaceae). *Journal of Ethnopharmacology*, 79: 369-372.

Berrougui, H., Herrera-Gonzalez, M.D., Marhuenda, E., Ettaib, A., Hmamouchi, M. (2002). Relaxant activity of methanolic extract from seeds of *Peganum harmala* on isolated rat aorta. *Therapie*, 57: 236-241.

Berrougui, H., Martín-Cordero, C., Khalil, A., Hmamouchi, M., Ettaib, A., Marhuenda, E., Herrera, M.D. (2006). Vasorelaxant effects of harmine and harmaline extracted from *Peganum harmala* L. seeds in isolated rat aorta. *Pharmacological Research*, 54: 150-157.

Bolton, T.B., Prestwich, S.A., Zholos, A.V., Gordienko, D.V. (1999). Excitation-contraction coupling in gastrointestinal and other smooth muscles. *Annual Review of Physiology*, 61: 85–115.

Bornia, E.C., Amaral., V., Bazotte, R.B., Alves-do-Prado, W. (2008). The reduction of arterial tension produced by stevioside is dependent on nitric oxide synthase activity when the endothelium is intact. *Journal of Smooth Muscle Research*, 44: 1-8.

Bryan, R.M., You, J., Golding, E.M., Marreli, S.P. (2005). Endothelium-derived hyperpolarizing factor: a cousin to nitric oxide and prostacyclin. *Anesthesiology*, 102: 1261-1277.

Butler, M.S. (2004). The role of natural product chemistry in drug discovery. *Journal of natural products*, 67: 2141-2153.

Calixto, J.B. (2005). Twenty-five years of research on medicinal plants in Latin America: a personal view. *Journal of Ethnopharmacology*, 100: 131-134.

Campos, M.G., Oropeza, M.V., Villanueva, T., Aguilar, M.I., Delgado, G., Ponce, H.A. (2000). Xanthorrhizol induces endothelium-independent relaxation of rat thoracic aorta. *Life Sciences*, 67: 327-333.

Chan, P., Xu, D., Liu,J.C., Chen, Y.J., Tomlinson, B., Huang, W.P., Cheng, J.T. (1998). The effect of stevioside on blood pressure and plasma catecholamines in spontaneously hypertensive rats. *Life Sciences*, 63: 1679-1684.

Chen, C.X., Kwan, C.Y. (2001). Endothelium-independent vasorelaxation by leonurine, a plant alkaloid purified from Chinese motherwort. *Life Sciences*, 68: 953-960.

Chericoni, S., Testai, L., Calderone, V., Flamini, G., Nieri, P., Morelli, I., Martinotti, E. (2003). The xanthones gentiacaulein and gentiakochianin are responsible for the vasodilator action of the roots of *Gentiana kochiana*. *Planta Medica*, 69: 770-772.

Chericoni, S., Testai, L., Campeol, E., Calderone, V., Morelli, I., Martinotti, E. (2004). Vasodilator activity of *Michelia figo* Spreng. (Magnoliaceae) by *in vitro* functional study. *Journal of Ethnopharmacology*, 91: 263-266.

Côrtes, S.F., Rezende, B.A., Corriu, C., Medeiros, I.A., Teixeira, M.M., Lopes, M.J., Lemos, V.S. (2001). Pharmacological evidence for the activation of potassium channels as the mechanism involved in the hypotensive and vasorelaxant effect of dioclein in rat small resistance arteries. *British Journal of Pharmacology*, 133: 849-858.

Côrtes, S.F., Valadares, Y.M., de Oliveira, A.B., Lemos, V.S., Barbosa, M.P., Braga, F.C. (2002). Mechanism of endothelium-dependent vasodilation induced by a proanthocyanidin-rich fraction from *Ouratea semiserrata*. *Planta Medica*, 68: 412-415.

Deyama, T., Nihibe, S., Nakazawa, Y. (2001). Constituents and pharmacological effects of *Eucommia* and Siberian ginseng. *Acta Pharmacologica Sinica*, 22: 1057-1070.

Dias, C.S., Barbosa-Filho, J.M., Lemos, V.S., Côrtes, S.F. (2002). Mechanisms involved in the vasodilator effect of curine in rat resistance arteries. *Planta Medica*, 68: 1049-1051.

Dias, K.L., da Silva, C.D., Barbosa-Filho, J.M., Almeida, R.N., de Azevedo, N.C., Medeiros, I.A. (2004). Cardiovascular effects induced by reticuline in normotensive rats. *Planta Medica*, 70: 328-333.

Dimo, T., Rakotonirina, S.V., Tan, P.V., Azay, J., Dongo, E., Cros, G. (2002). Leaf methanol extract of *Bidens pilosa* prevents and attenuates the hypertension induced by high-fructose diet in Wistar rats. *Journal of Ethnopharmacology*, 83: 183-191.

Dimo, T., Nguelefack, T.B., Tan, P.V., Yewah, M.P., Rakotonirina, S.V., Kamanyi, A., Bopelet, M. (2003). Possible mechanism of action of the neutral extract from *Bidens pilosa* L. leaves on the cardiovascular system of anaesthetized rats. *Phytotherapy Research*, 17: 1135-1139.

Dimo, T., Mtopi, O.S.B., Nguelefack, T.B., Kamtchouing, P., Zapfack, L., Asongalem, E.A., Dongo, E. (2007). Vasorelaxant effects of *Brillantaisia nitens* Lindau (Acanthaceae) extracts on isolated rat vascular smooth muscle. *Journal of Ethnopharmacology*, 111: 104-109.

Dongmo, A., Kamanyi, M.A., Tan, P.V., Bopelet, M., Vierling, W., Wagner, H. (2004). Vasodilating properties of the stem bark extract of *Mitragyna ciliata* in rats and guinea pigs. *Phytoterapy Research*, 18: 36-39.

Dongmo, A.B., Kamanyi, A., Franck, U., Wagner, H. (2002). Vasodilating properties of extracts from the leaves of *Musanga cecropioides* (R. Brown). *Phytotherapy Research*, 16: S6-S9.

El Bardai, S., Lyoussi, B., Wibo, M., Morel, N. (2001). Pharmacological evidence of hypotensive activity of *Marrubium vulgare* and *Foeniculum vulgare* in spontaneously hypertensive rat. *Clinical and Experimental Hypertension*, 23: 329-343.

El Bardai, S., Morel, N., Wibo, M., Fabre, N., Llabres, G., Lyoussi, B., Quetin-Leclercq, J. (2003a). The vasorelaxant activity of marrubenol and marrubiin from *Marrubium vulgare*. *Planta Medica*, 69: 75-77.

El-Bardai, S., Wibo, M., Hamaide, M.C., Lyoussi, B., Quetin-Leclercq, J., Morel, N. (2003b). Characterisation of marrubenol, a diterpene extracted from *Marrubium vulgare*, as an L-type calcium channel blocker. *British Journal of Pharmacology*, 140: 1211-1216.

El-Bardai, S., Hamaide, M.C., Lyoussi, B., Quetin-Leclercq, J., Morel, N., Wibo, M. (2004). Marrubenol interacts with phenylalkylamine binding site of the L-type calcium channel. *European Journal of Pharmacology*, 492: 269-272.

Engel, L.W., Straus, S.E. (2002). Development of therapeutics: opportunities within complementary and alternative medicine. *Nature Reviews Drug Discovery*, 1: 229-237.

Ettarh, R.R., Emeka, P. (2004). *Morinda lucida* extract induces endothelium-dependent and–independent relaxation of rat aorta. *Fitoterapia*, 75: 332-336.

Fallon, M.B., Abrams, G.A., Abdel-Razek, T.T., Dai, J., Chen, S.J., Chen, Y.F., Luo, B., Oparil, S., Ku, D.D. (1998). Garlic prevents hypoxic pulmonary hypertension in rats. *The American Journal of Physiology*, 275: 283-297.

Ferreira, H.C., Serra, C.P., Endringer, D.C., Lemos, V.S., Braga, F.C., Cortes, S.F. (2007a). Endothelium-dependent vasodilation induced by *Hancornia speciosa* in rat superior mesenteric artery. *Phytomedicine, 14:* 473-478.

Ferreira, H.C., Serra, C.P., Lemos, V.S., Braga, F.C., Cortes, S.F. (2007b). Nitric oxide-dependent vasodilation by ethanolic extract of *Hancornia speciosa* via phosphatidyl-inositol 3-kinase. *Journal of Ethnopharmacology, 109:* 161-164.

Ganado, P., Sanz, M., Padilla, E., Tejerina, T. (2004). An *in vitro* study of different extracts and fractions of *Allium sativum* (garlic): vascular reactivity. *Journal of Pharmacological Sciences*, 94: 434-442.

Ghayur, M.N., Gilani, A.H. (2006). Radish seed extract mediates its cardiovascular inhibitory effects via muscarinic receptor activation. *Fundamental and Clinical Pharmacology*, 20: 57-63.

Guedes, D.N., Silva, D.F., Barbosa-Filho, J.M., Medeiros, I.A. (2002a). Muscarinic agonist properties involved in the hypotensive and vasorelaxant responses of rotundifolone in rats. *Planta Medica*, 68: 700-704.

Guedes, D.N., Barbosa-Filho, J.M., Lemos, V.S., Côrtes, S.F. (2002b). Mechanism of the vasodilator effect of 12-O-methylcurine in rat aortic rings. *Journal of Pharmacy and Pharmacology*, 54: 853-858.

Guedes, D.N., Silva, D.F., Barbosa-Filho, J.M., Medeiros, I.A. (2004). Endothelium-dependent hypotensive and vasorelaxant effects of the essential oil from aerial parts of *Mentha x villosa* in rats. *Phytomedicine*, 11: 490-497.

Harauma, A., Moriguchi, T. (2006). Aged garlic extract improves blood pressure in spontaneously hypertensive rats more safely than raw garlic. *The Journal of Nutrition*, 136: 769S-773S.

Ho, H.M., Chen, R., Huang, Y., Chen, Z.Y. (2002). Vascular effects of a soy leaves (*Glycine max*) extract and kaempferol glycosides in isolated rat carotid arteries. *Planta Medica*, 68: 487-491.

Hu, C.M., Kang, J.J., Lee, C.C., Li, C.H., Liao, J.W., Cheng, Y.W. (2003). Induction of vasorelaxation through activation of nitric oxide synthase in endothelial cells by brazilin. *European Journal of Pharmacology*, 468: 37-45.

Kamanyi, A., Bopelet, M., Aloamaka, C.P., Obiefuna, P.C.M., Ebeigbe, A.B. (1991). Endothelium-dependent rat aortic relaxation to the aqueous leaf extract of *Musanga cecropioides*. *Journal of Ethnopharmacology*, 34: 283-286.

Kang, D.G., Oh, H., Cho, D.K., Kwon, E.K., Han, J.H., Lee, H.S. (2002). Effects of bulb of *Fritillaria Ussuriensis* Maxim. on angiotensin converting enzyme and vascular release of NO/cGMP in rats. *Journal of Ethnopharmacology*, 81: 49-55.

Kang, D.G., Yin, M.H., Oh, H., Lee, D.H., Lee, H.S. (2004). Vasorelaxation by amentoflavone isolated from *Selaginella tamariscina*. *Planta Medica*, 70: 718-722.

Kang, D.G., Lee, J.K., Choi, D.H., Sohn, E.J., Moon, M.K., Lee, H.S. (2005). Vascular relaxation by the methanol extract of *Sorbus* cortex via NO-cGMP pathway. *Biological and Pharmaceutical Bulletin*, 28: 860-864.

Kim, D., Yokozawa, T., Hattori, M., Kadota, S., Namba, T. (2000). Effects of aqueous extracts of *Apocynum venetum* leaves on spontaneously hypertensive, renal hypertensive and nacl-fed-hypertensive rats. *Journal of Ethnopharmacology*, 72: 53-59.

Kim, S.H., Kang, K.W., Kim, K.w., Kim, N.D. (2000). Procyanidins in crataegus extract evoke endothelium-dependent vasorelaxation in rat aorta. *Life Sciences*, 67: 121-131.

Koehn, F.E., Carter, G.T. (2005). The evolving role of natural products in drug discovery. *Nature Reviews. Drug Discovery*, 4: 206-220.

Koh, S.B., Kang, M.H., Kim, T.S., Park, H.W., Park, C.G., Seong, Y.H., Seong, H.J. (2007). Endothelium-dependent vasodilatory and hypotensive effects of *Crotalaria sessiliflora* L. in rats. *Biological and Pharmaceutical Bulletin*, 30: 48-53.

Kressman, S., Muller, W.E., Blume, H.H. (2002). Pharmaceutical Quality of Different *Ginkgo biloba* Brands. *Journal of Pharmacy and Pharmacology*, 54: 661-669.

Kubota, Y., Tanaka, N., Umegaki, K., Takenaka, H., Mizuno, H., Nakamura, K., Shinozuka, K., Kunitomo, M. (2001). *Ginkgo biloba* extract-induced relaxation of rat aorta is associated with increase in endothelial intracellular calcium level. *Life Sciences*, 69: 2327-2336.

Kubota, Y., Tanaka, N., Kagota, S., Nakamura, K., Kunimoto, M., Umegaki, K., Schinozuka, K. (2006). Effects of *Ginkgo biloba* extract on blood pressure and vascular endothelial response by acetylcholine in spontaneously hypertensive rats. *Journal of Pharmacy and Pharmacology*, 58: 243-249.

Kwan, C.Y. (1995). Vascular effects of selective antihypertensive drugs derived from traditional medicinal herbs. *Clinical and Experimental Pharmacology* and *Physiology*, 22: S297-S299.

Kwan, C.Y., Chen, C.X., Deyama, T., Nishibe, S. (2004a). Endothelium-dependent vasorelaxant effects of the aqueous extracts of the *Eucommia ulmoides* Oliv. leaf and bark: Implications on their antihypertensive action. *Vascular Pharmacology*, 40: 229-235.

Kwan, C.Y., Zhang, W.B., Deyama, T., Nishibe, S. (2004b). Endothelium-dependent vascular relaxation induced by *Eucommia ulmoides* Oliv. bark extract is mediated by NO and EDHF in small vessels. *Naunyn-Schmiedeberg's Archives of Pharmacology*, 369: 206-211.

Kwan, C.Y., Zhang, W.B., Sim, S.M., Deyama, T., Nishibe, S. (2004c). Vascular effects of Siberian ginseng (*Eleutherococcus senticosus*): endothelium-dependent NO–and EDHF-mediated relaxation depending on vessel size. *Naunyn-Schmiedeberg's Archives of Pharmacology*, 369: 473-480.

Kwan, C.Y., Zhang, W.B., Nishibe, S., Seo, S. (2005). A novel in vitro endothelium-dependent vascular relaxant effect of *Apocynum venetum* leaf extract. *Clinical and Experimental Pharmacology and Physiology*, 32: 789-795.

Lahlou, S., Carneiro-Leão, R.F., Leal-Cardoso, J.H., Toscano, C.F. (2001). Cardiovascular effects of the essential oil of *Mentha x villosa* and its main constituent, piperitenone oxide, in normotensive anaesthetised rats: role of the autonomic nervous system. *Planta Medica*, 67: 638-643.

Lahlou, S., Magalhães, P.J., Carneiro-Leão, R.F., Leal-Cardoso, J.H. (2002a). Involvement of nitric oxide in the mediation of the hypotensive action of the essential oil of *Mentha x villosa* in normotensive conscious rats. *Planta Medica*, 68: 694-699.

Lahlou, S., Carneiro-Leão, R.F., Leal-Cardoso, J.H. (2002b). Cardiovascular effects of the essential oil of *Mentha x villosa* in DOCA-salt-hypertensive rats. *Phytomedicine*, 9: 715-720.

Lam, F.F.Y., Yeung, J.H.K., Kwan, Y.W., Chan, K.M., Or, P.M.Y. (2006). Salvianolic acid B, an aqueous component of danshen (*Salvia miltiorrhiza*), relaxes rat coronary artery by inhibition of calcium channels. *European Journal of Pharmacology*, 553: 240-245.

Lam, F.F.Y., Yeung, J.H.K., Chan, K.M., Or, P.M.Y. (2007). Relaxant effects of danshen aqueous extract and its constituent danshensu on rat coronary artery are mediated by inhibition of calcium channels. *Vascular Pharmacology*, 46: 271-277.

Lam, F.F.Y., Yeung, J.H.K., Chan, K.M., Or, P.M.Y. (2008). Mechanisms of the dilator action of cryptotanshinone on rat coronary artery. *European Journal of Pharmacology*, 578: 253-260.

Lang, C., Liu, Z., Taylor, H.W., Baker, D.G. (2005). Effect of *Eucommia ulmoides* on systolic blood pressure in the spontaneous hypertensive rat. *The American Journal of Chinese Medicine*, 33: 215-230.

Lee, C.N., Wong, K.L., Liu, J.C., Chen, Y.J., Cheng, J.T., Chan, P. (2001). Inhibitory effect of stevioside on calcium influx to produce antihypertension. *Planta Medica*, 67: 796-799.

Lee, J.W., Roh, T.C., Rho, M.C., Kim, Y.K., Lee, H.S. (2002). Mechanisms of relaxant action of a pyranocoumarin from *Peucedanum japonicum* in isolated rat thoracic aorta. *Planta Medica*, 68: 891-895.

Lee, T.H., Wang, G.J., Lee, Y.H., Chou, C.H. (2002). Inhibitory effects of glycosides from the leaves of *Melaleuca quinquinerva* on vascular contraction of rats. *Planta Medica*, 68: 492-496.

Legssyer, A., Ziyyat, A., Mekh, H., Bnouham, M., Herrenknecht, C., Roumy, V., Fourneau, C., Laurens, A., Hoerter, J., Fischmeister, R. (2004). Tannins and catechin gallate mediate the vasorelaxant effect of *Arbutus unedo* on the rat isolated aorta. *Phytotherapy Research*, 18: 889-894.

Lemos, V.S., Côrtes, S.F., dos Santos, M.H., Ellena, J., Moreira, M.E., Doriguetto, A.C. (2006). Structure and vasorelaxant activity of floranol, a flavonoid isolated from the roots of *Dioclea grandiflora*. *Chemistry and Biodiversity*, 3: 635-645.

Li, Z., Nakaya, Y., Niwa, Y., Chen, X. (2001a). K_{Ca} channel-opening activity of *Ginkgo biloba* extracts and ginsenosides in cultured endothelial cells. *Clinical and Experimental Pharmacology and Physiology*, 28: 441-445.

Li, Z., Chen, X., Niwa, Y., Sakamoto, S., Nakaya,Y. (2001b). Involvement of Ca^{2+}-activated K^+ channels in ginsenosides-induced aortic relaxation in rats. *Journal of cardiovascular Pharmacology*, 37: 41-47.

Maciel, S.S., Dias, K.L., Medeiros, I.A. (2004). Calcium mobilization as the endothelium-independent mechanism of action involved in the vasorelaxant response induced by the aqueous fraction of the ethanol extract of *Albizia inopinata* G.P. Lewis (AFL) in the rat aorta. *Phytomedicine*, 11: 130-134.

Madeira, S.V.F., Resende, A.C., Ognibene, D.T., Sousa, M.A.V., Soares de Moura, R. (2005). Mechanism of the endothelium-dependent vasodilator effect of an alcohol-free extract obtained from a vinifera grape skin. *Pharmacological Research*, 52: 321-327.

Mahady, G.B. (2002). *Ginkgo biloba* for the prevention and treatment of cardiovascular disease: a review of the literature. *The Journal of Cardiovascular Nursing*, 16: 21-32.

Martin, H.B., Stofer, W.D., Eichinger, M.R. (2000). Kavain inhibits murine airway smooth muscle contraction. *Planta Medica*, 66: 601-606.

Martin, H.B., McCallum, M., Stofer, W.D., Eichinger, M.R. (2002). Kavain attenuates vascular contractility through inhibition of calcium channels. *Planta Medica*, 68: 784-789.

Mashour, N.H., Lin, G.I., Frishman, W.H. (1998). Herbal medicine for the treatment of cardiovascular disease: Clinical Considerations. *Archives of International Medicine*, 158: 2225-2234.

Matsuura, M., Kimura, Y., Nakata, K., Baba, K., Okuda, H. (2001). Artery relaxation by chalcones isolated from the roots of *Angelica keiskei*. *Planta Medica*, 67: 230-235.

Mishra, S.K., Abbot, S.E.,Chouldhury, Z., Cheng, M., Khatab, N., Maycock, N.J.R., Zavery, A., Aaronson. (2000). Endothelium-dependent relaxation of rat aorta and main pulmonary artery by the phytoestrogens genistein and daidzein. *Cardiovascular Research*, 46: 539-546.

Mitamura, M., Horie, S., Sakaguchi, M., Someya, A., Tsuchiya, S., Van de Voorde, J., Murayama, T., Watanabe, K. (2002). Mesaconitine-induced relaxation in rat aorta: involvement of Ca^{2+} influx and nitric-oxide synthase in the endothelium. *European Journal of Pharmacology*, 436: 217-225.

Moon, M.K., Kang, D.G., Lee, J.K., Kim, J.S., Lee, H.S. (2006). Vasodilatory and antiinflammatory effects of the aqueous extract of rhubarb via a NO-cGMP pathway. *Life Sciences*, 78: 1150-1557.

Morello, S., Vellecco, V., Alfieri, A., Mascolo, N., Cicala, C. (2006). Vasorelaxant effect of the flavonoid galangin on isolated rat thoracic aorta. *Life Sciences*, 78: 825-830.

Newman, D.J., Cragg, G.M., Snader, K. M. (2003). Natural products as sources of new drugs over the period 1981-2002. *Journal of Natural Products*, 66: 1022-1037.

Nguelefack, T.B., Dimo, T., Mbuyo, E.P.N., Tan, P.V., Rakotonirina, S.V., Kamanyi, A. (2005). Relaxant effects of the neutral extract of the leaves of *Bidens pilosa* Linn on isolated rat vascular smooth muscle. *Phytotherapy Research*, 19: 207-210.

Nicasio, P., Meckes, M. (2005). Hypotensive effect of the hydroalcoholic extract from *Jacaranda mimosaefolia* leaves in rats. *Journal of Ethnopharmacology*, 97: 301-304.

Nishida, S., Satoh, H. (2003). Mechanisms for the vasodilations induced by *Ginkgo biloba* extract and its main constituent, bilobalide, in rat aorta. *Life Sciences*, 72: 2659-2667.

Nishida, S., Satoh, H. (2004). Comparative vasodilating actions among terpenoids and flavonoids contained in *Ginkgo biloba* extract. *Clinica Chimica Acta*, 339: 129-133.

Odigie, I.P., Ettarh, R.R., Adigun, S.A. (2003). Chronic administration of aqueous extract of *Hibiscus sabdariffa* attenuates hypertension and reverses cardiac hypertrophy in 2K-1C hypertensive rats. *Journal of Ethnopharmacology*, 86: 181-185.

Oh, K.S., Han, W., Wang, M.H., Lee, B.H. (2007). The effects of chronic treatment with *Morus bombycis* Koidzumi in spontaneously hypertensive rats. *Biological and Pharmaceutical Bulletin*, 30: 1278-1283.

Ojewole, J., Kamadyaapa, D.R., Gondwe, M.M., Moodley, K., Musabayane, C.T. (2007). Cardiovascular effects of *Persea americana* Mill (Laureaceae) (avocado) aqueous leaf extract in experimental animals. *Cardiovascular Journal of South Africa*, 18: 69-76.

Ojewole, J.A. (2006). Vasorelaxant and hypotensive effects of *Sclerocarya birrea* (A Rich) Hochst (Anacardiaceae) stem bark aqueous extract in rats. *Cardiovascular Journal of South Africa*, 17: 117-123.

Orallo, F. (1996). Regulation of cytosolic calcium levels in vascular smooth muscle. *Pharmacology and Therapeutics*, 69: 153-171.

Orallo, F., Alzueta, A.F. (2001). Preliminary study of the vasorelaxant effects of (+)-nantenine, an alkaloid isolated from *Platycapnos spicata*, in rat aorta. *Planta Medica*, 67: 800-806.

Orallo, F. (2004). Acute cardiovascular effects of (+)-nantenine, an alkaloid isolated from *Platycapnos spicata*, in anaesthetised normotensive rats. Planta Medica, 70: 117-126.

Ouédraogo, S., Ranaivo, H.R., Ndiaye, M., Kaboré, Z.I., Guissou, I.P., Bucher, B., Andriantsitohaina, R. (2004). Cardiovascular properties of aqueous extract from *Mitragyna inermis* (wild). *Journal of Ethnopharmacology*, 93: 345-350.

Owolabi, M.A., Jaja, S.I., Coker, H.A.B. (2005). Vasorelaxant action of aqueous extract of the leaves of *Persea americana* on isolated thoracic aorta. *Fitoterapia*, 76: 567-573.

Parkington, H.C., Coleman, H.A., Tare, M. (2004). Prostacyclin and endothelium-dependent hyperpolarization. *Pharmacological Research*, 49: 509-514.

Persson, I.A.L., Dong,L., Persson, K. (2006). Effect of Panax ginseng extract (G115) on angiotensin-converting enzyme (ACE) activity and nitric oxide (NO) production. *Journal of Ethnopharmacology*, 105: 321-325.

Phillips, O.A., Mathew, K.T., Oriowo, M.A. (2006). Antihypertensive and vasodilator effects of methanolic and aqueous extracts of *Tribulus terrestris* in rats. *Journal of Ethnopharmacology*, 104: 351-355.

Pires, S.L., de Assis, T.S., de Almeida, R.N., Filho, J.M., Julien, C., de Medeiros, I.A. (2000). Endothelium-derived nitric oxide is involved in the hypotensive and vasorelaxant responses induced by the aqueous fraction of the ethanolic extract of the leaves of *Albizia inopinata* (harms) g.p. lewis in rats. *Phytomedicine*, 7: 91-98.

Ponce, H.M., Campos, M.G., Aguilar, I., Delgado, G. (1999). Effect of xanthorrhizol, xanthorrhizol glycoside and trachylobanoic acid isolated from Cachani complex plants upon the contractile activity of uterine smooth muscle. *Phytotherapy Research*, 13: 202-205.

Raimundo, J.M., Almeida, R.R., Velozo, L.S.M., Kaplan, M.A.C., Gattass, C.R., Zapata-Sudo, G. (2004). In-vitro vasodilatory activity of the hexanic extract of leaves and stems from *Piper truncatum* vell in rats. *Journal of Pharmacy and Pharmacology*, 56: 1-6.

Rhyu, M.R., Kim, E.Y., Kim, B. (2004). Nitric-oxide-mediated vasorelaxation by rhizoma *Ligustici wallichii* in isolated rat thoracic aorta. *Phytomedicine*, 11: 51-55.

Rocha, A.P.M., Carvalho, L.C.R.M., Sousa, M.A.V., Madeira, S.V.F., Sousa, P.J.C., Tano, T., Schini-Kerth, V.B., Resende, A.C., Soares de Moura, R. (2007). Endothelium-dependent vasodilator effect of *Euterpe oleracea* Mart. (ACaí) extracts in mesenteric vascular bed of the rat. *Vascular Pharmacology*, 46: 97-104.

Rodríguez-Cruz, M.E., Pérez-Ordaz, L., Serrato-Barajas, B.E., Juaréz-Oropeza, M.A., Mascher, D., Paredes-Carbajal, M.C. (2003). Endothelium-dependent effects of the ethanolic extract of the mistletoe *Psittacanthus calycatus* on the vasomotor responses of rat aortic rings. *Journal of Ethnopharmacology*, 86: 213-218.

Runnie, I., Salleh, M.N., Mohamed, S., Head, R.J., Abeywardena, M.Y. (2004). Vasorelaxation induced by common edible tropical plant extracts in isolated rat aorta and mesenteric vascular bed. *Journal of Ethnopharmacology*, 92: 311-316.

Salah-Abbès, J.B., Abbès, S., Ouanes, Z., Houas, Z., Abdel-Wahhab, M.A., Bacha, H., Oueslati, R. (2008). Tunisian radish extract (*Raphanus sativus*) enhances the antioxidant status and protects against oxidative stress induced by zearalenone in Balb/c mice. *Journal of Applied Toxicology*, 28: 6-14.

Schuldt, E.Z., Ckless, K., Simas, M.E., Farias, M.R., Ribeiro-do-Valle, R.M. (2000). Butanolic fraction from *Cuphea carthagenensis* Jacq McBride relaxes rat thoracic aorta through endothelium-dependent and endothelium-independent mechanisms. *Journal of Cardiovascular Pharmacology*, 35: 234-239.

Seya, K., Furukawa, K.I., Taniguchi, S., Kodzuka, G., Oshima, Y., Niwa, M., Motomura, S. (2003). Endothelium-dependent vasodilatory effect of vitisin C, a novel plant oligostilbene from *Vitis* plants (Vitaceae), in rabbit aorta. *Clinical Science*, 105: 73-79.

Sharifi, A.M., Darabi, R., Akbarloo, N. (2003). Study of antihypertensive mechanism of *Tribulus terrestris* in 2K1C hypertensive rats: Role of tissue ACE activity. *Life Sciences*, 73: 2963-2971.

Slish, D.F., Ueda, H., Arvigo, R., Balick, M.J. (1999). Ethnobotany in the search for vasoactive herbal medicines. *Journal of Ethnopharmacology*, 66: 159-165.

Slish, D.F., Arvigo, R., Balick. (2004). *Alseis yucatanensis*: a natural product from Belize that exhibits multiple mechanisms of vasorelaxation. *Journal of Ethnopharmacology*, 92: 297-302.

Soares de Moura, R., Costa Viana, F.S., Souza, M.A., Kovary, K., Guedes, D.C., Oliveira, E.P., Rubenich, L.M., Carvalho, L.C., Oliveira, R.M., Tano, T., Gusmão Correia, M.L. (2002). Antihypertensive, vasodilator and antioxidant effects of a vinifera grape skin extract. *Journal of Pharmacy and Pharmacology*, 54: 1515-1520.

Song-Lin, L., Li, P., Lin, G., Chan, S.W., Ho, Y.P. (2000). Simultaneous determination of seven major isosteroidal alkaloids in bulbs of *Fritillaria* by gas chromatography. *Journal of Chromatography A*, 873: 221-228.

Tahri, A., Yamani, S., Legssyer, A., Aziz, M., Mekhfi, H., Bnouham, M., Ziyyat, A. (2000). Acute diuretic, natriuretic and hypotensive effects of a continuous perfusion of aqueous extract of *Urtica dioica* in the rat. *Journal of Ethnopharmacology*, 73: 95-100.

Tenorio, F.A., del Valle, L., González, A., Pastelín, G. (2005). Vasodilator activity of the aqueous extract of *Viscum album*. *Fitoterapia*, 76: 204-209.

Testai, L., Chericoni, S., Calderone, V., Nencioni, G., Nieri, P., Morelli, I., Martinotti, E. (2002). Cardiovascular effects of *Urtica dioica* L. (Urticaceae) roots extracts: *in vitro* and *in vivo* pharmacological studies. *Journal of Ethnopharmacology*, 81: 105-109.

Testai, L., Chericoni, S., Ammar, B., Luisa, P., Vincenzom C., Martinotti, E. (2005). Vasorelaxant effects of the chloroformic crude extract of *Bupleurum fruticosum* L. (Umbelliferae) roots on rat thoracic aorta. *Journal of Ethnopharmacology*, 96: 93-97.

TibiriCá, E., Almeida, A., Cailleaux, S., Pimenta, D., Kaplan, M.A., Lessa, M.A., Figueiredo, M.R. (2007). Pharmacological mechanisms involved in the vasodilator effects of extracts from *Echinodorus grandiflorus*. *Journal of Ethnopharmacology*, 111: 50-55.

Tirapelli, C.R., Ambrosio, S.R., da Costa, F.B., de Oliveira, A.M. (2002). Inhibitory action of kaurenoic acid from *Viguiera robusta* (Asteraceae) on phenylephrine-induced rat carotid contraction. *Fitoterapia*, 73: 56-62.

Tirapelli, C.R., Ambrosio, S.R., da Costa, F.B., Coutinho, S.T., de Oliveira, D.C.R., de Oliveira, A.M. (2004). Analysis of the mechanisms underlying the vasorelaxant action of kaurenoic acid in the isolated rat aorta. *European Journal of Pharmacology*, 492: 233-241.

Trigueiro, F., Cortes, S.F., Almeida, R.N., Lemos, V.S. (2000). Endothelium-independent vasorelaxant effect of dioclein, a new flavonoid isolated from *Dioclea grandiflora*, in the rat aorta. *Journal of Pharmacy and Pharmacology*, 52: 1431-1434.

Umegaki, K., Shinozuka, K., Watarai, K., Takenaka, H., Yoshimura, M., Daohua, P., Esashi, T. (2000). Ginkgo biloba extract attenuates the development of hypertension in deoxycorticosterone acetate-salt hypertensive rats. *Clinical and Experimental Pharmacology and Physiology*, 27: 277-282.

Uncini Manganelli, R.E., Chericoni, S., Baragatti, B. (2000). Ethnopharmacobotany in Tuscany: the plants used as antihypertensive. *Fitoterapia*, 71: S95–S100.

Vanhoutte, P.M. (2004). Endothelium-dependent hyperpolarizations: the history. *Pharmacological Research*, 49: 503-508.

Wang, S.P., Zang, W.J., Kong, S.S., Yu, X.J., Sun, L., Zhao, X.F., Whang, S.X., Zheng, X.H. (2008). Vasorelaxant effect of isopropyl 3-(3, 4-dihydroxyphenyl)-2-hydroxipropanoate, a novel metabolite from *Salvia miltiorrhiza*, on isolated rat mesenteric artery. *European Journal of Pharmacology*, 579: 283-288.

Wang, Z.T., Lau, C.W., Chan, F.L., Yao, X., Chen, Z.Y., He, Z.D., Huang, Y. (2001). Vasorelaxant effects of cardamonin and alpinetin from *Alpinia henryi* K. Schum. *Journal of Cardiovascular Pharmacology*, 37: 596-606.

Wong, K.L., Chan, P., Yang, H.Y., Hsu, F.L., Liu, I.M., Cheng, Y.W., Cheng, J.Y. (2004). Isosteviol acts on potassium channels to relax isolated aortic strips of Wistar rat. *Life Sciences, 74:* 2379-2387.

Wongcome, T., Panthong, A., Jesadanont, S., Kanjanapothi,D., Taesotikul, T., Lertpraertsuke, N. (2007). Hypotensive effect and toxicology of the extract from *Coscinium fenestratum* (Gaertn.) Colebr. *Journal of Ethnopharmacology*, 111: 468-475.

World Health Organization (WHO): Traditional medicine. (2003). Fact Sheet n° 134.

Xie, Y.W., Ming, D.S., Xu, H.X., Dong, H., But, P.P. (2000). Vasorelaxing effects of *Caesalpinia sappan* involvement of endogenous nitric oxide. *Life Sciences*, 67: 1913-1918.

Yin, M.H., Kang, D.G., Choi, D.H., Kwon, T.O., Lee, H.S. (2005). Screening of vasorelaxant activity of some medicinal plants used in Oriental medicines. *Journal of Ethnopharmacology*, 99: 113-117.

Yuzurihara, M., Ikarashi, Y., Goto, K., Sakakibara, I., Hayakawa, T., Sasaki, H. (2002). Geissoschizine methyl ether, an indole alkaloid extracted from *Uncariae Ramulus* et Uncus, is a potent vasorelaxant of isolated rat aorta. *European Journal of Pharmacology*, 444: 183-189.

Ziyyat, A., Mekhfi, H., Bnouham, M., Tahri, A., Legssyer, A., Hoerter, J., Fischmeister, R. (2002). *Arbutus unedo* induces endothelium-dependent relaxation of the isolated rat aorta. *Phytotherapy Research*, 16: 1-4.

Medicinal Plants: Phytochemistry, Pharmacology and Therapeutics, Vol. 1 *Pages* **131–154**
Editors: **V.K. Gupta, G.D. Singh, Surjeet Singh and A. Kaul**
Published by: **DAYA PUBLISHING HOUSE, NEW DELHI**

Chapter 6

Scope of Chicory with Special Reference to its Medicinal Value

Yogendrasinh B. Solanki and Sunita M. Jain*
Department of Pharmacology, L.M. College of Pharmacy, Navrangpura, Ahmedabad – 380 009, India

ABSTRACT

Chicory is commonly known as a coffee substitute. In traditional ayurvedic system of medicine, it is known as 'Kasni' and employed in variety of diseases. Numbers of studies have documented the physiological activities of chicory. It contains a soluble fermentable dietary fiber–Inulin, which is having beneficial effects in hyperlipidemia, hyperglycemia, cancer, and bile acid related disorders. The bifidogenic, hypolipidemia, hypoglycemic, cholestatic and anticancer activities of chicory can be attributed to inulin directly or indirectly. The bitter principles and polyphenolic acids are responsible for antiinflammatory, hepatoprotective, antioxidant, cytotoxic and antiHIV activities. These justify the traditional uses of this folk medicine and specify the medicinal importance beyond its commercial values as a coffee substitute.

Keywords: *Chicory, Dietary fibers, Hyperlipidemia, Hyperglycemia, Inulin, Oligofructosaccharides, Sesquiterpene lactones.*

Introduction

Chicory (*Cichorium intybus* L.) roots were commonly used as a coffee substitute (Pazola, 1987). The roasted chicory roots are added into the coffee in varying proportion. Upon roasting, the inulin

* Corresponding Author: E-mail: sunitalmcp@yahoo.com; Phone: (O) +91-79-2630 2746; (R) +91-79-2741 3840; (M) +91-0-94261 73029.

present in chicory is converted to oxymethylfurfurol, a compound with a coffee like aroma. The oxymethylfurfural was found to give pleasantly bitter taste to the brew and reduce its stimulant effect. Due to variety of physiological effects, chicory is popularly used as folk remedy for number of disorders like: anorexia, arrhythmia, cancer, cholecystosis, hypercholesterolemia, hyperglycemia, insomnia, jaundice, nephrosis, inflammation, sore throat, swelling, water retention, etc. It acts as a tonifying and detoxifying agent for the liver and used in jaundice, hepatosis, liver enlargement and bile acid related disorders. The leaves were found to have antiinflammatory action and were used in inflammatory conditions, swelling, bruises, etc. The leaves were also used as salads in human diet and were reported to be stomachic (Franke, 1981; Baumann, 1982). The juice of leaves has been used in eye disorders. The infusion of chicory was believed to be good for the liver, kidney and stomach. The chicory seeds were employed as hepatoprotective. The chicory root contains a reserve polysaccharide carbohydrate: Inulin– a soluble fermentable dietary fiber. Recently, the soluble fermentable dietary fibers were reported to have protective effect in cardiovascular disease, hyperlipidemia, diabetes, and cancer (Jenkins *et al.*, 1995; Marlett, 2001). Since, inulin has a bland neutral flavor and contributes a fat-like texture and mouth-feel when added to some foods. Commercially inulin was used to replace the sugars in preparations such as chocolate, dairy products, table spreads, frozen desserts and baked goods. Recently, chicory has been studied for variety of physiological effects on humans and animals in order to support the beneficial role of this folk medicine in the treatment of various disorders. The present review article will focus on the scientific reports to establish the medicinal importance of chicory.

Botanical Description

Cichorium intybus L., is a biennial plant belonging to the family *Asteraceae*. Chicory is one of only two species that comprise the genus–cichorium, endive being the other. It is commonly known as– Succory, Wild succory, Wild chicory, Witloof chicory, Garden chicory, Garden endive, Belgium endive, Common endive, Curly endive, Blue sailors, Blue dandelion, Cikorie, Hendibeh, Hinduba, Hindiba, Kasani, Kasni, Kiku-Niga-Na, Watcher of the road, etc. The name "Succory" means "to run under" in Latin was applied to chicory because its roots run to great depths and it is very difficult to pull up.

Chicory is a biennial plant that produces a rosette following seeding (Rumball, 1986), with taproot like dandelion. The stems are 2-3 feet high with lateral branches, which are spreading, giving off at a very considerable angle from the central stem (Figures 6.1A and 6.B). The root stock is light-yellow outside, white inside and contains a bitter milky juice, which is somewhat apparent and slightly sedative. The stem bears lanceolate leaves that are coarsely toothed near the bottom of the plant. The size of leaves decrease progressively from stem base to apex (Doorenbos and Riemens, 1959). The leaves at the base of the plant are large, hairy and somewhat resemble those of dandelion. Hence, it is called as "blue dandelion". It bears light–blue to violet flowers (Figure 6.1C), sometimes white or pink. The bloom first appears in late spring and continues into mid fall, *i.e.* from July to September or October. The flowers are about 2.5 cm wide and rays have toothed tip.

There were commonly two varieties: wild chicory and cultivated chicory. It required neutral (pH: 6.6 to 7.5) to mildly alkaline soil (pH: 7.6 to 7.8). It can be sow by seedling. Since it is invasive, spacing of 18-24 inch (45-60 cm) should be provided. The fragile soil mixed with sawdust and composted manure is good for chicory cultivation. It requires moderate sunlight and water. It is drought-tolerant; suitable for xeriscaping. The plant is dormant during cold winter months and bolts under long days during the subsequent growing season (Gianquinto and Pimpini, 1989). The *Cichorium intybus* L. vr. Silvestre is mainly cultivated for roots while *Cichorium intybus* L. vr. Foliosum is mainly cultivated for use as greens in salads.

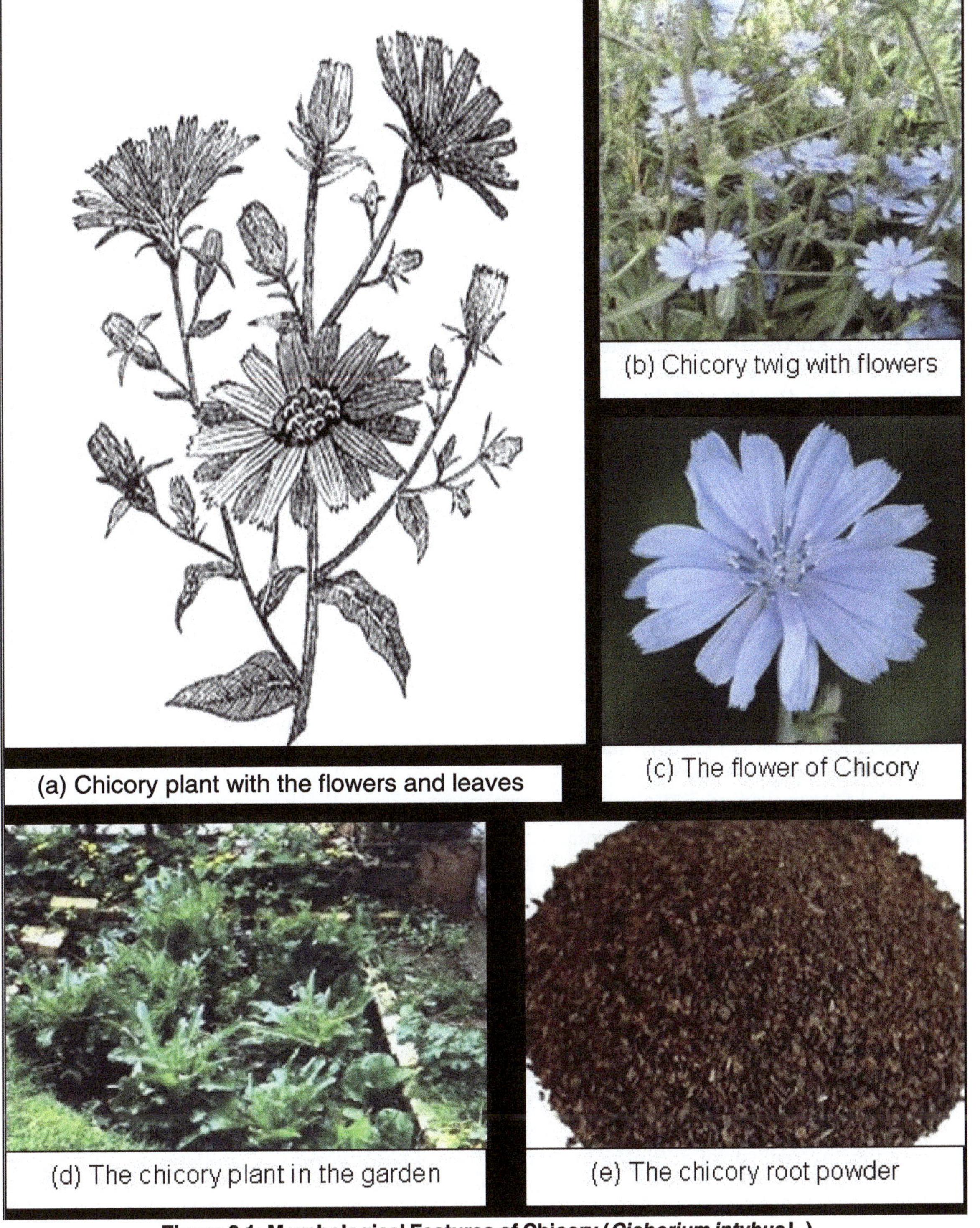

(a) Chicory plant with the flowers and leaves

(b) Chicory twig with flowers

(c) The flower of Chicory

(d) The chicory plant in the garden

(e) The chicory root powder

Figure 6.1: Morphological Features of Chicory (*Cichorium intybus* L.)

Chicory Production

Around 1960, the chicory roots were first used as a coffee substitute in Holland followed by many other countries like Sweden, France, etc. During 1806-1813, the cultivation and use of roasted chicory roots as coffee substitute have spreaded over the whole European continent. In the 19th century, the main centers of cultivation were north east France, Belgium, England, Russia, Holland, Australia, etc. Subsequently, it was cultivated in large scale in Poland, Hungary, Germany, Switzerland and India. However, presently efforts have been made for large scale cultivation in United States of America, Australia, New Zealand, etc. Presently over $^{1}/_{5}{}^{th}$ of world's consumption take place in eastern Europe especially in Poland (6 per cent), followed by Russia, Hungary, Romania, Czechoslovakia, and Germany. According to percentage, it was reported that 12 per cent to be consumed in South Africa, 9 per cent in India and 2 per cent in United States of America (Clarke and Macrae, 1987).

In India, chicory crop is mainly cultivated in Gujarat and Uttar Pradesh. It is mainly cultivated in the Jamnagar, Kheda, Anand, and Mehsana districts of Gujarat. These districts have about 40 per cent share in the total production of chicory used in the manufacturing of coffee. In Uttar Pradesh, it is cultivated in the districts of Etah, and Aligarh, where an area of about 4000 ha. has come under its cultivation during last four–five years. The estimated production of chicory (*Cichorium intybus* L. Sativum D.C.) in India is about 20000 metric tones in roasted form. The average productivity of the chicory roots ranges between: 30-32.5/ha. with an average sale price of Rs. 1500/tone. The cost of cultivation and net return per hector works out to be respectively Rs. 12000/ha and 47000/ha, with net profit of Rs. 35000/ha (Chandra and Kumari, 2005).

Phytochemical Constituents

Fresh chicory roots contained a considerable quantity of water (70-80 per cent). The roots were distinctive in containing the soluble dietary fiber–Inulin, a polymer of fructose with β-(2-1) glycosidic linkages (Figure 6.2); belonging to the fructans family (Mac Grogor and Greenwood, 1980). From the culinary viewpoint, the inulin is particularly interesting. Upon roasting, inulin is converted to oxymethylfurfurol, a compound with a coffee like aroma. During storage the inulin present in roots is converted into inulide and finally into fructose due to the presence of an enzymes inulocoagulase, which has been reported in the expressed root juice. Chicory roots also contain a cytokine, ribosylzeatin, a nucleotide sugar, uridine-5′-diphosphoglucose.

Besides inulin, the chicory also contains bitter sesquiterpene lactones (Figure 6.3), belonging to three major classes: Guaianolides, Eudesmanolides and Germacranolides (Table 6.1). The Sesquiterpene lactones occur throughout the plant, though at highest level in the roots (0.42 per cent dry weight). Among these, lactucopicrine and dihydrolactucopicrine were found to be more bitter than quinine hydrochloride (van Beek *et al.*, 1990). These bitter Sesquiterpene lactones were accumulated mainly as glycosides (Blaschek *et al.*, 1998; Kisiel and Zielinska, 2001). Some of the guaianolides isolated from chicory play a role in chemical defense of chicory plant as antifeedent (Ress and Harborne, 1985) and phytoalexins (Monde *et al.*, 1990; Grayer and Harborne, 1994). The (+)-Costunolide was considered as a parent compound, which on hydroxylation followed by cyclization converted into Germenacrene-A. The sesquiterpene lactones of chicory have been reported to have cytotoxic activity towards cultured cancer cells (Hladon′ *et al.*, 1978; Seto *et al.*, 1988). The chicory root extract showed antiinflammatory activity and hepatoprotective activity (Zafar and Ali, 1998; Ki *et al.*, 1999). Recently, a molecular mechanism of antiinflammatory action of sesquiterpene lactones via inhibition of transcription factors NF-kB have been proposed (Rungeler *et al.*, 1999; Han *et al.*, 2001). The

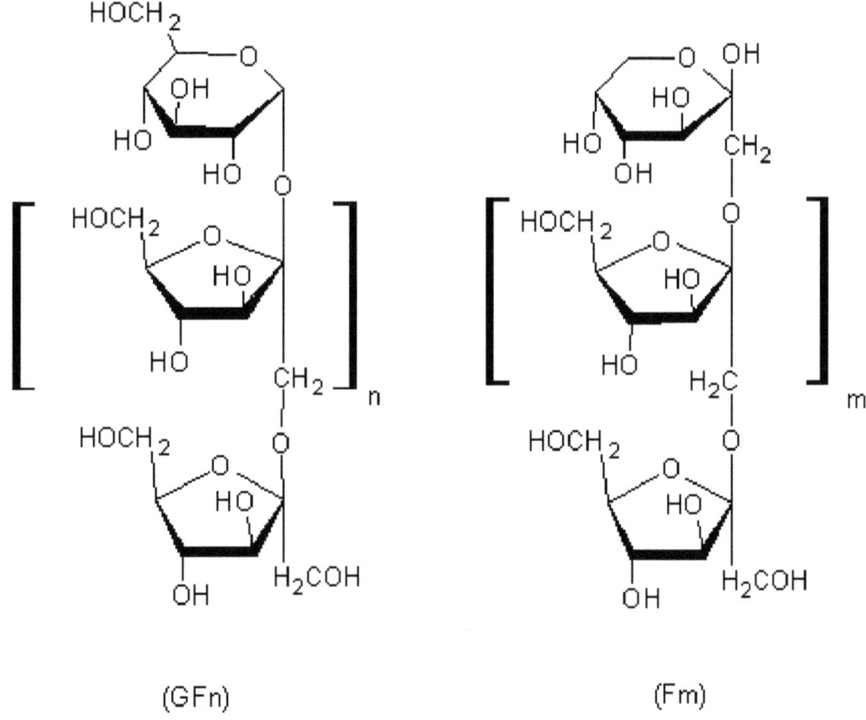

Figure 6.2: Chemical Structure of Inulin

accumulation of sesquiterpene lactones in hairy root cultures of chicory have been also studied (Malarz *et al.*, 2002).

Table 6.1: Major Sesquiterpene Lactones Reported in Chicory

Guaianolides	*Eudesmanolides*	*Germacranolides*
Lectucin,	Chicoriolide-A	Sonchuside-A,
8-deoxylectucin,	Sonchuside-C	Chicorioside-B,C
Lactucopicrin,		Germacrene-A
11(S),13-dihydrolectucin,		
11(S),13-dihydro-8-deoxylectucin		
11(S),13-dihydrolactucopicrin		

Phenolic acids having antioxidant activity were reported in the chicory roots such as L-chicoric acid, caffeic acid, dihydrocaffeic acid, chlorogenic acid, neochlorogenic acid, isochlorogenic acid, rosamaric acid, and ferulic acid (Figure 6.4). A number of flavonoids were reported namely esculatine, esculin, scopoletin, kaempferol, chicorin, jacquinelin, umbelliferone. Some other constituents reported are amino acids (lysine, leucine, methionine, threonine, tryptophan, isoleucine, histidine, arginine, valine, phenylalanine), vitamins (β-carotene, cholin, inositol, niacin, thiamine, riboflavine), and fatty acids (stearic acid, plasmatic acid, lenoleic acid, alpha-lenoleic acid, oleic acid, myristic acid) as well

Lactucin **8 - deoxylactucin** **Lactupicrin**

(A) Major guaianolide type of sesquiterpene lectones of Chicory

Sonchuside C **Cichoriolide A**

(B) Major eudesmanolide type of sesquiterpene lactones of Chicory

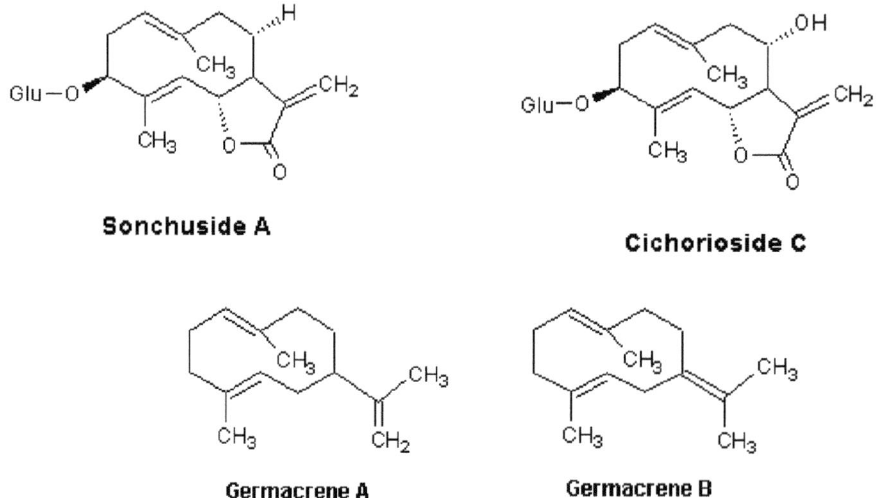

[Germacrene skeletones]

(C) Major germacranolide type of sesquiterpene lactones of Chicory

Figure 6.3: Chemical Structure of Sesqueterpene Lactones of Chicory

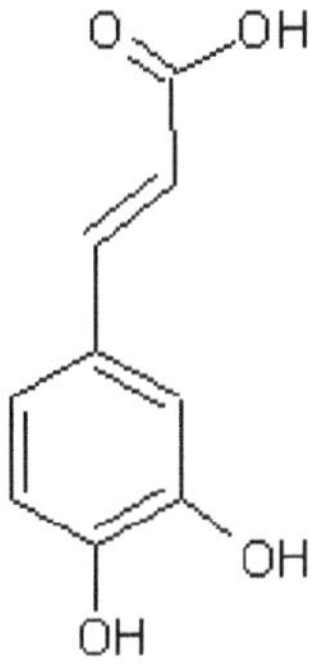

Caffeic acid
[3,4-dihydroxycinnamic acid]

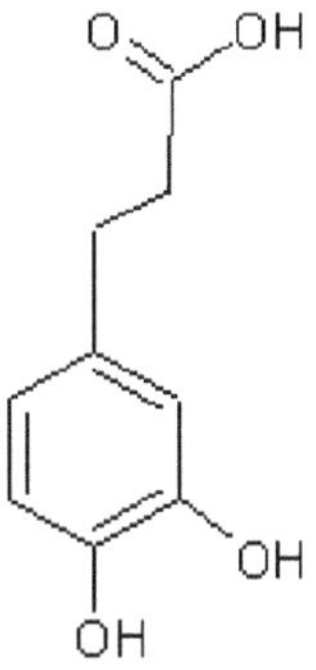

Dihydro-caffeic acid
[3,4-dihydroxy-dihydrocinnamic acid]

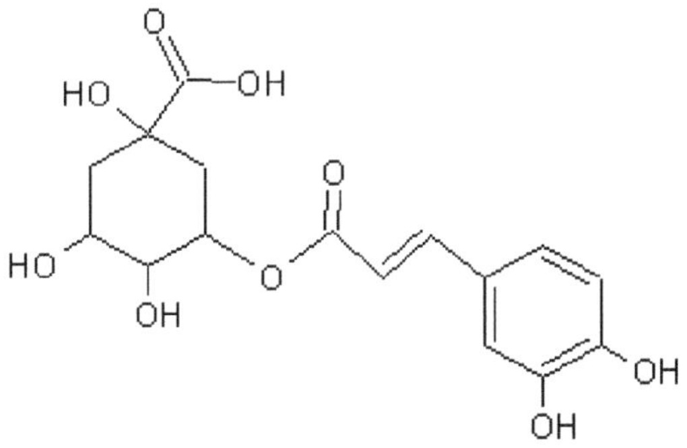

Chlorogenic acid

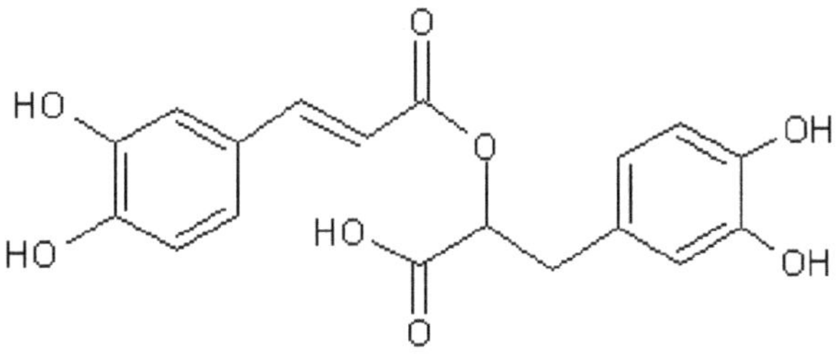

Rosamaric acid

Figure 6.4: Chemical Structure of Organic Acids Present in Chicory

as organic acids (valilic acid, p-hydroxybenzoic acid). Besides these, chicory also contains coumarins, occurring as glycosides. Hairy root culture of witloop chicory was found to produce coumarins, esculin and esculatin (Bais *et al.*, 1999).

Pharmacological Activities

Dietary Fibers and Lipid Lowering Activity

According to dietary fiber technical committee of the American association on cereal chemists (AACC), "*Dietary fiber is the edible part of plants or analogous carbohydrates that are resistant to digestion and absorption in the human small intestine with complete or partial fermentation on the large intestine. Dietary fiber includes polyssacharides, oligosaccarides, lignin and associated plant substances. Dietary fibers promote beneficial physiological effects including laxation and or blood cholesterol attenuation and/or blood glucose attenuation*". Some 36,000 plants from a variety of genera contain inulin as an energy source or as an osmoregulator assuring cold resistance. Many of commonly consumed foods were found to contain inulin (Table 6.2) (van Loo *et al.*, 1995). The food industries were able to utilize few plant species for large scale production of inulin such as Agave (*Agave azul tequllana*), Jerusalem artichoke (*Hellanthus tuberous*) and Chicory (*Cichorium intybus*). The major polysaccharide of chicory root extract was inulin–a polymer of fructose with β(2-1) glycosidic linkage, belonging to fructans family. Since inulin is soluble in water and not hydrolyzed by the digestive enzymes (Knudsen and Hessov, 1995), it was classified as a soluble dietary fiber (Roberfroid, 1993). *In vitro* hydrolysis of chicory inulin, yielded fructose and glucose. *In vitro* Inulin hydrolysis to fructose have been reported with variety of substances such as exo-inulinase or endo-inulinase (Yun *et al.*, 2000), catalysts (Motsumoto and Yurmazulkl, 1986), Zeolite (Jacob and Hinnekens, 1989; Abasaeed and Lee, 1995, 1996), activated carbon (Heinen *et al.*, 2001) or commercial inulinase (Obo'n *et al.*, 2000) like Fructozyme-L.

Table 6.2: Inulin Content (per cent of fresh weight) of Plants that are Commonly Used in Human Nutrition

Source	*Edible Parts*	*Dry solids Content*	*Inulin Content*
Onion	Bulb	6–12	2–6
Jerusalem artichoke	Tuber	19–25	14–19
Chicory	Root	20–25	15–20
Leek	Bulb	15–20	3–10
Garlik	Bilb	40–45	9–16
Artichoke	Leaves-heart	14–16	3–10
Banana	Fruit	24–26	0.3–0.7
Rye	Cereal	88–90	0.5–1
Barley	Cereal	NA	0.5–1.5
Dandelion	Leaves	50–55	12–15
Burdock	Root	21–25	3.5–4.0
Camas	Bulb	31–50	12–22
Murnong	root	25–28	8–13
Yacon	Root	13–31	3–19
Salsify	Root	20–22	4–11

NA: Data not available.

The hypolipidemic effects of soluble dietary fibers have been well established both in human (Glore *et al.*, 1994) and animals (Overtone *et al.*, 1994; de Deckere *et al.*, 1995; Tokunaga *et al.*, 1996; Roberfroid and Delzenne, 1998). The oligofructose was a non-digestible but fermentable oligomer of β-D-glucose obtained by enzymatic hydrolysis of the chicory inulin. Feeding a diet supplemented with 10 per cent oligofructose to rats have significantly lowered triglyceride (TG) and phospholipids in serum (Delzenne *et al.*, 1993; Fiordaliso *et al.*, 1995; Roberfroid and Delzenne, 1998). The hypolipidemic effects were likely due to decreased plasma VLDL levels (Fiordaliso *et al.*, 1995). Hepatocytes isolated from the oligofructose fed rats have significantly lowered capacity to esterify ($_{14}$C) palmitate into TG and a 40 per cent lower capacity to synthesize TG from ($_{14}$C) acetate (Fiordaliso *et al.*, 1995; Roberfroid and Delzenne, 1998). It has been suggested that there was a reduced *de novo* lipogenesis in liver which was a key even in reduction of VLDL triglyceride secretion in fructans fed rats. The activities of all the enzymes involved in lipogenesis like acety-CoA–carboxylase, fatty acid synthase (FAS), malic enzyme, ATP citrate lyase, glucose–6-phosphated dehydrogenase, were decreased by approximately 50 per cent in fructans fed rats. The enzyme FAS was believed to be regulated only through modification of protein and mRNA and it was the most sensitive to nutrients and hormones (Girard *et al.*, 1997). In fructans fed rats, the liver m-RNA for FAS were reduced suggesting that dietary fibers were likely to modify lipogenic enzymes gene expression and thereby produced antilipidemic effect. It has been further supported by the fact that chronic feeding of oligofructose to rats prevented triacylglycerol accumulation induced by fructose in the liver (Kok *et al.*, 1996).

When rats were fed with resistant starch, the serum TG level and FAS activity were reduced with concomitant lower post prandial insulinemia (Takase *et al.*, 1994). However, the effects of inulin type of fructans on glycemic and insulinemia were not yet fully studied. In one of study, it was observed that oligofructose given to rats at a dose of 10 per cent for 30 days have reduced post prandial glycemia and insulinemia by 7 per cent and 20 per cent respectively, suggesting that inulin type fructans reduces glucose and insulin concentration and thereby decreased induction of lipogenic enzymes gene expression (Bichard, 1997), which was mediated through insulin (Girard *et al.*, 1997). The streptozotocin-treated rats fed with a diet containing 20 per cent oligofructose for 2 months were found to show decrease in post prandial glycemia (Bichard, 1997).

Chicory inulin was fermented in large bowel into short chain carboxylic acid (SCCA) by bowel microbial flora. The production of SCCA in the large bowel of oligofructose fed rats was responsible for a more than 2 fold increase in the portal concentration of both acetate and propionate (Steinmetz and Porter, 1991; Girard *et al.*, 1997). The propionate was reported to inhibit fatty acid synthesis *in vitro* (Nishina and Freeland, 1990; Wright *et al.*, 1990; Lynn *et al.*, 1994) where as acetate was found to be lipogenic substrate. It has been suggested that the production of SCCA especially propionate by fermentation of inulin fructans was partly responsible for antilipidemic effects of oligofructose and fructans.

It was believed that the dietary fructans modify the physiology of the large bowel wall cells and thereby decreased the synthesis and release of GIP and Glucagon-like peptide-1(GLP-1) amide which in turn decreased insulin level in blood resulting in poor expression of gene coding all lipogenic enzymes and decreased *de novo* synthesis of triglycerol. GIP and Glucagon-like peptide-1(GLP-1) amide were the hormonal mediators found to be responsible for post prandial insulin release from pancreatic β-cells (Morgan, 1996) and have direct anabolic insulin like action on lipid metabolism and stimulated *de novo* lipogenesis and increase lipoprotein lipase activity (Oben *et al.*, 1991; Knapper *et al.*, 1995; Zampelas *et al.*, 1995). Thus, various mechanisms have been proposed for the hypolipidemic activity of inulin type of fructans and chicory root extract. However, none of the studies have suggested that any one mechanism was fully accounting for the hypolipidemic effect. Therefore, further investigation is required in this area, emphasizing the contribution of each mechanisms and behavior in presence of lipid lowering drugs.

Hypoglycemic Activity

Insufficient dietary fibers intake was associated with increased risk of diabetes (Trowell, 1972) or increased intake of dietary fibers reduced the risk of diabetes (Jenkins *et al.*, 1995; Chandalia *et al.*, 2000). Well fermented viscous fibers, either as a part of food or as a supplement, have reduced glycemic response (Jenkins *et al.*, 1977; Anderson *et al.*, 1987; Wolever, 1990; Jenkins *et al.*, 1999) and improved insulin sensitivity (Fukagawa *et al.*, 1990). Experimental evidence have demonstrated that the addition of viscous fibers in diet, slowed gastric emptying rates, reduced digestion and the absorption of glucose and thereby benefited immediate postprandial glucose metabolism (Kashimura *et al.*, 1996) and long-term glucose control (Buyken *et al.*, 1998; Vuksan *et al.*, 1999; Chandalia *et al.*, 2000) in individuals with diabetes mellitus. Long term ingestion of 50 g of dietary fibers per day for 24 weeks have improved glycemic control and reduced the number of hypoglycemic events in individual with type-I diabetes (Giacco *et al.*, 2000; Kalkwarf *et al.*, 2001). In pregnant women with type-1 diabetes, a higher fiber intake has been found to be associated with lower daily insulin requirement (Kalkwarf *et al.*, 2001). Studies in individuals with type-2 diabetes, have suggested that high fiber intake has diminished insulin demand (Revillese *et al.*, 1980; Simpson *et al.*, 1981). Oligofructose given to rats at a dose of 10 per cent for 30 days have reduced the post prandial glycemia and insulinemia by 77 per cent and 20 per cent respectively (Bichard, 1997). The mechanisms through which, dietary fibers affect insulin requirement or insulin sensitivity were not clear. Various mechanisms have been proposed for hypoglycemic action of dietary fibers like;

1. Change in the viscosity of small intestine after dietary fiber intake, leads to poor glucose absorption and thereby reduce immediate post prandial glucose levels.
2. Production of SCCA on fermentation of dietary fibers by microbial flora, affects the postprandial glucose levels and insulin release. Propionate is glucogenic in liver and increases blood sugar level.
3. Increased expression of the gut-derived proglucagon gene and secretion of proglucagon-derived peptides, including glucagons–like-peptide-1 (GLP-1) (Reimer and McBurney, 1996; Massimino *et al.*, 1998), which was found to reduce gastric emptying rates, promoted glucose uptake and disposal in the peripheral tissues, enhanced insulin-dependent glucose disposal, inhibited glucagon secretion and reduced hepatic glucose output in animals and humans (D'Alwessio, 2000).

Chicory inulin, being a soluble fermentable dietary fiber, was likely to improve glycemic control and reduce insulin requirement. However, experimental data on humans have shown that oral inulin did not modify insulin sensitivity (Dominique *et al.*, 2003) and in some cases even reduced insulin levels (Jackson *et al.*, 1999). However, these studies were carried out in subjects with obesity or dyslipidemia and not with the diabetes. Recently, it has been observed that dietary fibers like inulin and oligofructose have decreased the production of GLP-1 in the gut, which was further supported by the decreased lipogenic enzymes gene expression in liver. Limited data were available and some were contradictory regarding the effect of chicory inulin on glycemic control.

Anticancer Activity

Various historical observational and epidemiological studies have supported that high fiber intake protect against cancer incidences (Trock *et al.*, 1990; Steinmetz and Porter, 1991; Howe *et al.*, 1992). Prebiotic fiber sources, such as inulin, act as selective substrate for bacteria that produce specific SCFA (Green *et al.*, 1998) and can lower the intestinal pH. The butyrate has been shown to increase apoptosis in human colonic tumor cell lines (Hague *et al.*, 1993). Prebiotic cultures, such as lactic culture, have been shown to possess antimutagenic and anticarcinogenic properties (Goldin and Gorbach, 1980; Bodana and Rao, 1990; Lidbeck *et al.*, 1992). The bifidogenic and prebiotic role of chicory root extract was well established. The evidences have suggested that increased number of bifidobecteria in the colon and reduced intestinal pH have a direct impact on carcinogenesis in the large intestine (Goldin and Gorbach, 1980; Koo and Rao, 1991). Different mechanisms have been proposed for anticancer activities of dietary fibers like inulin:

1. A reduction in the production of carcinogenic substances by decreasing the amount of pathogenic bacteria in the colon (Rumney and Rowland, 1995).
2. Lowering of colonic pH to affect pH dependent enzymatic reactions, for example, secondary bile acid formation (Buddington *et al.*, 1996; Rowland *et al.*, 1998).
3. Reducing the amount of carcinogenic substances available to colonic mucosa by adsorption of the substances to the cell wall of the microbiota, by speeding up the gastrointestinal transit time and by increasing colonic content, by promoting SCFA-butyric acid (Hague *et al.*, 1993; Pool-Zobel *et al.*, 1993; Reddy and Rivenson, 1993; Verghese *et al.*, 1998).

Being bifidogenic and prebiotic, chicory was likely to be effective in colon cancer. However, no work has been reported regarding the potential of chicory root in colon cancer. The major phenolic acids present in chicory such as chicoric acid, caffeic acid and chlorogenic acid have antioxidants activities. Among these, caffeic acid and its derivative caffeic acid phenyl ester (CAPE) were strong and selective matrix metalloproteinase-9 activity and transcription inhibitors. They were found to inhibit MMP-2 and 9 selectively. Treatment of HepG2 Cells with caffeic acid (100 μg/ml) and CAPE (5 μg/ml) suppressed probol 12-Myristate 13-Acetate induced MMP-9 expression by inhibiting the function of NF-KB as well as MMP-9 catalytic activity (Chung *et al.*, 2004). NF-kB has been found to be a key transcription factor involved in the activation of genes that encode inflammatory cytokines such as the TNF-α and IL-1β. The NF-kB can induce the activation of MMP-9 and cyclooxygenase (COX-2) (Pahl, 1999; Garg and Aggarwal, 2002). Caffeic acid and CAPE were found to inhibit activities of certain enzymes such as lipoxygenase, cycloxygenase, glutathione-s-transferase and xanthin oxidase (Koshihara *et al.*, 1984; Schefferlie and van Bladeren, 1993; Mirzoeva *et al.*, 1996; Michaluart *et al.*, 1999).

Hence, the antitumor activity of chicory can be attributed to more than one mechanisms and active constituents. However, very few studies have been carried out using extract of chicory. The tumor-inhibitory effect of an ethanolic extract of chicory root was studied against ehrlich ascities carcinoma in mice and significant activity were obtained at dose from 300-700 mg/kg (Hazra *et al.*, 2002). However, the mechanism was yet not established. Aberrant crypt foci (ACF) were believed to be early indicators of colonic cancer, being preneoplastic lesions that could lead to the formation of colonic adenomas and carcinomas in humans and some animals (Reddy *et al.*, 1997). One study (Rao *et al.*, 1998) employed a colonic ACF assay to evaluate possible preventive properties of certain agents (eg. Coffee fiber, inulin and pectin) on colonic cancer and has demonstrated that inulin containing diet reduced the azoxymethane (AOM) induced effect on the number of ACF/cm^2 in the colon. Inulin was found to increase cecal sort chain fatty acids by 3-5 folds, which has been shown to increase apoptosis. The effect of *bifidobecterium longum* and inulin have been studied on ACF caused by the colon carcinogen AOM, by measuring the concentration of ammonia and urea, B-glucoranidase and B-glucoside (a known tumor promoters) and observed decrease in ammonia concentration and b-glucoranidase activity and decrease in ACF formation.

Antioxidant Activity

The inverse association between coffee intake and colon cancer was well established in some epidemiological studies (Baron *et al.*, 1994; Favero *et al.*, 1998; Giovannucci, 1998) which might be explained in part by antioxidant chlorogenic acid–an ester of caffeic acid and quinic acid, present in coffee. The chlorogenic acid and caffeic acid were found to have antioxidant activity *in vitro* (Castelluccio *et al.*, 1995, Rice-Evans *et al.*, 1996) and inhibited the formation of mutagenic and carcinogenic N-nitroso compounds *in vitro* (Kono *et al.*, 1995). The chlorogenic acid was also found to inhibit DNA damage *in vitro* (Shibata *et al.*, 1999; Kasai *et al.*, 2000). The mechanism of absorption of chlorogenic acids in humans was also well studied (Olthof *et al.*, 2001). The antioxidants activities of caffeic acid were well studied *in vitro* (Bors *et al.*, 2002; Nayeemunnisa and Kumuda Rani, 2003). Chicory roots contain caffeic acid and chlorogenic acid as major phenolic acids. Therefore, it might be expected to have antioxidant activities. However, only limited data were available. In one of the study, the cardio-protective effect of chicory leaves extract were studied on aging myocardium of albino rats and was found to activate catalase, lower lipid peroxidation and decrease taurine as well as glutathione (GSH) levels (Nayeemunnisa and Kumuda Rani, 2003).

The water soluble antioxidant properties of *cichorium intybus* var. Silvestre were investigated and evaluated *in vitro* and *ex vivo* as protective against rat liver cell microsome lipid peroxidation (Gazzani *et al.*, 2000). The effect of chicory decoction on lipid metabolism and antioxidant defend system, were studied on pancreatic functions of rats in experimental dyslipidemia (Kocsis *et al.*, 2003). The *in vitro* free radical scavenging property of chicory extract has been investigated with the help of chemiluminescence measurement and improvements were found in antioxidant status of pancreatic tissues.

Antiinflammatory Activity

Chicory is traditionally used in treatment of inflammatory conditions. However limited data were available regarding the antiinflammatory activity of chicory. Ethyl acetate extract of chicory root has produced a marked inhibition of prostaglandin E2 (PGE2) production in human colon carcinoma HT29 cells treated with the pro-inflammatory agent TNF-alpha. Two independent mechanisms of action were identified, first one is a drastic inhibition of the induction by TNF-alpha of cyclooxygenase-2 (COX-2) protein expression, and second one is a direct inhibition of COX enzyme activities with a significantly higher selectivity for COX-2 activity. The inhibition of TNF-alpha-dependent induction of COX-2 expression was mediated by an inhibition of NF-kB activation. A major sesquiterpene lactone of chicory root, the guaianolide 8-deoxylactucin, was identified as the key inhibitor of COX-2 protein expression present in chicory extract (Cavin *et al.*, 2005). However, the other constituents of chicory roots like chicoric acid and caffeic acid, were also reported to have antiinflammatory activities.

Hepatoprotective Activity

Traditionally, seeds of chicory were used for hepatic conditions and liver rejuvenation (Nadkarni, 1994). It has shown protective effects in mice with high levels of liver damaging enzymes (Gilani *et al.*, 1998). An alcoholic extract of the plant was found to be effective against chlorpromazine induced hepatic damage in adult albino rats. It also exhibited resorptive activity. In one of the study chicory roots were successively extracted with chloroform, methanol and water and subjected to preliminary phytochemical and hepatoprotective screening in rats against CCl_4 and paracetamol induced toxicity. It have been found that two components were active against CCl_4 and paracetamol induced liver toxicity (Gadgoli and Mishra, 1994). The antihepatotoxic effects of roots and root callas extract of chicory were studied in albino rats. Kasni or chicory is one of the important ingredient ofnumber of ayurvedic preparations such as Bonnisan, Geriforte, Herbolax, Liv-52, Liv-52 Digyton, Liv-52 vet, Geriforte Aqua, etc. put in to the market by Himalaya healthcare (P) Ltd. The hepatoprotective activity of herbal formulations–AV/LTP/15 and HD-03, containing chicory as one of the ingredient, have been well established (Mitra *et al.*, 1998; Agarwal, 1999).

AntiHIV Activity

Protease and reverse transcriptase (RT) inhibitors are presently used in combination for the treatments of HIV infection. However, resistance to these drugs has been reported. Hence, next target is HIV integrase. It has been found that dicaffeoylquinic acid and dicaffeyltartaric acid blocked HIV replication in tissue culture at non-toxic concentration (Robinson *et al.*, 1996a and 1996b). *In vitro* studies indicated that they were potent and selective inhibitors of HIV integrase (Robinson *et al.*, 1996a and 1996b; Mc Dougall *et al.*, 1998). These compounds exhibited 10 to 100 fold selectivity against HIV integrase over other HIV enzymes (Robinson *et al.*, 1996a). However, the mechanism of antiHIV activity was not clear. Several studies indicated that they act by inhibiting gp120 binding to CD_4 (Mahmood *et al.*, 1993) and RT (Nishizawa *et al.*, 1989; Nonaka *et al.*, 1990). L-Chicoric acid in tissue culture inhibits integrase by interacting at residues near the catalytic triad in the integrase active site (King and Robinson, 1998). The chicoric acid being one of the major phenolic acid present in chicory, it might be expected that chicory have beneficial effects in HIV–infection. However, no data were yet available.

Bile Acid Metabolism

Chicory is traditionally employed in the jaundice and for tonifying and detoxifying the livers. Chicory root extract has been reported to have mild choleretic effect. It works by increasing the flow of bile into the digestive tract and is therefore an appetizer and digestive aid (Bouhnik *et al.*, 1994). It was also found to promote bile acid excretion in stool (Kritchevsky, 1978; Kishimoto *et al.*, 1995; Trautwein *et al.*, 1998). The choleretic activity of chicory was partly attributed to polyphenolic and bitter principles and partly to inulin.

Prebiotic and Bifidogenic Activity

A prebiotic is *"a non-digestible food ingredient that beneficially affects the host by selectively stimulating the growth and/or activity of one or a limited number of bacteria in the colon that can improve the host health."* The fructans extracted from the root of *Cichorium intybus* L. were considered as a prebiotic and have been authorized as food ingredients in all European countries as well as in the U.S., Canada and Japan. These fructans–inulin and oligofructose were fermented in the large intestine and metabolized by enzymes from bacteria such as saccharolytic Clostridia, bacteroids and bigfidobacteria. The bifidobacteria is preferred target microorganism for prebiotic (Gibson *et al.*, 1995) as they comprised one of the dominant bacterial populations in the human large intestine and exerted a variety of effects beneficial to host health. *In vitro* fermentation of chicory inulin and oligofructose was well studied using human colonic bacteria (Wada, 1990; Wang, 1993; Wang and Gibson, 1993). The bifidogenic nature of chicory inulin and its hydrolysate was well studied *in vivo* using human volunteers (Kleessen *et al.*, 1994; Bouhnik *et al.*, 1996; Kleessen *et al.*, 1997). Volunteers fed a diet supplemented with 4, 8 or 12.5 g chicory oligosaccharides per day shown a significant increase in bifidobacteria in feces. However, most of the studies have utilized only the bifidobacterial count and did not give information on counts of other bacterial genera. The bifidogenic nature of chicory was partly accounted for variety of physiological effects like hypolipidemic, hypoglycemic, anticancer, etc.

Gastrointestinal Activities

The 1997 Commision E on phytotherapy and herbal substances of the German Federal Institute for Drugs recommended chicory, "the dried, above ground parts and / or roots" for loss of appetite and dyspepsia. It increases bile acid flow into the digestive tract and act as appetizer and digestive aid.

However, no firm data were available regarding the effects of chicory root extract on appetite and food consumption. It might be believed that the bitter principles of chicory root have stomachic action. However, the beneficial effects of chicory root extract on the irritable bowel syndrome were well reported.

It is known that chicory inulin and oligofructose affect bowel functions. Daily dose of inulin ranging between 4-15 g, did not affect the gastrointestinal transit time but increased stool frequency and have a faecal bulking effect, about 1.5 to 2 g per g of inulin ingested (Hond *et al.*, 2002). In elderly people, chicory inulin had a moderate laxative effect and relieving constipation with only mild discomfort (Kleessen *et al.*, 1997). Chicory inulin and oligofructose increased stool frequency especially when the initial stool frequency was low (Gibson *et al.*, 1995). Inulin has been found to increase bowel frequency by about 1.6 times (Tramonte *et al.*, 1997), but did not affect intestinal permeability (Sokotka *et al.*, 1997).

Table 6.3: Traditional Non-medicinal Uses of Chicory

Homeopathic	Used for Amblyopia, constipation, headache.
Veterinary	Has been used to calm nervous conditions; also for general debility, loss of appetite, liver problems, and jaundice.
Flower remedy	Chicory 'essence' is prepared from the flowers. A few drops of liquid have been used for 'crying jags' or for those who were overly possessive or critical of others, or just plain overbearing and controlling; also for those with 'martyr' syndrome.
Culinary	It is often found as a blanched winter vegetable in markets. The forced heads were placed in salt water for several minutes, then drained and added to a pot in water with a bit of butter; boiled gently for 1 hour, or until tender and served with white or cheese sauce. Young leaves picked before flowering were used fresh like spinach or in salad, stir fries and sautes. The stalks have been blanched while growing and eaten like celery. Flowers used raw in salads and for jelly; also candied and used for cake decoration. Root can also be eaten raw or dried and ground for flour (unroasted root); also as a tea made from the cut, dried root. The root has also been cooked and eaten like carrot.
Coffee substitute	Roots were dug, dried and ground and used as a coffee substitute or added to coffee Young spring roots were considered best by some while others prefer the fall dug root. They were washed, dried, then roasted in a slow oven at 200º to 225ºF for 1 to 4 hours, or until roots were thoroughly dry. They were then cooled and ground in a coffee grinder and stored and used as coffee or combined with coffee.
Cosmetic	An infusion of the flowering tops has been used as a skin cleanser.
Animal feed	Provides feed for livestock.
Gardening	Because of the unusual feature of opening and closing its petals at predictable times, it is used in Floral Clocks.
Dye	The leaves and blossoms produce mustard yellow with an alum mordant; brassy gold with chrome; yellow-green with copper; bright yellow with tin; forest green with iron; creamy beige with no mordant.

Miscellaneous Activities

Chicory was believed to have depressant effect on the CNS. It antagonized the stimulant effect of coffee. The bitter principles of chicory were believed to be responsible for these effects. However, no animal or human data were yet available. Chicory also has depressant effect on the myocardium and pressure effect on the blood pressure. It also modifies immune response and has antimicrobial activities.

Therapeutic Application

According to the traditional ayurvedic system of medicine; the plant is bitter, acrid, thermogenic, antiinflammatory, appetizer, digestive, stomachic, liver tonic, cholegogue, cardiotonic, depurative, diuretic, emmenagogue, febrifuge, alexeteric, and tonic. It is useful in vitiated conditions of *Kapha* and *pitta*, cephalalgia, hepatomegaly, inflammations, anorexia, dyspepsia, flatulence, colic, gout, burning sensation, allergic conditions of the skin, insomnia, jaundice, splenomegaly, hyperdipsia, skin diseases, Leprosy, strangury, amenorrhoea, chronic and bilious fevers, ophthalmia, pharyngitis, vomiting, diarrhea, arthralgia, lumbago, asthma and general debility (Prajapati *et al.*, 2004). Besides medicinal and commercial uses, it is also used traditionally for various purposes (Table 6.3).

Contraindications, Interactions and Side Effects

In proper therapeutic dosages, chicory is safe. Commission E reported contraindications of hypersensitivity to chicory and other Asteraceae and adverse effects of rare allergic skin reactions. Patients with bilestones or gallstones should first consult a physician. An occupational allergy to chicory has been found in vegetable wholesaler on oral, cutaneous or inhalatory exposure due to presence of allergenic protein. The carcinogens *viz.* 1,2-benzoperylene, 3,4-benzopyrone and floranthene occurred in chicory and their content increases on roasting, especially above 175°.

References

Abasaeed, A.E, and Lee, Y.Y. (1995). Inulin hydrolysis to fructose by a novel catalyst. *Chem. Eng. Tech.*, 18: 440-444.

Abasaeed, A.E, and Lee, Y.Y. (1996). Kinetics of inulin hydrolysis by zeolite LZ-M-8. *Hung. J. Indust. Chem.*, 24:149-153.

Agarwal, A. (1999). Therapeutic efficacy of AV/LTP/15 in hepatic dysfunction in dogs. *Ind. Veterinary Medical Journal*, 23(3): 245-247.

Anderson, J.W., Gustafson, N.J., Bryant, C.A., Tietyn, J.-C. (1987). Dietary fiber and diabetes: A comprehensive review and practical applications. *J. Amer. Diet. Asso.*, 87(9):1189-1197.

Bais, H.P., Sudha, G., and Ravishankar, G.A. (1999). Putrescine influences growth and production of coumarins in hairy root cultures of witloof chicory (*Cichorium intybus* L. cv. Lucknow local). *J. Plant Growth Regul.*, 18: 159-165.

Baron, J.A., Gerhardsson de Verdier, M., and Ekbom, A. (1994). Coffee, tea, tobacco, and cancer of the large bowel. Cancer Epidemiol. Biomark. Prev., 3: 565-570.

Baumann, H. (1982). Die griechische Pflanzenwelt in Mythos, Kunst und Literature, Hirmer, Munich, pp.82.

Bichard, S. (1997). Influence de measures nutritionnelles sur l'homeostasie glucidique du rat diabetique. Effects benefiques des fructo-oligosaccharides et du vanadium. PhD Thesis, Universite Catholique de Louvain, Belgium.

Blaschek, W., Hansel, R., Keller, K., Reichling, J., Rimpler, H., and Schneider, G. (1998). Hager handbuch der Pharmazcutischen Praxis. Vol: 1 Springer Publisher, Berlin, pp: 865-871.

Bodana, A.R., and Rao, D.R. (1990). Antimutagenic activity of milk fermented by Streptococcus thermophilus and Lactobacillus bulgaricus. *J. Dairy Sci.*, 73: 3379-3384.

Bors, W., Michel, C., Stettmaier, K., Lu, Y.R., and Foo, L.Y. (2002). Pulse radiolysis, EPR spectroscopy and theoretical calculations of caffeic acid oligomer radicals. *Biochim. Biophys. Acta.*, 1620: 97-107.

Bouhnik, Y., Flourié, B., Andrieux, C., Bisetti, N., Briet, F., and Rambaud, J.C. (1996). Effects of Bifidobacterium sp. fermented milk ingestion with or without inulin on colonic bifidobacteria and enzymatic activities in healthy humans. *Eur. J. Clin. Nutr.*, 50: 269-273.

Bouhnik, Y., Flourié, B., Ouarne, F., Riottot, M., Bisetti, N., Bornet, F. and Rambaud, J. C. (1994). Effects of prolonged ingestion of fructo-oligosaccharides (FOS) on colonic Bifidobacteria, faecal enzymes and bile acids in humans. *Gastroenterology.*, 106: A598.

Buddington, R.K., Williams, C.H., Chen, S.–C., and Witherly, S.A. (1996). Dietary supplement of neosugar alters the fecal flora and decreases activities of some reductive enzymes in human subjects. *Am. J. Clin. Nutr.*, 63: 709-716.

Buyken, A.E., Toeller, M., Heitkamp, G., Vitelli, F., Stehle, P., Scherbaum, W.A., Fuller, J.H., and The EURODIAB IDDM Complication Study Group. (1998). Relation of fiber intake to HbA1c and the prevalence of severe ketoacidosis and severe hypoglycemia. *Diabetologia*, 41:882-890.

Castelluccio, C., Paganga, G., Melikian, N., Bolwell, G.P., Pridham, J., Sampson, J., and Rice, E.C. (1995). Antioxidant potential of intermediates in phenylpropanoid metabolism in higher plants. *FEBS Lett.*, 368: 188-192.

Cavin, C., Delannoy, M., Malnoe, A., Debefve, E., Touche, A., Courtois, D., and Schilter, B. (2005). Inhibition of the expression and activity of cyclooxygenase-2 by chicory extract. *Biochem. Biophys. Res. Commun.*, 327(3): 742-749.

Chandalia, M., Garg, A., Lutjohann, D., von Bergmann, K., Grundy, S.M., and Brinkley, L.J. (2000). Beneficial effects of high dietary fiber intake in patients with type-2 diabetes mellitus. *N. Engl. J. Med.*, 342(19):1392-1398.

Chandalia, M., Garg, A., Lutjohann, D., vonBergmann, K., Grundy, S.M., and Brinkley, L.J. (2000). Beneficial effects pf high dietary fiber intake in patients with type-2 diabetes mellitus. *N. Eng. J. Med.*, 342:1392-1398.

Chandra, S., and Kumari, D. (2005). Chicory: a medicinal plant used as coffee substitute. *Agrobios Newsletter*, (5):53-55.

Chung, T., Lee, Y., and Kim, C. (2004). Hepatitis B viral HBx induces matrix mtalloproteinase-9 gene expression through activation of ERKs and PI-3K/AKT pathways: Involvement of invasive potential. *FASEB J.*, 18: 1123-1125.

Clarke, R. J., and R. Macrae, R. (1987). Coffee Related beverages. *vol.5*. Elsevier Applied Science Publishers. London and New York.

D'Alwessio, D. (2000). Glucagon–like peptide1 (GLP-1) in diabetes and aging. *J. AntiAging Med.*, 3: 329-333.

de Deckere, E.A., Kloots, W., and Van Amelsvoort, J.M. (1995). Both raw and retrograded starch decrease serum triacylglycerol concentration and fat accretion in the rat. *Br. J. Nutr.*, 73:287-298.

Delzenne, N., and Roberfroid, M.B. (1994). Physiological effects of nondigestible oligosaccharides. Lebensm. *Wiss. u. Technol.*, 27:1–6.

Delzenne, N., Kok, N., Fiordaliso, M., Deboyser, D., Goethals, F., and Roberfroid, M. (1993). Dietary fructo-oligosaccharides modify lipid metabolism in rats. *Am. J. Clin. Nutr.*, 57(S): 820S.

Dominique, L., Frédérique, D., and Michel, B. (2003). Addition of inulin to a moderately high-carbohydrate diet reduces hepatic lipogenesis and plasma triacylglycerol concentrations in humans. *Am. J. Clin. Nutr.*, 77: 559-564.

Doorenbos, J., and Riemens, P.C. (1959). Effect of vernalization and daylength on number and shape of leaves in chicory and endive. *Acta. Bot. Neerl.*, 8:63-67.

Favero, A., Francesch,i S., La Vecchia, C., Negri, E., Conti, E., and Montella, M. (1998). Meal frequency and coffee intake in colon cancer. *Nutr. Cancer*, 30: 182-185.

Fiordaliso, M., Kok, N., Desager, J.P., Goethals, F., Deboyser, D., Robersfroid, M., and Delzenne N. (1995). Dietary oligofructose lowers triacylglycerides, phospholipids and cholesterol in serum and VLDL of rats. *Lipids*, 30: 163-167.

Franke, W. (1981). *Nutzpflanzenkunde*, Thieme, Stuttgart.

Fukagawa, N.K., Anderson, J.W., Hageman, G., Young, V.R., and Minaker, K.L. (1990). High-carbohydrate, high-fiber diets increase peripheral insulin sensitivity in healthy young and old adults. *Am. J. Clin. Nutr.*, 52:524-528.

Gadgoli, C.H., and Mishra, S.H. (1994). Antihepatotoxic activity of *Cichorium intybus*. *J. Ethnopharmaco*, 58: 131-134.

Garg, A., and Aggarwal, B.B. (2002). Nuclear transcription factor-kappaB as a target for cancer drug development. *Leukemia*, 16: 1053-1068.

Gazzani, G., Daglia, M., Papetti, A., and Gregotti, C. (2000). *In vitro* and *ex vivo* anti and pro-oxidant components of Cichorium intybus. *J. Pharm. Biomed. Anal.*, 3: 127-133.

Giacco, R., Parillo, M., Rivellese, A.A., Lasorella, G., Giacco, A., D'Episcopo, L., and Riccardi, G. (2000). Long-term dietary treatment with increased amounts of fiber–rich low glycemic index natural foods improves blood glucose control and reduces the number of hypoglycemic events in type-1 diabetic patients. *Diabetes Care*, 23:1461-1466.

Gianquinto, G., and Pimpini, F. (1989). The influence of temperature on growth, bolting and yield of chicory cv. Rosso di chioggia (*Cichorium intybus* L.). *J. Hortic. Sci.*, 64:687-695.

Gibson, G.R., Beatty, E.R., Wang, X., and Cummings, J.H. (1995). Selective stimulation of bifidobacteria in the human colon by oligofructose and inulin. *Gatroenterology*, 108: 975-982.

Gilani, A.H., Janbaz, K.H., and Shah, B.H. (1998) Esculetin prevents liver damage induced by paracetamol and CCl_4. *Pharmacol. Rev.*, 37(1): 31-35.

Giovannucci, E. (1998). Meta-analysis of coffee consumption and risk of colorectal cancer. *Am. J. Epidemiol.*, 147: 1043-1052.

Girard, J., Ferr'e, P., and Foufelle, F. (1997). Mechanisms by which carbohydrates regulate expression of genes for glycolytic and lipogenic enzymes. *Ann. Rev. Nutr.*, 17: 325-352.

Girard, J., Ferr'e, P., and Foufelle, F. (1997). Mechanisms by which carbohydrates regulate expression of genes for glycolytic and lipogenic enzymes. *Ann. Rev. Nutr.*, 17: 325-352.

Glore, S.R.; Van Treeck, D.; Knehans, A.W., and Guild, M. (1994). Soluble fiber and serum lipids: a literature review. *J. Amer. Diet. Asso.*, 94(4):425-436.

Goldin, B.R., and Gorbach, S.L. (1980). Effect of *Lactobacillus acidophilus* dietary supplements on 1,2-dimethylhydrazine dihydrochloride-induced intestinal cancer in rats. *J. Natl. Cancer Inst.*, 64: 263-265.

Grayer, R.J., and Harborne, J.B. (1994). A survey of antifungal compounds from higher plants 1982-1993. *Phytochemistry*, 37:19-42.

Green, C.J., Van Hoeij, K.A., and Bindels, J.G. (1998). Short chain fatty acid (SCFA) and gas production of individual fiber sources and a mix typical to a normal diet using an *in vitro* technique. *J. Pediatr. Gastroenterol. Nutr.*, 26:591-597.

Hague, A., Manning, A.M., Hanlon, K.A., Hutschtscha, L.I., Hart, D., and Paraskeva, C. (1993). Sodium butyrate induces apoptosis in human colonic tumor cell lines in 53-independent pathway: implications for possible role of dietary fiber in the prevention of large bowel cancer. *Int. J. Cancer*, 55: 498–505.

Hague, A., Manning, A.M., Hanlon, K.A., Hutschtscha, L.I., Hart, D., and Paraskeva, C. (1993). Sodium butyrate induces apoptosis in human colonic tumor cell lines in 53-independent pathway: implications for possible role of dietary fiber in the prevention of large bowel cancer. *Int. J. Cancer*, 55: 498–505.

Han, J.W., Lee, B.G., Kim, Y.K., Yoon, J.W., Jin, H.K., Hong, S., Lee, H.Y., Lee, K.R., and Lee, H.W. (2001). Ergolide Sesquiterpene lactones from Inula Britannica, inhibits inducible nitric oxide synthase and cyclo-oxygenase-2 expression in RAW 264.7 macrophages through the inactivation of NF-kB. *Br. J. Pharmacol*, 133: 503-512.

Hazra, B., Sarkar, R., Bhuttacharya, S., and Roy, P. (2002). Tumor inhibitory activity of chicory root extract against ehrlich ascities carcinoma in mice. *Fitoterapia*, 73 (7-8): 730-733.

Heinen, A.W., Peters, J.A., and van Bekkam, H. (2001). Combined hydrolysis and hydrogenation of inulin catalyzed by bifunctional Ru:C. *Carbohydrate Research*, 330: 381-390.

Hladon', B., Drozdz, B., Holub, M., Szafarek, P., and Klimaszewska, O. (1978). Sesquiterpene lactones (SL) part XXIV. Further studies on cytotoxic activities of SL in tissues culture of human cancer cells. *Pol. J. Pharmacol. Pharm.*, 30: 611-620.

Hond, E.D., Geypens, B., and Ghosse, Y. (2002). Effect of high performance chicory inulin on constipation. *Nutrition. Research*, 20(5): 731-736.

Howe, G.R., Benito, E., and Castello, R. (1992). Dietary intake of fiber and decreased risk of cancers of the colon and rectum: evidence from the combined analysis of 13 case-control studies. *J. Natl. Cancer Inst.*, 84:1887-1896.

Jackson, K.G., Taylor, G.R., Clohessy, A.M., and Williams, C.M. (1999). The effect of the daily intake of inulin on fasting lipid, insulin and glucose concentrations in middle-aged men and women. *Br. J. Nutr.*, 82(1):23-30.

Jacob, P.A., and Hinnekens, H. (1989). Single step catalytic process for the direct conversion of polysaccharides to polyhydric alcohols. *European Patent*, EP329923.

Jenkins, D.J.A., Jenkins, A.L., Wolever, T.M.S., Vuksan, V., Rao, A.V., Thompson, L.U., and Josse, R.G. (1995). Dietary fiber, carbohydrate metabolism and diabetes. *In: Dietary Fiber in Health and Disease.* Ed. By Kritchevsky, D., Bonfield, C., and Anderson, J.W., NY: Plenum Press, New York, pp.137–145.

Jenkins, D.J.A., Jenkins, A.L., Wolever, T.M.S., Vuksan, VRao, A.V., Thompson, L.U., and Josse, R.G. (1995). Dietary fibers, carbohydrate metabolism and diabetes. *In: Dietary fibers in health and disease,*Ed. By Kritchevsky, D., and C. Bonfield, C., MN: Egan Press, St. Paul, pp.137-145.

Jenkins, D.J.A., Jenkins, A.L., Wolver, T.M.S., Vuksan, V. (1999). Fiber and physiological and potentially therapeutic effects of slowing carbohydrate absorption. *In: New development in dietary fiber: Physiological, physiocochemical, and Analytical aspects.* Ed. By Ivan Furda and Charles J.B., NY: Plenum Press, New York, pp. 129-134.

Jenkins, D.J.A., Leeds, A.R., Gassull, M.A., Cochet, B., and Alberti, K.G.M.M. (1977). Decrease in postprandial insulin and glucose concentrations by guar and pectin. *Ann. Int. Med.,* 86:20-23.

Kalkwarf, H.J., Bell, R.C., Khoury, J.C., Gouge, A.L., and Miodovnik, M. (2001). Dietary fibers intakes and insulin requirements in pregnant women with type–1 diabetes. *J. Am. Diet. Assoc.,* 101:305-310.

Kasai, H., Fukada, S., Yamaizumi, Z., Sugie, S., and Mori, H. (2000). Action of chlorogenic acid in vegetables and fruits as an inhibitor of 8-hydroxydeoxyguanosine formation *in vitro* and in a rat carcinogenesis model. *Food Chem. Toxicol.,* 38: 467-471.

Kashimura, J., Kimura, M., and Itokawa, Y. (1996). The effects of isomaltulose, isomalt, and isomaltulose-based oligomers on mineral absorption and retention. *Bio. Trace. Elem. Res.,* 54:349-350.

Ki, C.-G., Yim, D.-S., and Lee, S.Y. (1999). Biological activities of the root of *Cichorium intybus* L. *Nat. Prod. Sci.,* 5:155-158.

King, P.J., and Robinson, W.E.Jr. (1998). Resistance to the AntiHuman Immunodeficiency Virus Type 1 Compound L-Chicoric Acid Results from a Single Mutation at Amino Acid 140 of Integrase. *J. Virology,* 72(10): 8420-8424.

Kishimoto, Y., Wakabayashi, S., and Takeda, H. (1995). Hypocholesterolemic effect of dietary fiber: relation to intestinal fermentation and bile acid excretion. *J. Nutr. Sci. Vitaminol.,* 41(1): 151-161.

Kisiel, W., and Zielinska, K. (2001). Guaianolides from *Cichorium intybus* and structure revision of Cichorium sesquiterpene lactones. *Phytochemistry.* 57: 523-527.

Kleessen, B., Sykura, B., Zunft, H. J., and Blaut, M. (1994). Effect of inulin on colonic Bifidobacteria of elderly man. *FASEB J.,* 8: A185.

Kleessen, B., Sykura, B., Zunft, H. J., and Blaut, M. (1997). Effects of inulin and lactose on faecal microflora, microbial activity, and bowel habit in elderly constipated persons. *Am. J. Clin. Nutr.,* 65: 1397-1402.

Knapper, J.M.E., Puddicombe, S.M. and Morgan, L.M. (1995). Enteroinsular hormones glucose dependent insulinotropic polypeptide and glucagons-like peptide-1 (7-36) amide; effects on lipoprotein lipase activity in explants of rat adipose tissue. *J. Nutr.,* 125:183-188.

Knudsen, K.E.B., and Hessov, I. (1995). Recovery of inulin from Jerusalem artichoke (*Helianthus tuberous* L.) in the small intestine of man. *Br. J. Nutr.,* 74:101-113.

Kocsis, I., Hagymasi, K., Kery, A., Szoke, E., and Blazovics, A. (2003). Effect of chicory on pancreatic status of rats in experimental dyslipidemia. *Acta Biologica. Szegediensis,* 47(1-4): 143-146.

Kok, N., Roberfroid, M., and Delzenne, N. (1996). Dietary OFS modifies the impact of fructose on hepatic triacylglycerole metabolism. *Metabolism,* 45: 1547-1550.

Kono, Y., Shibata, H., Kodama, Y., and Sawa, Y. (1995). The suppression of the N-nitrosating reaction by chlorogenic acid. *Biochem. J.*, 312: 947-953.

Koo, M., and Rao, A.V. (1991). Long-term effect of Bifidobacteria and neosugar on precursor lesions of colonic cancer in CF1 mice. *Nutr. Cancer*, 16: 249-257.

Koshihara, Y., Neichi, T., Murota, S., Lao, A., Fujimoto, Y., and Tatsuno, T. (1984). Caffeic acid is a selective inhibitor for leukotriene biosynthesis. *Biochim. Biophys. Acta.*, 792: 92-97.

Kritchevsky, D. (1978). Influence of dietary fiber on bile acid metabolism. *Lipids*, 13(12): 982-985.

Lidbeck, A., Nord, C.E., Gutafsson, J.-A. and Rafter, J. (1992). Lactobacilli, anticarcinogenic activities and human intestinal microflora. *Eur. J. Cancer Prev.*, 1: 341-353.

Lynn, M.E., Mathers, J.C., and Parker, D.S. (1994). Increasing luminal viscosity stimulates crypt cell proliferation throughout the gut. *Proc. Nutr. Soc.*, 3: 227A.

Mac Grogor, E.A., and Greenwood, C.T. (1980). Polymers in nature. John Wiley and Sons, New York.

Mahmood, N., Moore, P.S., De Tommasi, N., De Simone, F., Colman, S., Hay, A.J., and Pizza, C. (1993). Inhibition of HIV infection by Caffeoylquinic acid derivatives. *Antimicrob. Agents Chemother.*, 4: 235-240.

Malarz, J, Stajakowska, A., and Kisiel, W. (2002). Sesquiterpene lactones in a hairy root culture of *cichoriyum intybus. Z. Naturforsch.*, 57c:994-997.

Marlett, J.A. (2001). Dietary fibers and cardiovascular disease. *In:* Hand book of dietary fibers. Ed. By Cho, S.S., Dreher, M.L., Marcel Dekker, Inc., New York, pp.17-30.

Massimino, S.P., McBurney, M.I., Field, C.J., Thomson, A.B.R., Pospisil, L., Keelan, M., Hayek, M.G., and Sunvold, G.D. (1998). Fermentable fiber increases GLP-1 secretion and improves glucose homeostasis despite increased intestinal glucose transport capacity in healthy dogs. *J. Nutr.*, 128:1786-1793.

Mc Dougall, B., King, P.J., Wu, B.W., Hostomasky, Z., Reinecke, M.G., and Robinson, W.E. Jr. (1998). Dicaffeoylquinic and dicaffeoyltartatic acids are selective inhibitors of human immunodeficiency virus type-1 integrase. *Antimicrob. Agents Chemother.*, 42: 140-146.

Michaluart, P., Masferrer, J.L., Carothers, A.M., Subbaramaiah, K., Zweifel, B.S., Koboldt, C., Mestre, J.R., Grunberger, D., Sacks, P.G., Tanabe, T., and Dannenberg, A.J. (1999). Inhibitory effects of caffeic acid phenethyl ester (CAPE) on the activity and expression of cyclooxygenase-2 in human oral epithelial cells and in a rat model of inflammation. *Cancer Res.*, 59: 2347-2352.

Mirzoeva, O.K., Yaqoob, P., Knox, K.A., Calder, P.C. (1996). Inhibition of ICE family cysteine proteases rescues murine lymphocytes from lipoxygenase inhibitor-induced apoptosis. *FEBS Lett.*, 396: 266-270.

Mitra, S.K., Venkataranganna, M.V., Sundaram, R., and Gopumadhavan, S. (1998). Protective effect of HD-03, a herbal formulation, against various hepatotoxic agents in rats. *J. Ethnopharmacol.*, 63(3): 181-186.

Monde, K., Oya, T., Shira, A., and Takasugi, M. (1990). A guaianolide phytoalexin, cichoralexin from *Cichorium intybus. Phytochemistry*, 29:3449-3451.

Morgan, L.M. (1996). The metabolic role of GIP: physiology and pathology. *Biochem. Soc. Trans.*, 24:585-591.

Motsumoto, K., and Yurmazulkl, H. (1986). Production of fructose syrups. *US Patent* US4613377.

Nadkarni, A.K. (1994). Indian material medica, vol: 1, popular prakashan, Bombay, pp. 313-314.

Nayeemunnisa, and Kumuda Rani, M. (2003). Cytoprotective effects of C. intybus in ageing myocardium of albino rats. *Current Science*, 84(7): 941-943.

Nishina, P., and Freeland, R. (1990). Effects of propionate on lipid biosynthesis in isolated hepatocytes. *Hepatology*, 16: 1350-1356.

Nishizawa, M., Yamagishi, T., Dutschman, G.E., Parke, W.B., Bonder, A.J., Kilkuskie, R.E., Cheng, Y.C., and Lee, K.H. (1989). AntiAIDS agents, 1, isolation and characterization of four new tetragalloylquinic acids as a new class of HIV reverse transcriptase inhibitors from tannic acid. *J. Nat. Prod.*, 52: 762-768.

Nonaka, G.I., Nishizawa, M., Yamagishi, T., Kashiwada, Y., Dutschman, G.E., Bonder, A., Kilkuskie, RE., Cheng, Y.-C., and Lee, K.-H. (1990). AntiAIDS agents, 2, inhibitory effects of tannins on HIV reverse transcriptase and HIV replication in Hg lymphocyte cells. *J. Nat. Prod.*, 53: 589-595.

Oben, J., Morgan, L.M., Fletcher, J., and Marks, V. (1991). Effect of the entero-pancreatic hormones, gastric inhibitory polypeptide and glucagon-like polypeptide-1(7-36) amide on fatty acid synthesis in explants of rat adipose tissue. *J. Endocrinol.*, 130:267-272.

Obo'n, J.M., Castellar, M.R., Iborra, J.L., and Manjon. (2000) B-Galactosidase immobilized for milk lactose hydrolysis a simple experimental and midelling study of batch and continuous reactors. *Biochemical Education*, 28:164-168.

Olthof, M.R., Hollman, P.C.H., and Katan, M.B. (2001). Chlorogenic acid and caffeic acid are absorbed in humans. *Journal of Nutrition*, 131: 66-71.

Overtone, P., Furlonger, N., Beety, J., *et al.* (1994). The effects of dietary sugar-beet fiber and guar gum on lipid metabolism in wistar rats. *Br. J. Nutr.*, 72:385-395.

Pahl, H.L. (1999). Activators and target genes of Rel/NF-kappaB transcription factors. *Oncogene*, 18(49): 6853-6866.

Pazola, Z. (1987). The chemistry of chicory and chicory product beverages. *In:* Coffee. Vol. 5: *Related Beverages*. Ed. By Clarke R.J., and Macrae, R., NY: Elsevier Applied Sciences Publishers; New York, pp.19-57.

Pool-Zobel, B.L., Bertram, B., Knoll, M., Lambertz, R., Neudecker, C., Schillinger, U., Schmezer, P., and Holzapfel, W.H. (1993). Antigenotoxic properties of lactic acid bacteria *in vivo* in the gastrointestinal tract of rats. *Nutr. Canc.*, 20: 271-281.

Prajapati, N.D., Purohit, S.S., Sharma, A., and Kumar, T. (2004). Section–II: Medicinal plants A to Z., *In: A Handbook of Medicinal Plants*. Agrobios, Jodhpur, India, pp. 139-140.

Rao, C.V., Chou, D., Simi, B., Ku, H., and Reddy, B.S. (1998). Prevention of colonic aberrant cript foci and modulation of large bowel microbial activity by dietary coffee fiber, inulin and pectin. *Carcinogenesis*, 19:1815-1819.

Reddy, B.S., and Rivenson, A. (1993). Inhibitory effect of Bifidobacterium longum on colon, mammary and liver carcinogenesis induced by 2-amino-3-methylimidazo [4,5f] quinoline, a food mutagen. *Cancer Res.*, 53: 3914-3918.

Reddy, B.S., Hamid, R., and Rao, C.V. (1997). Effect of dietary oligofructose and inulin on colonic preneoplastic aberrant cript foci inhibition. *Carcinogenesis,* 18: 1371-1374.

Reimer, R.A., and McBurney, M.I. (1996). Dietary fiber modulates intestinal proglucagon mRNA and postprandial secretion of GLP-1 and Insulin in Rats. *Endocrinol.,* 137: 3948-3956.

Ress, S.B. and Harborne, J.B. (1985). The role of Sesquiterpene lactones and phenolics in the chemical defense of the chicory plant. *Phytochemistry,* 24:2225-2231.

Revillese, A., Riccardi, G., Giacco, A., Pacioni, D., Genovese, S., Mattioli, P., and Mancini, M. (1980). Effect of dietary fiber on glucose control and serum lipoprotein in diabetic patients. *Lancet,* ii :447-477.

Rice-Evans, C.A., Miller, N.J., and Paganga, G. (1996). Structure-antioxidant activity relationships of flavonoids and phenolic acids. *Free Radic. Biol. Med.,* 20: 933–956.

Roberfroid, M.B. (1993). Dietary fiber, Inulin and Oligofructose: a review comparing their physiological effects. *Crit. Rev. Food. Sci. Technol.,* 33:103-148.

Roberfroid, M.B., and Delzenne, N.M. (1998). Dietary fructans. *Annu. Rev. Nutr.,* 18:117-143.

Robinson, W.E.Jr., Cordeiro, M., Abdel-Malek, S., Jia, Q., Chow, S.A., Reinecke, M.G., and Mitchell, W.M. (1996a). Dicaffeoylquinic acid inhibitors of human immunodeficiency virus (HIV) integrase: inhibition of the core catalytic domain of HIV integrase. *Mol. Pharmacol.,* 50: 846-855.

Robinson, W.E.Jr., Reinecke, M.G., Abdel-Malek, S., Jia, Q. and Chow, S.A. (1996b). Inhibitors of HIV-1 replication that inhibit HIV integrase. *Proc. Natl. Acad. Sci. USA.,* 93: 6326-6331.

Rowland, I.R., Rumney, C.J., Coutts, J.T., and Lievense, L.C. (1998). Effect of Bifidobacterium longum and inulin on gut bacterial metabolism and carcinogen-induced aberrant crypt foci in rats. *Carcinogenesis,* 19: 281-285.

Rumball, W. (1986).Grasslands Puna Chicory (*Cichorium intybus* L.) *N.Z.J. Exp. Agric.* 14:105-107.

Rumney, C., and Rowland, I.R. (1995). Nondigestible oligosaccharides–potential anticancer agents? *BNF Nutr. Bull.,* 20: 194-203.

Rungeler, P., Castro, V., Mora, G., Goren, N., Vichnewski, W., Pahl, H.L., Merfort, I., and Schmidt, T.J. (1999). Inhibition of transcription factor NF-kB by Sesquiterpene lactones: a proposed mechanism of action. *Bioorg. Med. Chem.,* 7:2343-2352.

Schefferlie, J.G., and van Bladeren, P.J. (1993). *In vitro* and *in vivo* reversible and irreversible inhibition of rat glutathione S-transferase isoenzymes by caffeic acid and its 2-S-glutathionyl conjugate. *Food Chem. Toxicol.,* 31: 475-482.

Seto, M., Miyase, T., Umehara, K., Ueno, A., Hirano, Y., and Otani, N. (1988). Sesquiterpene lactones from *Cichorium endivia L* and *C. intubus L.* and cytotoxic activity. *Chem. Pharm. Bull.,* 36: 2423-2429.

Shibata, H., Sakamoto, Y., Oka, M., and Kono, Y. (1999). Natural antioxidant, chlorogenic acid, protects against DNA breakage caused by monochloramine. *Biosci. Biotechnol. Biochem.,* 63: 1295-1297.

Simpson, H.C.R., Simpson, R.W., Lously, S., Carter, R.D., Geekie, M., and Hockaday, T.D.R. (1981). A high carbohydrate leguminous fiber diet improves all aspects of diabetic control. *Lancet,* i: 1-15.

Sokotka, L., Bratova, M., Slemrova, M., Manak, J., and Zadak, Z. (1997). Inulin as the soluble fiber in liquid enteral nutrition. *Nutrition,* 13: 21-25.

Steinmetz, K.A., and Porter, J.D. (1991). A review of vegetables, fruits, and cancer. *1. Epidemiol. Cancer Caus. Contr.*, 2:325-357.

Takase, S., Goda, T., and Watanabe, M. (1994). Monostearylglycerol–Strach complex: its digestibility and effects on glycemic and lipogenic responses. *J. Nutr. Sci Vitaminol.*, 40: 23-36.

Tokunaga, T., Oku, T., and Hosoya, N. (1996). Influence of chronic intake of a new sweetener fructo-oligosaccharide (Neosugar) on growth and gastrointestinal function of the rat. *J. Nutr. Sci. Vitaminol.*, 32:111-121.

Tramonte, S.M., Brand M.B., Mulrow, C.D., Amato, M.G., O'Keefe, M.E., and Ramirez, G. (1997). The treatment of chronic constipation in adults. A systemic review. *J. Gen. Intern. Med.*, 12: 15-24.

Trautwein, E.A., Rieckhoff, D., and Erbersdobler, H.F. (1998). Dietary Inulin Lowers Plasma Cholesterol and Triacylglycerol and Alters Biliary Bile Acid Profile in Hamsters. *The Journal of Nutrition*, 128 (11): 1937-1943.

Trock, B., Lanza, E., and Greenwald, P. (1990). Dietary Fiber, Vegetables, and Colon Cancer: Critical Review and Meta-analyses of the Epidemiologic Evidence. *J. Natl. Cancer Inst.*, 82(8):650-66.

Trowell, H. (1972). Ischemic heart disease and dietary fiber. *Am. J. Clin. Nutr.*, 25:926-934.

van Beek, T.A., Mass, P., King, B.M., Leelereq, E., Voragen, A.G.J., and de Groot, A. (1990). Bitter Sesquiterpene lactones from chicory roots. *J. Agri. Food and Chem.*, 38:1035-1038.

van Loo, J., Coussement, P., De Leenheer, L., Hoebregs, W., and Schaafsma, G. (1995). On the presence of inulin and oligofructose as natural ingredients in the western diet. *Crit. Rev. Food Sci. Nutr.*, 35(6): 525-552.

Verghese, M., Chawan, C.B., Williams, L., and Rao, D.R. (1998). Dietary inulin suppresses azoxymethane-induced preneoplastic aberrant crypt foci in rat colon. *In: Proceedings of the Nutritional and Health Benefits of Inulin and Oligofructose Conference*, Md. Pennsylvania State Univ., Bethesda, pp: 55.

Vuksan, V., Jenkins, D.J.A., Spadafora, P., Sievenpiper, J.L., Owen, R., Vidgen, E., Brighenti, F., Josse, R., Leiter, L.A., and Bruce-Thompson, C. (1999). Konjac-mannan (Glucomannan) improves glycemia and other associated risk factors for coronary heart disease in type-2 diabetes: A randomized controlled metabolic trial. *Diabetes Care*, 22:913-919.

Wada, K. (1990). *In Vitro* fermentability of Oligofructose and Inulin by Some Species of Human Intestinal Flora. Technical Report by Calpis Intestinal Flora Laboratory, available from ORAFTI, Aandorenstraat 1-B3300 Tienen, Belgium.

Wang, X. (1993). Comparative Aspects of Carbohydrate Fermentation by Colonic Bacteria. Doctoral thesis, University of Cambridge, Cambridge, U.K.pp.1-123

Wang, X., and Gibson, G.R. (1993). Effects of the in vitro fermentation of oligofructose and inulin by bacteria growing in the human large intestine. *J. Appl. Bacteriol.* 75: 373-380.

Wolever, T.M.S. (1990). Relationship between dietary fiber content and composition in foods and glycemic index. *Am. J. Clin. Nutr.*, 51:72-75.

Wright, R.S., Anderson, J.W., and Briges, S.R. (1990). Propionate inhibits hepatocyte lipids synthesis. *Proc. Soc. Exp. Biol. Med.*, 195: 26-29.

Yun, J.W., Park, J.P., Song, J.P., Lee, C.Y., Kim, J.H., and Song, S.K. (2000). Continuous production of inulo-oligosaccharides from chicory juice by immobilized endoinulinase. *Bioprocess. Enginerring,* 22:189-194.

Zafar, R., and Ali, S.M. (1998). Antihepatotoxic effects of Roots and root callus extract of *Cichorium intybus L. J. Ethanopharmacol.,* 63: 227-231.

Zampelas, A., Morgan, L., Furlonger, N., Williams, C. (1995). Effects of dietary fatty acid composition on basal and hormone-stimulated hepatic lipogenesis and on circulating lipids in the rat. *Br. J. Nutr.,* 74:381-392.

Medicinal Plants: Phytochemistry, Pharmacology and Therapeutics, Vol. 1 *Pages* **155–177**
Editors: **V.K. Gupta, G.D. Singh, Surjeet Singh and A. Kaul**
Published by: **DAYA PUBLISHING HOUSE, NEW DELHI**

Chapter 7

Role of Curcuminoids, the Yellow Colored Phenols of Turmeric, in Disease Prevention and Health Maintenance

Somepalli Venkateswarlu and Gottumukkala V. Subbaraju*
Laila Research Centre, Unit I, Phase III, Jawahar Autonagar
Vijayawada – 520 007, India
Aptuit Laurus Pvt. Ltd., ICICI Knowledge Park,
Turkapally, Shameerpet, Hyderabad – 500 078, India

ABSTRACT

Curcuminoids are the yellow coloured phenolic diarylheptanoids found in turmeric and other plants of *Curcuma* genus. Turmeric powder is one of the well-known ingredients in Ayurveda, the Indian system of medicine and it is also used as a food additive and food preservative. It is one of the most valued spices in the Indian food. Curcuminoids possess therapeutic profile as antioxidants, antiinflammatory agent, anticancer compounds and antimicrobials and have excellent safety profile. This review summarizes the importance of curcuminoids in health maintenance and as disease preventive agents.

Keywords: *Anticancer, Antiinflammatory, Antimicrobial, Antioxidants, Curcuminoids, Turmeric.*

* Corresponding Author: E-mail: subbaraju.gv@aptuitlaurus.com.

Introduction

The question of whether the medicines discovered today are safer, more efficacious, and more affordable than generic medicines or medicines that are centuries old could be answered "no" for most of the modern medicines. If so, then it is logical to revisit and revive these age-old medicines for the welfare of mankind. Turmeric is one such age-old medicine. Its history dates back over 5000 years, to the heyday of Ayurveda (which means the science of life). Turmeric derived from the rhizome of the plant, *Curcuma longa* has been used by the people of the Indian subcontinent for centuries with no known side effects, not only as a component of food but also to treat a wide variety of ailments.

Curcuma longa is a rhizomatous herbaceous perennial plant of the ginger family, Zingiberaceae which is native to tropical South Asia. It belongs to the genus *Curcuma* that consists of hundreds of spices of plants that possess rhizomes and underground root like stems.

Its rhizomes are boiled for several hours in water and then dried in hot ovens, after which they are ground into a deep orange-yellow powder commonly used as a spice in curries and other South Asian cuisine. Sangli, a town in the southern part of the Indian state of Maharashtra, is the largest and most important trading centre for turmeric in Asia or perhaps in the entire world. Turmeric was highly esteemed by the ancient Indo-European people for its golden-yellow dye resembling sunlight. This culture, known as Arya, worshiped the solar system. The married women apply turmeric on their cheeks in the evening, in anticipation of a visit by the goddess, Lakshmi, at that time. Turmeric became of special importance to man with the discovery that its powdered rhizome, when added to various food preparations, preserved their freshness and nutritive value. Turmeric, which belongs to a group of aromatic spices, was originally used as a food additive in curries to improve the shelf life of the food. Long before the time of cheaper synthetic food preservatives, spices like turmeric played a vital role as food additives and were valued more than gold and precious stones.

Traditional Uses

In Ayurvedic medicine, turmeric is thought to have many medicinal properties and many in India use it as a readily available antiseptic for cuts, burns, bruises and many other applications. In Ayurveda, turmeric has been used internally as a stomachie, tonic and blood purifier, and externally in the prevention and treatment of skin diseases. Half to one gram, twice a day, was given for flatulence and dyspepsia. It has been prescribed in liver diseases, and particularly for jaundice and urinary tract diseases. In chronic catarrh and coryza, the inhalation of the fumes of burning turmeric causes copious mucous discharge and gives instant relief. Boiled with milk and sugar, turmeric has been a traditional remedy for colds. Turmeric and alum powder in the proportion of one-to-20 are applied into the ear in chronic otorrhea. Turmeric has been described as useful in skin diseases, *e.g.*, the juice of the fresh rhizome is used in parasitic skin infections, and turmeric powder rubbed down with oil has been applied to soften rough skin. In combination with lime and saltpeter, turmeric has also been applied to bruises, sprains, cuts, wounds, infected wounds and inflammations. In pemphigus (an allergic and inflammatory skin conditions) and shingles, after applying a thick coat of mustard oil, turmeric powder is sprinkled to alleviate pain, inflammation and to speed up healing. In smallpox and chickenpox, a coat of turmeric is applied to facilitate the process of scabbing. Mixed with borax as a paste, turmeric is applied to reduce tissue swelling due to inflammation. A decoction of turmeric is prepared (one ounce of turmeric to 20 ounces of water), and applied as a cooling eye wash and a lotion to relieve burning in purulent ophtalmia known in India as "country sore eye".

Turmeric exemplifies an herb for which clinical applications have evolved over time. Until recently, this perennial herb, widely cultivated in tropical regions of Asia, particularly in India, was valued primarily as a commercial item for imparting a lively color and also a part of most curry powders. In India, it is preferred for dyeing purposes and flavoring purposes. The long-established image of turmeric as a commercial dyestuff and component of curry was partly responsible for overshadowing its importance as a medicinal herb.

Turmeric: Botanical Aspects

Like other members of the family Zingiberaceae, *Curcuma longa* L. is a typical herbaceous plant (Figure 7.1) with thick and fleshy rhizomes and leaves in sheaths. The plants reach a height of up to one meter. Leaves, alternate, obliquely erect or subsessile are oblong, lanceolate and dark green, surmounting leaf sheaths tapering near the leaf and broadening near the base, enveloping the succeeding shoot. Inflorescence is terminal on leafy spurious stems appearing between the sheaths. Flowers, which are occasionally seen on cylindrical spikes bearing numerous greenish white bracts, are narrow, yellowish-white in color. Most cultivated varieties are sterile triploids, but fruits are stray and inconspicuous.

The underground rhizome (Figure 7.2), which is processed into the turmeric of commerce, consists of two distinct parts.

1. The egg-shaped primary or mother rhizome, which is an extension of the stem and forms the bulbs, *C. rotunda* of Western commerce.
2. Several ovate, oblong or pyriform or cyclindrical multi branched rhizomes growing downward from the primary rhizome which form the *C. longa* of commerce.

The significance of turmeric in medicine has changed considerably since the discovery of the antioxidant properties of naturally occurring phenolic compounds. The same ground, dried rhizome of *Curcuma longa*, which has been used for centuries as a spice, food preservative and a coloring agent, has been found to be a rich source of phenolic compounds called curcuminoids. Three main

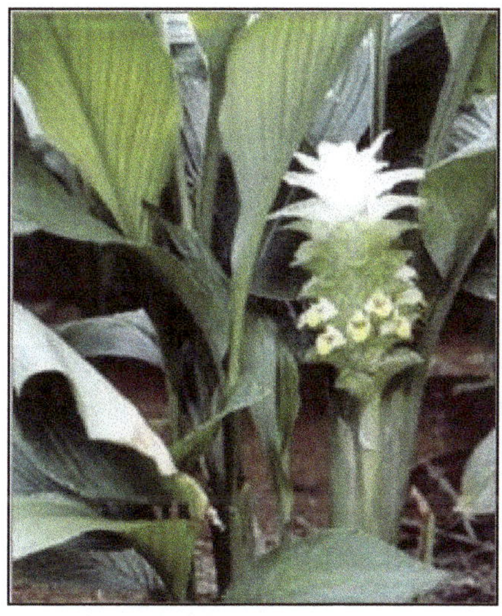

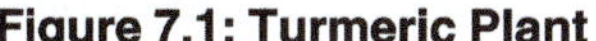

Figure 7.1: Turmeric Plant

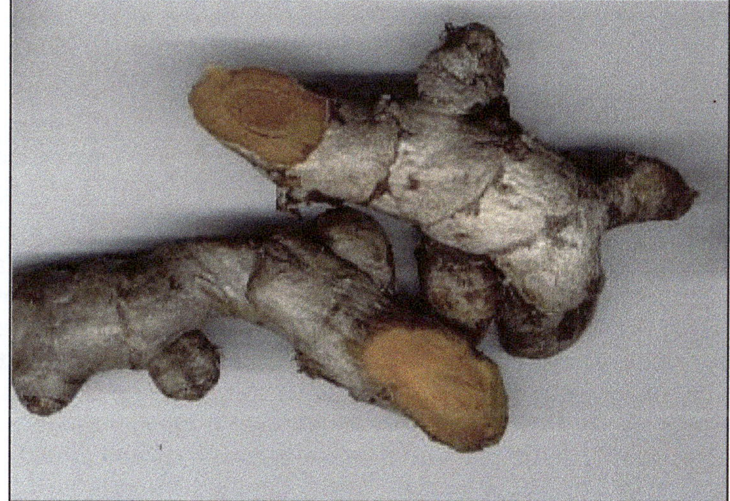

Figure 7.2: Turmeric Rhizome

curcuminoids were isolated from turmeric: curcumin, demethoxycurcumin, and bisdemethoxycurcumin. All the three impart the hallmark yellow pigmentation to its rhizomes (Majeed *et al.*, 1995) and particularly the powdered turmeric (Figure 7.3).

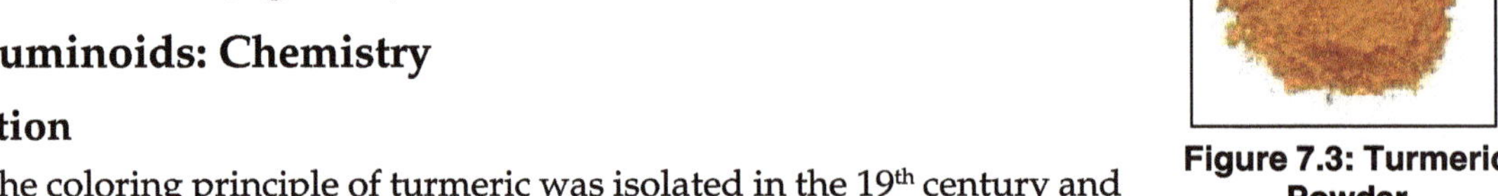

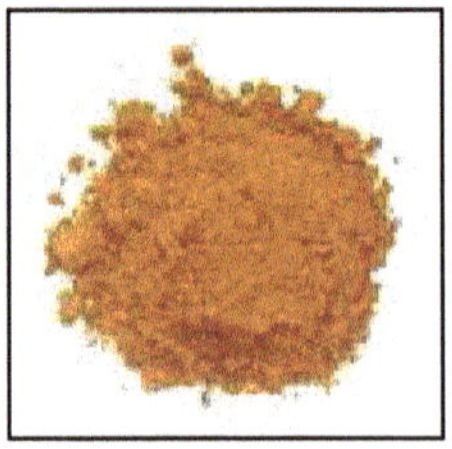

Figure 7.3: Turmeric Powder

Curcuminoids: Chemistry

Isolation

The coloring principle of turmeric was isolated in the 19th century and called curcumin. Curcuminoids now refer to a group of phenolic compounds present in turmeric, which are chemically related to its principal ingredient curcumin. Three curcuminoids were isolated from turmeric *viz.*, curcumin, demethoxycurcumin and bisdemethoxycurcumin (Figure 7.4) (Chattopadhyay *et al.*, 2004).

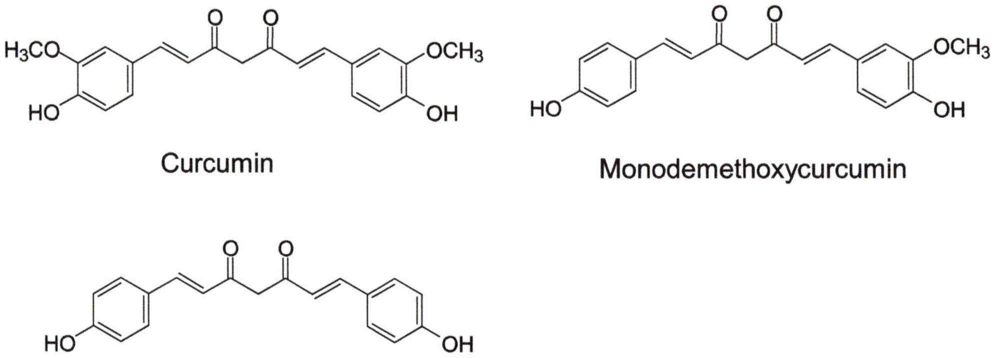

Curcumin

Monodemethoxycurcumin

Bisdemethoxycurcumin

Figure 7.4: Chemical Structures of Major Curcuminoids from *C. longa*

Curcumin, demethoxycurcumin, and bisdemethoxycurcumin have also been isolated from *Curcuma managga* (Abas *et al.*, 2005), *Curcuma zedoaria* (Syu *et al.*, 1998), *Curcuma xanthorrhiza* (Aggarwal *et al.*, 2007), *Curcuma aromatica*, *Curcuma phaeocaulis* (Tohda *et al.*, 2006), and other herbs like *Costus speciosus* (Aggarwal *et al.*, 2007), *Etlingera elatior* (Mohamad *et al.*, 2005), *and Zingiber cassumunar* (Aggarwal *et al.*, 2007).

Considering the various biological activities of curcuminoids, attempts were made by several researchers in the past to isolate curcuminoids from turmeric rhizomes.

Rhizomes were extracted by using various techniques such as hydro-distillation, low-pressure solvent extraction, Soxhlet, and supercritical extraction using carbon dioxide. Extraction of curcuminoids involved prior extraction of rhizomes with hexane to remove much of the volatile and fatty components and then extracting with benzene. The concentrate was further purified by crystallization from ethanol to yield orange-yellow needles. But, the yield of curcuminoids was poor. The hot and cold percolation extraction methods gave good yields with a high recovery of curcuminoids. Alternatively, curcuminoids were extracted as insoluble lead salt (Jayaprakasha *et al.*, 2005). Recently, extraction of curcuminoids using supercritical carbon dioxide modified by 10 per cent ethanol was also reported (Baumann *et al.*, 2000). Although supercritical fluid extraction is known to be a clean technology giving acceptable yields and purity, its major disadvantage lies in its high operating pressures. The scale up problems could also be severe when the extraction is to be done in large scale. To avoid all these problems microwave assisted extraction (MAE) technique for selective and rapid extraction of curcuminoids is reported recently. Turmeric powder was irradiated with microwave showed marginally higher extraction of curcuminoids in 60 min by acetone. The feasibility of this technique has to be studied further for industrial applicability (Dandekar and Gaikar, 2002; Manzan *et al.*, 2003).

Isolation of pure curcumin from plant material is time consuming and curcumins sold in the market is therefore, a purified extract containing a mixture of the three curcuminoids *i.e,* curcumin (75–81 per cent), demethoxycurcumin (15–19 per cent) and bisdemethoxycurcumin (2.2–6.6 per cent). The standardized *C. longa* extract or turmeric extract in the market is 95 per cent of all the three curcuminoids and much of the biological studies were on this extract (Composition).

Structure

Curcumin, $C_{21}H_{20}O_6$, mp 184–185°C was isolated as early as 1815. It is insoluble in water but soluble in ethanol and acetone. Daube obtained it in crystalline form. The structure of curcumin as a diferuloylmethane was confirmed by the degradative work and synthesis by Lampe in 1910 (Roughley and Whiting, 1973).

On boiling with alkali, curcumin gave vanillic acid and ferulic acids whose structures were established. Fusion with alkali yielded protocatechuic acid and oxidation with potassium permanganate yielded vanillin. On hydrogenation, mixtures of hexahydro–and tetrahydro-derivative were obtained and on acetylation gave diacetyl derivative. Based on these, the structure of curcumin was established as diferuloylmethane (Figure 7.4).

Synthesis

Heller isolated two products by condensation of acetyl acetone with vanillin in the presence of ethanolic hydrogen chloride. These two products differed by the reaction of boric acid and ferric chloride. Heller came to the conclusion that normal curcumin which gives deep reddish brown color with ferric chloride has the keto-enol structure, while the two products which gave only pale yellowish

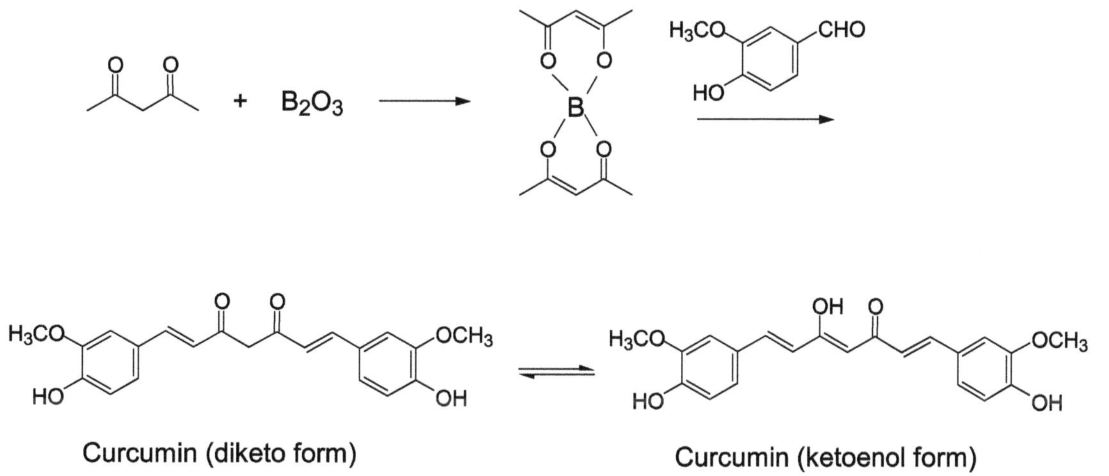

+ B_2O_3 → ; H_3CO, CHO, HO →

Curcumin (diketo form) ⇌ Curcumin (ketoenol form)

Figure 7.5: Synthesis of Curcuminoids

brown color have diketone structures and these forms being stereo isomers of the same structure. Recently, curcuminoids were synthesized in good yield from acetyl acetone and vanillin using boric oxide (Pabon, 1964; Pedersen *et al.*, 1985; Babu and Rajasekharan, 1994).

Other Curcuminoids

Besides these major curcuminoids such as curcumin, demethoxycurcumin and bisdemethoxycurcumin five minor constituents are also isolated. One of these is cyclocurcumin, which was isolated from the mother liquor of *Curcuma longa* extract by repeated purification, as yellow gum (Kiuchi *et al.*, 1993). 1-(4-Hydroxy-3,5-dimethoxyphenyl)-7-(4-hydroxy-3-methoxyphenyl)-1,6-heptadiene-3,5-dione has been isolated from rhizomes of *Curcuma xanthorrihiza* (Masuda *et al.*, 1992; Venkateswarlu *et al.*, 2004) (Figure 7.6).

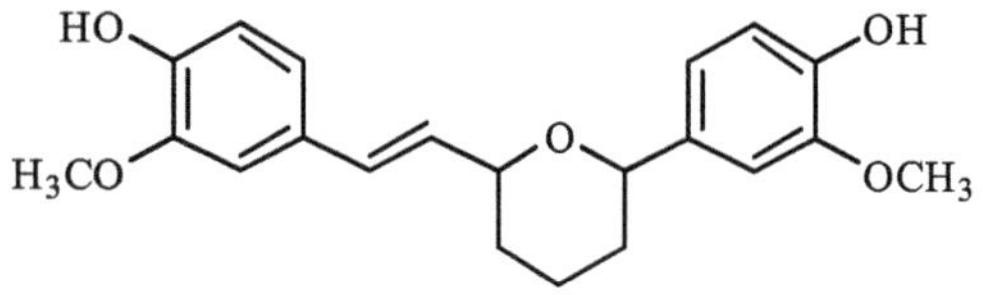

Cyclocurcumin

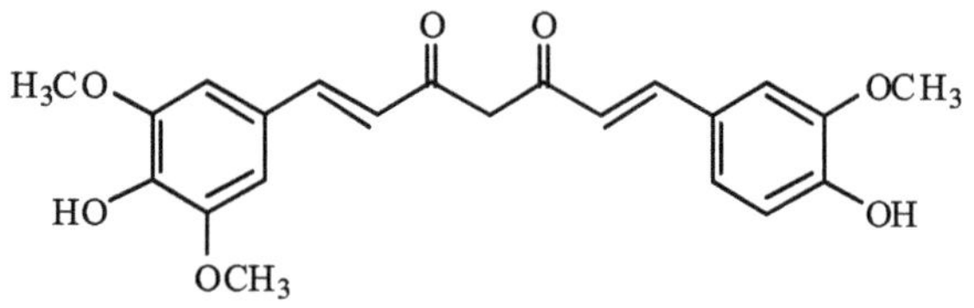

1-(4-Hydroxy-3,5-dimethoxyphenyl-
7-(4-hydroxy-3-methoxyphenyl)-
1,6-heptadiene-3,5-dione

Figure 7.6: Minor Curcuminoids from *C. longa*

Bisdemethylated curcumin was also present as minor constituent in the *C. longa* extract (Akio *et al.*, 1993). Monodemethylated curcumin was isolated from *Curcuma domestica* (Nakayama *et al.*, 1993). Recently, demethylated monodemethoxycurcumin (Figure 7.7) was also isolated from *Curcuma longa* as minor natural product (Jiang *et al.*, 2006). The NCI group has synthesized bisdemethylated curcumin from curcumin and found that it is having good antiHIV activity than curcumin (Mazumder *et al.*, 1997). Very recently, the curcumin mixture or standardized *C. longa* extract is converted into demethylated curcuminoid mixture having bisdemethylated curcumin (70–80 per cent by wt.), monodemethylated curcumin (2–8 per cent by wt.), demethylated monodemethoxycurcumin (10–20

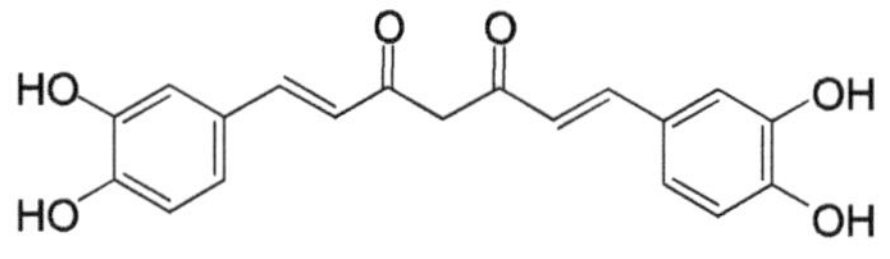

Bisdemethylcurcumin

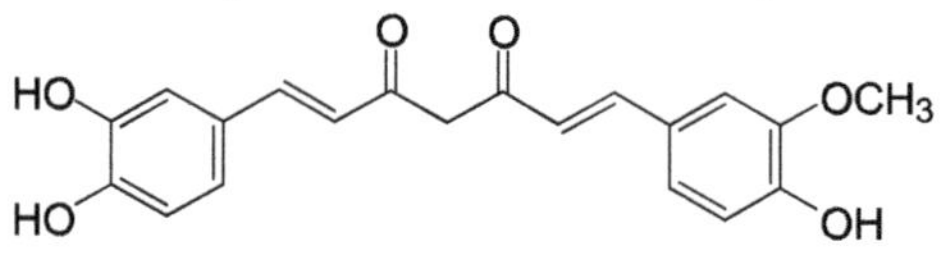

Monodemethylcurcumin

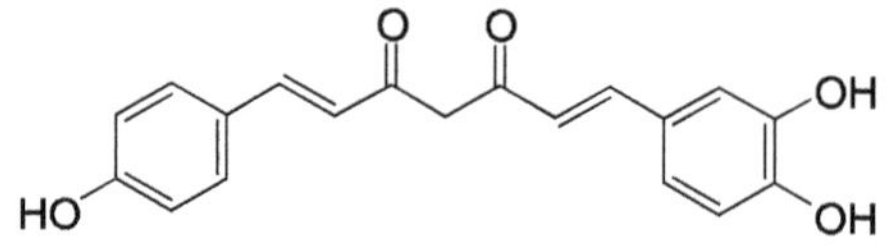

Demethylmonodemethoxycurcumin

Figure 7.7: Demethylated Analogs of Cucurminoids

per cent by wt.) and bisdemethoxycurcumin (0.5–2 per cent by wt.) by a simple procedure (Ganga Raju *et al.*, 2007). They also found that this enriched demethylated curcuminoid mixture has strong antioxidant activity and has several fold potent activity than the curcuminoid mixture. Moreover, this demethylated curcuminoid mixture also exhibits potent 5-lipoxygenase inhibitory activity and has also several fold potent activity than the curcumin mixture.

Biological Activities

The use of *Curcuma longa* to treat a variety of inflammatory, biliary and respiratory disorders, has generated scientific interest in the curative properties of the turmeric rhizome. Much of the work has focused on the use of dried extracts, the volatile oil and the active principles, the curcuminoids.

Antioxidant Activity

Oxidation is the transfer of electrons from one atom to another and represents an essential part of aerobic life and in our metabolism, since oxygen is the ultimate electron acceptor in the electron flow system that produces energy in the form of ATP (Adenosine triphospate). The oxygen molecule is very stable in the ground state, but it is changed into reactive oxygen species (ROS), namely, superoxide ion (O_2^{-1}), peroxide radical (?OOH), hydroxyl radical (?OH) and nitric oxide (NO?) by the environmental pollutants, radiolysis, UV and the reduction pathway to H_2O in the living tissues. These free radicals play a major role in the initiation and progression of a wide range of pathological diseases like cancer, Alzheimer's, Parkinson's and cardiovascular diseases. In the food industry, free radicals have been found to be responsible in the deterioration of foods during processing and storage. In view of this, considerable attention has been given to the addition of antioxidants in foods and supplementation of antioxidants to biological systems to scavenge free radicals.

The aging process exemplifies the cumulative result of deterioration of individual cells, tissues and organs, promoted by free radicals. The human body has built-in mechanisms to counteract free radicals. These mechanisms are collectively known as the body's antioxidant defense mechanism. Unfortunately, in most instances, the antioxidant defense is gradually overwhelmed by the aging process, or a disease, or both. The inflammatory processes associated with microbial or viral infections and the progression of cancer are just a few disease conditions which contribute to depletion of the antioxidant defense system of the body. Therefore, it is important to preserve the body's defenses against damages by free radicals. Some vitamins, minerals, and natural compounds such as phenolics, flavonoids and carotenoids, have the ability to counteract free radical damage by scavenging or neutralizing the free radicals. These diversified groups of nutrients, micronutrients and food supplements belong to a category of biologically important substances known as "antioxidants'.

The antioxidative compounds can be classified into two types: phenolics and β-diketones. Phenolic compounds exert their antioxidant activity by acting primarily as hydrogen atom donators, thereby inhibiting the propagation of radical chain reactions. Antioxidant potential of the phenolics depends on the number and arrangement of phenolic hydroxyl groups, as well as the nature of the other substituents on the aromatic rings. Few natural products, like curcuminoids have both phenolic and β-diketone groups in the same molecule and thus became potential antioxidants (Halliwell and Gutteridge, 1985; Larson, 1988).

Curcuminoids exhibit potent antioxidant properties and recent studies provide convincing evidence for the antioxidant properties of curcuminoids.

Both turmeric and curcuminoids inhibited generation of potent free radicals like superoxide and hydroxyl radicals (Reddy and Lokesh, 1992). The antioxidant properties of curcumin in prevention of lipid peroxidation, another process that generates free radicals, is well recognized (Sharma, 1976). Studies on spice principles as antioxidants in the inhibition of lipid peroxidation of rat liver microsomes revealed that curcumin was a potential antioxidant. Among the spice principles tested, curcumin showed the highest ability to prevent lipid peroxidation. Curcumin, in this study, was found to be eight times more potent than vitamin E.

Animals fed with curcumin showed decreased levels of lipid peroxides and subsequent reduction in the chemically induced inflammation (Sreejayan Rao, 1994). Thus, it is obvious from these studies that curcumin prevents the production of tissue-damaging free radicals. Also, under *in vitro* conditions, in tissue culture, rat and mouse liver cells incubated in the presence of micromolar concentrations of curcumin reduced the generation of lipid peroxides (Sharma *et al.*, 1972). Curcumin also prevented the oxidative damage and alteration of the DNA genetic material in cultured fibroblasts (Shih and Lin, 1993).

A potential role of curcumin in preventing oxidative damage to the arterial wall has been studied. Cardiovascular disease is caused by the progressive narrowing of the arterial walls. This is essentially due to the deposition of cholesterol plaque inside the arterial walls resulting from high levels of oxidized cholesterol in the blood. Oxidation of blood cholesterol is evaluated in clinical studies by measuring blood levels of lipid peroxides. Administration of 500 mg of curcuminoids daily to healthy humans for seven days lowered the levels of blood lipid peroxides by 33 per cent, as well as the levels of blood cholesterol by 29 per cent. The authors of this study indicated possible use of curcuminoids in the prevention of cardiovascular disease (Soni and Kuttan, 1992).

An important corollary of the antioxidant action of curcuminoids in their potential use as natural food additives to prevent the oxidation and resultant rancidity of oils and fats during storage and heating.

In a recent research report (Sreejayan Rao, 1994), the inhibitory effect of lipid peroxidation by various curcuminoids was compared against a well-known antioxidant, vitamin E (α-tocopherol). In this investigation, the lipid peroxidation in the biological materials was induced by the addition of ferrous sulfate (Fe^{+2}), ferric chloride (Fe^{+3}), Fe^{+3}-ADP-ascorbate complex or Fe^{+3}-ADP-NADPH complex. The results revealed that the curcuminoids were more potent inhibitors of experimentally induced lipid peroxidation than vitamin E α-tocopherol. All the three curcuminoids tested, curcumin, demethoxycurcumin, and bisdemethoxycurcumin were almost equally active. Very recently, curcuminoids and bisdemethylcurcumin were studied for their antioxidant activity by superoxide free radical (NBT) and DPPH free radical scavenging methods and found that curcuminoids are potent antioxidants when compared with the natural antioxidants like vitamine E, BHA, BHT and vitamin C. Interestingly, the bisdemethylcurcumin is several times more potent than the curcuminoids (Venkateswarlu *et al.*, 2005).

The antioxidant mechanism of curcuminoids may include one or more of the following interactions:

1. Scavenging or neutralizing the free radicals
2. Interacting with oxidative cascade, and preventing its outcome
3. Oxygen quenching, and making it less available for oxidative reactions
4. Inhibition of oxidative enzymes like cytochrome P-450, and
5. Chelating or disarming oxidative properties of metal ions such as iron (Fe).

In conclusion, turmeric and its active constituents, curcumins or curcuminoids have antioxidant properties and effectively inhibit the free radical damage to biomolecules both *in vitro* and *in vivo* conditions. The fact that curcuminoids act as antioxidants by prevention and intervention processes, makes them very unique disease preventive agents (Anto *et al.*, 1996).

Antiinflammatory A

Inflammation results from the complex series of actions and reactions triggered by the body?s immunological response to tissue damage. Many diseases as well as physical trauma, including surgery, induce inflammatory reactions. These reactions, although necessary to start the healing process, too often create an unbearably painful condition, which may even perpetuate the disease. Several inflammatory mediators, such as, histamine, eicosanoids, platelet activating factor, TNF etc are involved in the inflammation process.

Inflammation is an active part of many chronic disease states. Steroidal drugs like cortisone, and non-steroidal antiinflammatory drugs (NSAID) like phenylbutazone and indomethacin, are used in clinical practice to subdue the inflammation. Some of the antiinflammatory drugs inhibit the lipoxygenase pathway, and the other by cyclooxygenase pathway resulting in different potency and clinical applications for the antiinflammatory drugs. Two of the factors that are very active mediators in the inflammatory process are both derived from the fatty acid, arachidonic acid.

These are the leukotrienes, produced by 5-lipoxygenase (5-LOX) and the prostaglandins, produced by cyclooxygenase (COX). Currently, NSAID's (non steroidal antiinflammatory drugs) are the primary therapy for many inflammatory diseases, *e. g.* rhematoid arthritism, osteoarthritis, periodontal disease etc. Unfortunately regular use of NSAID's produce dangerous side effects such as changes in blood pressure levels and increases the development of ulcers of the stomach and duodenum (Samuelsson, 1983; Srimal and Dhawan, 1973).

Curcuminoids and other constituents of turmeric are well known for their antiinflammatory activity. Turmeric is one of the oldest antiinflammatory drugs used in Ayurvedic medicine. In fact, it

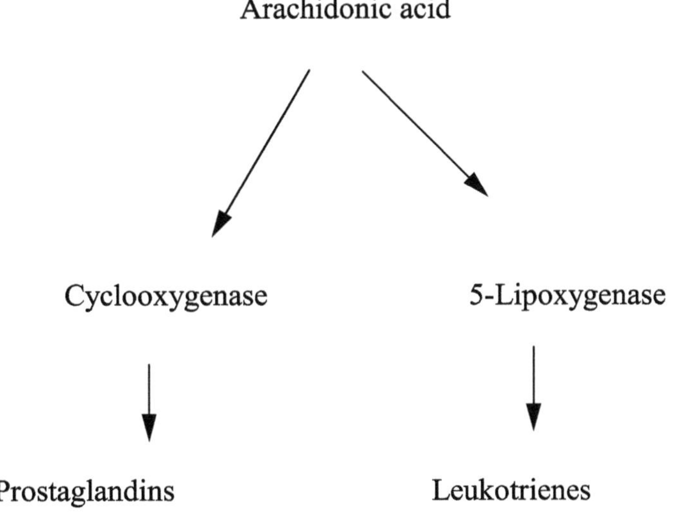

Figure 7.8: Arachidonic Acid and Cascade

was in India that the research on the antiinflammatory properties of turmeric was initiated. Turmeric extract, volatile oil from turmeric and curcuminoids were reported to possess antiinflammatory activity in different experimental models of inflammation in mice, rats, rabbits and pigeons. The antiinflammatory activity of turmeric and curcuminoids was evaluated in inflammatory reactions induced by chemical or physical irritants like carrageenin, cotton pellets, formaldehyde, and granuloma pouch technique.

The antiinflammatory properties of curcuminoids were studied in carrageenin induced foot paw edema in mice and rats. The oral doses of curcumin required to reduce the inflammatory edema, or tissue swelling, to half the size (ED_{50}–a dose effective in reducingedema by 50 per cent) are indicated below:

Species	ED_{50} *Curcumin*	ED_{50} *Cortisone*
Mice	48 mg/Kg	45 mg/Kg
Rats	100.2 mg/Kg	78 mg/Kg

Utilizing cotton pellet and granuloma pouch tests in rats, both curcumin and non-steroidal drug, phenylbutazone, were effective at ED_{50} dose of 48 mg/Kg (Srinivas and Prabhakaran, 1989).

The antiinflammatory activity of curcumin was evaluated in a group of patients who underwent surgery or suffered from trauma. A double-blind placebo controlled trial in which three groups of patients received curcumin (400 mg), a placebo (250 mg of lactose powder) or phenylbutazone (100 mg) respectively, three times a day for five consecutive days after surgery (for hernia or hydrocele). The treatment with curcumin resulted in reduced inflammation and was as equally effective as the treatment with phenylbutazone. Turmeric has also been evaluated in the treatment of inflammation associated with various forms of arthritis. Oral administration of curcumin at a dose of 3 mg/kg and sodium curcumin at a dose of 0.1 mg/kg inhibited formalin-induced arthritis in rats. Curcumin was comparably effective to phenylbutazone in arresting formalin-induced arthritis in rats.

The antirheumatic properties of curcuminoids were tested in a double-blind clinical trial in 49 patients with diagnosed rheumatoid arthritis. Curcumin administered at a dose of 1200 mg/per day for five to six weeks, produced a significant improvement in all patients. All patients showed overall improvement in morning stiffness, and physical endurance. The therapeutic effects were comparable to those obtained with phenylbutazone (Majeed *et al.*, 1995).

Turmeric was also used to treat patients with chronic respiratory disorders, with resulting subjective improvement of the condition and significant relief in symptoms like cough and dyspnea. Eye drops prepared from the decoction of turmeric, known as "Haridra Eye Drops", were used in 25 cases of an inflammatory condition of the eye, bacterial conjunctivitis. Clinical symptoms such as eye redness or burning sensation, started subsiding from the third day of treatment. The cure rate evaluated during the six-day treatment was 23 out of 25 patients completely relieved from the condition (Ammon *et al.*, 1993).

Curcumin and its four synthetic analogs were examined for antiinflammatory potential in carrageenin induced foot paw edema and cotton pellet granuloma models of inflammation on rats. The antiinflammatory potency of tested curcummin, curcumin analogs and phenylbutazone were established in the following order: sodium curcumin> tetrahydrocurcumin> curcumin> phenylbutazone and triethylcurcumin. Sodium salt of curcumin was effective at half the dose of the parent compound, curcumin. Comparison of curcumin and its analogs in acute and subacute models of inflammation revealed that curcumin analogs are more active in alleviating acute inflammation (Majeed *et al.*, 1995).

One of the mechanisms understood for the antiinflammatory action of curcumins is its inhibition of cyclooxygenase and lipoxygenase enzymes (Huang *et al.*, 1991). These enzyme inhibitions may be a result of diminishing inflammatory products of the arachidonic acid metabolism, *e.g.*, prostaglandins and leukotrienes. Curcumin has similar action as that of aspirin and aspirin-like antiinflammatory agents. However, there is an important advantage of curcumin over aspirin, since curcumin, unlike aspirin, selectively inhibits synthesis of inflammatory prostaglandin thromboxane, while not affecting the synthesis of prostacyclin. Prostacyclin is an important factor preventing vascular thrombosis, and any drug that affects its synthesis, particularly if used in large dose, may increase the risk of vascular thrombosis. Curcumin may therefore, be preferable in patients who, for example, are prone to vascular thrombosis and require antiinflammatory and antiarthritic therapy (Rao *et al.*, 1993, 1995).

Anticancer Activity

Cancer is a group of diseases in which cells are aggressive (grow and divide without respect to normal limits), invasive (invade and destroy adjacent tissues), and sometimes metastatic (spread to other locations in the body). These three malignant properties of cancers differentiate them from benign tumors, which are self-limited in their growth and don't invade or metastasize (although some benign tumor types are capable of becoming malignant). Cancer may affect people at all ages, even fetuses, but risk for the more common varieties tends to increase with age. Cancer causes about 13 per cent of all deaths. According to the American Cancer Society, 7.6 million people died from cancer in the world during 2007. Apart from humans, forms of cancer may affect other animals and plants.

Nearly all cancers are caused by abnormalities in the genetic material of the transformed cells. These abnormalities may be due to the effects of carcinogens, such as tobacco smoke, radiation, chemicals, or infectious agents. Other cancer-promoting genetic abnormalities may be randomly acquired through errors in DNA replication, or are inherited, and thus present in all cells from birth. Complex interactions between carcinogens and the host genome may explain why only some develop cancer after exposure to a known carcinogen. New aspects of the genetics of cancer pathogenesis, such as DNA methylation, and microRNAs are increasingly being recognized as important.

Turmeric extracts and curcuminoids have been found to be cancer preventing compounds in different tumor models, as well as in limited human studies (Nagabhusan and Bhide, 1992). Supplementation of 1 per cent turmeric in the daily diet inhibited benzopyrene-induced stomach tumors and also spontaneous mammary tumors in mice. Oral administration of turmeric water extract or curcumin inhibited benzopyrene-induced stomach tumors in mice (Azuine *et al.*, 1992). In another study, mice fed 0.5 per cent, 1 per cent and 2 per cent curcumin in daily diet at initiation and post initiation stages of benzopyrene-induced stomach cancer, showed reduction in rate of benign and malignant tumor development. Rats fed with 0.2 per cent of curcumin in daily diet showed inhibition of azoxymethane-induced colon precancerous lesions and also reduced the development of colon carcinoma (Rao *et al.*, 1995; Duvoix *et al.*, 2005; Soudamini and Kuttan, 1992).

Turmeric extract applied to mouse skin prevented dimethylbenzanthracene (DMBA) and methylcholanthrene induced skin tumors (Dhillon *et al.*, 2008). Skin painting with curcumin also prevented DMBA induced skin tumors in mice (Azuine *et al.*, 1992). This study confirmed that curcuminoids inhibit cancer at initation, promotion and progression of development.

In clinical studies, curcumin 0.5 per cent ointment applied topically on skin cancerous lesion in 62 patients, was found to reduce foul smell, itching, pain and exudates in majority of the patients. Foul smell was considerably reduced in more than 90 per cent, pain and itching in 50 per cent and exudates was reduced in 70 per cent of cases (Azuine and Bhide, 1992).

Turmeric extract alone or in combination with betel leaf extract was effective against methyl acetoxy methyl nitrosamine induced oral tumors in hamster buccal pouch (Tanaka *et al.*, 1994). Curcumin also inhibited 4-nitroquinoline induced oral tumors in rats. In a study done in India, anticarcinogenic effectiveness of curcumin was tested in patients with oral cancer. One hundred patients were given 500 mg of curcumin three times a day for 30 days. Some patients responded with a dramatic clinical improvement within 15 days, while others responded gradually, during the 30-day treatment.

Clinical studies in a variety of cancer cell lines including breast, cervical, colon, gastric, hepatic, leukemia, oral epithelial ovarian, pancreatic, and prostate have consistently shown that curcumin possesses anticancer activity *in vitro* and in pre-clinical animal models. The robust activity of curcumin in colorectal cancer has led to five phase I clinical trials, showing the safety and tolerability of curcumin. Every clinical trial has concluded that curcumin is safe and poses minimal adverse effects. Dose up to 8000 mg per day of curcumin were well tolerated. The success of these trials has led to the development of phase II trials that are currently enrolling patients (Jhonson and Mukhtar, 2007).

Antimicrobial Activity

The antibacterial effects of alcoholic extract of turmeric, curcumin and oil from turmeric have been studied. An alcoholic extract of turmeric at a dose of 50 mg/mL showed *in vitro* bactericidal activity. Turmeric oil was found to possess bacteriostatic action *in vitro* in dilutions of up to 1:1000. The essential oil at a dose of 4.5 to 90 ml/100mL was found effective *in vitro* against variety of microorganisms. Curcumin at concentration of 2.5 to 50 mg/100 mL inhibited *in vitro* growth of *Staphylococcus aureus*. Sodium curcuminate was found effective *in vitro* against Micrococcus pyogenes in a dilution of one part per million (Bhavanishankar and Srinivasa Murthy, 1979; Banerjee and Nigam, 1978; Dahl *et al.*, 1989).

Interestingly, the antibacterial and antiviral activities of curcumin were significantly enhanced by illumination with visible light. The light-enhanced toxicity of the curcumin molecule to microorganisms has been found to be oxygen-dependent. It is mediated through curcumin generated superoxide, hydrogen peroxide and hydroxyl radicals. These experimental data support the potential use of curcumin combined with light therapy (phototherapy) in the treatment of some bacterial and viral infections (Kunchandy and Rao, 1990; Misra and Sahu, 1977).

The crude ether and chloroform extracts of turmeric stem showed fungistatic activity against several dermatophytes *in vitro*. The aqueous and alcoholic extracts of turmeric as well as curcumin inhibited production of aflatoxins by *Aspergillus parasiticus in vitro*. Aflatoxin is a metabolic of mold, which grows on food and contaminates various foods stored in unsanitary, humid conditions. Aflatoxins ingested with food, for example with moldy peanuts, may, over a long term, cause liver damage and cancer. The modifying effects of turmeric extract and curcumin on aflatoxin induced liver damage were studied in ducklings.

Aflatoxin-treated ducklings showed a decrease in body weight and white blood cell counts. They also had elevated levels of serum and liver glutamate pyruvate transaminase activity. Feeding turmeric extract and curcumin to ducklings which were exposed to aflatoxin, prevented the loss of body weight and decrease the damage to white blood cells. The glutamate pyruvate transaminase activity in turmeric extract and curcumin fed animals was normalized to the control levels (Soni *et al.*, 1992).

AntiHIV Activity

Human immunodeficiency virus (HIV) is a retrovirus that can lead to acquired immunodeficiency syndrome (AIDS), a condition in humans in which the immune system begins to fail, leading to life-threatening opportunistic infections. Previous names for the virus include human T-lymphotropic virus-III (HTLV-III), lymphadenopathy-associated virus (LAV), and AIDS-associated retrovirus (ARV).

Infection with HIV occurs by the transfer of blood, semen, vaginal fluid, pre-ejaculate, or breast milk. Within these bodily fluids, HIV is present as both free virus particles and virus within infected immune cells. The four major routes of transmission are unprotected sexual intercourse, contaminated needles, breast milk, and transmission from an infected mother to her baby at birth. Screening of blood products for HIV has largely eliminated transmission through blood transfusions or infected blood products in the developed world.

HIV infection in humans is now pandemic. As of January 2006, the Joint United Nations Programme on HIV/AIDS (UNAIDS) and the World Health Organization (WHO) estimate that AIDS has killed more than 25 million people since it was first recognized on December 1, 1981, making it one of the most destructive pandemics in recorded history. It is estimated that about 0.6 per cent of the world's population is infected with HIV. In 2005 alone, AIDS claimed an estimated 2.4–3.3 million lives, of which more than 570,000 were children. A third of these deaths are occurring in sub-Saharan Africa, retarding economic growth and increasing poverty. According to current estimates, HIV is set to infect 90 million people in Africa, resulting in a minimum estimate of 18 million orphans. Antiretroviral treatment reduces both the mortality and the morbidity of HIV infection, but routine access to antiretroviral medication is not available in all countries.

Turmeric was studied as a potential antiviral agent against HIV. The infection with HIV is characterized by a complex command system which results in virus activation or inactivation. The essential structural part of that command system in HIV is called long terminal repeat (LTR). Drugs that interfere with LTR may be of potential therapeutic value in delaying active HIV infection and progression of AIDS. Curcumin has been found to effectively inhibit activation of the LTR and to decrease HIV replication (Li *et al.*, 1993).

In a controlled clinical study, a group of 18 HIV-seropositive patients with CD-4 cell counts ranging from 5 to 615 and CD-8 cell counts ranging from 283 to 1467, took an average of 2 g of curcuminoids per day for an average of 127 days. This regimen resulted in the increase of CD-4 and CD-8 cell counts as compared to control treatment. No adverse effects of the treatment were noted. However, further studies are required to confirm the usefulness of these curcuminoids in AIDS management (Majeed *et al.*, 1995).

Hepatoprotective Activity

Hepatotoxicity (from hepatic toxicity) implies chemical-driven liver damage. The liver plays a central role in transforming and clearing chemicals and is susceptible to the toxicity from these agents. Certain medicinal agents when taken in overdoses and sometime even when introduced within therapeutic ranges may injure the organ. Other chemical agents such as those used in laboratories and industries, natural chemicals (*e.g.* microcystins) and herbal remedies can also induce hepatotoxicity. Chemicals that cause liver injury are called hepatotoxins.

More than 900 drugs have been implicated in causing liver injury and it is one of the common reasons for a drug to be withdrawn from the market. Chemicals often cause subclinical injury to liver which manifests only as abnormal liver enzyme tests. Drug induced liver injury is responsible for 5 per cent of all hospital admissions and 50 per cent of all acute liver failures. Hepatoprotection or antihepatotoxicity is the ability to prevent damage to the liver.

Curcumin and turmeric have been shown to protect liver against a variety of toxicants *in vitro* as well as *in vivo*. They include carbon tetrachloride, aflatoxin B-1, paracetamol, iron and cyclophosphamide in mouse, rat and duckling (Sardjoko and Vermeulen, 1990; Yoshinobu *et al.*, 1983). It has been found a dose of 30 mg/kg/day for 10 days of curcumin to be protective. More than 80 per cent inhibition of mutagenesis induced by aflatoxin B-1 in *Salmonella thyphimurium* tester strains TA98 and TA100 by turmeric and curcumin at a concentration of 2 µg/plate was reported (Soni *et al.*, 1997). Turmeric in the diet (5 and 10 per cent) has been found to stimulate enzymes (arylhydrocarbon hydroxylase, UDPglucuronyl transferase, glutathione-S-transferase) which metabolize xenobiotics. The effect of turmeric (4.0 g/kg/day) and curcumin (0.4 g/kg/day) on the hepatic levels of glutathion-S-transferase, acid soluble sulfhydryl (-SH), cytochrome b_5 and cytochrome P-450 enzymes after 14 or 21 days of administration in lactating dams and translactationally exposed F-1 pups were studied. All the enzymes examined were significantly elevated in lactating dams as well as in pups. Curcumin has been reported to strongly inhibit cytochrome 4501A in liver, an isoenzyme involved in the bioactivation of several toxins including benzo[a]pyrene (Singh *et al.*, 1995).

Effect on Gastrointestinal Tract

Several reports suggest that curcumin as well as turmeric increase bile flow. In a report, they found that sodium curcuminate decreased the amount of solids in the bile in low doses but increase the excretion of bile salts, bilirubin and cholesterol in high doses. The regression of established cholesterol gall stones in mice by curcumin was reported. The same authors had earlier reported the preventive action of curcumin on the formation of cholesterol gall stones in mice and hamsters. The gastric secretion was found to be reduced after 3 h in conscious rabbits by aqueous and methanolic extracts of turmeric. While the aqueous extract reduced the acid output, methanolic extract mainly decreased the pepsin output. In another study, gastric mucin content was found to be increased. The gastric and duodenal antiulcer properties of curcumin as well as turmeric, in high doses, are also documented. An oral dose of 500 mg/Kg of ethanolic extract of turmeric produced significant antiulcer effect in a variety of models in rat (Ramprasad and Sirsi, 1957; Srimal, 1997).

Effect on Respiratory System

Among quadrupeds, the respiratory system generally includes tubes, such as the bronchi, used to carry air to the lungs, where gas exchange takes place. A diaphragm pulls air in and pushes it out. Respiratory systems of various types are found in a wide variety of organisms.

In humans and other mammals, the respiratory system consists of the airways, the lungs, and the respiratory muscles that mediate the movement of air into and out of the body. Within the alveolar system of the lungs, molecules of oxygen and carbon dioxide are passively exchanged, by diffusion, between the gaseous environment and the blood. Thus, the respiratory system facilitates oxygenation of the blood with a concomitant removal of carbon dioxide and other gaseous metabolic wastes from the circulation. The system also helps to maintain the acid-base balance of the body through the efficient removal of carbon dioxide from the blood.

In humans and other animals, the respiratory system can be conveniently subdivided into an upper respiratory tract (or conducting zone) and lower respiratory tract (respiratory zone), trachea and lungs.

The respiratory tract is constantly exposed to microbes due to the extensive surface area, which is why the respiratory system includes many mechanisms to defend itself and prevent pathogens from entering the body.

In a clinical trial conducted with volatile oil of *Curcuma* in patients with bronchial asthma and found encouraging results. This is in accord with the ancient literature. Clinical trial in other respiratory disorders is warranted. In another study, they have reported the protective effect of curcumin (200 mg/kg for 7 days) on rat lung against the toxicity induced by cyclophosphamide. Antiallergic activity of *Curcuma* extract has also been reported (Venkatesan and Chandrasekaran, 1995).

Wound Healing Property

In medicine, a wound is a type of physical trauma where in the skin is torn, cut or punctured (an open wound), or where blunt force trauma causes a contusion (a closed wound). In pathology, it specifically refers to a sharp injury which damages the dermis of the skin. To heal a wound, the body undertakes a series of actions collectively known as the wound healing process. Tissue repair and wound healing are complex processes that involve inflammation, granulation and tissue remodeling. Injury initiates a complex series of events that involves interactions of multiple cell types, various cytokines, growth factors, their mediators and the extra-cellular matrix proteins (ECM).

Local application of turmeric is a household remedy in India for several conditions such as skin diseases, insect bites and chicken pox. The wound healing properties of turmeric was investigated long back and its local application was found to be effective. Curcumin was studied for the enhancement of wound healing by thickness punch wound model. Curcumin treated wound biopsies showed a large number of infiltrating cells such as macrophage, neutrophils and fibroblasts as compared to untreated wound. The presence of myofibroblast in curcumin treated wound demonstrated faster wound contraction (Sidhu *et al.*, 1998). Migration of various cells represents potential sources of growth factors required for the regulation of biological processes during wound healing. Transforming growth factor (TGF-b1) is important in wound healing as it stimulates the expression of fibronectin (FN) and collagen by fibroblasts and increases the rate of formation of granulation tissue *in vivo* (Varga *et al.*, 1987). Curcumin treatment resulted in enhanced fibrinectin (FN) and collagen expression. Further more, the treatment led to an increased formation of granulation tissue including greater cellular content, neo-vascularization and a faster re-epithelialization of wound in both diabetic as well as hydrocortisone impaired wounds by regulating the expression of TGF-b1, its receptors and nitric oxide synthase during wound healing (Mani *et al.*, 2002). Other studies involving systemic administration of curcumin have shown its beneficial effects by the enhancement of muscle regeneration after trauma by modulating NF-kB activity (Thaloor *et al.*, 1999). Recent studies have suggested that curcumin inhibited the damage caused by hydrogen peroxide in human keratinocytes and fibroblasts suggesting the antioxidant role in enhanced wound repair (Toan-Thang *et al.*, 2001). Similarly, curcumin incorporated collagen matrix treatment showed increased wound reduction, enhanced cell proliferation and efficient free radical scavenging as compared with control and collagen treated rats (Gopinath *et al.*, 2004). Curcumin pretreatment enhanced the synthesis of collagen, hexosamine, DNA, nitrile, and histologic assessment of wound biopsy specimens showed improved collagen deposition and an increase in fibroblast and vascular densities suggesting that curcumin may be able to improve radiation-induced delay in wound repair (Chandra and Krishnamurthy, 2005). These studies clearly suggested that curcumin treatment resulted in faster closure of wounds, better regulation of granulation tissue formation and induction of growth factors (Maheswari *et al.*, 2006).

Curcuminoids: Toxicology and Safety

Toxicology is the study of the adverse effects of chemicals on living organisms. It is the study of symptoms, mechanisms, treatments and detection of poisoning, especially the poisoning of people and the relationship between dose and its effects on the living organism. The chief criterion regarding the toxicity of a chemical is the dose, *i.e.* the amount of exposure to the substance. Recent concerns regarding the safety of selective enzyme inhibitors in large-scale chemoprevention trials emphasis the importance of carefully evaluating any potential toxicity of agents at the preclinical and early clinical trial levels. It cannot be assumed that diet-derived agents will be innocuous when administered as pharmaceutical formulations at doses likely to exceed those consumed in the dietary matrix.

For centuries, turmeric has been used as a food additive, medicinal agent, cosmetic and fabric dye, without harboring known side effects. This record of safety has been one of the deciding factors that allowed the FAO/WHO expert committee on food additives to approve curcuminoids as natural food coloring substance. Turmeric is listed by the US FDA as an herb generally recognized as safe (GRAS) for its intended use a spice, seasoning and flavoring agent.

Studies of curcumin in animals have confirmed a lack of significant toxicity since an early report in which doses up to 5 g/kg were administered orally to Sprague-Dawley rats. In another report suggested that dietary consumption of turmeric up to 1.5 g per person per day, equating to a maximum of 150 mg/day of curcumin, are not associated with adverse effects in humans. Systematic preclinical studies funded by the Prevention Division of the US National Cancer Institute did not discover adverse effects in rats, dogs or monkeys of doses up to 3.5 g/kg body weight (BW) administered for up to 3 month (Huang *et al.*, 1997). One report of dietary curcumin suggested ulcerogenic activity in the stomach of the albino rat, but this finding has not been confirmed in subsequent studies. In more recent preclinical studies of curcumin, no toxicity has been observed from 2 per cent dietary curcumin (approximately 1.2 g/kg, BW) administered to rats for 14 days or from 0.2 per cent dietary curcumin (approximately 300 mg/kg, BW) administered to mice for 14 weeks (Sharma *et al.*,, 2001).

Administration of 1.2-2.1 g of oral curcumin daily to patients with rheumatoid arthritis in India for 2-6 weeks did not result in any reported adverse effects. In a study of high dose oral curcumin in Taiwan, Cheng and colleagues administered up to 8 g daily of curcumin for 3 months to patients with pre-invasive malignant or high risk pre-malignant conditions, stating that no toxicity was observed. In patients with advanced colorectal cancer treated in the UK, curcumin was well tolerated at all dose levels up to 3.6 g daily for up to 4 months (Sharma *et al.*, 2004, 2005).

Genotoxicity and Tetratogenic Studies

Turmeric and curcumin were tested for tetratogenic effects *in vitro* and *in vivo*. In the Ames test and the Micronucles test in mice, turmeric and curcumin proved to be nongenotoxic (Azuine *et al.*, 1992). Rats maintained on diets containing 0.5 per cent turmeric and 0.15 per cent curcumin for 12 weeks did not show any increase in chromosomal damage, as compared to the control animals. Some animals within the treated and control groups were mated. The rate of pregnancy, egg implantation and mean number of live and dead fetus were similar in curcumin-receiving and the untreated control animals. No embryo toxicity, skeletal or visceral abnormalities of the new-born were observed as a result of pregnant rats and rabbits receiving 0.6 and 1.6 g/kg curcumin in a diet (Vijayalakshmi, 1980).

Curcuminoids: Pharmacokinetics

Pharmacokinetics is a branch of pharmacology dedicated to the determination of the fate of substances administered externally to a living organism. In practice, this discipline is applied mainly to drug substances, though in principle it concerns itself with all manner of compounds ingested or otherwise delivered externally to an organism, such as nutrients, metabolites, hormones, toxins, etc. Pharmacokinetics is often divided into several areas including, but not limited to, the extent and rate of Absorption, Distribution, Metabolism and Excretion. This sometimes is referred to as the ADME scheme. Absorption is the process of a substance entering the body. Distribution is the dispersion or dissemination of substances throughout the fluids and tissues of the body. Metabolism is the irreversible transformation of substances and its daughter metabolites. Excretion is the elimination of the substances from the body. In rare cases, some drugs irreversibly accumulate in a tissue in the body.

Pharmacokinetic studies in rats indicate that the absorption of pure curcumin from the gastrointestinal tract is about 60-65 per cent after administration of a single oral dose of 400 mg/kg. About 40 per cent of the administered dose was recovered unchanged in the faeces over a period of 5 days with a peak after 3 days. Free curcumin was not detected in urine but excretion of glucuronic acid and sulfate conjugates was observed from day 1 to day 7, suggesting an enterohepatic circulation (Ammon *et al.*, 1992). This result was confirmed by *in vitro* experiments using intestine of rat and [^{3}H]-curcumin. About 30-80 per cent of the labeled compound disappeared from the mucosal side but could not be detected on the serosal side, indicating that it undergoes transformation during absorption (Flynn *et al.*, 1986). Studies with [^{3}H]-curcumin *in vivo* confirmed that absorption from gastrointestinal tract remained between 60-66 per cent irrespective of the dose, but the duration of retention of label was dose-dependent (Ravindranath and Chandrasekhara, 1982).

The low availability of oral curcumin is well established. Phase I clinical trials have shown that curcumin is safe even at high doses (12 g/day) in humans but exhibit poor bioavailability. Typically, quantifiable serum levels are not achieved until doses of up to 3600 mg are used. Major reasons contributing to the low plasma and tissue levels of curcumin appear to be due to poor absorption, rapid metabolism, and rapid systemic elimination. Curcumin is a large lipophilic molecule that undergoes extensive gastrointestinal and hepatic metabolism after oral dosing. Phase I metabolism is through a reduction reaction forming tetrahydrocurcumin, hexahydrocurcumin, and hexahydrocurcuminol. Phase II metabolism consists of glucouronidation and sulfation by O-conjugation to form curcumin glucuronide and curcumin sulfate and rapidly excreted. The majority of curcumin elimination is via alcohol dehydrogenase to form hexahydrocurcumin in fecal matter (Agarwal *et al.*, 2003).

To improve the bioavailability of curcumin, numerous approaches have been undertaken. The alkaloid piperine from the Piper species is a known inhibitor of glucouronidation in the liver and small intestine and has been studied to assess the modulation of curcumin bioavailability (Atal *et al.*, 1985). Ten healthy volunteers received 2000 mg of curcumin with and without 20 mg of piperine in a randomized controlled fashion (Shoba *et al.*, 1998). An increase in bioavailability of 2000 per cent was seen with a curcumin and piperine combination compared to curcumin alone ($p<0.001$). Employing liposome drug delivery technology has also successfully been performed *in vitro* and *in vivo* studies to enhance bioavailability (*i.e* murine model). Another drug delivery system successfully used curcumin encased in natural biodegradable polymers (bovine serum albumin and chitosan) in Wistar rats and formulated with β-cyclodextrin to enhance bioavailbility (Anand *et al.*, 2007).

Conclusions

In view of excellent safety profile and disease preventive properties of curcuminoids, the components of turmeric, could be considered as ideal nutraceuticals. Inexpensive nature and availability of unlimited quantity of curcuminoids both from natural sources and synthetic approaches have made them accessible to all humans, poor and rich alike. Attractive color and antimicrobial properties led to the use of curcuminoids as common food additives.

Ability to cure dreaded diseases like cancer made curcuminoids as lead compounds for the development of pharmaceuticals. Non-habit forming and absence of side effects allow long time use to address chronic diseases like rheumatism. Balanced modulation of competing enzymes like leukotrienes and cyclooxygenases by curucminoids provide pain relief without side effects.

However, oral administration of curcuminoids are poorly bioavailable. Combining curcuminoids with piperine enhanced the bioavailability, but, proper structural modification could lead to the discovery of a wonder drug.

Acknowledgements

The authors thank Dr. G. Ganga Raju, Chairman, Laila Group and Dr. C. Satyanarayana, CEO, Aptuit Laurus, for their encouragement.

References

Abas, F., Lajis, N.H., Shaari, K., Israf, D.A., Stanslas, J., Yusuf, U.K., and Raof, S.M. (2005). A labdane diterpene glucoside from the rhizomes of *Curcuma mangga. Journal of Natural Products*, 68: 1090–1093.

Aggarwal, B.B., Kumar, A., and Bharti, A.C. (2003). Anticancer potential of curcumin: Preclinical and clinical studies. *Anticancer Research*, 23: 363–398.

Aggarwal, B.B., Sundaram, C., Malani, N., and Ichikawa, H. (2007). Curcumin: the Indian solid gold. *Advances in Experimental Medicine and Biology*, 595: 1–75.

Akio, M.F., Yoshimasa, T.N., and Toshihiko, O.N. (1993). Method for making tetrahydrocurcumin and a substance containing the antioxidative substance tetrahydrocurcumin. US 5,266,344.

Ammon, H.P.T., Anazodo, M.I., Safayhi, H., Dhawan, B.N., and Srimal, R.C. (1992). Curcumin: A potent inhibitor of leukotriene B_4 formation in rat peritoneal polymorphonuclear neutrophils (PMNL). *Planta Medica*, 58: 226.

Ammon, H.P.T., Safayhi, H., Mack, T., and Sabieraj, J. (1993). Mechanism of antiinflammatory actions of curcumin and boswellic acids. *Journal of Ethnopharmacology*, 38: 105–112.

Anand, P., Kunnumakkara, A.B., Newman, R.A., and Aggarwal, B.B. (2007). Bioavailability of Curcumin: Problems and Promises. *Molecular Pharmaceutics*, 4: 807–818.

Anto, R.J., Kuttan, G., Babu, K.V.D., Rajasekharan, K.N., and Kuttan, R. (1996). Antitumour and free radical scavenging activity of synthetic curcuminoids. *International Journal of Pharmaceutics*, 131: 1–7.

Atal, C.K., Dubey, R.K., and Singh, J. (1985). Biochemical basis of enhanced drug bioavailability by piperine: Evidence that piperine is a potent inhibitor of drug metabolism. *Journal of Pharmacology and Experimental Therapeutics*, 232: 258–262.

Azuine, M.A., and Bhide, S.V. (1992). Protective single/combined treatment with betel leaf and turmeric against methyl (acetoxymethyl) nitrosamine-induced hamster oral carcinogenesis. *International Journal of Cancer*, 51: 412–415.

Azuine, M.A., Kayal, J.J., and Bhide, S.V. (1992). Protective role of aqueous turmeric extract against mutagenicity of direct acting carcinogens as well as benzo[alpha]pyrene induced genotoxicity and carcinogenicity. *Journal of Cancer Research and Clinical Oncology*, 118: 447–452.

Babu, K.V.D., and Rajasekharan, K.N. (1994). Simplified condition for the synthesis of curcumin 1 and other curcuminoids. *Organic Preparations and Procedures International*, 26: 674–676.

Banerjee, A., and Nigam, S.S. (1978). Antimicrobial efficacy of the essential of *Curcuma longa*. *Indian Journal of Medical Research*, 68: 864–866.

Baumann, W., Rodrigues, S.V., and Viana, L.M. (2000). Pigments and their solubility in and extractability by supercritical CO_2: The case of curcumin. *Brazilian Journal of Chemical Engineering*, 17: 323–328.

Bhavanishankar, T.N., and Srinivasa Murthy, V. (1979). Effect of turmeric (*Curcuma longa*) fractions on the growth of some intestinal and pathogenic bacteria in vitro. *Indian Journal of Experimental Biology*, 17: 1363–1366.

Chandra, J.G., and Krishnamurthy, R.G. (2005). Curcumin treatment enhances the repair and regeneration of wounds in mice exposed to hemibody[gamma]-irradiation. *Plastic and Reconstructive Surgery*, 115: 515–528.

Chattopadhyay, I., Biswas, K., Bandyopadhyay, U., and Banerjee, R.K. (2004). Turmeric and curcumin: Biological actions and medicinal applications. *Current Sci*ence, 87: 44–53.

Dahl, T.A., McGowan, W.M., Shand, M.A., and Srinivasan, V.S. (1989). Photokilling of bacteria by the natural dye curcumin. *Archives of Microbiology*, 151: 183–185.

Dandekar, D.V., Gaikar, V.G. (2002). Microwave assisted extraction of curcuminoids from *Curcuma longa*. *Separation Science and Technology*, 37: 2669–2690.

Dhillon, N., Aggarwal, B.B., Newmann, R.A., Wolf, R.A., Kunnumakkara, A.B., Abbruzzese, J.L., Ng, C.S., Badmaev, V., and Kurzrock, R. (2008). Phase II trial of curcumin in patients with advanced pancreatic cancer. *Clinical Cancer Research*, 14: 4491–4499.

Duvoix, A., Blasius, R., Delhalle, S., Schnekenburger, M., Morceau, F., Henry, E., Dicato, M., and Diederich, M. (2005). Chemopreventive and therapeutic effects of curcumin. *Cancer Letters*, 223: 181–190.

Flynn, D.L., Rafferty, M.F., and Boctor, A.M. (1986). Inhibition of 5-hydroxy-eicosatetraenoic acid (5-HETE) formation in intact human neutrophils by naturally-occurring diarylheptanoids: inhibitory activities of curcuminoids and yakuchinones. *Prostaglandins Leukotriens Medicine*, 22: 357–360.

Ganga Raju, G., Rama Raju, G., Subbaraju, G.V., and Venkateswarlu, S. (2007). Process for producing enriched fractions of tetrahydroxycurcumin and tetrahydrotetrahydroxycurcumin from the extracts of *Curcuma longa*. PCT: WO 2007043058.

Gopinath, D., Ahmed, M.R., Gomathi, K., Chitra, K., Sehgal, P.K., and Jayakumar, R. (2004). Dermal wound healing processes with curcumin incorporated collagen films. *Biomaterials*, 25: 1911–1917.

Halliwell, B., and Gutteridge, J.M.C. (1985). *Free Radicals in Biology and Medicine;* Oxford University press, Oxford, New York.

Huang, M.T., Lysz, T., Ferraro, T., Abidi, T.F., Laskin, A.J.D., and Conney, A.H. (1991). Inhibitory effects of curcumin on *in vitro* lipoxygenase and cyclooxygenase activities in mouse epidermis. *Cancer Research*, 51: 813–819.

Huang, M.-T., Newmark, H.L., and Frenkel, L. (1997). Inhibitory effects of curcumin on tumorigenesis in mice. *Journal of Cellular Biochememistry*, 67: 26–34.

Jayaprakasha, G.K., Jagan Mohan Rao, L., and Sakariah, K.K. (2005). Chemistry and biological activities of *Curcuma longa. Trends in Food Science and Technology*, 16: 533–548.

Jiang, H., Timmermann, B.N., Gang, D.R. (2006). Use of liquid chromatography–electrospray ionization tandem mass spectrometry to identify diarylheptanoids in turmeric (*Curcuma longa* L.) rhizome. *Journal of Chromatography A*, 1111: 21–31.

Johnson, J.J., and Mukhtar, H. (2007). Curcumin for chemoprevention of colon cancer. *Cancer Letters*, 255: 170–181.

Kiuchi, F., Goto, Y., Sugimoto, N., Akao, N., Kondo, K., and Tsuda, Y. (1993). Nematocidal activity of turmeric: synergistic action of curcuminoids. *Chemical and Pharmaceutical Bulletin*, 41: 1640–1643.

Kunchandy, E., and Rao, M.N.A. (1990). Oxygen radical scavenging activity of curcumin. *International Journal of Pharmaceutics*, 58: 237–240.

Larson, R.A. (1988). The antioxidants of higher plants. *Phytochemistry*, 27: 969–978.

Li, C.J., Zhang, L.J., Dezube, B.J., Crumpacker, C.S., and Pardee, A.B. (1993). Inhibitors of type 1 human immunodeficiency virus long terminal repeat-directed gene expression and virus replication. *Proceedings of the National Academy of Sciences*, (USA), 90: 1839–1842.

Maheswari, R.K., Singh, A.K., Gaddipati, J., and Srimal, R.C. (2006). Multiple biological activities of curcumin: a short review. *Life Sciences*, 78: 2081–2087.

Majeed, M., Badmaev, V., Shivakumar, U., and Rajendran, R. (1995). Curcuminoids: antioxidant phytonutrients, Nutriscience Publishers, Piscataway, New Jersey.

Mani, H., Sidhu, G.S., Kumari, R., Gaddipati, J.P., Seth, P., and Maheswari, R.K. (2002). Curcumin differentially regulates TGF-B1, its receptors and nitric oxide synthase during impaired wound healing. *BioFactors*, 16: 29–43.

Manzan, A.C.C.M., Toniolo, F.S., Bredow, E., and Povh, N.P. (2003). Extraction of essential oil and pigments from *Curcuma longa* [L.] by steam distillation and extraction with volatile solvents. *Journal of Agricultural and Food Chemistry*, 51: 6802–6807.

Masuda, T., Isobe, J., Jitoe, A., and Nakatani, N. (1992). Antioxidative curcuminoids from rhizomes of *Curcuma xanthorrhiza*. *Phytochemistry*, 31: 3645–3647.

Mazumder, A., Neamati, N., Sunder, S., Schulz, J., Pertz, H., Eich, E., and Pommier, Y. (1997). Curcumin analogs with altered potencies against HIV-1 integrase as probes for biochemical mechanisms of drug action. *Journal of Medicinal Chemistry*, 40: 3057–3063.

Misra, S.K., and Sahu, K.C. (1977). Screening of some indigenous plants for antifungal activity against dermatophytes. *Indian Journal of Pharmacology*, 9: 269–272.

Mohamad, H., Lajis, N.H., Abas, F., Ali, A.M., Sukari, M.A., Kikuzaki, H., and Nakatani, N. (2005). Antioxidative constituents of *Etlingera elatior*. *Journal of Natural Products*, 68: 285–288.

Nagabhusan, M., and Bhide, S. V. (1992). Curcumin as an inhibitor of cancer. *Journal of American College of Nutrition*, 11: 192–198.

Nakayama, R., Tamura, Y., Yamanaka, H., Kikuzaki, H., and Nakatani, N. (1993). Two curcuminoid pigments from *Curcuma domestica*. *Phytochemistry*, 33: 501–502.

Pabon, H.Y.Y. (1964). A synthesis of curcumin and related compounds. *Recueil des Travaux Chimiques des Pays-Bas*, 83: 379–386.

Pedersen, U., Rasmussen, P.B., and Lawesson, S.-O. (1985). Synthesis of naturally occurring curcuminoids and related compounds. *Liebigs Annalen der Chemie*, 1557–1569.

Ramprasad, C., and Sirsi, M. (1957). *Curcuma longa* and bile secretion-quantitative changes in the bile constituents induced by sodium curcuminate. *Journal of Scientific and Industrial Research*, 16C: 108–110.

Rao, C.V., Rivenson, A., Simi, B., and Reddy, B.S. (1995). Chemoprevention of colon carcinogenesis by dietary curcumin naturally occurring plant phenolic compound. *Cancer Research*, 55: 259–266.

Rao, C.V., Simi, B., and Reddy, B.S. (1993). Inhibition by dietary curcumin of azoxymethane-induced ornithine decarboxylase, tyrosine protein kinase, arachidonic acid metabolism and aberrant crypt foci formation in the rat colon. *Carcinogenesis*, 14: 2219–2225.

Ravindranath, V., and Chandrasekhara, N. (1982). Metabolism of curcumn-studies with [^{3}H]curcumin. *Toxicology*, 22: 337–344.

Reddy, A.C.P., and Lokesh, B.R. (1992). Studies on spice principles as antioxidants in the inhibition of lipid peroxidation of rat liver microsomes. *Molecular and Cellular Biochemistry*, 111: 117–124.

Roughley, P.J., and Whiting, D.A. (1973). Experiments in the biosynthesis of curcumin. *Journal of the Chemical Society, Perkin Transactions 1*, 2379–2388.

Samuelsson, B. (1983). Leukotrienes: mediators of immediate hypersensitivity reactions and inflammation. *Science*, 220: 568–575.

Sardjoko, I.A.D., and Vermeulen, N.P.E. (1990). Cytotoxic and cytoprotective activities of curcumin: Effects on paracetamol-induced cytotoxicity, lipid peroxidation and glutathione depletion in rat hepatocytes. *Biochemical Pharmacology*, 39: 1869–1875.

Sharma S.C., Mukhtar, H., Sharma, S.K., and Krishna Murty, C.R. (1972). Lipid peroxide formation in experimental inflammation. *Biochemical Pharmacology*, 21: 1210–1214.

Sharma, O.P. (1976). Antioxidant activity of curcumin and related compounds. *Biochemical Pharmacology*, 25: 1811–1812.

Sharma, R.A., Euden, S.A., Platton, S.L., Cooke, D.N., Shafayat, A., Hewitt, H.R., Marczylo, T.H., Morgan, B., Hemingway, D., Plummer, S.M., Pirmohamed, M., Gescher, A.J., and Steward, W. (2004). Phase I clinical trial of oral curcumin: biomarkers of systemic activity and compliance. *Clinical Cancer Research*, 10: 6847–6854.

Sharma, R.A., Gescher, A.J., and Steward, W.P. (2005). Curcumin: The story so far. *European Journal of Cancer*, 41: 1955–1968.

Sharma, R.A., Ireson, C.R., Verschoyle, R.D., Hill, K.A., Williams, M.L., Leuratti, C., Manson, M.M., Marnett, L.J., Steward, W.P., and Gescher, A. (2001). Effects of Dietary Curcumin on Glutathione *S*-Transferase and Malondialdehyde-DNA Adducts in Rat Liver and Colon Mucosa: Relationship with Drug Levels. *Clinical Cancer Research*, 7: 1452–1458.

Shih, C.A., and Lin, J.K. (1993). Inhibition of 8-hydroxydeoxyguanosine formation by curcumin in mouse fibroblast cells. *Carcinogenesis*, 14: 709–712.

Shoba, G., Joy, D., Joseph, T., Majeed, M., Rajendran, R., and Srinivas, P.S.S.R. (1998). Influence of piperine on the pharmacokinetics of curcumin in animals and human volunteers. *Planta Medica*, 64: 353–356.

Sidhu, G.S., Singh, A.K., Thaloor, D., Banaudha, K.K., Patnaik, G.K., Srimal, R.C., and Maheswari, R.K. (1998). Enhancement of wound healing by curcumin in animals. *Wound Repair and Regeneration*, 6: 167–177.

Singh, A., Singh, S.P., and Bamezai, R. (1995). Postnatal modulation of hepatic biotransformation system enzymes via translactational exposure of F_1 mouse pups to turmeric and curcumin. *Cancer Letters*, 96: 87–93.

Soni, K.B., and Kuttan, R. (1992). Effect of oral curcumin administration on serum peroxides and cholesterol levels in human volunteers. *Indian Journal of Physiology and Pharmacology*, 36: 273–275.

Soni, K.B., Lahiri, M., Chackradeo, P., Bhide, S.V., and Kuttan, R. (1997). Protective effect of food additives on aflatoxin-induced mutagenicity and hepatocarcinogenicity. *Cancer Letters*, 115: 129–133.

Soni, K.B., Rajan, A., and Kuttan, R. (1992). Reversal of aflatoxin induced liver damage by turmeric and curcumin. *Cancer Letters*, 66: 115–121.

Soudamini, K.K., and Kuttan, R. (1992). Chemoprotective effect of curcumin against cyclophosphamide toxicity. *Indian Journal of Pharmaceutical Sciences*, 54: 213–217.

Sreejayan Rao, M.N.A. (1994). Curcuminoids as potent inhibitors of lipid peroxidation. *Journal of Pharmacy and Pharmacology*, 46: 1013–1016.

Srimal, R.C. (1997). Turmeric: a brief review of medicinal properties. *Fitoterapia*, LXVIII: 483–493.

Srimal, R.C., and Dhawan, N. (1973). Pharmacology of diferuloyl methane (curcumin), a non-steroidal antiinflammatory agent. *Journal of Pharmacy and Pharmacology*, 25: 447–452.

Srinivas, C., and Prabhakaran, K.V.S. (1989). Harida (*Curcuma longa*) and its effect on abhisayanda (conjunctivitis). *Ancient Science of Life*, 8: 279–283.

Syu, W.J.; Shen, C.C.; Don, M.J.; Ou, J.C.; Lee, G.H.; and Sun, C.M. (1998). Cytotoxicity of curcuminoids and some novel compounds from *Curcuma zedoaria*. *Journal of Natural Products*, 61: 1531–1534.

Tanaka, T., Makita, H., Ohnishi, M., Hirose, Y., Wang, A., Mori, H., Satoh, K., Hara, A., and Ogawa, H. (1994). Chemoprevention of 4-nitroquinoline 1-oxide-induced oral carcinogenesis by dietary curcumin and hesperidin: comparison with the protective effect of β-carotene. *Cancer Research*, 54: 4653–4659.

Thaloor, D., Miller, K.J., Gephart, J., Mitchell, P.O., and Pavlath, G.K. (1999). Systemic administration of the NF-kB inhibitor curcumin stimulates muscle regeneration after traumatic injury. *American Journal of Physiology-Cell Physiology*, 277: C320–C329.

Toan-Thang, P., Patrick, S., Seng-Teik, L., and Sui-Yang, C. (2001). Protective effects of curcumin against oxidative damage on skin cells *in vitro*: its implication for wound healing. *Journal of Trauma-Injury, Infection and Critical Care*, 51: 927–931.

Tohda, C., Nakayama, N., Hatanaka, F., and Komatsu, K. (2006). Comparison of antiinflammatory activities of six *Curcuma* rhizomes: a possible curcuminoid-independent pathway mediated by *Curcuma phaeocaulis* extract. *Evidence Based Complementary and Alternative Medicine*, 3: 255–260.

Varga, J., Rosenbloom, J., and Jimenez, S.A. (1987). Transforming growth factor beta (TGF beta) causes a persistent increase in steady-state amounts of type I and type III collagen and fibronectin mRNAs in normal human dermal fibroblasts. *Biochemical* Journal, 247: 597–604.

Venkatesan, N., and Chandrakasan, G. (1995). Modulation of cyclophosphamide-induced early lung injury by curcumin, an antiinflammatory antioxidant. *Molecular and Cellular Biochemistry*, 142: 79–87.

Venkateswarlu, S., Ramachandra, M.S., and Subbaraju, G.V. (2004). Synthesis and antioxidant activity of 5'-Methoxycurcumin: an yellow pigment from *Curcuma xanthorrhiza*. *Asian Journal of Chemistry*, 2: 827–830.

Venkateswarlu, S., Ramachandra, M.S., and Subbaraju, G.V. (2005). Synthesis and biological evaluation of polyhydroxycurcuminoids. *Bioorganic and Medicinal Chemistry*, 13: 6374–6380.

Vijayalakshimi, (1980). Genetic effects of turmeric and curcumin in mice and rats. *Mutation Research/ Genetic Toxicology*, 79: 125–132.

Yoshinobu, K., Yuriko, S., Noriko, W., Yoshiteru, O., and Hiroshi, H. (1983). Antihepatotoxic principles of *Curcuma longa* rhizomes. *Planta Medica*, 49: 185–187.

Medicinal Plants: Phytochemistry, Pharmacology and Therapeutics, Vol. 1 *Pages 178–191*
Editors: **V.K. Gupta, G.D. Singh, Surjeet Singh and A. Kaul**
Published by: **DAYA PUBLISHING HOUSE, NEW DELHI**

Chapter 8

Opioid Activity of the Ethanol Extract from *Psychotria carrascoana* Delprete and E. B. Souza Leaves in Mice

Cláudia Ferreira Santos[1], Antonia Torres Dávila Pimenta[2], Adriana Sousa Barros[1], Victor Martins Gomes[1], Natália Rocha Celedônio[1], Marta Regina Kerntopf[1], Silvânia Maria Mendes Vasconcelos, Ana Maria Sampaio Assreuy[1], Elnatan B. de Souza[3], Mary Anne Sousa Lima[2], Edilberto Rocha Silveira[2], Francisco Arnaldo Viana[4] and Nilberto Robson Falcao do Nascimento[1]*

[1]Curso de Mestrado Acadêmico em Ciências Fisiológicas, Instituto Superior de Ciências Biomédicas, Universidade Estadual do Ceará, Fortaleza-Ce, Brasil
[2]Curso de Pós-GraduaCao em Química Orgânica, Departamento de Química Orgânica e Inorgânica, Centro de Ciências, Universidade Federal do Ceará, CP 12 200, 60451-970, Fortaleza-Ce, Brasil
[3]Universidade Vale do Acaraú, Sobral-CE, Brasil
[4]Universidade do Estado do Rio Grande do Norte, Mossoró-RN, Brazil

ABSTRACT

The antinociceptive effect of the ethanolic extract (EEPc) obtained from the leaves of *Psychotria carrascoana* Delprete and E. B. Souza (Rubiaceae) was evaluated in models of nociception *in vivo* and for opioid-like activity, *in vitro*. EEPc was injected in mice at 10, 30 or 100 mg/kg doses,

* Corresponding Adress: Av. Paranjana, 1700, Itaperi, Fortaleza, Ceará; E-mail: nilberto@uece.br; Phone: 558531019836; Fax: 558531019810

before stimuli (writing test, formalin and hot plate tests) or added (0.1-300.0 mg/mL) into organ baths with isolated vas deferens under electrical field stimulation. EEPc inhibited the writhing test response with maximal effect at 100 mg/kg (97 per cent). In addition, EEPc blocked both phases of the formalin test, being more effective in the inflammatory phase with maximal inhibition (86 per cent) at 100 mg/kg. EEPc enhanced the reaction time to thermal stimuli at all times analyzed (30, 60 and 90 min): at 30 mg/kg (76, 78 and 25 per cent) and 100 mg/kg (76, 76 and 64 per cent), respectively. This effect was blocked by naloxone. Animal motor performance was not altered by EEPc. EEPc (0.1-300mg/mL) inhibited neurogenic contraction with maximal effect at 300 mg/mL by 89.5±3.6 per cent (IC_{50}= 17.8 [9.7-25.9] mg/ml). This effect was reversed (64.4±9.7 per cent of control before EEPc) by post-treatment and prevented (89.5±3.6 per cent EEPc–38.7±4.6 per cent EEPc+NLX by pretreatment) with naloxone. The EEPc antinociceptive action may occurs by direct agonist action on pre-synaptic opioid receptors and by probably by its antiinflammatory activity. Qualitative HPLC analysis for the ethanol extract indicated the presence of the pirrolidinoindole alkaloid calycosidine.

Keywords: *Opioide-like antinociception, Psychotria carrascoana leaves, Vas deferens.*

Introduction

Psychotria (Rubiaceae) is one of the largest genera of flowering plants with 1650 species distributed in tropical regions. This genus is easily encountered in the State of Ceará, Brazil as in other states, where spontaneously grows in areas such as pasture, beside roads and in empty grounds. Although considered as a weed for agricultural purposes (Lorenzi and Matos, 2002), species of this genus are used in traditional medicine against dizziness, hallucination, dementia and rubella (Joly *et al.*, 1987). *P. viridis* and *P. carthagenensis* are often spoken in the literature in relation to the hallucinogenic beverage ayahuasca, widespread throughout the Amazon where it is known as Santo Daime, and used for religious, medicinal and social purposes (Rivier *et al.*, 1972). Elisabettsky *et al.* (1995) described that in the North and Northeast of Brazil this plant is also used in folk medicine in the treatment of pain disorders, for which purpose it is prepared from the plant leaves and roots as infusions.

The genus *Psychotria* has been regarded as a promising source of alkaloids, mainly of the polypirrolidinoindoline type (Elisabetsky *et al.*, 1997). It has being demonstrated that alkaloids obtained from *Psychotria* spp show diverse pharmacological actions, such as inhibition of human platelet aggregation (Beretz *et al.*, 1985) and opiate-like analgesic effects in behavioral tests (Elisabetsky *et al.*, 1997). Psychotridina, an alkaloid isolated from *P. colorata* showed dose-dependent antinociceptive response both in chemical and thermal models of nociception, suggesting the participation of N-methyl-D-aspartate (NMDA) receptors in this effect (Amador *et al.*, 2001). Other alkaloid, psychollatine (formerly known as umbellatine) isolated from *Psychotria umbellata* Vell. was shown to have analgesic activity by modulating NMDA, 5-HT and opioid receptors (Both *et al.*, 2006). Kodanko *et al.* (2007) recently described the synthesis of steroisomers of hodgkinsine and demonstrated its opioid-like activity in the tail flick and capsaicin pain models.

The present study was undertaken in order to demonstrated the antinociceptive action of the ethanol extract obtained from leaves of the specie *Psychotria carrascoana* Delprete and E. B. Souza, that has been described recently (Delprete and Souza, 2004). For this, classical *in vivo* models of nociception (acetic acid-induced abdominal constrictions–writing test, formalin and hot plate tests) and the motor performance test (Rota Rod) were used. The electrical stimulated mouse vas deferens (Hughes *et al.*, 1974), was also used for examining the potential opioid-like activity of the *P. carrascoana* extract. In addition, the qualitative HPLC analysis of the ethanol extract indicated the presence of calycosidine, a pyrrolidinoindoline alkaloid with antinociceptive activity.

Materials and Methods

Animals

Male Swiss mice (25–30g) were obtained from the central animal house of Federal University of Ceará and maintained in a controlled 12/12 h light/dark cycle, temperature of 22±5 °C with free access to water and food. Investigations were conducted in accordance with international guidelines (NIH publication N°85-23, revised 1985) and the experimental protocols approved by the Institutional Animal Care and Use Committee of the State University of Ceara–UECE, Fortaleza-CE, Brazil.

Plant Material

Leaves of *P. carrascoana* native from Crato-County, Araripe's Plateau, Ceará, Northeast Brazil and were identified by Dr. Elnatan B. de Souza (Vale do Acaraú University). A voucher specimen (# 32531) has been deposited at the Herbário Prisco Bezerra (Biology Department, Federal University of Ceara–UFC, Fortaleza,Ceará, Brazil.

Ethanol Extract Preparation

Air dried young leaves (0.7 kg) of *P. carrascoana* were extracted with ethanol at room temperature. The solvent was removed under reduced pressure yielding a dark brown semi-solid mass (101.4 g). This material was further dissolved in a vehicle (NaCl 0.9 per cent containing 1 per cent dimethylsulfoxide-DMSO) to adequate concentrations before administration into animals.

HPLC

The ethanol extract from leaves of *P. carrascoana* was compared with a original sample of the alkaloid calycosidine, previously isolated from the stems. Chromatography was performed using a Shimadzu system (Kioto-Japan) consisting of two pumps model LC-10ATvp, membrane degasser Model DGU-14A, photodiode array detector (Model SPD-M10Avp), dynamic chamber mixing, manual injector Model 7725i with loop of 20 µl, controlled by means of Class–VP 6.1 software for data processing. All solvents used were of HPLC grade (Merck, Germany).

The analytical separation and identification of the calycosidine in the ethanol extract was carried out a room temperature on Shim-Pack LC8 reverse phase column (PN–228-17874-91)(150 mm x 4,6 mm; 5 µm) using the solvents H_2O–HCOOH 0.1 per cent (A) and MeOH (B) as mobile phase. The gradient consisted of linear gradient from 10 per cent B to 80 per cent B for 10 min, followed by 10 min of isocratic elution. The flow rate was 0.5 ml min^{-1}, aliquot of 20 µl were injected, monitored at 254 nm and UV spectra were recorded in the range 190–370 nm.

Identification of calycosidine standard alkaloid was possible by comparison of the retention time (5,8 min) in the extract, and confirmed by co-injection of calycosidine with the plant extract.

Drugs and S

Acetic acid was purchased from Vetec Química Farm. Ltda, formaldehyde from Reagen Quimibrás Ind. Química S. A. (both companies from Rio de Janeiro, RJ, Brazil), naloxone, yohimbine, noradrenaline, ATP and morphine were purchased from Sigma Chemical Company (St Louis, MO). Yohimbine was dissolved by using 0.5 per cent ethanol in saline (V/V). All other drugs were dissolved in distilled water. Control was done with vehicle (1 per cent DMSO in saline V/V).

Acetic Acid-Induced Writhing in Mice

Mice (n= 6-12 per group) were injected i.p. with 0.8 per cent acetic acid (0.1 mL/10g; body weight) and after 10 min, the number of abdominal constrictions was registered for 20 min (Koster *et al.*, 1959). Animals were treated by intraperitoneal route with the ethanol extract of *Psychotria carrascoana* leaves (EEPc) at the doses of 10, 30 or 100 mg/kg (0.1 ml/10 g body weight), 30 min before acetic acid administration. Control animals were injected with similar volume of vehicle.

Formalin Test

In this test, 25 ml of 2.5 per cent formaldehyde was administered (n = 9-12 per group) in the mice right hind paws and the licking time was registered from 0 to 5 min (phase 1–neurogenic) and from 15 to 30 min after the intraplantar injection of formalin (phase 2–inflammatory) (Hunskaar *et al.*, 1985; Tjolsen *et al.*, 1992). Mice were treated with the EEPc (10, 30 or 100 mg/kg; i.p; 0.1 ml/10 g body weight), 30 min before formalin administration. Control animals were injected with similar volume of vehicle. A experimental positive control group was treated with morphine (5m/kg; s.c) 30 min before formalin injection.

Hot Plate Test

Animals previously selected were submitted to the plate heated at 55.5 °C. Three groups of n=8-12 mice each were treated with the EEPc (10, 30 or 100 mg/kg; i.p; 0.1 mL/10 g body weight) and the control group received the same volume of vehicle. In another experiment, animals were treated with naloxone (2 mg/kg; i.p.) 15 min before EEPc (100mg/kg). Two experimental groups treated with morphine (5mg/kg; s.c) or with naloxone (2 mg/kg; i.p) 15 minutes before morphine (5mg/kg; s.c) were used as positive controls. Measurements were performed at time zero (0 time) and 30, 60 or 90 min after administration, with a cut-off time of 40 s to avoid animal paw lesion (Woolfe and McDonald, 1944).

Motor Performance Test

Animals (n= 8-10) were selected 24h before to the test by eliminating those mice that did not remain on the bar of the Rota Rod for two consecutive period of 60s. Mice were treated with the EEPc (30 and 100mg/kg; i.p.) or vehicle 30min before submitted to test. The evaluation was made by placing animals in the Rota-rod (UGO BASILE, model-DS 37) during 60 s, 15, 30 or 60 min after injection (Duham and Miya, 1957).

Vas Deferens Model

The whole vas deferens was dissected from mature male mice (35–40 g) killed by cervical dislocation. Each vas deferens was stripped of adhering fat and mesenteric investment. Strips of prosthatic segments, approximately 15 mm long, were suspended vertically in 5mL organ bath containing Krebs solution (composition in mM: NaCl 118, KCl 4.75, $NaHCO_3$ 24, $CaCl_2$ 54, KH_2PO_4 0.93, glucose 11, EDTA 0.027 and ascorbic acid 0.1) gassed in 5 per cent CO_2/95 per cent O_2 at 37°C for isometric recording of mechanical activity. Following tissue preparation (resting tension of 0.25 g for 40 min), the vas deferens was submitted to electrical field stimulation (EFS; 30V pulse, 0.5ms duration, 0.1Hz frequency) and thereafter a concentration-response curve of EEPc (0.1, 0.3, 1.0, 3.0, 10.0, 30.0 or 300.0 mg/mL) was performed alone or after 30 min incubation with yohimbine (10mM) or naloxone (10mM). The contractions were recorded with an isometric force displacement transducer coupled to a four-channel Narco-Biosystems physiograph (Narco, Houston, TX, USA). The inhibition of the EFS-contraction response was expressed as percentage of control contractions, *i.e.*, before administration of the extract (Henderson *et al.*, 1972). In other set of experiment, to test whether EEPc inhibitory activity in the vas deferens would have a post-synaptic mechanism, we probed this extract against 10 mM noradrenaline or 30 mM adenosine triphosphate (ATP)-induced contractions in mice vas deferens. The peak contraction attained in the presence of the vehicle of EEPc was compared with the peak contraction obtained in the presence of 300 mg/mL of this extract (a concentration that almost abolishes neurogenic contraction).

Statistical Analysis

The data were expressed as mean±S.E.M. and subjected to ANOVA followed by Tukey or Dunnett's comparison test $P<0.05$ was considered significant.

Results

The ethanol extract (EEPc) of *Psychotria carrascoana* leaves significantly and dose-dependently decreased the number of the acetic acid-induced abdominal constrictions in mice at the two higher doses used. The maximal inhibitory effect was observed at 100 mg/kg (97 per cent) which was followed by the dose of 30 mg/kg (57 per cent), compared to control group (Figure 8.1).

In the formalin test, EEPc inhibited at 30 and 100 mg/kg (37.7 per cent and 57.7 per cent, respectively) the first phase of the test (neurogenic) and also showed significant analgesic effect in the second phase (inflammatory) at doses of 10, 30 or 100 mg/kg, reduced the time in which animals showed nociception responses by 40, 64 and 86 per cent, respectively. Similarly, morphine (5 mg/kg; s.c) induced a potent antinociceptive activity in both phases with 85.1±4.8 per cent and 97.2±7.6 per cent inhibition, respectively (Figure 8.2).

Animals treated with EEPc and assayed in the hot plate test enhanced the reaction time to thermal stimuli at all times analyzed. The dose of 30 mg/kg increased this latency by 76, 78 and 25 per cent after 30, 60 and 90 min, respectively, followed EEPc administration. At the dose of 100 mg/kg the increase in latency showed to be around 76, 76 and 64 per cent in the same time analyzed (Figure 8.3a). The antinociceptive effect of EEPc was completely blocked by naloxone pretreatment. Morphine induced an increase in latency after 30 min of 90.8±8.1 per cent which was also blocked by naloxone (Figure 8.3b).

Intraperitoneal treatment with EEPc did not alter the animals motor performance at any doses tested (Table 8.1). This result validates the nociceptive effect previously described in all models of nociception used.

Table 8.1: Effect of Treatment with *Psychotria carrascoana* Ethanolic Extract (i.p.) in Rota-Rod Test in mice

Treatments	*Dose (mg/Kg)*	*Motor Performace on the Rota-Rod (s)*
Vehicle	0	107±13.0
EEPc	30	94±16.2
EEPc	100	90±19.3

Values are reported as means±SEM, n=8-10.

In the vas deferens model, EEPc, dose dependently (0.1-300mg/ml), inhibited electrical field-induced contraction with maximal effect observed at 300 mg/ml by 89.5±3.6 per cent (IC_{50}= 17.8 [9.7-25.9] mg/ml) (Figures 8.6 and 8.5a). In another set of experiments, tissue pre-treatment with naloxone blocked the maximal inhibitory response induced by EEPc (EEPC alone–89.5±3.6 per cent vs. EEPc+NLX–16.7±4.6 per cent; p<0.001; n=12) (Figures 8.6 and 8.5b). This inhibitory effect was also reversed by 64.4±9.7 per cent after addition of naloxone (Figure 8.5c) with a similar profile of the reversion attained when morphine was used as agonist (Figure 8.5d). However, tissue pre-treatment with yohimbine (α-2-receptor antagonist) did not affect the maximal inhibitory response evoked by EEPc (EEPc alone 89.4±3.6 per cent vs. EEPC+ YOH–97.5±1.9 per cent) (Figure 8.6). Accordingly,

Figure 8.1: HPLC Chromatogram of Fresh Extract Compared with Calycosidine.

Chromatographic conditions are as described in the material and methods section. Identification of calycosidine standard alkaloid was possible by comparison of the retention time (5.8 min) in the extract, and confirmed by co-injection of calycosidine with the plant extract.

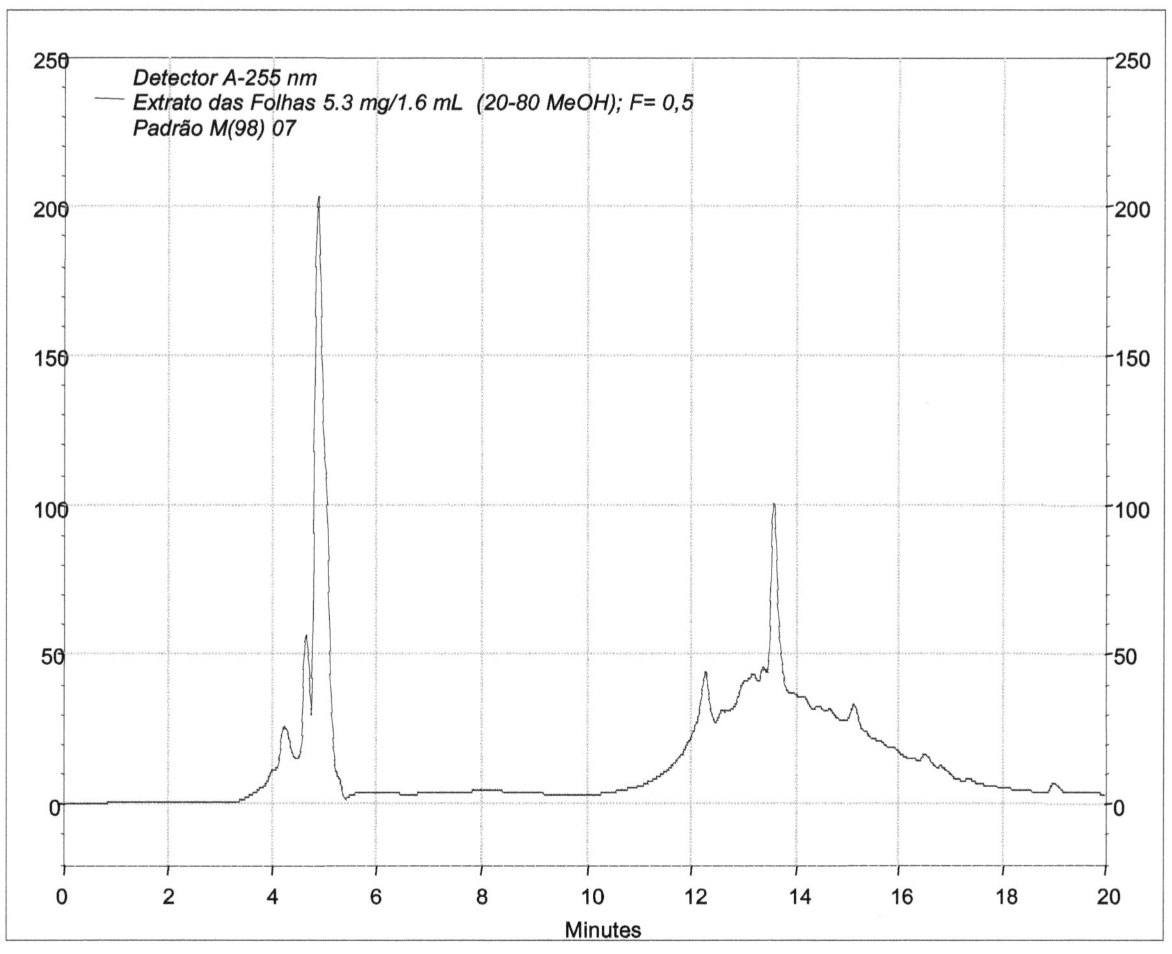

(a) Standard of Calycosidine

Contd...

Figure 8.1–Contd...

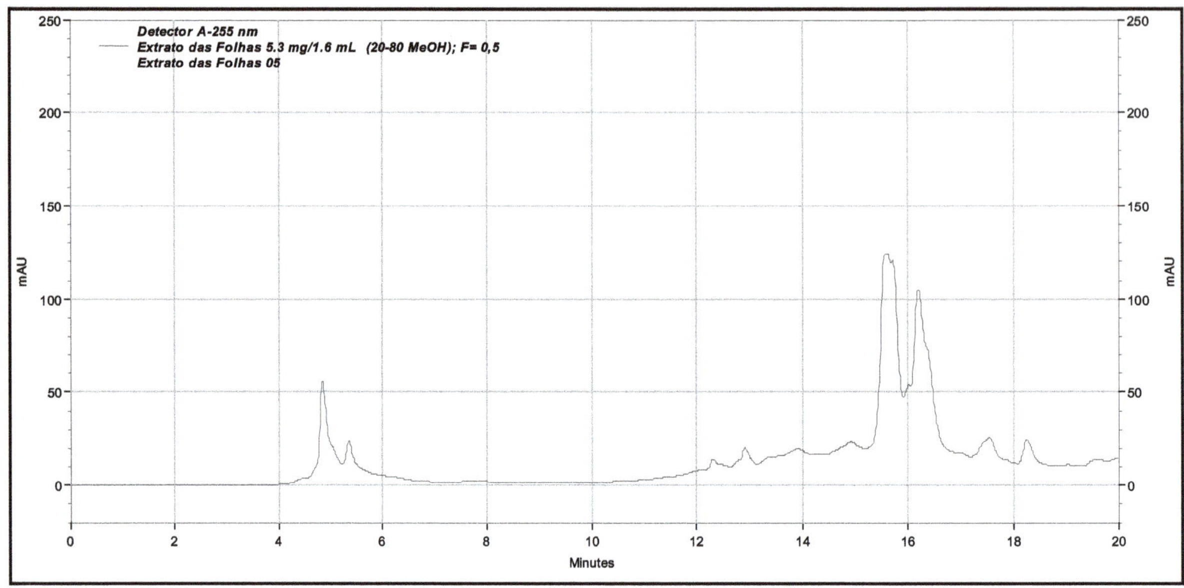

(b) Ethanol Extract from Leaves of *P. carrascoana*

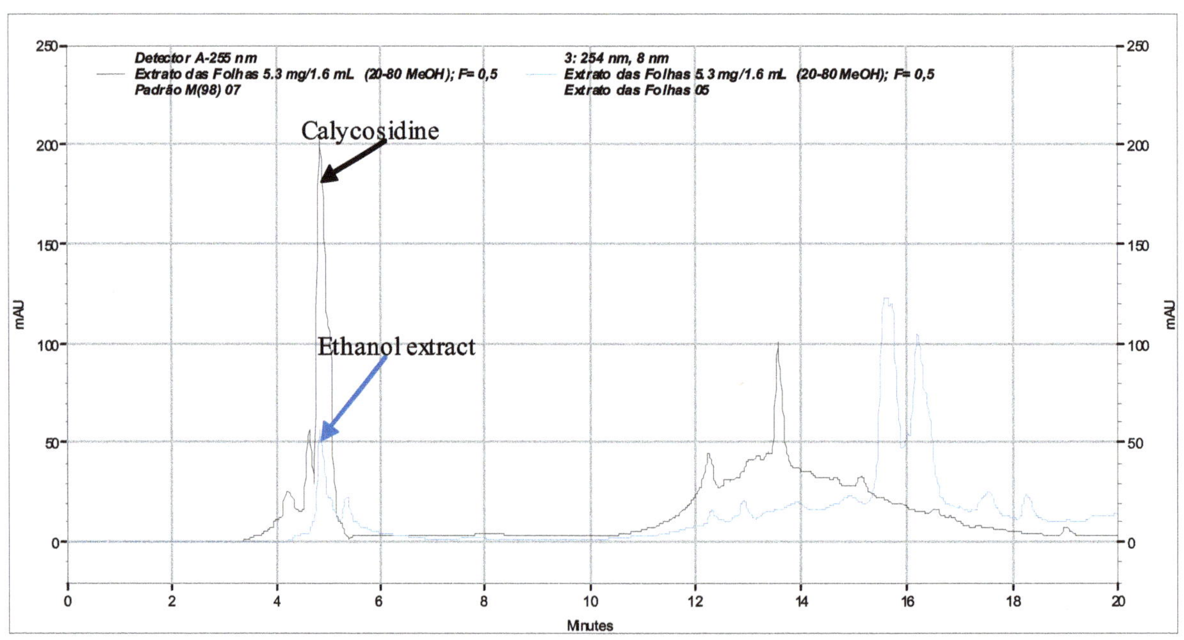

(c) HPLC Chromatogram Depicting Co-injection of Calycosidine with the Plant Extract

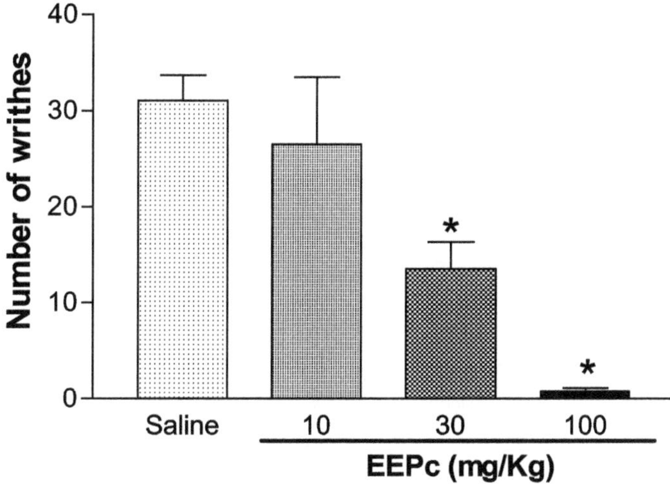

Figure 8.2: The Ethanolic Extract of *Psychotria carrascoana* Leaves Inhibits the Acetic Acid-induced Abdominal Constrictions in Mice.

Animals were treated i.p. with EEPc at 10 (n=6); 30 (n=10); or 100 (n=6) mg/kg or vehicle (n=12), 30 min before i.p. injection of 0.8 per cent acetic acid. Ten minutes later, the number of constrictions was registered for 20 min. Values are reported as means±SEM. *p<0.05 compared to vehicle.

incubation of EEPc for 5 min did not inhibit contractions promoted by 10mM of the exogenous agonists noradrenaline and ATP (Figure 8.7).

Discussion and Conclusions

Species from the *Psychotria* genus have being popularly used for pain treatment (Elisabetsky *et al.*, 1995). Various investigations have being demonstrating a relashionship between the plant analgesic effect and presence of alkaloids with opioide-like activity. *In vivo*, Elisabetsky and collaborators (1995) described that alkaloids presented in leaves and flowers of *Psychotria colorata* have marked opiate-like analgesic effects; *In vitro*, Amador and collaborators (1996) showed an inhibitory effect of *P. colorata* flower alkaloids on [^{3}H]naloxone binding in rat striata, as well a decrease in adenylate cyclase basal activity.

Pharmacological studies conducted using isolated *Psychotria* alkaloids have shown mixed mechanisms for its analgesic action: Hodgkinsine, a trimeric pyrrolidinoindoline type alkaloid present as a major constituent of *Psychotria spp*, has shown to produce dose-dependent, naloxone reversible, analgesic effect in thermal models of nociception and in the capsain-induced pain. In addition, *in vivo* assays have demonstrated that calycosidine has the same analgesic profile of hodgkinsine (Verotta *et al.*, 2002). On the other hand, psycotridine presented a dose-dependent analgesic effect in the tail flick model of nociception that was not reversed prior treatment with naloxone. Additionally, this substance decreased capsain-induced pain and inhibited binding to cortex membranes. These results ruled out the psycotridine opioid activity and strongly suggested participation of NMDA receptors (Amador *et al.*, 2001).

In the present study we demonstrated the analgesic effect of *P. carrascoana* in mice. Intraperitoneal treatment with its ethanol extract (EEPc) in mice caused a dose-dependent antinociceptive effect in the three classical experimental models of nociception (acetic acid-induced abdominal-constrictions, 1st

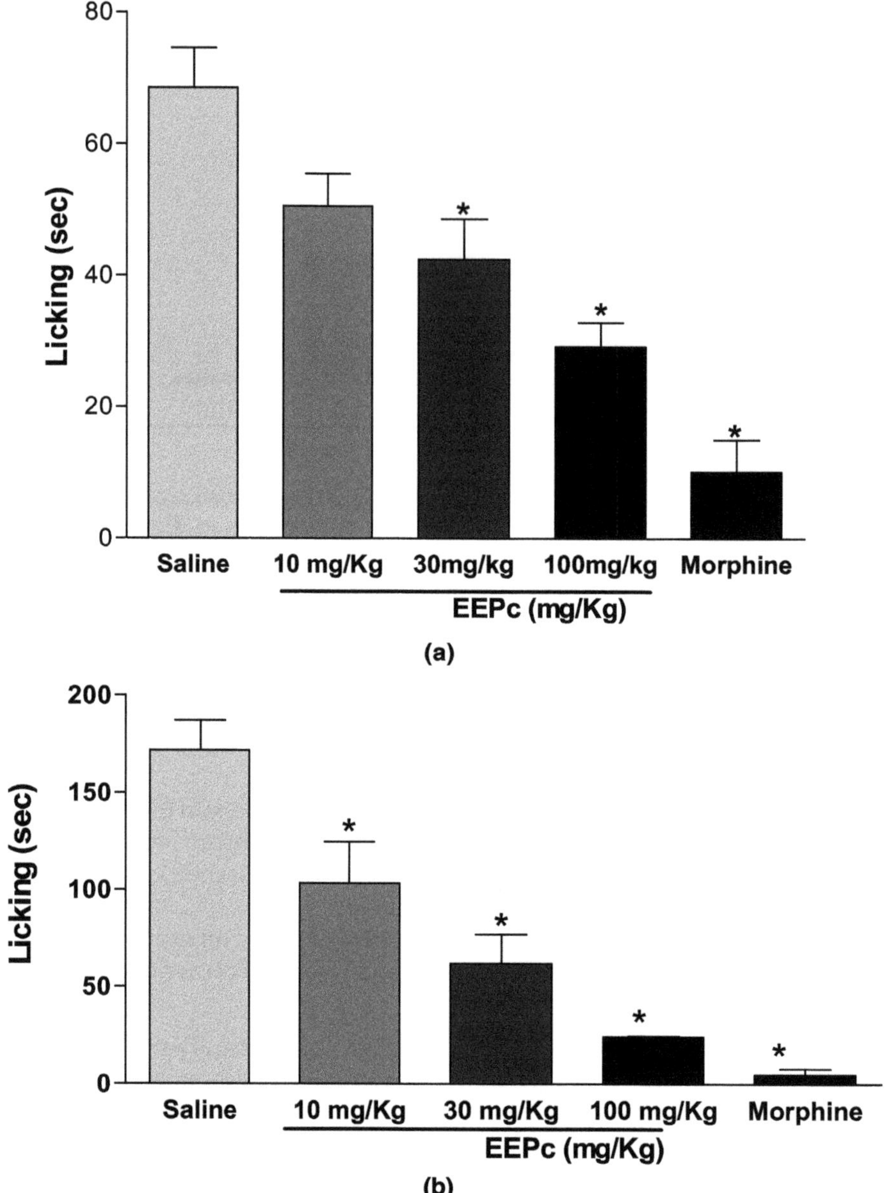

Figure 8.3: The Ethanolic Extract of *Psychotria carrascoana* Leaves Inhibits the Neurogenic (a) and the Inflammatory Phase (b), of the Formalin Test.

Animals were treated with EEPc at 10 (n=10), 30 (n=9) or 100 (n=10) mg/kg; i.p. or vehicle (n=12), 30 min before intraplantar injection of 2.5 per cent formaldehyde. The licking time was registered from 0 to 5 min (phase 1, neurogenic) and from 15 to 30 min after formalin (phase 2, inflammatory). Control animals were injected with similar volume of vehicle. Morphine (5mg/Kg; s.c) 30 minutes before formalin challenge was used as positive control. Values are reported as means±SEM. *p<0.05 compared to vehicle.

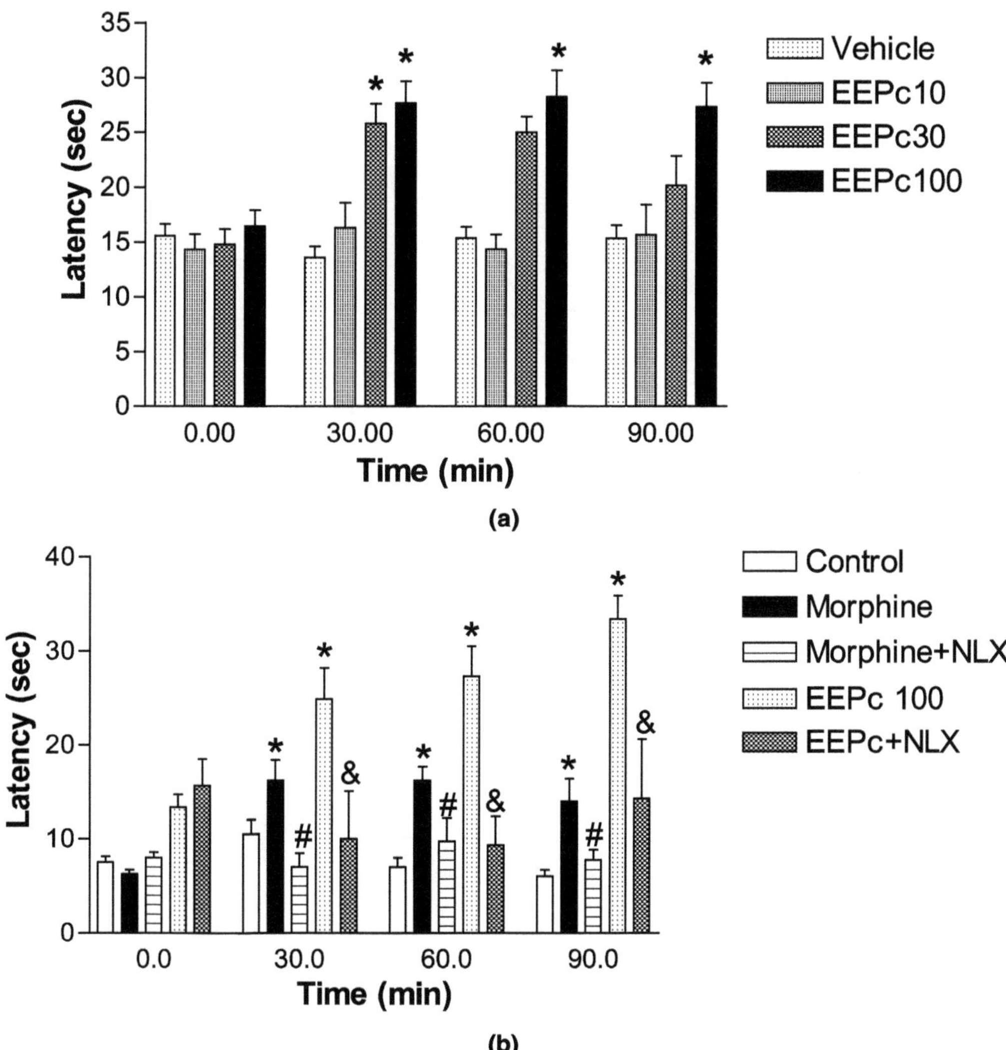

Figure 8.4: Antinociceptive Effect of the Ethanolic Extract of *Psychotria carrascoana* Leaves in the Hot Plate Test.

(a) Animals were treated i.p. with EEPc at 10 (n=12), 30 (n=8) or 100 (n=12) mg/Kg or vehicle (n=12); (b) Animals were treated i.p with naloxone (NLX; 2mg/kg) 30min before EEPc (100mg/kg) or morphine (5mg/Kg; s.c). Measurements were performed at time zero (0 time) and 30, 60 and 90 min after treatment, with a cut-off time of 40 s to avoid animal paw lesion. Values are reported as means±SEM. *p<0.05 compared to control. #p<0.05 compared to Morphine alone. and p<0.05 compared to EEPc 100 alone.

and 2[snd] phase of formalin test and hot plate test) tested. This data demonstrated that the ethanol extract of *P. carrascoana* has central and peripherally mediated antinociceptive activities. In the hot plate test the *Psychotria* antinociceptive effect was reversed by prior treatment of animals with naloxane,

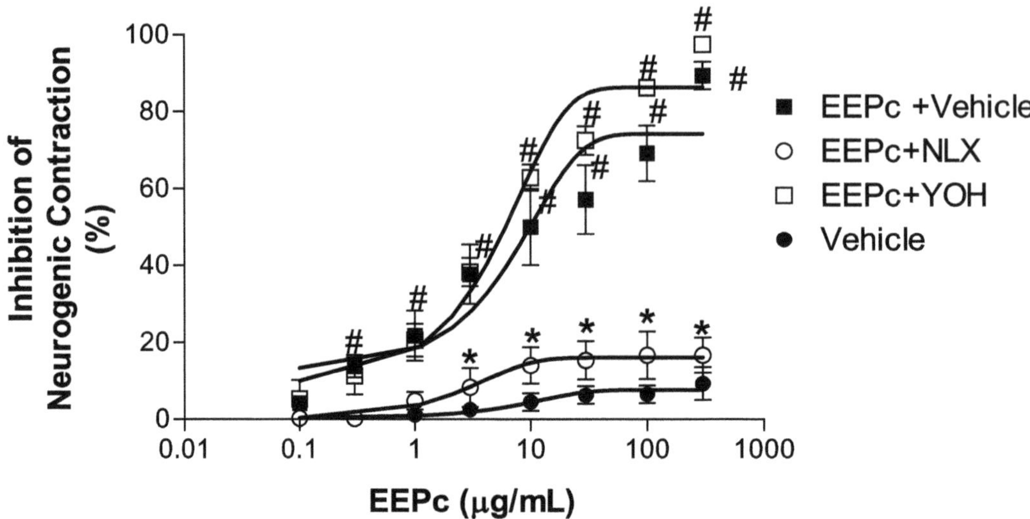

Figure 8.5: Effect of the Ethanolic Extract of *Psychotria carrascoana* Leaves (EEPc) in Neurogenic Contractions in MVD in the Absence or Presence of 10 mM Naloxone or Yohimbine. Values are reported as means±SEM. *p<0.05 compared to EEPc plus naloxone (NLX;30mM). #p<0.05 vs. Vehicle

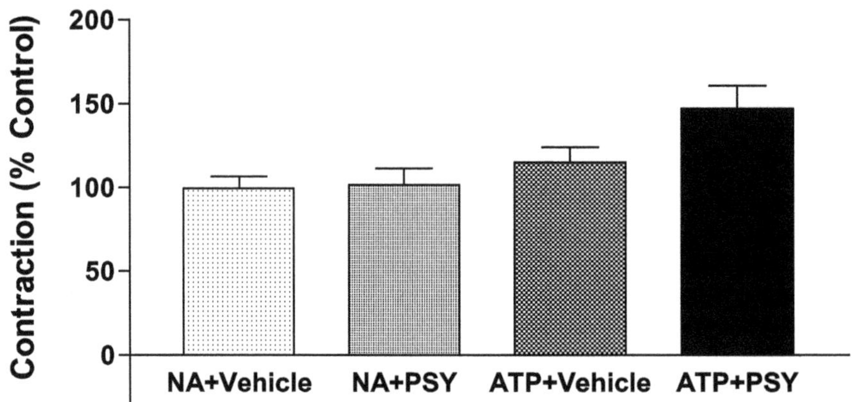

Figure 8.6: Lack of Effect of the Ethanolic Extract of *Psychotria carrascoana* Leaves (EEPc) in Pharmacological Contractions in MVD Evoked by Exogenous Administration of Noradrenaline (NA; 10 mM) or Adenosine Triphosphate (ATP;30 mM) in the Absence or Presence of 300 mg/ml EEPc (PSY). Values are reported as means±SEM (n=9 and 12, respectively).

suggesting an opioid activity. The peripheral action may be due to its antiinflammatory activity, but this has to be tested properly in specific inflammatory models.

In order to evaluate the possible non-specific muscle-relaxant or sedative effects of EEPc its activity was also evaluated in the rota rod test. It was observed that motor performance was not altered by any dose used. The mouse vas deferens has served as a useful bioassay for examining the properties of opiate receptors (Henderson *et al.*, 1972). In this model the EEPc showed to inhibit the electrical field-

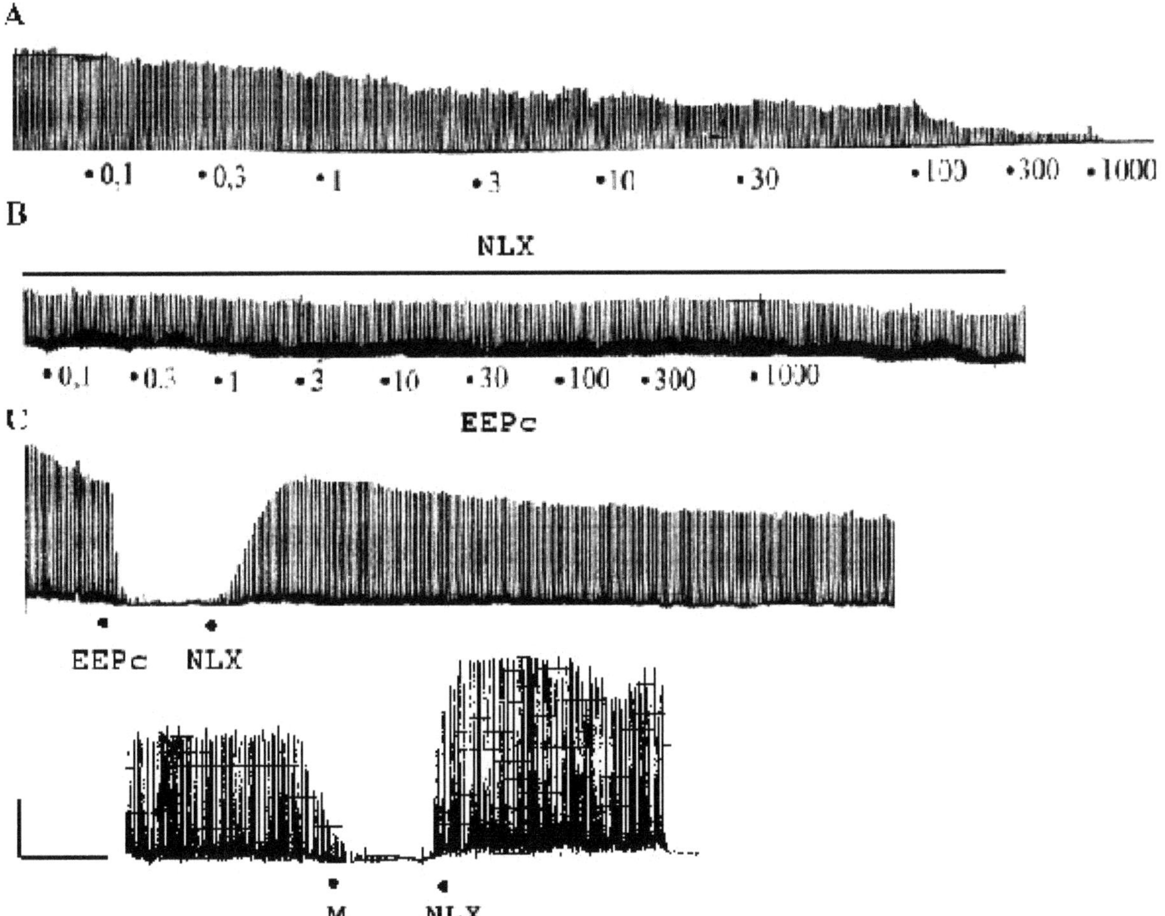

Figure 8.7: Typical Physiographic Recordings Showing the Effect of the Ethanolic Extract of *Psychotria carrascoana* Leaves (EEPc) in Neurogenic Contractions in MVD in the Absence (A) or Presence of 10 mM Naloxone (NLX) (B). Panel (C) Shows the Pre-synaptic Inhibition of Neurotransmission Induced by EEPc and its s Rapid Reversion Induced by Naloxone (10 mM). The Positive Control Experiment done with Morphine (M) is Shown in Panel (D).

induced contraction, an effect that was reversed and also prevented by naloxone. The direct effect in opiod recetor was shown both by the prevention of the inhibitory effect of EEPc in neurogenic contraction by naloxone and also by the prompt reversion induced by naloxone of this inhibitory activity.This data reinforces the opioid effect demonstrated in the hot plate model. Furthermore, EEPc did not alter the contractions evoked by noradrenaline or ATP pointing to a pre-synaptic activity.

These data all together do indicate that antinociceptive action of EEPc occurs via inhibition of nociception by direct action on pre-synaptic opioid receptors. Nevertheless, the data obtained *in vivo* must be due, besides the direct opioid activity demonstrated in this study, to other effects such as interaction with NMDA and 5-HT receptor in the central nervous systems. This mechanism should be considered in further investigations.

The direct effect in opiod receptor was shown both by the prevention of the inhibitory effect of EEPc in neurogenic contraction by naloxone and also by the prompt reversion induced by naloxone of this inhibitory activity. This data reinforces the opioid effect demonstrated in the hot plate model.

The opioid–like activity of the ethanolic extract of *P. carrascoana* is demonstrated by the reversion as well as blockade by the opioid antagonist naloxone. The presence of the alkaloid calycosidine may contribute to the analgesic activity described in this report. Calycosidine is a derivative of Hodgkinsine and these compounds share its analgesic effect with same pharmacological profile. Nevertheless, other non-identified compounds present in the extract may contribute to the antinociceptive activity described herein as well as the antiinflammatory activity related to the second phase of the formalin test.

The analysis of the ethanol extract obtained from leaves of *P. carrascoana* by HPLC showed the presence of the alkaloid calycosidine as constituent of the extract and in further studies this alkaloid will be used in order to compare its antinociceptive activity with the crude extract. The antinociceptive activity described in this study confirms the validity of the ethnopharmacological approaches in the search for new analgesic drugs.

References

Amador T.A, Elisabestky,E.Souza, D.O. (1996). Effects of *Psychotria colorata* alkaloids in brain opioid system. *Neurochemitry Research,* 21(1): 97-102.

Amador T.A, Verotta L., Nunes, D.S.,Elisabestky,E. (2001). Involvment of NMDA receptors in the analgesic properties of psychotridine. *Phytomedicine,* 8(3):202-206.

Both FL, Meneghini L, Kerber VA, Henriques AT, Elisabetsky E. (2006). Role of glutamate and dopamine receptors in the psychopharmacological profile of the indole alkaloid psychollatine. *J Nat Prod.,* 69(3):342-345.

Beretz A., Roth-Georger A., Corre G., Kuballa B., Anton R., Cazenave J.P. (1985). Polyindolinic alkaloids from *Psychotria forsteriana*. Potent inhibitors of the aggregation of human platelets. *Planta Medica,* 4: 300-303.

Delprete, P. G.; Souza, E. O. (2004). *Psychotria carrascoana,* a new species from the carrasco vegetation of Northeastern Brazil. *Novon,*14: 158-162.

Duham, N.W.; Miya, T.S. (1957). A note on a simple apparatus for detecting neurological deficit in rats and mice. *Journal of American Pharmacists Association,* 46: 208-209.

Elisabetsky E., Amador T.A., Albuquerque R.R., Nunes D.S., Carvalho A. C. (1995). Analgesic activity of *Psychotria colorata* (Willd. ex R. and S.) Muell. Arg. alkaloids. *Journal of Ethnopharmacology,* 48: 77-83.

Elisabetsky, E.; Amador, T.A.; Leal, M.B.; Nunes, D.S.; Carvalho, A.C.T. and Verotta,L. (1997). Merging ethnopharmacology with chemotaxonomy: an approach to unveil bioactive natural products. The case of Psychotria alkaloids as potential analgesics. *Ciencia e Cultura,* 49(5/6):378-409.

Henderson G., Hughes J., Kosterlitz H.W. (1972). A new example of a morphine-sensitive neuro-effector junction: adrenergic transmission in the mouse vas deferens. *British Journal of Pharmacology,* 46(4): 764-766.

Hughes J, Kosterlitz HW, Leslie FM. (1974). Proceedings: Assessment of the agonist and antagonist activities of narcotic analgesic drugs by means of the mouse vas deferens.*Br J Pharmacol.,* 51(1): 139-140.

Hunskaar S, Fasmer OB, Hole K. (1985). Formalin test in mice, a useful technique for evaluating mild analgesics. *Journal of Neuroscience Methods,* 14(1): 69-76.

Joly, L.G., Guerra S., Septimo R., Solis P.N., Correa M., Gupta M., Levy S., Sandberg F. (1987). Ethnobotanical inventory of medicinal plants used by the Guaymi Indians in western Panama. Part I. *Journal of Ethnopharmacology,* 20(2): 145-171.

Koster, R., Anderson, M., De Beer, E. J. (1959). Acetic acid for analgesic screening. *Federation Proceedings,* 18: 412.

Lorenzi, H.; Matos, F.J.A. (2002). Plantas medicinais no Brasil: nativas e exóticas cultivadas. Nova Odessa, SP: *Instituto Plantarum,*: 158-159.

Rivier, L., Lindgren, J. E. (1972). Ayahuasca, the South American hallucinogenic drink: an ethnobotanical and chemical investigation. *Economic Botany,* 26: 101-129.

Tjolsen A, Berge OG, Hunskaar S, Rosland JH, Hole K. (1992).The formalin test: an evaluation of the method. *Pain,* 51(1): 5-17.

Verotta L, Orsini F, Sbacchi M, Scheildler MA, Amador TA, Elisabetsky E. (2002). Synthesis and antinociceptive activity of chimonanthines and pyrrolidinoindoline-type alkaloids. *Bioorganic and Medical Chemistry,* 10(7): 2133-2142.

Woolfe, G.; Mac Donald, A. D. (1944). The evalution of the analgesic action of pethidine hydrochloride (Demerol). *Journal of Pharmacological Experimental Therapeutics,* 80: 300-307.

Medicinal Plants: Phytochemistry, Pharmacology and Therapeutics, Vol. 1 *Pages* ***192–201***
Editors: **V.K. Gupta, G.D. Singh, Surjeet Singh and A. Kaul**
Published by: **DAYA PUBLISHING HOUSE, NEW DELHI**

Chapter 9

Comparative Effects of Soybean, Sunflower, Olive and Sugar Cane Wax Oils and their Respective Fatty Acids in Cutaneous Inflammation

N. Ledón*, A. Casacó, S. Rodríguez, A. Gonzalez, N. Merino, O. Ancheta, V.J. Rodriguez, J. Cruz, R. González, A. Capote, M. Cano, Z. Tolon, E. Rojas and R. González
Molecular Immunology Center, 216 esq 17 C, Habana, Cuba

ABSTRACT

The interest in some kind of oils for treating psoriasis has been increased in the last years. It has been shown that cutaneous signs and symptoms of psoriasis can be reversed by the dermal application of vegetable oils. Taking into account that psoriasis does not occur in animals and it is not possible to induce the disease in laboratory animals; the antiinflammatory effects of soybean (*Glycine max* L), sunflower (*Helianthus annuus* L), olive (*Olea europaea* L) and sugar cane wax (*Saccharum officinarum* L) oils and their respective fatty acids were studied in the following experimental models: the 12-O-tetradecanoylphorbol-13–acetate, arachidonic acid-induced inflammation and in the mouse tail test of psoriasis.

In general, our results have shown, that fatty acids exert a better antiinflammatory and antipsoriatic effects and a lower polymorphonuclear leukocyte infiltration than their respective

* Corresponding Author: E-mail: nuris@cim.sld.cu.

oils on topical application. The best results were obtained with the fatty acids from sugarcane oil. Qualitative and quantitative differences in the chemical composition of the oils provide explanation of our results.

Keywords: *Cutaneous inflammation, Fatty acids, Olive oil, Sugarcane oil, Sunflower oil, Soybean oil.*

Introduction

Fatty acids have a wide range of biological roles and cellular functions. They are important components of the phospholipid bilayers of cellular membranes, which affect membrane fluidity and lipid-protein interactions. Thus, fatty acids can influence transport of proteins and cellular receptors for hormones and neurotrasmitters (Galli *et al.*, 1994). They affect the production of many biologically active compounds, including lipid-derived cellular mediators such as platelet-activating factor, eicosanoids, and cytokines (Roche, 1999). Fatty acids also have the ability to affect the expression of genes encoding for enzymes which are involved in lipids metabolism and to interact with nuclear receptor proteins that bind to DNA, therefore fatty acids can alter the transcription of regulatory genes (Sessler and Ntambi, 1998).

However, all oils and their constitutive fatty acids have not the same effects on cellular functions. The purpose of the present study is to compare the antiinflammatory effect of soybean, sunflower, olive and sugar cane oils and their respective fatty acids with different composition in two models of inflammation and in the mouse tail test of psoriasis.

Materials and Methods

Chemicals, Materials and Animals

Sugar cane wax oil (FAM) was obtained from a sugar factory, whereas, soybean, olive and sunflower oils from a extraction oil factory. Fatty acids and oils at different concentrations were evaluated in different models. All reagents not specifically described were purchased from Sigma Chemical (St Louis. MO). Male OF1 mice (20-22g) were obtained from the National Center for Production of Laboratory Animals (CENPALAB, Havana, Cuba). The experiments were carried out in accordance with the ethical guidelines for investigations in laboratory animals.

Chemical Composition of Oils and their Fatty Acids

The samples for determination of oils and fatty acid mixtures components to be tested in the experiments were obtained by a saponification and further filtration process in order to eliminate the unsaponified matter and the acid released. Gas Chromatographic analysis of fatty acids were performed on a SHIMADZU G-C-14A equipment which has a double flame ionization detector and a 3.1 meter column full with cromazor-w coated with 7 per cent of polyethylene glycol succinate. The argon carrier gas flow rate was 8 ml/min. The oven temperature program was 90-195°C, 6°C/min. and the injector was at 270°C. The composition of fatty acid mixture after being methylated with n-methyl-n-nitroso-p-toluensulfonamid was determined (Table 9.1).

Arachidonic Acid (AA) and 12-O-tetradecanoylphorbol-13-acetate (TPA) Induced Ear Edema in Mice

Tested substances or indomethacin (1mg/ear) plus AA (0.5mg/ear) or triamcinolone (1 mg/ear) plus TPA (4 mg/ear) dissolved in acetone (20ml) or the inflammatory substances plus the vehicle or only acetone were applied to the ears of mice. At appropriate time (1h for AA and 6h or 18h for TPA treatment), the animals were killed by cervical dislocation and a 6mm diameter disc from each ear was removed with a metal punch. The antiedematous effect of test substance was expressed as percentage inhibition of the ear swelling compared with the edema produced by AA or TPA (Puignero and Queralt, 1997).

Table 9.1: Qualitative and Quantitative (per cent) Composition of Fatty Acid Mixtures

Fatty Acids	*Oils*			
	Sugarcane	*Sunflower*	*Soybean*	*Olive*
Capric (C10)	0.33	–	–	–
Lauric (C12)	0.45	–	–	–
Miristic (C14)	0.56	–	0.34	–
Pentadecanoic (C15)	0.03	–	–	–
Palmitic (C16)	29.40	15.41	13.91	18.44
Palmitoleic (C16:1)	0.02	–	–	2.65
Estearic (C18)	3.73	3.23	4.06	2.59
Oleic (C18:1)	14.88	26.36	23.56	65.25
Linoleic (C18:2)	42.20	55.00	52.74	11.07
Linolenic (C18:3)	8.03	–	5.39	–
Araquidic (C20)	0.10	–	–	–
Dodeicosanoic (C22)	0.12	–	–	–
Trieicosanoic (C23)	0.02	–	–	–
Tetraeicosanoic (C24)	0.11	–	–	–
Pentaicosanoic (C25)	0.02	–	–	–

Assay of PLA_2 activity

Ear tissues from mice killed 18 hours after TPA treatment were homogenized in 0.5 ml homogenizing buffer (100 mM KCl, 10 mM tris-HCl, pH 7.4 (buffer A). Homogenates were centrifuged for 15 min at 3500g and 4°C and pellet was eliminated. 50 ml of each sample (20-25 mg of protein) were incubated at 24°C, 15 min with buffer A plus 2 mM $CaCl_2$, and with fluorescence substrate 1 acyl-2-[6-[(7-nitro-1,2,3 benzoxadiazol-4-il)amino]-caproil]phosphatidilcoline ($5x10^{-6}$ M) (Molecular Probes, Eugene, OR). Fluorescence excitation was at 470nm and emission at 540 nm. Titers were based on comparisons with standard curves obtained with bovine pancreas phospholipase A_2 of known activity and the determination were performed in a spectrofluorimeter (Wittenauer *et al.*, 1984).

Mieloperoxidase Assay

Ear tissues from mice killed 6 hours after TPA treatment were homogenized in 50 mM K_2HPO_4/ KH_2PO_4 buffer (pH 6) containing 0.5 per cent of hexadecyl trimethylammonium bromide using a polytron homogenizer. After freeze-thawing 3 times, the samples were centrifuged at 2500g for 30 min at 4°C and the resulting supernatant assayed spectrophotometrically for MPO as described before (Romay *et al.*, 1998).

Psoriasis Tail Test

The modified mouse tail test established by Bosman *et al.* (1992) was used. Mice tails were treated locally with 0.1 ml of the tested substances (4.02 mg) or with paraffin (negative control group) on its proximal part or non treated. Animals were treated weekly twice daily, for 3 weeks. Another group of animals was orally treated with 0.01 mg/kg per day, with a suspension of retinoic acid in water and was considered as positive control group. At the end of the treatment, animals were killed and longitudinal sections of tails of about 5 mm thickness were prepared and stained with hematoxylin-eosin for histological examination. Smaller pieces were taken for ultrastructural processing.

Histological Examination

Ten sequential scales were examined for the presence of a granular layer induced in the previously parakeratotic skin areas. The induction of orthokeratosis in those parts of the adult mouse tail which have normally a parakeratotic differentiation is quantified measuring the length of the granular layer (A) and the length of the scale (B). The proportion (A/B) x 100 represents the per cent orthokeratosis per scale, and the drug activity (DA) was calculated as follows: DA=[(mean OK of treated group–mean OK of control group)/100-mean OK of control group]x 100 where OK=orthokeratosis. The measurements were carried out at the border of the scale with a semiautomatic image evaluation unit (Rodríguez, 1992).

Ultrastructural Processing

Skin tail pieces were fixed in 5 per cent glutaraldehyde for 24 h and postfixed in 1 per cent osmium tetroxide for about 8 h, buffered in 1 mol/l sodium cacodylate buffer (pH 7.4). Fixed pieces were dehydrated in graded concentrations of acetone and embedded in Spurr resin. Semithin sections for recognizing scale (interfollicular) regions, before preparing ultrathin sections in these areas. Sections were stained with uranyl acetate and lead citrate and studied under a JEOL JEM 100 S transmission Electron Microscope (Ancheta, 1996).

Statistical Analysis

Data are presented as means±standard deviation. Due to a non-gaussian distribution of orthokeratosis values (100 per cent is the maximal effect) the Kruskal-Wallis test was used. For the rest of the experiments statistical significance among groups was analyzed by ANOVA one way and Duncan's multiple-range test. Values of $p < 0.05$ were considered to be significant.

Results

Inflammatory response of the mouse ear skin was characterized by various methods: oedema by ear punch weight, by MPO activity, by PLA_2 activity and by histophatology studies in the TPA induced inflammation in mouse ear, oedema by ear punch weight in arachidonic acid-induced inflammation and orthokeratosis induction in mouse tail test of psoriasis.

When different vegetable oils or their fatty acids were co-applied with TPA or arachidonic acid, marked and dose dependent anti–inflammatory activity was observed in the animals (Figures 9.1 and 9.3). Better inhibitory activity was observed with the free fatty acids than with their original oils. The free fatty acids from sugar cane oil showed the best results. Evaluated histologically, 18 hours after TPA treatment showed acanthosis, edema and a prominent cellular infiltrate comprised predominantly of neutrophils (Figure 9.2A) compared to fatty acids (Figure 9.2B). When treated topically with vegetable oils or their fatty acids, this inflammatory response was largely abrogated.

Figure 9.1: Effect of Tested Substances on Edema, and MPO and PLA_2 Activities on TPA Induced Ear Inflammation Values having the Different Letters are Statistically Significant at $p<0.05$ ($X \pm S.D$, n=10/group)

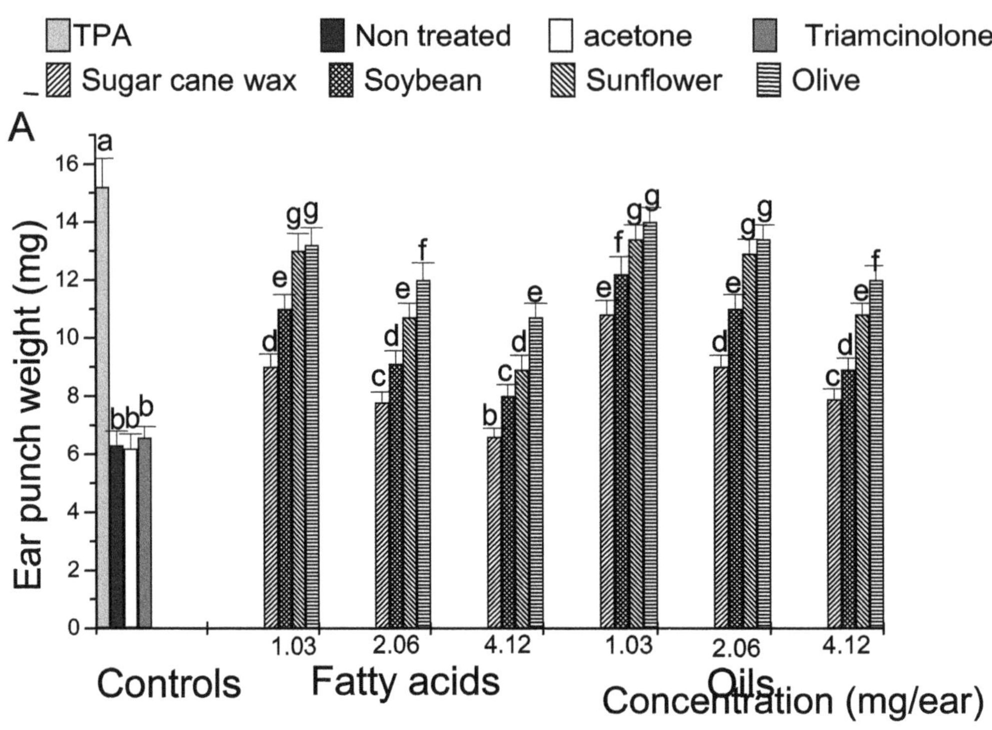

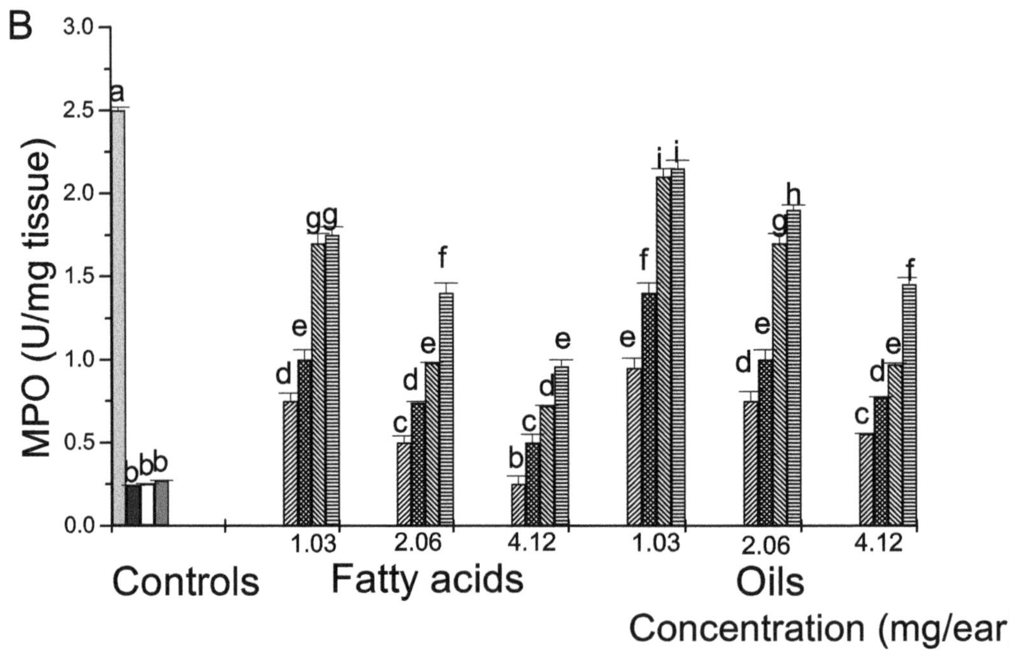

Contd...

Figure 9.1–Contd...

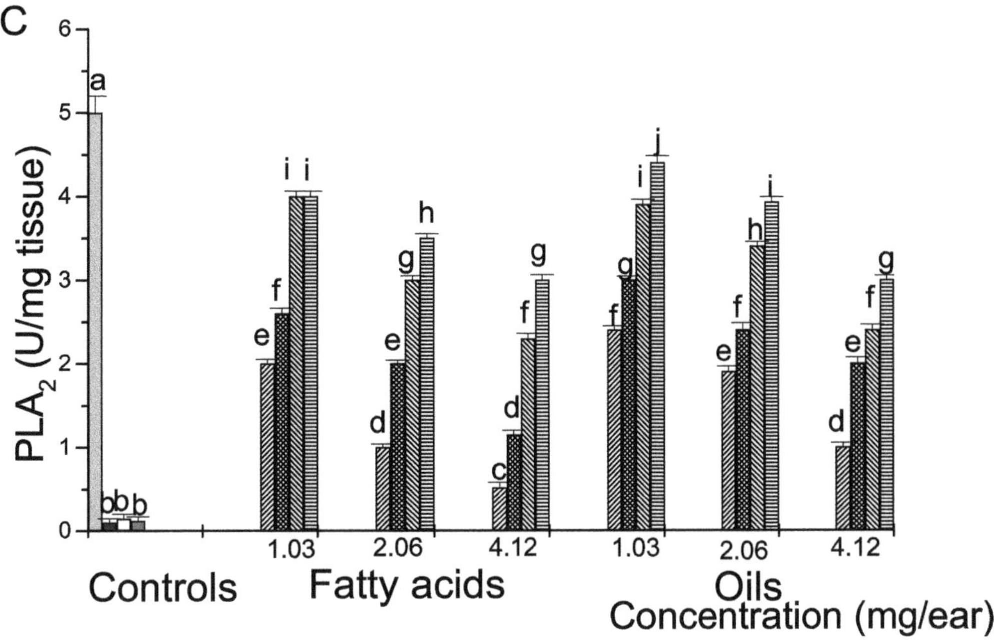

Figure 9.4 shows that all oils and their fatty acids have an important drug activity in the mouse tail test. The figure represents the orthokeratotic values showing that fatty acids have a better induction of granular layer than their respective oils. All oils and their fatty acids showed an important antiinflammatory activity. Sugar cane wax oil and their fatty acids showed the best inhibitory activity.

Table 9.1 shows the quantitative and qualitative composition of the four vegetable oils studied. In this table, it could be noted that the linoleic/linolenic ratio for sugar cane is 5; and 9.8 for soybean, whereas sunflower and olive oils have not detectable linolenic acid.

Discussion

It has been suggested that botanical lipids have antiinflammatory actions due to their ability to reduce the phospholipase A_2 activity, with the subsequent reduction of synthesis of those oxygenation products of arachidonic acid which are potent mediators of inflammation and also blocking the leukotriene B_4 receptors (Zurier 1993, Yagaloff *et al.*, 1994,Ledón *et al.*, 2007). Essential fatty acids also play an important role in the structure and physiology of the skin and the cutaneous effects of its deficiency in rats and humans have been reversed by application of linoleic acid (Ledón *et al.*, 2005). They are also important for the cutaneous eicosanoids metabolism (Ledón *et al.*, 2003).

The main barrier of the skin is the stratum corneum. Topically applied drugs must first penetrate this barrier in order to reach their site of action and the clinical usefulness of drugs is frequently hampered by their inability to pass. Our results have shown that topical applications of fatty acids exert a better antiinflammatory effect than their respective oils. These results could be explained due to the possibility of fatty acids to increase skin permeability by disrupting the ordered lamellar structure of the biolayers in the stratum corneum, leading to increased fluidization of the intracellular medium.

Evaluated histologically, after TPA treatment showed acanthosis, edema and a prominent cellular infiltrate comprised predominantly of neutrophils (Figure 9.2A) compared to fatty acids (Figure 9.2B)

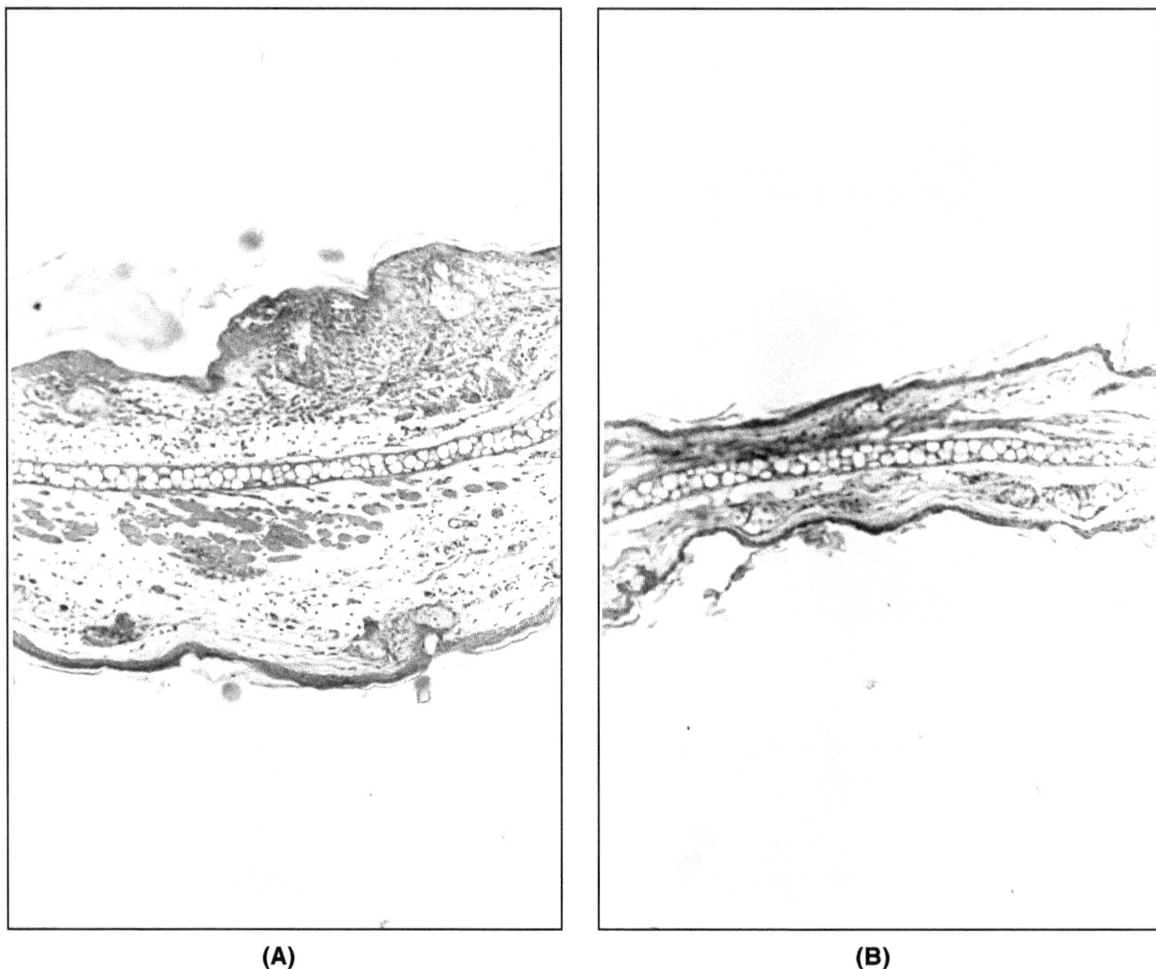

(A) (B)

Figure 9.2: (A) Histopathology of an Ear Mouse 18 Hours After Treatment with TPA, showed Acanthosis, Edema and a Prominent Cellular Infiltrate Comprised Predominantly of Neutrophils. Hematoxilin-eosin staining. 50X. (B) Histopathology of an Ear Mouse 18 Hours After Topical Treatment with the Fatty Acid Mixture from Sugarcane Wax Oil. Its present the normal characteristics of this kind of tissue. Hematoxilin-eosin staining. 50X.

Loftsson *et al.* (1995) showed that addition of pure cod-liver oil to propylene glycol vehicle did not increase the permeability but their fatty acids did it. So, they concluded that unsaturated fatty acids must be in the free way in order to be able to act as skin penetration enhancers (Loftsson, 1995). Therefore, it is possible to assume that the better effect of the fatty acids compared to their original oils depend on their more efficient penetration for reaching their site of action.

Special considerations must be taken with sugar cane oil and its fatty acids that showed very interesting orthokeratotic and antiinflammatory properties. These results could be related to an

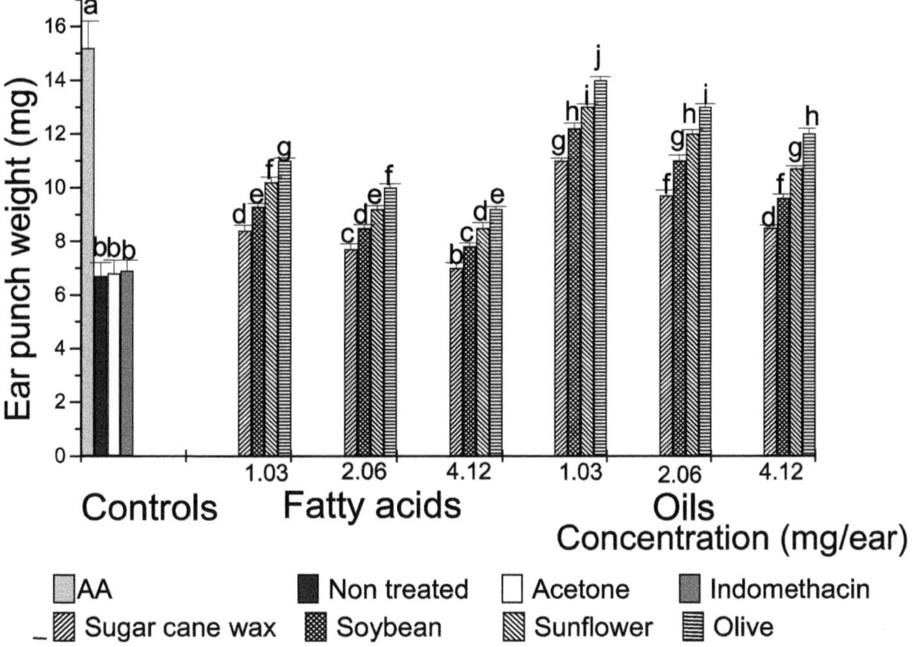

Figure 9.3: Effect of Tested Substances on Edema in AA Induced Ear Inflammation. Values having the Different Letters are Statistically Significant at p<0.05 (X±S.D, n=10/group)

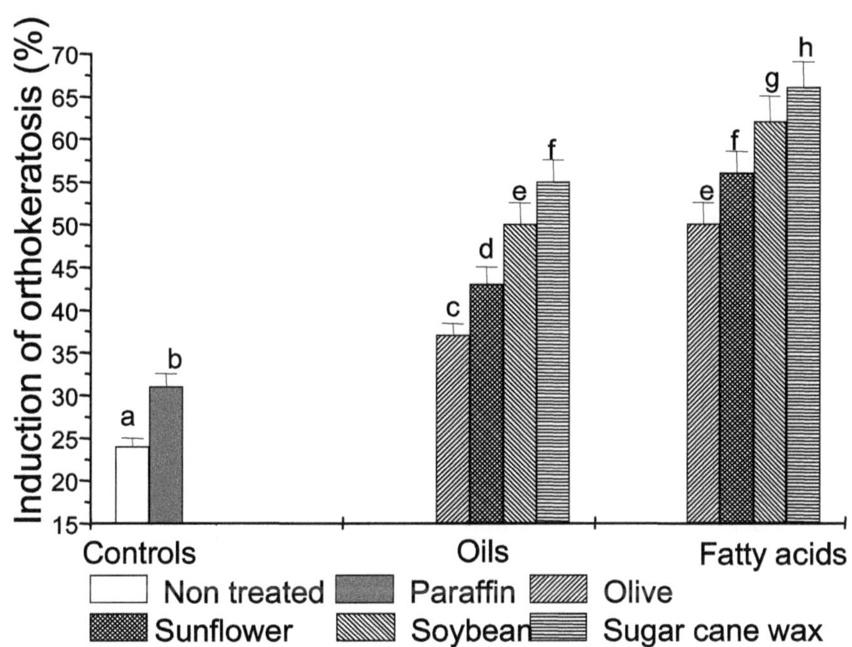

Figure 9.4: Effect of Tested Substances on Mouse Tail Test of Psoriasis. Values having the different letter are statistically significant at p<0.05(X±S.D, n=10/group).

appropriate n-6/n-3 fatty acid ratio in the sugar cane oil, (see table 1, per cent of linoleic acid/per cent linolenic acid=5). The essential fatty acids belong to the n-6 and n-3 families of polyunsaturated acids, derived from linoleic acid and linolenic acid. Since both linoleic and linolenic acids are substrates of the same enzyme, competition occurs among the 2 essential fatty acids. Too high concentration of linolenic acid can decrease the conversion of linoleic acid into higher polyunsaturated n-6 fatty acids. Conversely, if it is too high the intake of linoleic is likely to impair synthesis of eicosapentanoic acid from linolenic acid. Therefore, n-6 and n-3 essential fatty acids should be provided in balanced proportion. An n-6/n-3 fatty acid ratio comprised among 4 and 6 is generally recommended as the most beneficial (Bezard *et al.*, 1994; Roche, 1999).

References

Ancheta, O., Ramos, M.E., De la Rosa, M.C., Rodríguez, S.(1996). Metodología para el procesamiento de tejido vegetal en microscopía electrónica de transmisión. *Biotecnología aplicada.*, 13: 195-196.

Bezard, J., Blond, J.P., Bernard, A., Clouet, P. (1994). The metabolism and availability of essential fatty acids in animal and human tissues. *Reprod Nutr Dev.*, 34: 539-568.

Bosman, B., Matthiesen, T., Hess, V, Friderichs, E. (1992) A quantitative method for measuring antipsoriatic activity of drugs by the mouse tail test. *Skin Pharmacol.*, 5: 41-48

Galli, C., Simopoulus, AP., Tremoli, E. (1994). Effects of fatty acids and lipids in health and disease. *Word Rev. Nutr. Diet.*, 76: 1-149.

Ledón, N., Casacó, A., Rodríguez, V., Cruz, J., González, R., Tolón, Z., Cano, M., Rojas, E. (2003) Antiinflammatory and analgesic effects of a mixture of fatty acids isolated and purified from sugar cane wax oil..*Planta Med.*, 69:367-369.

Ledón, N., Romay, Ch., Rodríguez, V., Cruz, J., Rodríguez, S., Ancheta, O., González, A., González, R., Tolón, Z., Cano, M., Rojas, E., Capote, A., Valdes, T. (2005) Further studies on a mixture of fatty acids from sugar cane (Saccharum officinarum) wax oil in animal models of hypersensitivity. *Planta Med.*, 71:126-129.

Ledón, N., Casacó, A., Remirez, D., González, A., Cruz, J., González, R., Capote, A., Tolón, Z., Rojas, E., Rodríguez, V.J., Merino, N., Rodríguez, S., Ancheta, O., Cano, M.C (2007) Effects of a mixture of fatty acids from sugar cane (Saccharum officinarum L.) wax oil in two models of inflammation: zymosan-induced arthritis and mice tail test of psoriasis. *Phytomedicine,* 14 :690-695.

Loftsson, T., Gudmundsdottir, T.K., Fridriksdottir, H. (1995) Fatty acids from cod-liver oil as skin penetration enhancers. *Pharmazie.*, 50: 188-190.

Puignero, V. Queralt, J. (1997) Effect of topically applied cyclooxygenase 2 selective inhibitors on arachidonic acid and tetradecanoylphorbol acetate induced dermal inflammation in the mouse. *Inflammation*, 21: 433-440.

Roche, H.M. (1999). Unsaturated fatty acids. *Proc. Nutr. Soc.*, 58: 397-401

Rodríguez, R., Fernandez, B.J., Wong, R., Campos, R., Falcon, L. (1992) MADIP, Morfometria Analítica y Digitalización en Patologia. Software para diagnostico e investigación en patología. *Rev Cubana Invest Biomed.*, 11: 126-128.

Romay, C., Ledon, N., Gonzalez, R. (1998) Further studies on antiinflammatory activity of phycocyanin in some animals models of inflammation. *Inflamm. Res.*, 47:334-338.

Sessler, A.M., Ntambi, J.M.(1998). Polyunsaturated fatty acid regulation of gene expression. *J. Nutr.*, 128: 923-926.

Wittenauer, L.A., Shirai, K. Jackson, R.L., Johnson, J.D. (1984) Hydrolysis of a fluorescent phospholipid substrate by Phospholipase A_2 and lipoprotein lipase. *Biochem. Biophys. Res. Comm.*, 118: 894-901.

Yagaloff, K,A, Franco, L., Simko, B., Burghardt, B. (1995) Essential fatty acids are antagonists of the leukotriene B-4 receptor. *Prost. Leuk. and Essential Fatty acids*, 52: 293-297.

Zurier, R.B.(1993) Fatty acids, inflammation and immune responses. *Prostaglandins Leukotrienes and Essential Fatty.*, 48: 57-62.

Medicinal Plants: Phytochemistry, Pharmacology and Therapeutics, Vol. 1 (2010) *Pages* **202–214**
Editors: **V.K. Gupta, G.D. Singh, Surjeet Singh and A. Kaul**
Published by: **DAYA PUBLISHING HOUSE, NEW DELHI**

Chapter 10

Mitochondrial Protection was Involved in the Effect of *Limonium sinense* Extract Against APAP-Induced Toxicity

J. Gao[1]*, Y.H. Tang[2], L.Z. Xu[2], X.H. Tang[3] and X.N. Zhao[2]
[1]School of Pharmacy, Jiangsu University, Zhenjiang, 212013, P.R. China
[2]School of Medicine, Nanjing University, Nanjing, 210093, P.R. China
[3]Jiangsu Provincial Key Laboratory of Coastal Wetland Bioresources and Environmental Protection, Yancheng Teachers College, Yancheng, 224002, P.R. China

ABSTRACT

The present study was undertaken to investigate the hepatoprotective activity of aqueous extracts of *Limonium sinense* (Girard) Ktze root (LSE) against acetaminophen (APAP)-induced liver damage and to elucidate the possible mechanisms underlying the hepatoprotection. The serum alanine aminotransferase (sALT), serum aspartate aminotransferase (sAST) activity and serum glutathione (GSH) content were detected, and the histopathology of liver was observed. The mitochondrial swelling, mitochondrial membrane potential (MMP) and transcription of voltage-dependent anion channels (VDAC) gene were also investigated. It was found that 100 mg/kg, 200 mg/kg and 400 mg/kg LSE can restore the APAP-induced changes on mice liver in a dose-dependent manner. And the mechanisms underlying its hepatoprotection might be related to the protection on liver mitochondria, especially on VDAC, the most important protein on outer membrane of mitochondria.

Keywords: *Acetaminophen, Hepatoprotection, Limonium sinense (Girard) Ktze, Mitochondria, Voltage-dependent anion channels.*

* Corresponding Author: E-mail: jinggao@ujs.edu.cn; Phone: +86-511-88791552; Fax: +86-511-88791552.

Introduction

Liver is the central organ in the metabolism and detoxification of drugs and toxins, so it is more frequently affected by drugs and placed in the risk of toxic damage than any other organ. Abnormalities in liver function lead to different types of liver injury, including fibrosis, alcoholic liver disease and hepatitis (Wissam Bleibel *et al.*, 2007). Liver injury depends initially on the development of hepatocyte stress, which can finally lead to activation of cell death programs for apoptosis or necrosis(Gunawan *et al.*,2007). Mitochondria are known as "gatekeeper" in cell life and death, and they have three most important functions: regulation of energy metabolism, reactive oxygen species (ROS) production and initiation of apoptosis and necrosis. Thus mitochondria dysfunction is usually involved in a wide range of diseases such as the cancer, diabetes, hepatitis, and the age-related neurodegenerative diseases (Armstrong, 2007). The voltage-dependent anion channel (VDAC), a very abundant protein in the outer membrane of mitichondria, plays an important role in the mitochondria associated apoptosis (Tsujimoto *et al.*,2002).

Recently herbs have become more and more attractive as health-beneficial foods and as a source material for the development of medicine(Ha *et al.*,2005). Herbal medicines derived from plant extracts are utilized progressively for the treatment of various clinical diseases, but their modes of action are relatively little known (Matthews *et al.*,1999). *Limonium sinense* (Girard) Ktze is a kind of herb mainly distributed along seashores and salts marshes in southern China, Ryukyus (Japan) and western Taiwan, and has been used traditionally for treating bleeding, piles, fever, hepatitis, diarrhoea, bronchitis and other disorders(Li,1978). Recently, the hepatoprotective activity of *Limonium sinense* (Girard) Ktze root extracts (LSE) against carbon tetrachloride (CCl_4) and D-galactosamine (D-GalN) intoxication in rats has already been reported (Chaung *et al.*, 2003), and the mechanisms underlying its protective effects on CCl_4-induced hepatotoxicity are supposedly related to the mitochondrial protection(Tang *et al.*, 2007). Keeping these facts in view, the present study was undertaken to evaluate the protective effect of LSE on acetaminophen (APAP)-induced hepatotoxicity and to elucidate the possible mitochondrial mechanisms underlying the hepatoprotective activity.

Materials and Methods

Plant Material

The whole plant of *Limonium sinense* was collected from the Yancheng seabeach in China and identified by Mr. Yao Gan (Institute of Botany of Jiangsu Province, Chinese Academy of Sciences) in December 2005. The dried *Limonium sinense* root (100 g) was cut and mixed with water, and subjected to continuous hot extraction. The resulting extract was filtered and subsequently concentrated with a water bath until it evaporated to 32.89 g (yield: 32.89 per cent w/w) of crude LSE. The concentration used in the research was based on the dry weight of the extracts.

Chemicals

APAP was purchased from Sigma-Aldrich Co. (St. Louis, MO, USA). Rhodamine123 (Rh123) and succinate were purchased from Sigma Chemical (St. Louis, MO, USA). RNAiso reagent, dNTP, Taq polymerase and 100bp DNA Marker were from TaKaRa Biotechnology (Dalian) Co., Ltd. (Dalian, P.R.China). Rever Tra Ace reverse transcriptase were from ToYoBo Biotechnology (Shanghai) Co., Ltd. (Shanghai, P.R.China), Oligo$(dT)_{15}$ were from Invitrogene Co. (Carlsbad, CA, USA), and RNase inhibitor were from Promega Biotechnology Co., Ltd. (Beijing, P.R.China). All other chemicals were of high purity from commercial sources.

Animals

Male ICR mice weighed 18-22 g were from Experiment Animal Center of Yangzhou University, Yangzhou, P.R.China (Certificate No. SCXK 2003-0002). The animals were fed with standard laboratory diet and water *ad libitum* and maintained at a controlled temperature (20°C–25°C) with a 12 h dark/light cycle. All animals received humane care and the study protocols complied with the guidelines of Nanjing University. All mice were randomly assigned and acclimatized for 2 days before the experiment.

APAP-induced Hepatotoxicity in Mice

The mice were divided into five groups each consisting of eight animals as follows: the normal group was injected with single saline (0.9 per cent NaCl, 0.02 ml/g body weight) intraperitoneally. APAP group received a single intraperitoneal dose of 160 mg/kg APAP (APAP was applied in saline solution at a concentration of 16 mg/ml at 70°C, then cooled to 37°C for administration). LSE100, LSE200, LSE400 groups were administered with 100, 200, 400 mg/kg of LSE via the intragastric route once daily for 5 consecutive days and received a single intraperitoneal dose of 160 mg/kg APAP at the sixth day, respectively. The animals were sacrificed 12 h after the APAP application.

Assay of Serum Enzyme Activities and Serum Glutathione (GSH) Content

Blood collected was clotted and centrifuged at 3,000 g at 4°C for 20 min to separate serum and the sALT and sAST activities were measured with a spectrophotometric diagnostic kit from Changchun Huili, Biotech Co.Ltd. The GSH content in serum was measured with a GSH diagnostic kit from Nanjing Jiancheng, Bioengineering Co.Ltd.

Histological Examinations

The liver tissues were fixed in 10 per cent phosphate buffered formalin for 24 h, then dehydrated in gradual ethanol (30-100 per cent) and cleared in n-butanol. After embedded in paraffin, liver tissues were chopped into slices and stained with hematoxylin and eosin for histological observation.

Isolation of Liver Mitochondria

Liver mitochondria were isolated by differential centrifugation according to the method of Apprille (Aprille *et al.*,1977). In brief, mouse livers were excised and homogenized in isolation buffer containing 225 mM D-mannitol, 75 mM sucrose, 0.05 mM EDTA and 10 mM Tris-HCl (pH 7.4) at 4°C, centrifuged at 600 g for 5 min, and the supernatant and crude mitochondrial fraction was centrifuged for 10 min at 8,800 g. The mitochondrial pellet was enriched (8,800 g for 10 min, twice) and resuspended in isolation medium. Mitochondrial protein was determined with a protein assay kit Coomassie Brilliant Blue(Bradford,1976) on a spectrophotometer.

Measurement of Mitochondrial Swelling

Mitochondrial swelling was assessed by measuring the changes in absorbance of their suspension at 540 nm by using a 752 spectrophotometer. Liver mitochondria isolated from each group of mice were dissolved in 3 mL of the assay buffer (0.5 mg protein/ml) containing 125 mM sucrose, 50 mM KCl, 2 mM KH_2PO_4, 10 mM HEPES and 5 mM succinate. 100 μM of Ca^{2+} was added to the assay buffer to initiate the mitochondrial swelling and the absorbance (A) at 0.5, 1, 2, 3, 4, and 5 minutes were measured. The swelling rate of mitochondrial swelling was calculated as follows: $(\Delta A_{APAP} - \Delta A_{drug}) / (\Delta A_{Control} - \Delta A_{APAP}) \times 100$ per cent, $\Delta A = A_{0\,min} - A_{5\,min}$.

Determination of Mitochondrial Membrane Potential

Mitochondrial membrane potential (MMP) was measured according to Emaus (Emaus *et al.*,1986) using Rh123 as a probe for membrane potential. Rh123, a cationic fluorescent dye whose mitochondrial fluorescence intensity decreased quantitatively in response to dissipation of the MMP, was used to evaluate perturbations in MMP(Wu *et al.*,1990). Briefly, the assay was carried out at 37°C in a medium (pH 7.4) containing 225 mM mannitol, 70 mM sucrose and 5 mM HEPES (N-2-hydroxyethylpiperazine-N-2-ethanesulfonic acid). Mitochondria isolated from liver homogenates (0.5 mg/mL) were added to the reaction medium. Changes in fluorescence were measured with a Hitachi 850 spectrophotofluorometer at 505 nm excitation wavelength and then 534 nm emission wavelength after adding 0.3 μM Rh123. The MMP calculated was based on Nernst equation: $\Delta\Psi m$ (in mV)=–59 log $[Rh123]_{in}/[Rh123]_{out}$, accounting for the distribution of Rh123 between mitochondria and medium.

Evaluation of VDAC mRNA level by RT-PCR Assay

Total RNA was extracted from liver homogenates using RNAiso reagent. Reverse transcription was started with 5 μg of total RNA at 42°C for 20 min in a 20 μl reaction mixture containing 40 U RNase inhibitor, 0.25 mM each of dNTP, 0.5 μg Oligo$(dT)_{15}$ and 200 U Rever Tra Ace reverse transcriptase. The reaction was terminated by incubation at 99°C for 5 min. PCR amplification was performed with 4 μl cDNA by adding 5 mM $MgCl_2$, 2.5 U Taq polymerase, 0.25 mM each dNTP, and 5′–and 3′–sequence-specific oligonucleotide primers for VDAC and β-actin in 10×Taq polymerase reaction buffer, respectively. β-actin was used as a loading control. The whole PCR process comprised 30 cycles and each cycle contained 94°C, 1 min; 50°C, 1min; 72°C, 1 min; and finally 72°C, 4 min. The amplified fragments were detected by agarose gel electrophoresis and visualized by ethidium bromide (EB) staining. The oligonucleotide primers used were: for VDAC, sense 5′–GGC TAC GGC TTT GGC TTA AT–3′ and antisense 5′–CCC TCT TGT ACC CTG TCT TGA–3′, yielding a deduced amplification product of 301 bps; while, for β-actin, sense 5′–AGT GTG ACG TTG ACA TCC GTA–3′ and antisense 5′–GCC AGA GCA GTA ATC TCC TTC T–3′ yielding a deduced amplification product of 112 bps.

Statistical Analysis

Statistical significance was analyzed by one-way analysis of variance (ANOVA) followed by SNK-q test. P value < 0.01 or < 0.05 were considered statistically significant.

Results

Inhibory Effect of LSE on the Elevation of sALT and sAST Level Induced by APAP

LSE made a comparatively rapid recovery of the serum enzyme activities from APAP-induced hepatotoxicity (Figure 10.1). Mice pretreated with 100 mg/kg LSE inhibited the elevation of both sALT and sAST levels induced by APAP. While pretreatment of 200 mg/kg and 400 mg/kg LSE helped to maintain the serum enzyme activities closely to the level of normal group.

Effect of LSE on APAP–Induced Serum GSH Depletion

The serum GSH depletion induced by APAP was illustrated in Figure 10.2. Serum GSH content in the APAP treatment group decreased to 52.9 per cent of the normal level. While 100, 200 and 400 mg/kg LSE blocked the depletion and restored the GSH levels to 63.5 per cent, 82.6 per cent and 88.7 per cent, respectively.

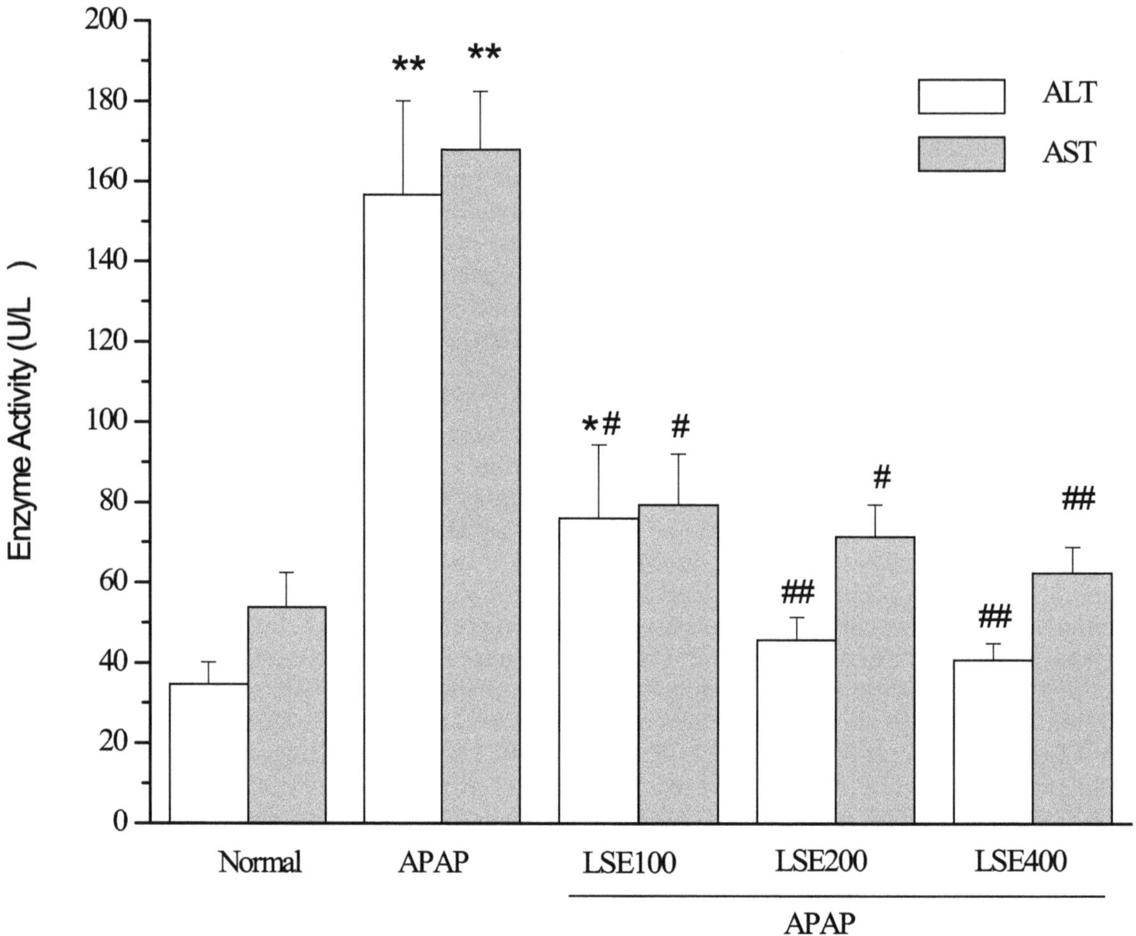

Figure 10.1: Inhibition of LSE on the Elevation of sALT and sAST Level Produced by 160mg/kg APAP. Mean ± SD for eight mice. *P<0.05 , **P<0.01 *vs* normal group; #P <0.05, ##P<0.01 *vs* APAP group.

Preventive Effect of LSE Against APAP-induced Liver Histopathological Changes

Histopathological changes occurred in the APAP treatment group (Figure 10.3B). Hepatocytes around the central veins were eosinophilic in appearance particularly, and showed cytoplasmic vacuolization with the presence of necrotic areas in the centrilobular regions. When 100 mg/kg LSE was given to mice prior to the APAP treatment (Figure 10.3C), the liver damage was reduced to some extent with less eosinophilia, but there were still swollen hepatocytes surrounding the central veins. With 200 mg/kg LSE and 400 mg/kg (Figures 10.3Dand 10.3E), the area of liver damage was further reduced.

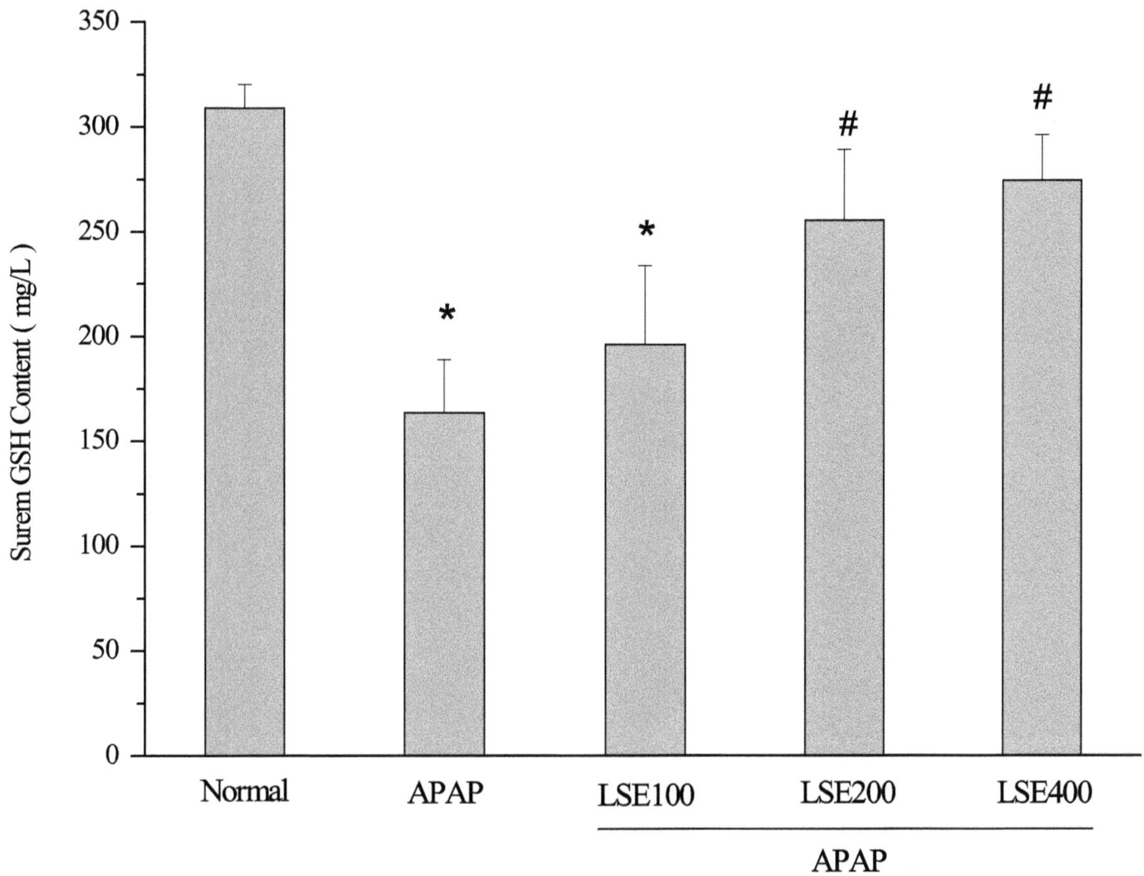

Figure 10.2: Protective Effect of LSE on APAP-Induced Decrease of Serum GSH Content. Mean ± SD for eight mice. *P<0.05 vs. normal group; #P<0.05 vs. APAP group.

Reversed Ca^{2+}-induced Mitochondrial Swelling Ability Following the Treatment of LSE

As shown in Figure 10.4, 100 µM Ca^{2+} induced the swelling of normal liver mitochondria, which was greatly attenuated in mice with pretreatment of 160 mg/kg APAP. LSE at a dose of 100 mg/kg blocked the attenuation induced by APAP to some extent, and the inhibitive rate was about–18.8 per cent, while at the doses of 200 mg/kg and 400 mg/kg, the inhibitive rates were up to –67.2 per cent and –72.7 per cent, respectively.

Protective Effect of LSE Against APAP-Induced Dissipation of MMP

Compared with the MMP of normal mice (–172.6±13.6 mV), MMP in APAP treatment group was decreased to –114.2±10.3 mV (Figure 10.5), which was reverted to–132.9±6.3 mV, –138.2±12.4 mV and –154.9±12.8 mV, respectively, following preadministration of LSE at doses of 100, 200 and 400 mg/kg. Although it seemed difficult to entirely recuperate the dissipation of MMP induced by APAP, the restoring trend was definite.

Figure 10.3: Effects of LSE Pretreatment on APAP-Induced Liver Damage in Mice

(A) Liver from mice in normal group; (B) liver from mice treated with APAP; (C–E) liver from mice treated with APAP plus 100 C200 or 400 mg/kg LSE respectively.

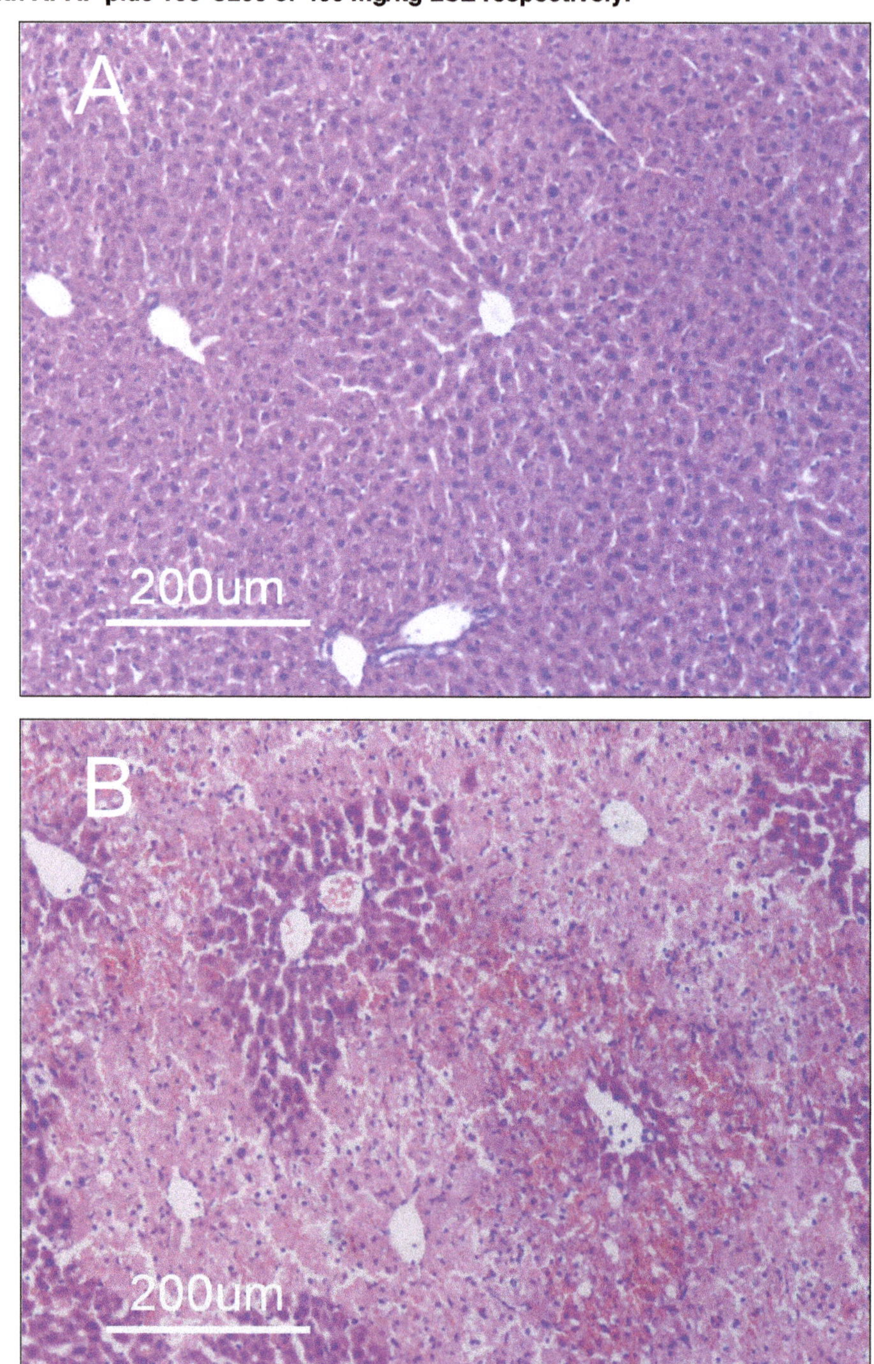

Contd...

Figure 10.3–Contd...

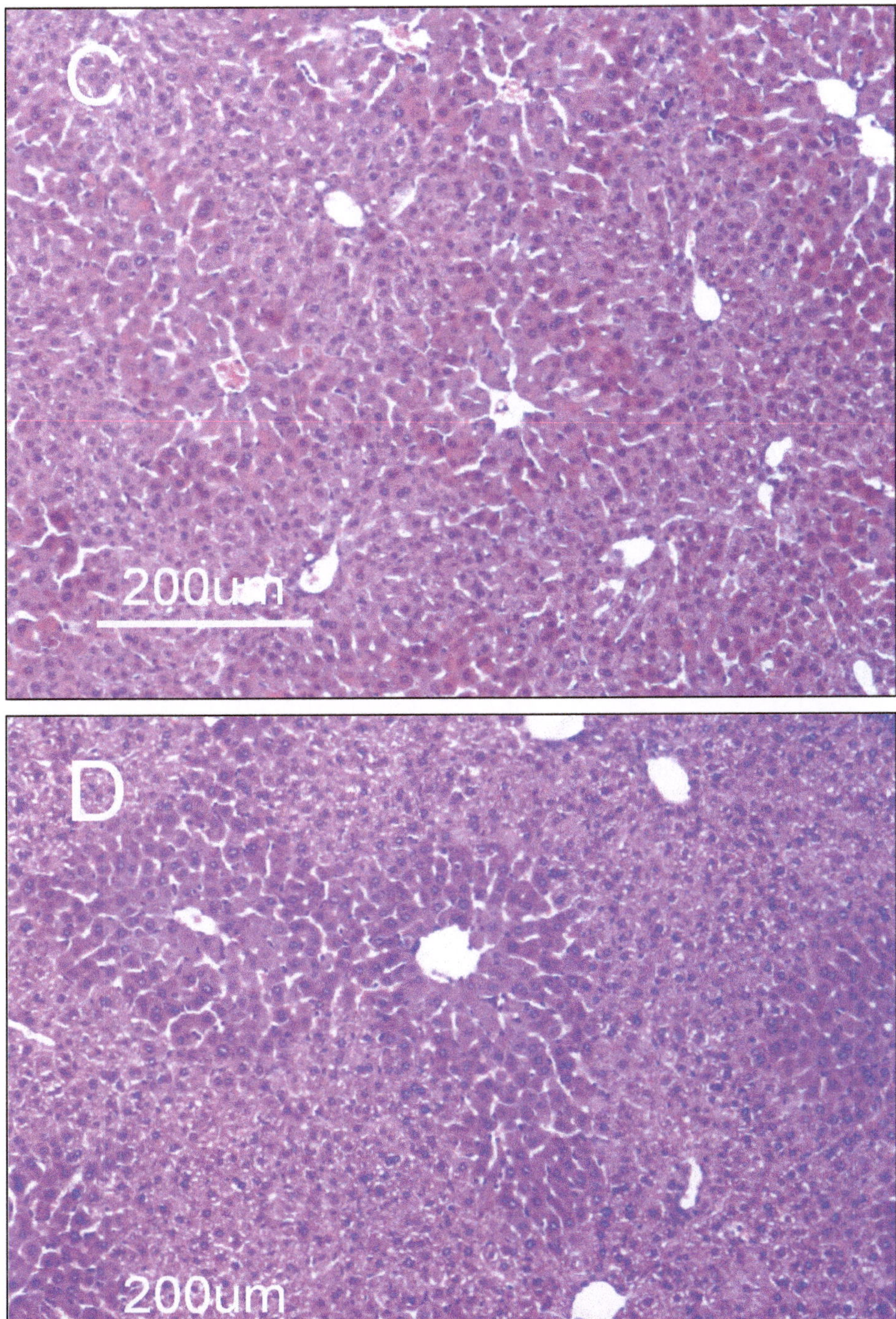

Contd...

Figure 10.3–Contd...

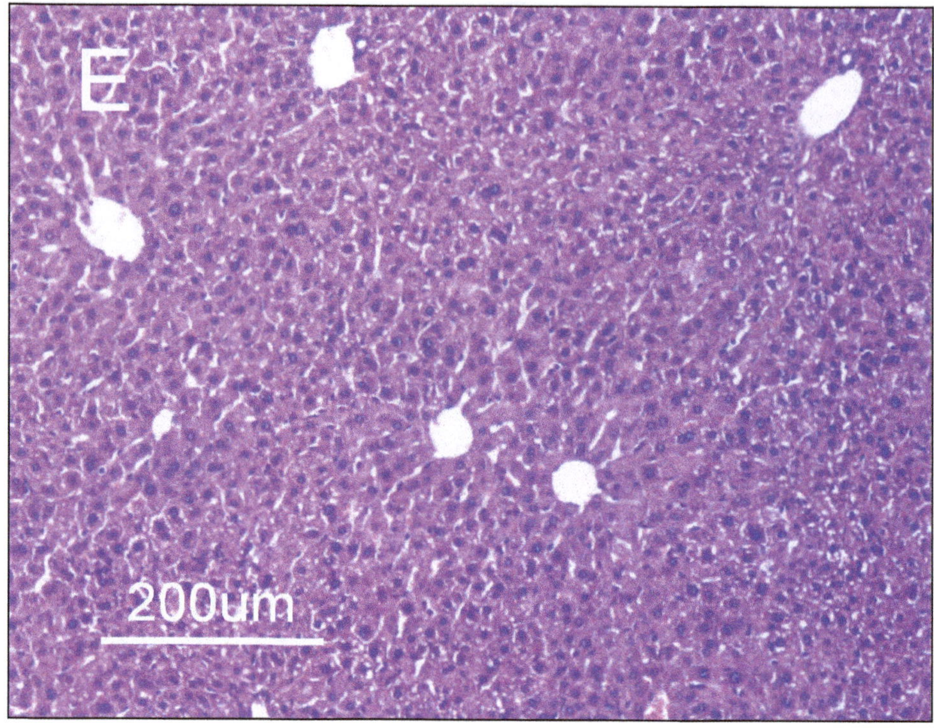

Effect of LSE on the Transcription of Liver VDAC Gene

To assess the transcription of VDAC, RT-PCR was performed using total RNA isolated from mice liver homogenates. As shown in Figure 6, the VDAC mRNA level in the liver homogenates of APAP treatment group was significantly elevated, against that of normal group. However, the expression of VDAC was down-regulated when mice were pretreated with 100 mg/kg, 200 mg/kg and 400 mg/kg LSE.

Discussion

In the present study, we used APAP, a widely used analgesic and antipyretic, to make the liver injury model(Mitchell *et al.*,1973). Mitochondrial dysfunction plays an important role in the mechanisms of APAP hepatotoxicity. N-acetyl-p-benzoquinone imine (NAPQI), a reactive metabolite of APAP by the P450 system, depletes GSH *in vivo* and covalently binds to cellular proteins causing functional deficits within the cell(Jaeschke *et al.*,2006; Mitchell *et al.*,1973). These early events cause mitochondrial dysfunction with reactive oxygen and peroxynitrite formation (Jaeschke *et al.*,2003). The oxidant stress then triggers the opening of mitochondrial membrane permeability transition pores (MPTP) and results in mitochondrial swelling and the collapse of MMP(Don *et al.*,2004; Masubuchi *et al.*,2005). All these things lead to necrosis in hepatocytes(Piret *et al.*,2004).

The increased sAST and sALT levels following APAP treatment indicated the liver injury. While the inhibitive effects on APAP-induced elevation of sAST and sALT by various dosage of LSE (100,

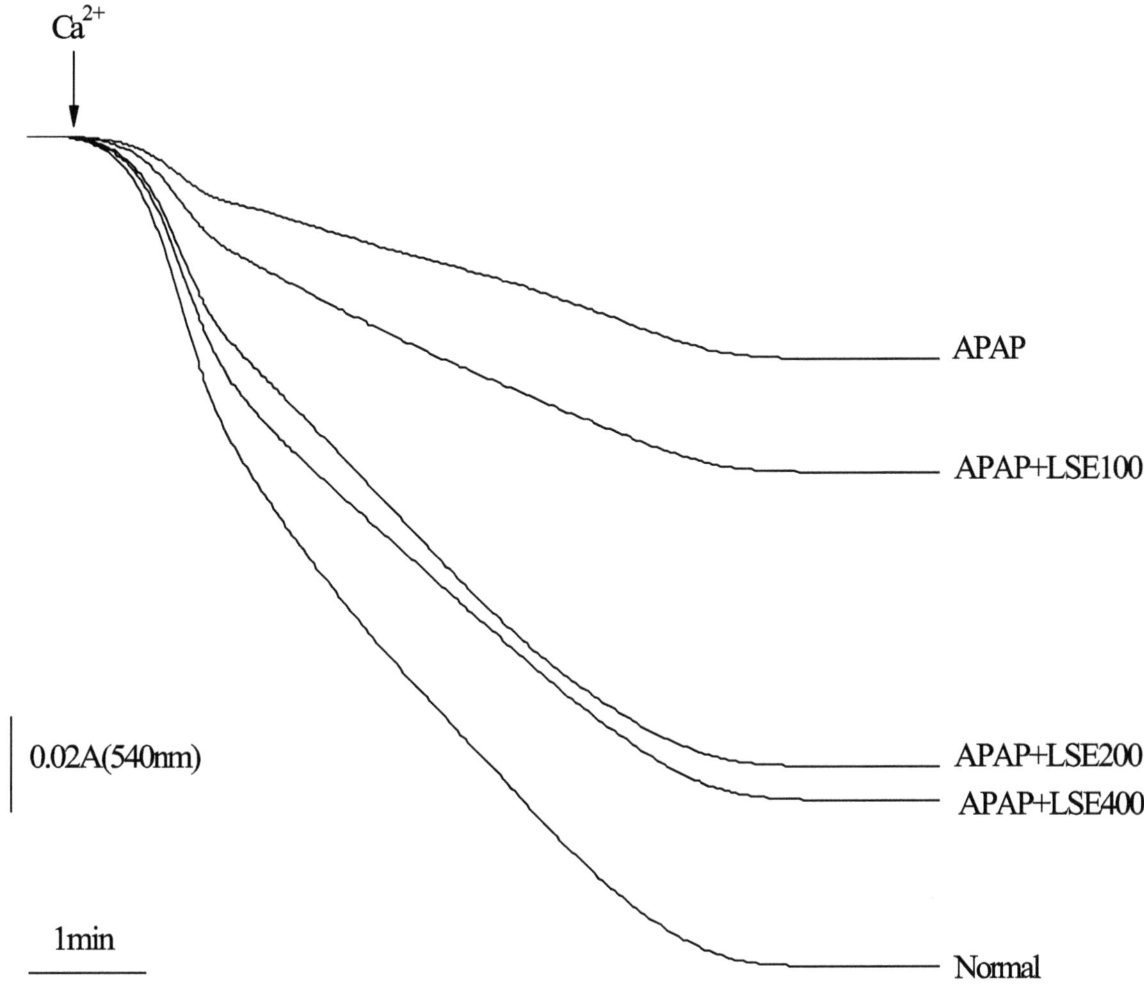

Figure 10.4: Effect of LSE on Ca^{2+}-induced Mitochondrial Swelling.
100, 200, 400 mg/kg LSE prohibited Ca^{2+}-induced mitochondrial swelling. The curves represent typical recordings from experiments of at least three different mitochondrial preparations.

200, 400 mg/kg) afforded a good hepatoprotection, which was confirmed by the changes in the liver histopathology. Previous studies on the mechanisms of APAP-induced hepatotoxicity had shown that GSH played a key role in the detoxification of its reactive toxic metabolites, and the liver necrosis began when GSH stores were markedly depleted (Mitchell *et al.*,1973; Mitchell *et al.*,1973). Our results showed that pretreatment with LSE significantly reduced APAP-induced hepatic GSH depletion, and this protective effect turned out to be dose-dependent.

Then we focused on the mitochondria function analysis by detecting the mitochondrial swelling and MMP. Ca^{2+}-induced mitochondrial swelling is a behavior of mitochondrial susceptibility. Normal

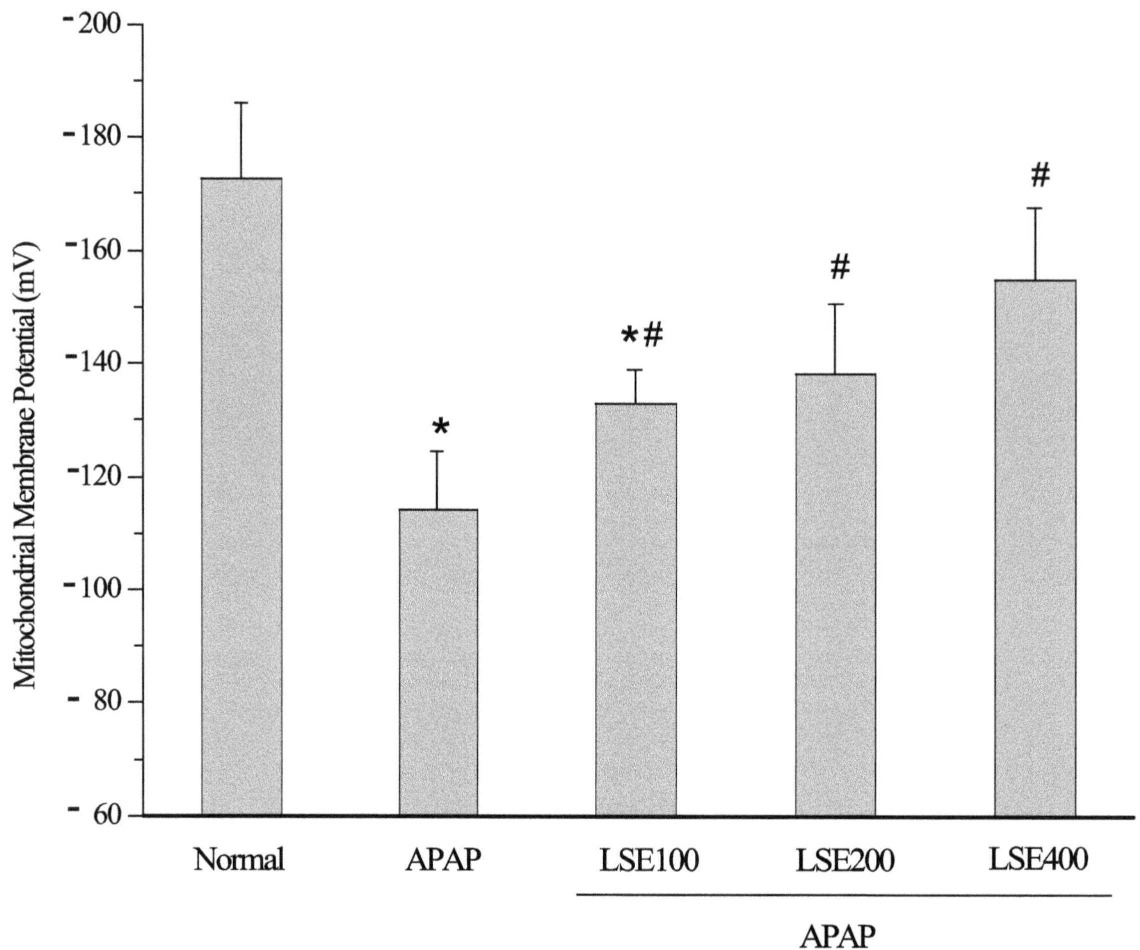

Figure 10.5: Inhibition of LSE on the Dissipation of Mitochondrial Membrane Potential. Mean ± SD for eight mice. *P<0.05 vs normal group; #P<0.05 vs APAP group.

mitochondria are susceptive to 100 μM Ca^{2+} and swell very obviously in a short time (5 min in our study), while decreased swelling capability indicates mitochondrial dysfunction. MMP is one of the earliest biochemical manifestations of cell death. The results indicated that both the depression of mitochondrial swelling and the dissipation of MMP occurred on the APAP treated group, and LSE pretreatment at dosages from 100 mg/kg to 400 mg/kg significantly restored the mitochondrial function to some extent insulted by APAP.

Finally, we paid more attention on the voltage-dependent anion channel (VDAC), one of the most important proteins on the mitochondria outer membrane regarding the process of apoptosis (Premkumar *et al.*,2002; Tsujimoto *et al.*,2002). It was found that APAP caused an elevation of liver mitochondrial VDAC transcription, which was significantly blocked in the LSE pretreated groups, especially in the 200 and 400 mg/kg LSE groups. In our previous study, it was found that both VDAC mRNA and protein levels could be increased following the treatment of CCl_4, which could be prevented by LSE (Tang *et al.*,2007).

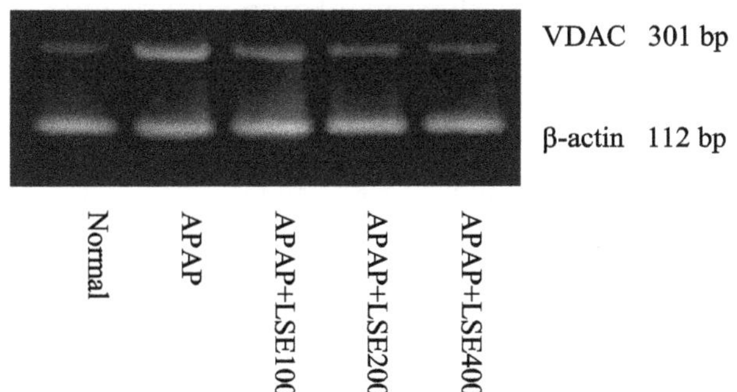

Figure 10.6: Regulation of LSE on the Transcription of Mitochondrial VDAC in Mice Liver. 100, 200, 400 mg/kg LSE prohibited APAP-induced elevation of VDAC mRNA level.

In summary, the findings of the current study illustrate that LSE has a dose-dependent protective effect against APAP-induced hepatotoxicity, and this protective effect is probably related to mitochondrial protection. The above data suggest that the protective effect of LSE on liver mitochondria might be related to down-regulation of the expression of mitochondrial VDAC which could be elevated by hepatoxicity induction. But the mitochondrial mechanisms underlying LSE hepatoprotection and the active components of LSE await further study.

Acknowledgements

This work was financially supported by the Natural Science Foundation of Education Department of Jiangsu Province (Key Project No. 07KJA18017) and the Foundation of Jiangsu Provincial Key Laboratory of Coastal Wetland Bioresources and Environmental Protection (No. JLCBE05011). We would like to thank Mr. Yao Gan, an engineer of Institute of Botany of Jiangsu Province, Chinese Academy of Sciences, for the identification of the plant *Limonium sinense* (Girard) Ktze. We also gratefully acknowledge Professor Zu Xuan Zhang, School of Medicine, Nanjing University and Xian Chong Tao, Center of Modern Analysis Nanjing University for their support and assistance during this study.

References

Aprille, JR, Hom, JA, Rulfs, J.(1977). Liver and skeletal muscle mitochondrial function following burn injury. *J. Trauma.*, 17: 279-287.

Bradford, MM.(1976). A rapid and sensitive method for the quantitation of microgram quantities of protein utilizing the principle of protein-dye binding. *Analytical Biochemistry*, 72: 248-254.

Chaung, SS, Lin, CC, Lin, J.(2003). The hepatoprotective effects of *Limonium sinense* against carbon tetrachloride and beta-D-galactosamine intoxication in rats. *Phytother Res.*, 17(7): 784-791.

Don, AS, Hogg, PJ.(2004). Mitochondria as cancer drug targets. *Trends in Molecular Medicine*, 10: 372-378.

Emaus, RK, Grunwald, R, Lemasters, JJ.(1986). Rhodamine 123 as a probe of transmembrane potential in isolated rat-liver mitochondria: spectral and metabolic properties. *Biochimica et Biophysica Acta (BBA)–Bioenergetics*, 850: 436-448.

Gunawan, BK, Kaplowitz, N.(2007). Mechanisms of drug-induced liver disease. *Clinics in Liver Disease*, 11: 459-475.

Ha, KT, Yoon, SJ, Choi, DY, Kim, DW, Kim, JK, Kim, CH.(2005). Protective effect of Lycium chinense fruit on carbon tetrachloride-induced hepatotoxicity. *Journal of Ethnopharmacology*, 96: 529-535.

J.S.Armstrong.(2007). Mitochondrial Medicine: Pharmacological targeting of mitochondria in disease. *British Journal of Pharmacology*, 151: 1154–1165.

Jaeschke, H, Cover, C, Bajt, ML.(2006). Role of caspases in acetaminophen-induced liver injury. *Life Sciences*, 78: 1670-1676.

Jaeschke, H, Knight, TR, Bajt, ML.(2003). The role of oxidant stress and reactive nitrogen species in acetaminophen hepatotoxicity. *Toxicology Letters*, 144: 279-288.

Li, HL.(1978). Plumbaginaceae, Flora of Taiwan. *Editorial Committee of the Flora of Taiwan. Edited and Published, Taipei*, Vol.IV: 90-93.

Masubuchi, Y, Suda, C, Horie, T.(2005). Involvement of mitochondrial permeability transition in acetaminophen-induced liver injury in mice. *Journal of Hepatology*, 42: 110-116.

Matthews, HB, Lucier, GW, Fisher, KD.(1999). Medicinal herbs in the United States: Research needs. *Environmental Health Perspectives*, 107: 773-778.

Mitchell, JR, Jollow, DJ, Potter, WZ.(1973). Acetaminophen-induced hepatic necrosis: I. Role of drug metabolism. *J.Pharmacol.Exp.Ther.*, 187: 185-194.

Mitchell, JR, Jollow, DJ, Potter, WZ.(1973). Acetaminophen-induced hepatic necrosis:IV. Protective role of glutathione. *J.Pharmacol.Exp.Ther.*, 187: 211-217.

Piret, J-P, Arnould, T, Fuks, B, Chatelain, P, Remacle, J, Michiels, C.(2004). Mitochondria permeability transition-dependent tert-butyl hydroperoxide-induced apoptosis in hepatoma HepG2 cells. *Biochemical Pharmacology*, 67: 611-620.

Premkumar, A, Simantov, R.(2002). Mitochondrial voltage-dependent anion channel is involved in dopamine-induced apoptosis. *J. Neurochem.*, 82(2): 345-352.

Tang, XH, Gao, J, Chen, J, Xu, L, Tang, Y, Dou, H, Yu, W, Zhao, X.(2007). Expression of VDAC Regulated by Extracts of *Limonium sinense* Ktze root Against CCl_4-induced Liver Damage. *Int. J. Mol. Sci.*, 8: 204-213.

Tsujimoto, Y, Shimizu, S.(2002). The voltage-dependent anion channel: an essential player in apoptosis. *Biochimie*, 84: 187-193.

Wissam Bleibel, Kim, S, D'Silva, K, Lemmer, ER.(2007). Drug-induced liver injury: review article. *Dig.Dis.Sci.*, 52: 2463-2471.

Wu, EY, Smith, MT, Bellomo, G.(1990). Relationships between the mitochondrial transmembrane potential, ATP concentration,and cytotoxicity in isolated rat hepatocytes. *Arch Biochem Biophys.*, 282: 358-362.

Medicinal Plants: Phytochemistry, Pharmacology and Therapeutics, Vol. 1 *Pages* **215–227**
Editors: **V.K. Gupta, G.D. Singh, Surjeet Singh and A. Kaul**
Published by: **DAYA PUBLISHING HOUSE, NEW DELHI**

Chapter 11

Multi-Targeted Approaches for Polygenic Disorders Using Medicinal Plants: A New Battle Against Old Adversaries

V.S. Muthusamy and B.S. Lakshmi*
Centre for Biotechnology, Anna University, Chennai – 600 025, India

ABSTRACT

A tremendous interest exists in plants and plant based products with rapidly increasing commercial and scientific value. Till now, the concept of herbal therapy using poly herbal combinations is appreciated with its superior efficacy and lesser side effects in comparison with either single isolated constituents of plant or a commercially available drug. Comparably the concept has also been criticised for the complex nature, indefinite mechanisms and poor pharmacokinetic properties. The greater interaction between traditional systems of medicine with modern biotechnological tools has opened up the possibility to analyse the insight mechanism of herbals. In this review, the beneficial effects of herbals were examined with respect to the multi-target action of plants and phytoprinciples on a molecular level with suitable examples. In addition, the rational of multi-target selection, screening strategy and the preliminary assay methodologies are also discussed. Progress in the field of multi–target approach with plant extracts and their compounds may open the probability to use extract combinations for the treatment of diseases that were previously reserved for chemotherapeutics only.

***Keywords**: Polygenic disorders, Multi-target approaches, Medicinal plants.*

---

* Corresponding Author: E-mail: lakshmibs@annauniv.rdu.

Introduction

The survival of living beings including human relies on plants, which fuels the creatures by converting carbon dioxide and water to sugars and nitrogen to amino acid. The identification and usage of plants by human for medicinal and other purposes has commenced in primitive times. Plant derived medicines are used in all civilizations and cultures and, always played a key role in health care systems worldwide. Nowadays, traditional medicine is the first choice healthcare treatment for 60–80 per cent of the world's population for the treatment of common ailments and diseases (Farnsworth *et al.*, 1985; World Health Organization, 2002). Traditional Medicine is defined by the World Health Organisation (WHO 1978a) as

> "The sum total of knowledge or practices whether explicable or inexplicable, used in diagnosing, preventing or eliminating a physical, mental or social disease which may rely exclusively on past experience or observations handed down from generation to generation, verbally or in writing. It also comprises therapeutic practices that have been in existence often for hundreds of years before the development of modern scientific medicine and are still in use today without any documented evidence of adverse effects".

Although traditional medicines have been used for thousands of years, for most such medicines, neither the active component nor their molecular targets have been well identified. Complex nature, indistinct mechanism of action, herbal-drug interaction and quality assurance are the main disputes of herbal therapy. However, ethnopharmacological observation in the past has resulted in the discovery of several important drugs. In pharmaceutical research, ranging from Digoxin to Prostratin (a drug candidate for treatment of human immunodeficiency virus) the ethnobotanical approach to drug discovery has proved successful. 61 per cent of all the new drugs introduced worldwide during 1981 to 2002 can be traced to or were inspired by Natural Products (Newman *et al.*, 2003).

Inflammatory and autoimmune diseases, including rheumatoid arthritis, inflammatory bowel diseases, cancer, diabetes, multiple sclerosis, psoriasis and asthma, provide tremendous challenge to current drug discoverers. The precise causes of these diseases are not known, but they, in general, can be considered as 'gene expression diseases' in which the proinflammatory gene program of the organism is aberrantly activated (Patrick, 1998). Wide varieties of therapeutic agents are now being examined for autoimmune disorders by targeting single target. But, in most of the cases it becomes difficult to maintain the redundant side effects and drug resistance with monotherapy. In current drug discovery approaches, combination drugs and multi-targeted molecules are preferable choices to control complex diseases like cancer, diabetes and inflammation (Zhang and Meier, 2006). The combination drugs are less prone to drug resistance because that influences multiple targets simultaneously.

Botanicals are thought of offering strong therapeutical efficacy with minimal side affects particularly against autoimmune and metabolic disorders since most of their efficacies are from a mixture of active molecules acting at the same time (Muthusamy *et al.*, 2008). The rapid growth of robust biotechnological and analytical techniques gives a ray of hope in plant based drug discovery approach (Kroll and Cordes, 2006). In this review, we discuss the biological rationale for multi target therapeutics, strategy to screen the medicinal plants for multi-targeted lead discovery, review some existing plant based molecules and present a systematic approach to identify interactions between molecular cascades that could be leveraged for therapeutic benefit.

Need of Multi-Targeted Therapy

The rapid improvement in molecular biology over the last decade has led to the identification of the bio markers of many diseases, thereby providing plenty of novel targets for therapeutic intervention. Polygenic diseases such as cancer or multifactorial diseases that affect various tissues or cell types such as diabetes and inflammatory disorders are not completely controlled by the drugs devised to act on single molecular target (Thomas *et al.*, 2007). The heterogeneity of the affected cells, tissues and organs as well as redundancy of defensive mechanisms favour the development of drugs that affect multiple pathways (Figure 11.1). Since multiple gene products have been identified at the sites of inflammation, there has been a surge of interest in identifying intracellular signaling targets, including transcription factors that control inflammatory gene expression and which are amenable to drug discovery.

Introducing modern drug discovery tools for the exploration of natural values can help to minimise the search efforts of the multi-targeted molecules on drug discovery and to nullify the so-called flaws

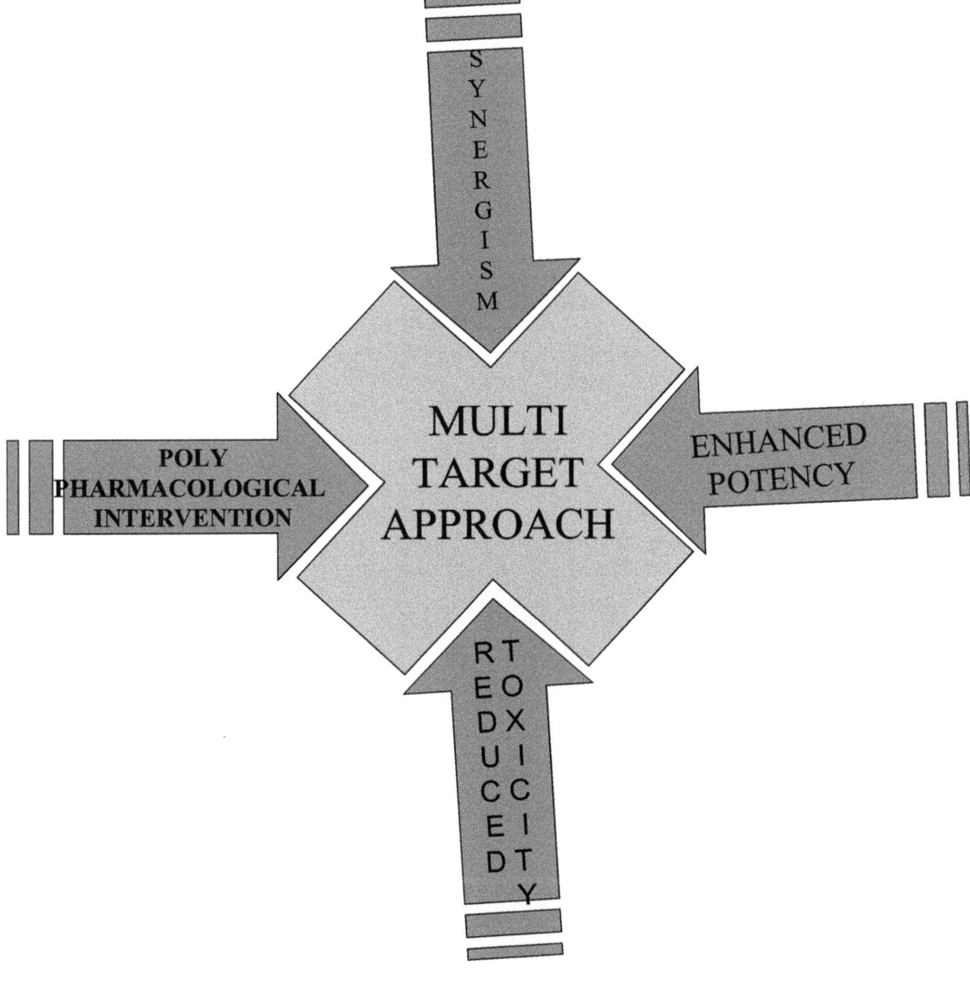

Figure 11.1

of herbal therapy. Subramanian *et al.*(2008) postulated the multi-target therapy advantages of *Alpinia officinarum* in treating Enteropathogenic *Escherichia coli* (EPEC) induced diarrhea via its bactericidal and antiinflammatory activities than conventional antibiotic monotherapy which only controls bacterial growth not the reactive inflammation caused by killed microbes. Multi targeted therapies act synergistically, and expected to lead enhanced potency with minimal doses, and controls dose limiting toxicities. Jun Wang *et al.*(2006) observed the similar synergism between Artimisinin–a plant based anti malarial compound with commercially available antibiotics in the protection of EPEC induced diarrhea through suppression of pro inflammatory cytokines.

Rational Multi Target Selections

Target selection plays vital role and considered to be a heart of the drug discovery programme. Reynold and Elliot (2006) reported that the combined genetic and molecular studies and lawful use of whole animal models with properly performed epidemiology analysis are mandatory to select the appropriate targets.

Duscica Pavlovic *et al.* (2007) reported that genes involved in redox modification is a key mechanism in mediating pathological process such as inflammation, tumor formation, diabetes, atherosclerosis, aging, etc. and stressed the importance of antioxidant therapy with existing monotherapies. Figure 11.2 described the cross talk between genes involved in oxidative stress, cancer,

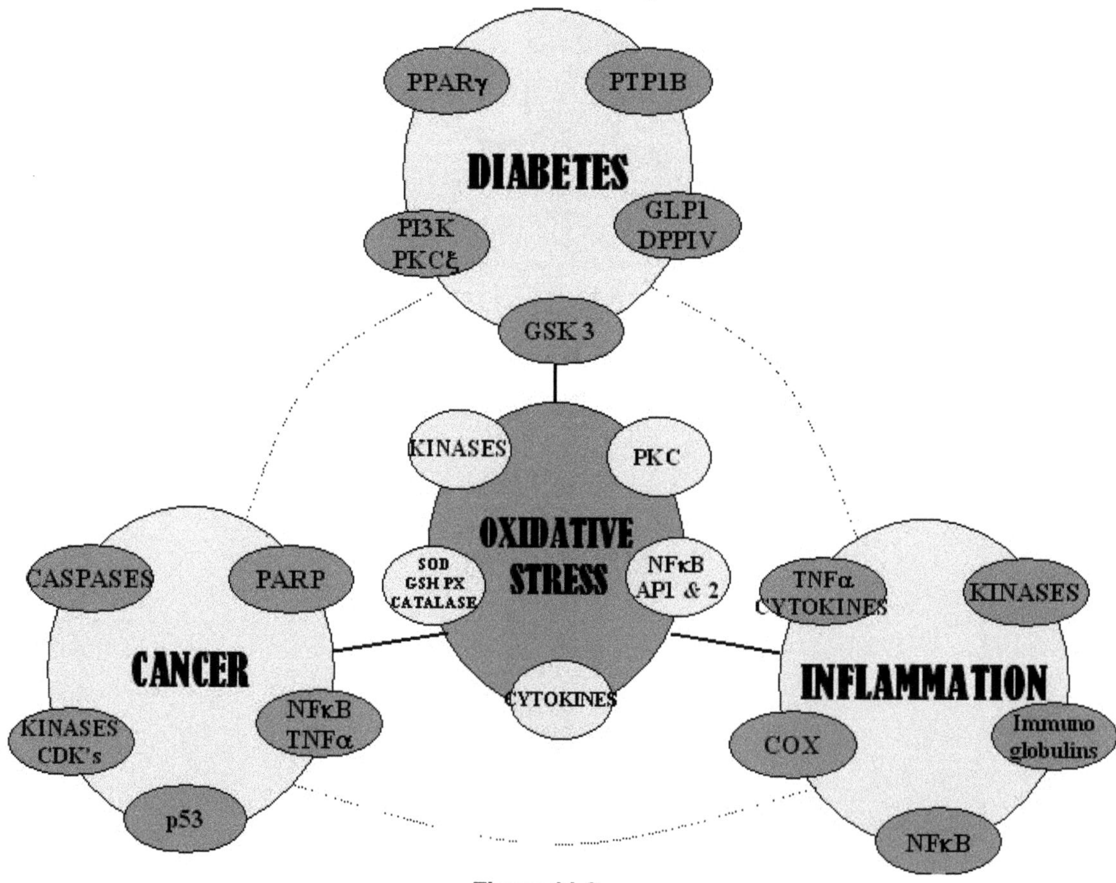

Figure 11.2

diabetes and inflammation. The activation of NF-κB–a transcription factor has been associated with a wide variety of human diseases, including cancer, AIDS, rheumatoid arthritis, diabetes, asthma, atherosclerosis, osteoporosis, and Alzheimer's disease (Kwang and Aggarwal, 2005). Kinases are primary regulators of many vital processes in intricate signaling pathways to control every aspect of cellular function cells. There are approximately 500 different kinases encoded in the human genome, and many human diseases have been linked to these enzymes including all forms of autoimmune disorders. Cyclin Dependent Kinases in cancer and Glycogen synthase kinases in diabetes are the successful models of anti kinase approach in current drug discovery programme (Baier *et al.*, 2007). In summary, target selection in drug discovery is a complex scientific, strategic concern and it needs thorough understanding of cell signaling pathways, and the key mediators involved in the diseases.

An Appraisal of Herbal as Multi-Targeted Therapy

Free radicals are the main cause of many deleterious reactions in the pathogenesis of auto-immune diseases. Oxygen free radicals are not only generated during diabetes, ischemia, tissue damage, cancer, inflammation and aging conditions but also from exogenous sources such as UV light, pollution, life style changes and various medications (Atawodi, 2005). Protection of cellular constituents is one of the most important targets for modern medicine. Nowadays, plant-based products are widely commercialized as a nutrition supplement by rationalizing its antioxidant potential. Tannins, polyphenols and flavonoids are the main antioxidants present in most of the plants and their significance in treating various diseases like cancer (Cicilio *et al.*, 2003), diabetes (Xueqing Liu *et al.*, 2005), etc are well documented. Since, most of the plants exhibit anti oxidant activity it can be used as one of the target in multi targeting approach of autoimmune diseases.

Apart from antioxidant potential, herbals also play specific role in managing autoimmune disorders. Extensive studies have been carried out on evaluation of multi functional potential of medicinal plants. A classical example is *Pterocarpus marsupium* a well-studied plant for Diabetes (Figure 11.3). The constituents isolated from this plant are an antioxidant (-) epicatechin, which causes an ATP dependent enhancement of glucose, stimulated insulin secretion from islets (Hii *et al.*, 1984), Myricetin and Quercetin which shows similar activity with protein tyrosine kinase inhibition (Robert *et al.*, 1989). In addition, the phenolics isolated from this plant are Marsupsin, Pterosupin and Pterostilbene which enhances insulin secretion (Manickam *et al.*, 1997) and an isoflavone namely 7-O-α-l-rhamnopyranosyl oxy-4′-methoxy-5-hydroxy which activates Glut-4, PPARg and PI3 kinase (Anandharajan *et al.*, 2005).

Most of the chemopreventive agents currently being studied are natural products or their derivatives. Many natural compounds, particularly plant products and dietary constituents, have been found to exhibit cancer chemopreventive activities both *in vitro* and *in vivo* (Lee *et al.*, 2001) (Figure 11.4). Podophyllotoxin from *Podophyllum peltatum* was the first natural product anticancer compound isolated in the year 1947. Though Podophyllotoxin is too toxic for use as an anticancer agent, etoposide and teniposide, which are modifications of an analog, 4′–demethylepi-podophyllotoxin, are used clinically to treat certain solid tumors (Hartwwll and Shear, 1947). The 'vinca alkaloids', vinblastine and vincristine from the Madagascan periwinkle, *Catharanthus roseus* are considered antimitotic drugs because they inhibit cell division. They act by binding to tubulin and preventing it from polymerizing into microtubules and found to be very effective in the treatment of Hodgkin's disease and childhood leukemia, respectively (Dewick, 1997). Later Paclitaxel, a blockbuster drug, was isolated from Pacific yew tree, *Taxus brevifolia* (Wani *et al.*, 1971). Though Paclitaxel acts as an antimitotic drug, it is the first anticancer drug discovered that stabilized microtubules and thus

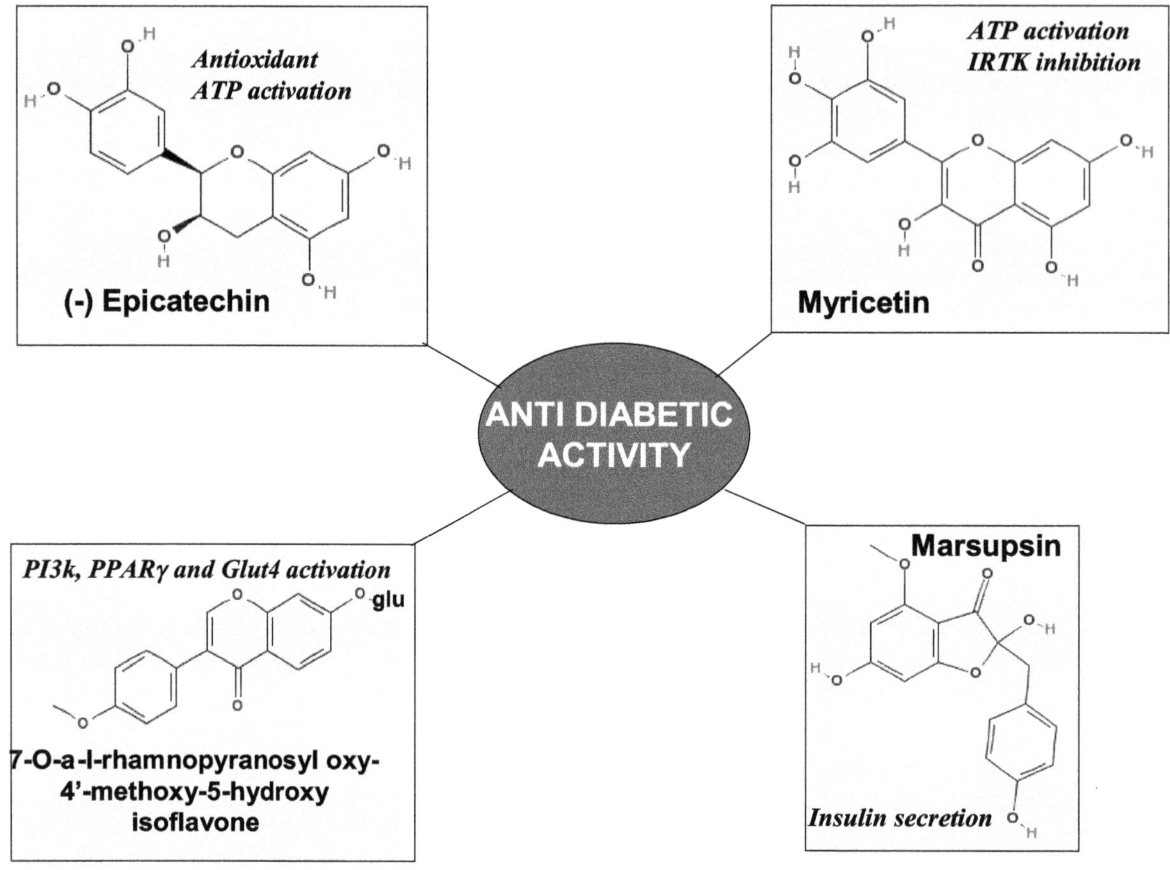

Figure 11.3

promotes their polymerization and used in the treatment of lung, ovarian, and breast cancer and Kaposi's sarcoma (Shu, 1998)). Hayley and Susan (2001) demonstrated the beneficial multi-targeted mechanisms of paclitaxel on modulating various kinases and transcription factors involved in apoptosis. Undoubtedly, more effort is needed to search for new cancer drugs with the aid of better screening methods from plants and other natural sources either in the form of crude extracts or as components isolated from them.

Evaluations of medicinal plants for inflammatory disorders provide us so many successful molecules like curcumin from *Curcuma longa*, andrographolide from *Andrographis paniculata*, etc. Ramanathan *et al.* (2006) described the mode of action and possible multi targeted mechanisms of Curcumin. Curcumin inhibits cytokine with increasing an index of phagocytosis. Curcumin abrogated the expression of cytokines (TNF-alpha and IL-1beta) and chemokines (MIP-1beta, MCP-1and IL-8) in both peripheral blood monocytes (Yang, 2005). It is also observed that curcumin inhibited MAP kinase activation and the phosphorylation of ERK–1/2 and its downstream target Elk-1. (Giri *et al.*, 2004). Curcumin down-regulates the expression of COX2, lipooxygenase, nitric oxide synthase inhibitors and inhibits the activity of c-Jun-N-terminal kinase, protein tyrosine kinases and protein serine/threonine kinases (Lin and Lin-Shiau, 2001) to produce potent anti-inflammatory activity. In

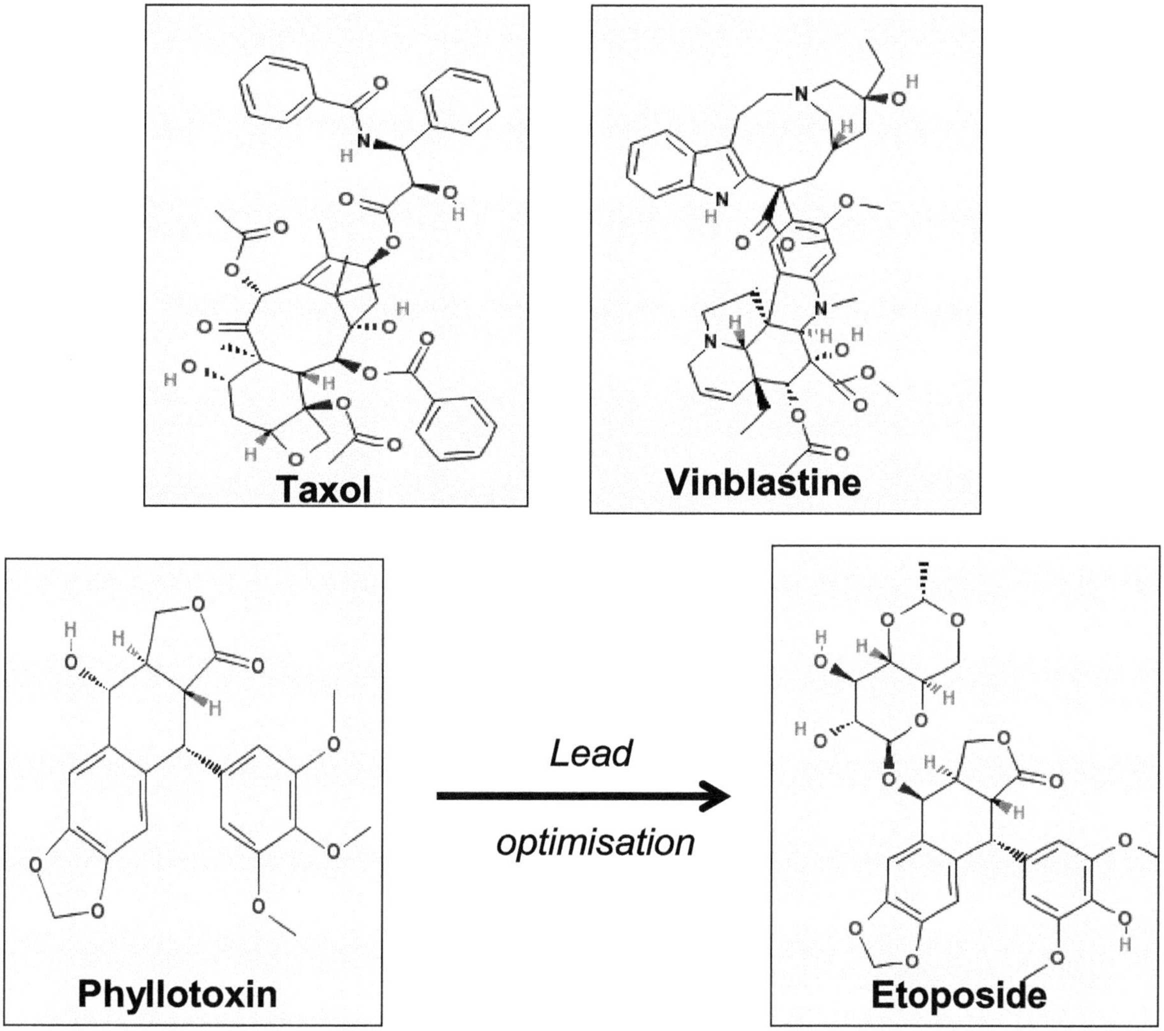

Figure 11.4

addition curcumin modifies the expression of MMP-9, uPA, chemokines, cell surface adhesion molecules, cyclin D1, growth factor receptor EGFR (Nishino *et al.*, 2004) to yield an effective anti tumor activity. These studies clearly show that curcumin can act on multiple targets thereby exhibit therapeutic and prophylactic activities on the treatment of polygenic disorders. The structural resemblance of Curcumin with Diarylheptanoids from *Alpinia officinarum*, and Gingerol from *Zingiber officinale* illustrates the similarity in biological activity of these compounds (Figure 11.5).

Multi-Targeted Approach: Screening Strategy

Mechanism-based assays look for activity using isolated systems such as enzymes, receptors, etc. or simply the molecular markers that play a significant role in the signaling cascade of pathogenesis of disease. The correlation of animal data and human response with *in vitro* data, time factor, and the

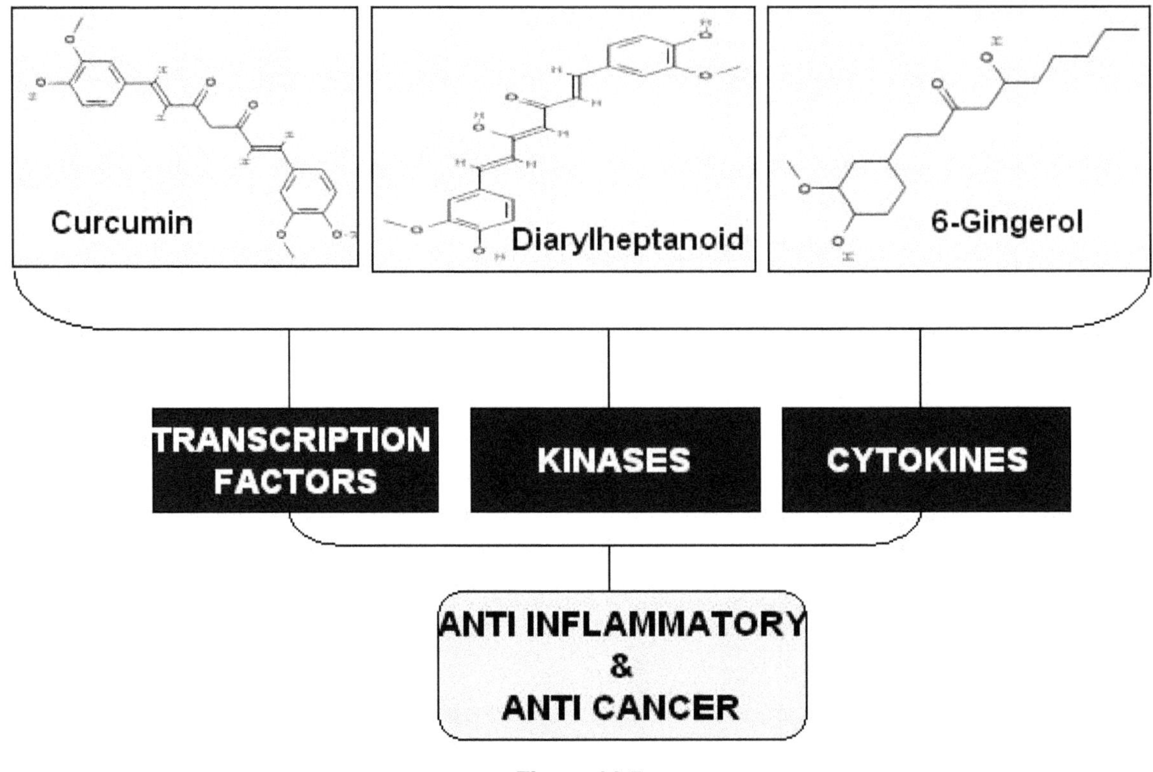

Figure 11.5

need of sophisticated assays that give multi-endpoint data are the major factors driving the development of *in vitro* and *ex vivo* assays (Grant *et al.*, 2007). A simple strategy to screen medicinal plants for multi-targeted assay is given in Figure 11.6.

Screening of Medicinal Plants for Diabetes

Skeletal muscle and adipocytes are the tissues where the major energy homeostasis takes place. Hence, the skeletal muscle (L6) and adipocyte cell lines (3T3–L1) are the preferred choice for the primary screening of compounds for diabetes *in vitro*. Usage of 2-deoxy-D-^{3}[H] glucose for the evaluation of glucose uptake profile of compounds in L6 and 3T3–L1 cells were well reported (Anandarajan *et al.*, 2005, 2006; Muthusamy *et al.*, 2008). The cells grown in 24-well plate were subjected to differentiation as described. After differentiation induction for the stipulated period, the cells were incubated with extracts for 24 hours. After experimental incubation, cells were stimulated with Insulin (100nM) for 20 min followed by rinsing with Krebs Ringer phosphate HEPES (KRPH) solution (118mM NaCl, 5mM KCl, 1.3mM $CaCl_2$, 1.2mM $MgSO_4$, 1.2mM KH_2PO_4 and 30mM HEPES–pH 7.4). The cells were subsequently pulsed for 20 min in KRPH solution containing 0.5mCi/ml 2-deoxy-D-^{3}[H] glucose. By aspirating medium, the glucose uptake terminated. Finally, the cells were washed thrice with ice-cold KRPH solution and then were lysed in 0.1 per cent SDS. The lysate was transferred to 96-well plate (Packard) with glass fiber paper and air dried overnight. The radioactivity of the samples was measured using a Top count liquid scintillation counter. Results were expressed as per cent glucose uptake with

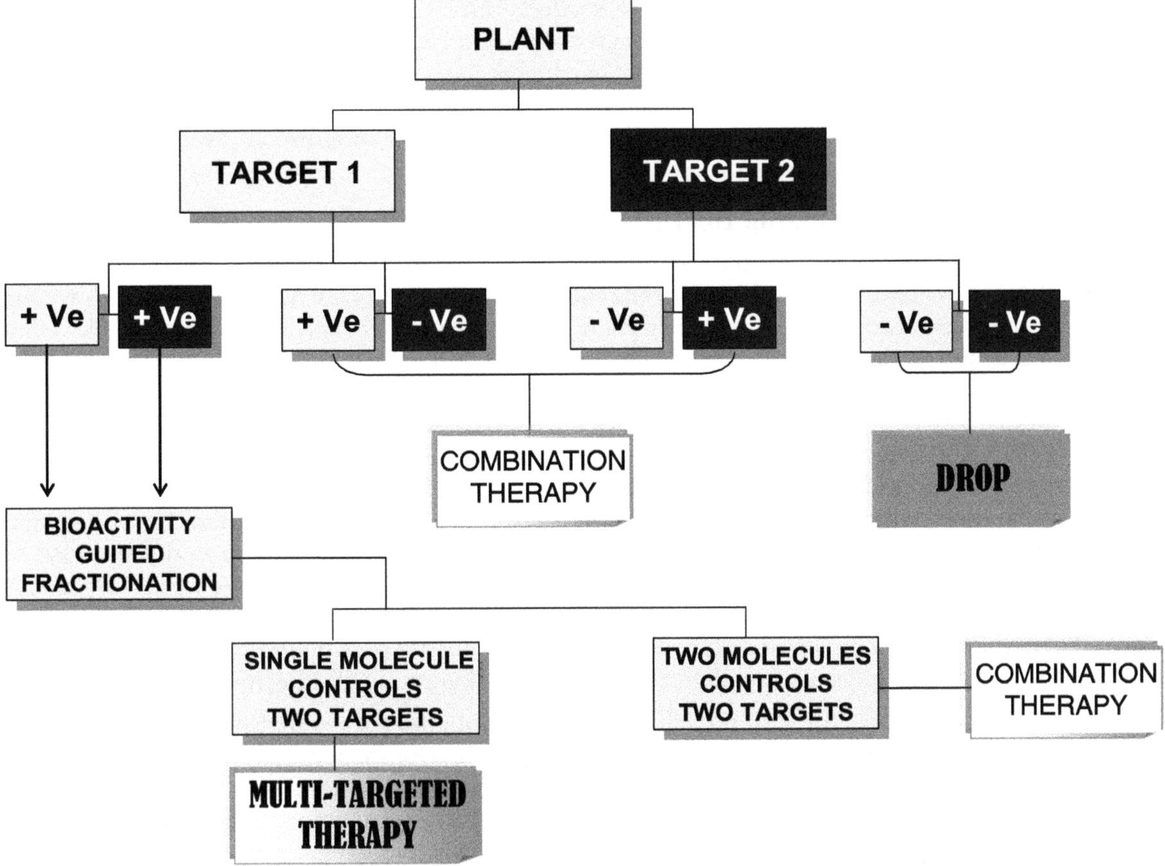

Figure 11.6

respect to solvent control. Rosiglitazone (50 mM) was used as the positive control. Further the mechanism used by the extracts and compounds were assessed by analyzing the expression profile of key genes involved in diabetes like IR, IRS, PTP1B, PI3k, Akt, PKCx, GLUT4, etc., using reverse transcriptase and immuno blotting methodologies.

Screening of Medicinal Plants for Cancer

Cellular assays for screening medicinal plants for cancer can be divided into cytotoxicity assays and other assay types that include morphological assays. Human cancer cell lines obtained from different organ systems, including lung, colon, breast, and other refractory, solid tumors, were used for the cell based primary screening. The simplest cytotoxicity assay is to measure the concentration of sample needed to inhibit cell growth by 50 per cent against a single cell line (Giridharan *et al.*, 2002). The major advantage of cytotoxicity assay is that all potential mechanisms concerning cellular proliferation are monitored simultaneously. Apart from the cytotoxic assay, ^{3}H radiolabelled thymidine incorporation assay is also used as prescreening and screening the plant extracts for identifying its antiproliferative nature. The uptake of thymidine for synthesizing DNA by the proliferating cancer cells in the treated group are measured and compared with the untreated control cells. Thymidine incorporation assay was done in a 24-well plate, seeded with 1×10^6 cells and treated with the extracts and compounds for the stipulated time points (Senthil *et al.*, 2007). Thymidine incorporation was detected by addition of 1mCi of [3H]-thymidine, 24 h before the harvest time point. The radioactivity of the samples was measured using a Top count liquid scintillation counter. DNA fragmentation assay, mRNA and protein expression analysis, and flow cytometry techniques can be adapted for the mechanism evaluation of apoptosis process.

Screening of Medicinal Plants for Inflammation

Human peripheral blood mononuclear cells (PBMC), macrophage cells (RAW 264.7 and J774 A.1–NFkB dependent cell line), and monocytic cells (U 937 and THP1) are normally used cells for the screening evaluation of compounds for inflammation. The cell proliferation assay using radiolabelled thymidine coupled with cell cytotoxicity assay were used as a primary screening methodology for inflammation (Gayathri *et al.*, 2007). In brief, PBMC in 200 µl were cultured in triplicate samples in 96 well U bottom micro titer plates at 2×105 cells/well in RPMI medium containing 10 per cent FCS, and 1 µg/ml of PHA (Phytohemagglutinin). The cells were incubated for 3 days with different concentrations of extracts and compounds. The cell proliferation was measured in a liquid scintillation counter after the cells were pulsed with 1 µCi/well of [3H] thymidine for the last 16 h of incubation. To confirm that the suppressive effect of extract and compound on lymphocyte proliferation is not because of cytotoxicity, the supernatants were also assayed for the enzyme Lactate dehydrogenase (LDH). This stable cytosolic enzyme, which is released upon cell lysis, was measured using the CytoTox 96™ assay. To assess the mechanism of action, measurement of nitrite production using Griess reagent, cytokine expression and kinases activation using RT-PCR and immuno blotting methods were applied.

There is a growing need for standardized, validated *in vitro* assays that provide dependable, predictive safety data for the broad range of products in the development and discovery of drugs. The assays having selectivity, sensitivity combined with good reproducibility and high sample throughput is preferred for multi target screening programs in drug discovery. A major advantage of the *in vitro* assays is that the fastness of total assay time for data analysis and decision-making. Utilization of these assay systems and monitoring the aftermath effects should help in the identification of unique natural products that can be compared with known currently available drugs. These aspects, combined with the ultimate goal to minimize animal testing, serve as incentive for net drug discovery programme.

Conclusion

The process of developing a new drug to treat an infirmity is long, costly and uncertain. Being chemically diverse and the ability to modulate several targets of complex system simultaneously, the importance of natural products in drug discovery is gaining increased attention. The search for a molecule to modify a multiple key factors in a disease process than a single key factor for many complex diseases is the current trend in drug discovery. Herbal extracts represent combinatorial chemistry of nature with vast range of chemical entities that have a complex effect on numerous cellular components and functions. They have great potential in the multi-target approach to diseases. However, potential of herbal drugs is diluted by the difficulty in standardization, pharmacodynamics and pharmacokinetics of these multi-component mixtures. To conclude, integration of ancient traditional knowledge in to the modern analytical and biotechnological sciences is needed to understand the profound mechanism of herbals and phytoprinciples thereby enhancing the significance of herbal therapy.

References

Anandharajan, R., Pathmanathan, K., Shankernarayanan, N. P., Ram A. Vishwakarma, and Arun Balakrishnan. (2005). Upregulation of Glut-4 and PPAR gamma by an isoflavone from *Pterocarpus marsupium* on L6 myotubes: a possible mechanism of action. *Journal of Ethnopharmacology*, 97: 253–260

Atawodi, S. E. (2005). Antioxidant potential of African medicinal plants. *African Journal of Biotechnology*, 4 (2): pp. 128-133.

Baier. G, Schraven. B, Zugel. U and Von Bonin. A. (2007). Kinases as Molecular Signaltransducers and Pharmacological Drug Targets in Inflammation. *In*: Sparking Signals. 3: pp. 1–28

Cecilia Matito, Foteini Mastorakou, Josep J. Centelles, Josep L. Torres and Marta Cascante. (2003). Antiproliferative effect of antioxidant polyphenols from grape in murine Hepa-1c1c7. *European Journal of Nutrition*, 42(1): 43–49.

David J. Newman, Gordon M. Cragg, and Kenneth M. Snader. (2003). Natural Products as Sources of New Drugs over the Period 1981-2002. *Journal of Natural Products*, 66 (7): pp 1022–1037.

Dewick, P. M. (1997). *In*: Medicinal Natural Products: A Biosynthetic Approach. John Wiley and Sons, Inc., New York, 329-330.

Dusica Pavlovic, Vidosava Dordevic, and Gordana Kocic. (2002). A "Cross-Talk" Between Oxidative Stress and Redox Cell Signaling. In: Facta Universitatis, Series: Medicine and Biology, 9(2): pp. 131–137.

Farnsworth, N.R., Akerle, O., Bingle, A.S., Soejarto, D.D., and Guo, Z. (1985). Medicinal plants in therapy. *In*: Bulletin of the World Health Organization 63, 965–981.

Gayathri, B., Manjula, N., Vinaykumar, K. S., Lakshmi, B. S. Balakrishnan, A. (2007). Pure compound from *Boswellia serrata* extract exhibits antiinflammatory property in human PBMCs and mouse macrophages through inhibition of TNFα, IL-1β, NO and MAP kinases. *International Immunopharmacology*, 7: 473–482.

Giri, R.K, V. Rajagopal and V.K. Kalra. (2004). Curcumin, the active constituent of turmeric, inhibits amyloid peptide-induced cytochemokine gene expression and CCR5-mediated chemotaxis of THP-1 monocytes by modulating early growth response-1 transcription factor. *Journal of Neurochemistry*, 91(5): 1199-210.

Giridharan, P., Somasundaram, S. T., Perumal, K., Vishwakarma, R. A., Karthikeyan, N. P., Velmurugan, R., and Balakrishnan, A.. (2002). Novel substituted methylenedioxy lignan suppresses proliferation of cancer cells by inhibiting telomerase and activation of c-myc and caspases leading to apoptosis. *British Journal of Cancer*, 87: 98–105.

Grant R. Zimmermann, Joseph Lehar and Curtis T. Keith. (2007). Multi-target therapeutics: when the whole is greater than the sum of the parts. *Drug Discovery Today*, 7: 34-42.

Hartwell, J. L., and Shear, M. J. (1947). Chemotherapy of cancer. Classes of compounds under investigation and active components or podophyllin. *Cancer Research*. 7: 716-717.

Hayley M. Mcdaid and Susan Band Horwitz. (2001). Selective Potentiation of Paclitaxel (Taxol)-Induced Cell Death by Mitogen-Activated Protein Kinase Kinase Inhibition in Human Cancer Cell Lines. *Molecular Pharmacology*, 60: 290–301.

Hii, C. S, and Howell, S. L. (1984). Effects of epicatechin on rat islets of Langerhans. *Diabetes*, 33: 291–296.

Jun Wang, Hong Zhou, Jiang Zheng, Juan Cheng, Wei Liu, Guofu Ding, Liangxi Wang, Ping Luo, Yongling Lu, Hongwei Cao[2] Shuangjiang Yu, Bin Li, and Lezhi Zhang (2006). The Antimalarial Artemisinin Synergizes with Antibiotics To Protect against Lethal Live *Escherichia coli* Challenge by Decreasing Proinflammatory Cytokine Release. *Antimicrobial Agents and Chemotherapy*, 50(7): 2420-2427

Kroll, U, and Cordes, C. (2006). Pharmaceutical prerequisites for a multi-target therapy. *Phytomedicine*, 13: 12–19

Kwang Seok Ahn, and Bharat B. Aggarwal. (2005). Transcription Factor NF-κB: A Sensor for Smoke and Stress Signals. *Annals of the New York Academy of Sciences*, 1056 (1): 218–233

Lee, M. L., and Schneider, G. (2001). Scaffold architecture and pharmacophoric properties of natural products and trade drugs: application in the design of natural product-based combinatorial libraries. *Journal of Combinatorial Chemistry*, 3: 284-289.

Lin, J.K and S.Y. Lin-Shiau. (2001). Mechanisms of cancer chemoprevention by curcumin. *Proc. Natl. Sci. Counc. Repub. China. B.* 25(2): 59-66.

Manickam, M, Ramanathan, M, Farboodniay Jahromi, M. A, Chansouria, J. P. N, and Ray, A. B. (1997). Antihyperglycemic Activity of Phenolics from *Pterocarpus arsupium*. *Journal of Natural Products*, 60: pp 609–610

Muthusamy, V. S, Anand, S, Sangeetha, K. N, Sujatha, S, Arun Balakrishnan, and Lakshmi, B. S. (2008). Tannins present in *Cichorium intybus* enhances glucose uptake and inhibits adipogenesis through PTP1B inhibition. *Chemico Biological Interaction*, doi:10.1016/j.cbi.2008.04.016.

Nishino, H., H. Tokuda, Y. Satomi, M. Masuda, Y. Osaka, S. Yogosawa, S. Wada, X.Y. Mou, J. Takayasu, M. Murakoshi, K. Jinnno and M. Yano. (2004). Cancer prevention by antioxidants. *Biofactors*, 22 : 57-61.

Patrick A. Baeuerle. (1998). Pro-inflammatory signaling: Last pieces in the NF-κB puzzle? *Current Biology*, 8(1): R19–R22.

Ramanathan, M, Muthusamy, V. S, Saravanan, S, Chandrasekaran, A. K. (2007). Turmeric an Indian Curry–Its Phytochemical and Pharmacological Perspective with Special Reference to Antiinflammatory Action. *In:* Recent Progress in Medicinal Plants, Vol. 17, Ed. By Govil, J.N Singh, V.K., and Ahmad Khalil, Studium Press LLC, USA, pp.1-20.

Reynold Spector, and Elliot S. Vesell. (2006). The Heart of Drug Discovery and Development: Rational Target Selection. *International Journal of Experimental and Clinical Pharmacology*, 77(2): 85–92.

Robert L. Geahlen, Nuphavan M. Koonchanok, Jerry L. McLaughlin, and Dan E. Pratt. (1989). Inhibition of Proteiin-Tyrosine Kinase Activity by Flavanoids and Related Compounds. *Journal of Natural Products*, 52: pp 982–986.

Senthil, V., Ramadevi, S., Venkatakrishnan, V., Giridharan, P., Lakshmi, B. S., Vishwakarma, R. A., and Balakrishnan, A. (2007). Withanolide induces apoptosis in HL-60 leukemia cells via mitochondria mediated cytochrome c release and caspase activation. *Chemico Biological Interaction*, 167: 19-30.

Shu, Y. Z. (1998). Recent Natural Products Based Drug Development: A Pharmaceutical Industry Perspective. *Journal of Natural Products*, 61: 1053-1071.

Subramanian Krishnan, Selvakumar Chinnasamy, Meenakshisundaram Shankaranarayanan, Arun Balakrishnan, Baddireddi Subhadra Lakshmi. Extract of *Alpinia officinarum* Suppresses Enteropathogenic. *Escherichia coli* (EPEC) Lipopolysaccharide (LPS) Induced. Inflammation in J774 A.1 Macrophages. *Journal of Helath Sciences*, 54(1): 112–117.

Thomas Efferth, Yu-jie Fu, Yuangang Zu, Gunter Schwarz, Venkata Sai Badireenath Konkimalla and Michael Wink. (2007). Molecular target-guided tumor therapy with natural products derived from traditional chinese medicine. *Current Medicinal Chemistry*, 14: 1–9.

Wani, M. C., Taylor, H. L., Wall, M. E., Coggon, P., and McPhail, A. T. (1971). The Isolation and Structure of Taxol, a Novel Antileukemic and Antitumor Agent from *Taxus brevifolia*. *Journal of American Chemical Society*, 93: 2325-2327.

Xueqing Liu, Jae-kyung Kim, Yunsheng Li, Jing Li, Fang Liu, and Xiaozhuo Chen. (2005). Tannic acid stimulates glucose transport and inhibits adipocyte differentiation in 3T3-L1 cells. *Journal of Nutrition*, 135(2): 165-71.

Yang, F., G.P. Lim, A.N. Begum, O.J. Ubeda, M.R. Simmons, S.S. Ambegaokar, P.P. Chen, R. Kayed, C.G. Glabe, S.A. Frautschy and G.M. Cole. (2005). Curcumin inhibits formation of amyloid beta oligomers and fibrils, binds plaques and reduces amyloid *in vivo*. *Journal of Biological Chemistry*, 280(7): 5892-901

Zhang, Z., and Meier, K. E. (2006). New assignments for multitasking signal transduction inhibitors. *Molecular Pharmacology*, 69:1510–1512.

Medicinal Plants: Phytochemistry, Pharmacology and Therapeutics, Vol. 1 *Pages 228–237*
Editors: **V.K. Gupta, G.D. Singh, Surjeet Singh and A. Kaul**
Published by: **DAYA PUBLISHING HOUSE, NEW DELHI**

Chapter 12

Safety Assessment of *Orthosiphon stamineus* Benth Methanol Leaf Extract: Drug Interaction and Oral Toxicity Study in Rats

Jin Han Chin[1]* and Abas Hj Hussin[2]
[1]School of Pharmacy, University College Sedaya International, UCSI Height, No. 1, Jalan Menara Gading, 56000. Kuala Lumpur, Malaysia
[2]School of Pharmaceutical Sciences, Universiti Sains Malaysia, 11800, Penang, Malaysia

ABSTRACT

Orthosiphon stamineus Benth. (Famili: Lamiceae) is commonly used to treat diabetes mellitus and bladder problems. Scientific studies reported on the toxicity and drug interaction of *O. stamineus* are limited. This study aims to examine the possible drug interactions and oral toxic effect of standardised methanol leaf extract of *O. stamineus* in female Sprague Dawley (SD) rats. The possible acute oral toxic effect of methanol extract of *O. stamineus* on rats was examined by measuring several serum parameters such as alanine aminotransferase (ALT), aspartate aminotransferase (AST), alkaline phosphatase (ALP), urea, creatinine, total cholesterol and triacylglycerol. Determination of the effect of one day and fourteen days treatment of methanol extract of *O. stamineus* extract on hepatic aminopyrine metabolism was done using isolated SD female rat hepatocytes. Aminopyrine-N-demethylase activity was determined by measuring

* Corresponding Author: E-mail: jinhanchin@hotmail.com.

the quantity of formaldehyde formed at 415 nm by microplate reader according to the colourimetric method of Nash. From the results obtained, no significant change on aminopyrine N-demethylase activity was observed in those SD rats treated with one day and fourteen days of methanol extract of *O. stamineus*. Any adverse signs and lethality was not observed in the toxicity study. Serum urea, creatinine and total cholesterol levels obtained from normal young female SD rats treated with 5 g/kg ($P<0.01$) of standardised methanol extract of *O. stamineus* were significantly lower than the control group. In conclusion, treatment with methanol extract of *O. stamineus* would not cause any significant interaction on aminopyrine metabolism in rat hepatocytes. Practically no toxic effect of methanol extract of *O. stamineus* was detected in rats. The oral LD_{50} of methanol extract of *O. stamineus* was shown to be greater than 5 g/kg.

Keywords: *Aminopyrine N-demethylase, Drug interaction, Hepatocytes, LD_{50}, Lethality, Oral toxicity, Orthosiphon stamineus.*

Introduction

Orthosiphon stamineus Benth. (Famili: Lamiceae) is a beautiful flowering plant, flower conspicuous, white and arranged in a terminal raceme (Wiart, 2002). Stamens of *O. stamineus* are long, expanding and shaped like cat's whiskers and its leaves are simple, without stipules and secussate, diamond-shaped, dark green above and paler below. *O. stamineus* Benth. is easily found in the countries such as Thailand, Indonesia and Europe. In these countries, *O. stamineus* is also known as yaa Nuat Maeo, Rau Meo or Cay Bac (Thailand), Misai Kucing (Malaysia), Kumis Kucing or Remujung (Indonesia), moustaches de chat (French) and Java Tea and Kidney Tea (European). *O. stamineus* has become popular natural medicine for the treatment of diabetes and hypertension in Malaysia (Indubala and Ng, 2000). It also used in many countries as a remedy to treat various diseases such as catarrh of the bladder, gout, jaundice and rheumatism (Wiart, 2002). *O. stamineus* contains several chemically active constituents such as terpenoids (diterpene and triterpene), polyphenols (lipophilic flavonoids and phenolic acids) and sterols (Tezuka *et al.*, 2000). Four compounds, identified as rosmarinic acid, eupatorin, sinensitin and 3'-hydroxy-5,6,7,4'-tetramethoxyflavone were isolated from the methanol leaf extract of *O. stamineus* collected from Kepala Batas, Penang, Malaysia (Akowuah *et al.*, 2004). In our continuing study on the bioactive constituents of *O. stamineus*, the oral administration of methanol leaf extract of *O. stamineus* has been shown to confer antioxidant property by inducing the activity of catalase, superoxide dismutase and glutathione peroxidase and the oral LD_{50} of the *O. stamineus* extract was shown to be greater than 5 g/kg in the young male SD rats (Chin *et al.*, 2008). However, safety concerns have arisen over the oral toxicity and concurrent use of *O. stamineus* extract with other modern drugs, moreover using female animals as subject. Hence, this paper aims to further examine the extent of drug interactions with methanol extract of *O. stamineus* and to evaluate the possible adverse/toxic effects could be attributed by the oral administration of methanol extract of *O. stamineus* extract in female SD rats.

Materials and Methods

Chemicals

All chemical used were of standard analytical purity grade. Aminopyrine was purchased from Sigma Chemical Co., St. Louis, MO. All other chemicals and reagents were obtained from local suppliers.

Experimental Animals

The albino rats weighing 100±10 g from Sprague Dawley (SD) strain bred in The Animal House Unit of Universiti Sains Malaysia, Penang were used throughout the experiment. All rats had free access to water and food. The animals were kept in the animal room (25±2 °C) under 12 h–light/dark cycle. Animals were maintained and handled according to the recommendations of the USM ethical committee which approved the design of the animal experiments. All rats were acclimatized for one week before used.

Extract Preparation

The leaves of the plant were collected in the late afternoon, from 30–45 days old white flowered plants. The leaves were chopped and dried at approximately 40°C for three days. Methanol extract of *O. stamineus* was prepared using a proportion of 10 g dried leaves in 100 mL of methanol by warming for four hours at 40°C. The solution was filtered through filter paper (Whatman No.1), concentrated and spray-dried to obtain the crude methanol extract (Akowuah *et al.*, 2004).

Herb-drug Interaction Study

Herb-drug interaction studies were divided into acute (one day treatment) and sub-chronic (fourteen days treatment). A total of 30 rats were used for each experiment. 30 young female SD rats were randomly assigned into five groups. Each group consists of six animals (n=6). First group was served as control group and received only distilled water. The 2nd, 3rd, 4th and 5th group were orally fed with a single dose daily of 5 mg/kg, 31.25 mg/kg, 125 mg/kg and 500 mg/kg of methanol extracts of *O. stamineus* respectively according to their treatment duration *i.e.*, 1 day treatment in the acute study and repeated dosed up to 14 days in the sub-chronic study. All rats were sacrificed 24 hours post-administration of the last dose. Liver samples of hepatocytes was prepared by the collagenase perfusion technique (Hussin and Skett, 1988). Assay for hepatocytes viability was conducted by using trypan blue exclusion. Only hepatocytes samples with the percentage of cell viability above 85 per cent were used to assay the aminopyrine N-demethylase activity.

Assay for Aminopyrine N-demethylase Activity

Freshly isolated hepatocytes (6000 cells) obtained from control rats and treatment rats were suspended in incubation medium which later were incubated in the presence of aminopyrine (25 mM) for 18 minutes at room temperature (27±1°C). The reaction was terminated by adding 25 per cent (w/v) $ZnSO_4$ and followed by saturated $Ba(OH)_2$. The sample was then centrifuged by table top centrifuge machine (Eppendorf®) at 1000 rpm for 5 minutes. 1 ml of supernatant was added to 2 ml of Nash reagent and incubated at 60 °C for 30 minutes in a waterbath shaker. Aminopyrine-N-demethylase activity was determined by measuring the quantity of formaldehyde formed at 415 nm by microplate reader (Powerwave X-340®; Biotek) according to the colourimetric method of Nash (1953).

Acute Oral Toxicity Study

Fixed dose procedures (FDP) (OECD guideline 420, 2001d) was followed in this acute oral toxicity study. 60 young female SD rats were randomly assigned into six groups (n =10). First group was served as negative control (untreated) group. Second group was served as positive group which was treated with vehicle *i.e.*, distilled water only. Group 3-6 were treated with a single dose of 0.5, 1.0, 3.0 and 5.0 g/kg body weight of methanol extract of *O. stamineus* respectively. The rats were observed closely at the first four hour to examine any toxic symptoms caused by methanol extract of *O. stamineus* (Chan and Hayes, 1994). All treated rats and control rat groups were fasted overnight (at least for 16 h prior to blood collection). Blood was taken via cardiac puncture and used to prepare blood serum for clinical biochemical analyses (Levine, 1995). Blood serum samples analysis was conducted by using Roche (Intergra 700®) machine. Serum biochemical parameters such as aspartate transaminase (AST), alanine transaminase (ALT), alkaline phosphatase (ALP), urea, creatinine, total cholesterol and triacylglycerol were selected for the analysis. Half of the survived rats (n=5) were sacrificed to obtain relative weight of organs such as liver, kidney, heart, lung and spleen and examine for any abnormalities in the organ.

Half of the survived rats (n=5) were then returned back to their own cage and kept for another 14 days observation period. During this period, rats had free access to commercial food pellets and water *ad libitum*. These groups of rats were observed two times daily to examine any occurrence of delay toxic symptoms. Food consumption, water intake and body weight gained were recorded at day-7 and–14 during the recovery period. Survived rats were then sacrificed and necropsy was carried out to see any organ damage and to obtain relative organ weight of liver, kidneys, lungs, heart and spleen.

Data Analysis

The values was shown as mean±standard deviation (S.D). Analysis was done using Dunnett's multiple comparison test. The levels of significant were set at $P<0.05$ and $P<0.01$.

Results

Effect on Aminopyrine N-demethylase Activity

Results obtained from the acute and sub-chronic study indicated no significant difference in the hepatic aminopyrine N-demethylase activity obtained from normal young female SD rats after being treated with 5 mg/kg, 31.25 mg/kg, 125 mg/kg and 500 mg/kg of methanol extract of *O. stamineus* compared to the control group (Figure 12.1).

Acute Oral Toxicity Study

During the experimental period, no lethality was seen within 24 hours post administration of methanol extract of *O. stamineus*. General observable toxic symptoms and adverse effects such as tremor, righting reflex and ataxia were not seen in normal young female SD rats. As seen in the Table 12.1, the serum urea, creatinine and total cholesterol levels of rats treated with 5 g/kg ($P<0.01$) of methanol extract of *O. stamineus* were significantly lower when compared to the control group. No significant changes in colour and relative organ weight *i.e.*, liver, kidney, heart, spleen and lung was observed in normal young female SD post-24 hours of dose administration as compared to positive control group (Table 12.2).

The body weight, food consumption, water intake and relative organ weight of normal young female SD rats treated with extract did not show any significant change when compared to control group during the fourteen days recovery period (Tables 12.3 and 12.4).

Discussion

Although evidence obtained from human and animal experiments support the hypothesis that natural products promote health, it is possible that interactions with other modern drugs may override any subtle benificial effects of natural products in humans. Most reports of toxic effects due to the use of herbal medicines are associated with hepatotoxicity which ranged from mild elevations of liver enzymes to liver failure requiring liver transporting (Saad *et al.*, 2006). The liver is the major organ responsible for the metabolism in most species (Gibson and Skett, 1994). The induction of hepatic

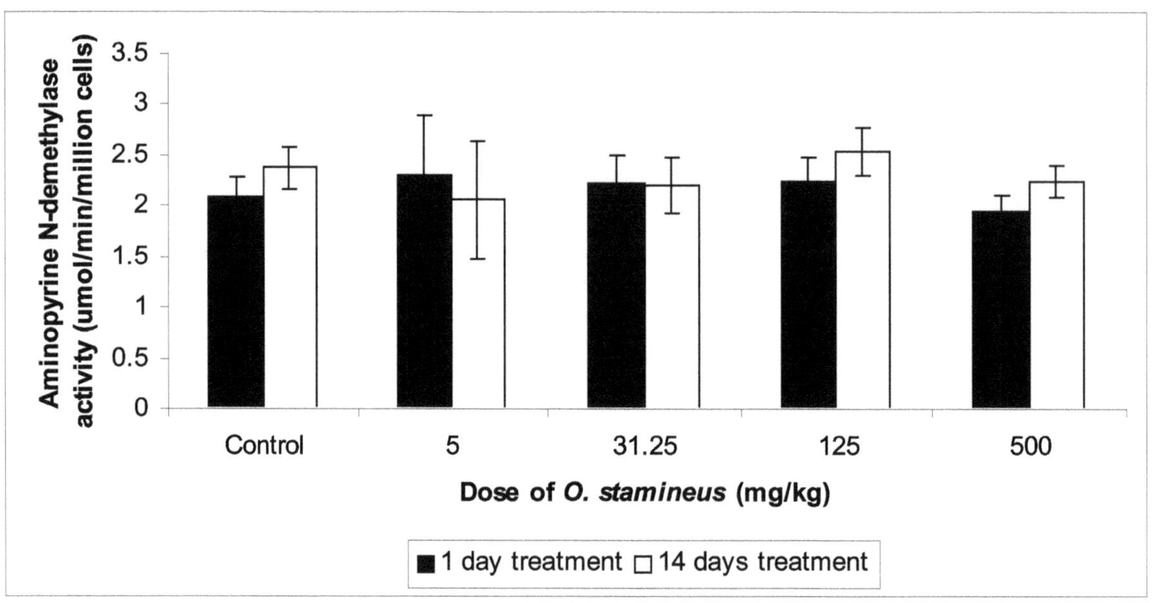

Figure 12.1: Effect of Acute (one day) and Sub-chronic (fourteen days) Oral Administration of Methanol Extract of *O. stamineus* on Aminopyrine N-demethylase Activity in Young Female SD Rat Hepatocytes
Results are analysed using Dunnett test; n=6; Value = mean±standard deviation.

metabolising enzymes plays a substantial role and has profound implications in clinical pharmacology especially metabolic interactions. In human liver the first step of biotransformation is mainly mediated by cytochrome P450 system. Among all isoforms of CYPs, CYP 3A4 needs particular attention in drug interactions. CYP 3A4 is involved in biotransformation of over 50 per cent of drugs in use today (Guengerich, 1996). For the safe use of methanol extract of *O. stamineus*, it is important to clarify CYP 3A4-mediated interaction between methanol extract of *O. stamineus* with the other modern drugs and the time course of methanol extract of *O. stamineus*-induced hepatic drug metabolising enzymes after a certain duration of treatment.

Model drug used in this study, aminopyrine is mainly N-demethylated by CYP P450 3A and 2B in rats and CYP 2C *i.e.*, CYP 2C19 in humans although many other isoforms of cytochrome P450 are also involved (Kamataki, 1993; Timbrell, 2000). Aminopyrine N-demethylase enzyme is categorised as N-dealkylation reaction which belongs to one of the oxidation processes in the phase I hepatic drug metabolism reaction (Hodgson and Goldstein, 2001). Many natural compounds are identified as inhibitors or inducers for cytochrome P450 systems (Zou *et al.*, 2002). Flavonoids induce direct stimulation of gene expression CYPs via a specific receptor *e.g.* aryl hydrocarbon receptor (AhR) or modulate enzymatic activities of CYP (Havsteen, 1983). As seen in Figure 12.1, it is suggested that methanol extract of *O. stamineus* may not cause any significant influence on the levels of CYP3A and CYP2B in normal young female SD rats which gave insignificant interaction with hepatic aminopyrine metabolism. The possible explanation could be due to the poor absorption of active chemical constituents in methanol extract of *O. stamineus* via gastrointestinal tract and are of insufficient amounts to possess significant interaction with the hepatic cytochrome P450 enzyme system in rats. Oral administration of rats with 15 mg/kg, 21 mg/kg and 5 mg/kg respectively of sinensitin, eupatorin and 3′-hydroxy-5,6,7,4′-tetramethoxyflavone has been reported to have a low absorption to about 10 per cent of sinensitin and below 2 per cent for both eupatorin and 3′-hydroxy-5,6,7,4′-tetramethoxyflavone (Loon *et al.*, 2004). By prolonging the treatment of duration and increasing the dose may change the whole scenario.

Table 12.1: Effect of Oral Administration of *O. stamineus* Leaf Extract on Biochemical Parameters in Young Female SD Rats

Dose of O. stamineus (g/kg body weight)	*Normal Young Female SD Rats (7 weeks old±1 week old)*			
	AST (U/L)	*ALT (U/L)*	*ALP (U/L)*	*Urea (μmol/L)*
Negative control	62.0±4.2	35.3±3.8	81.1±5.8	2.7±0.2
Positive control	59.0±5.0	36.0±5.0	81.3±11.0	2.5±0.6
0.5	57.7±5.5	35.0±5.0	80.3±4.5	2.5±0.5
1.0	69.0±12.1	42.0±13.1	83.3±18.2	2.3±0.3
3.0	68.7±12.7	38.0±2.0	86.0±5.3	3.0±0.
5.0	65.3±9.5	33.3±5.9	89.0±19.0	1.7±0.3**

	Creatinine (μmol/L)	*TC (μmol/L)*	*TAG (μmol/L)*
Negative control	13.2±2.5	0.76±0.10	0.33±0.03
Positive control	14.0±2.7	0.79±0.06	0.32±0.02
0.5	13.0±1.0	0.70±0.12	0.30±0.06
1.0	12.7±1.2	0.80±0.05	0.40±0.05
3.0	16.3±1.5	0.70±0.04	0.30±0.06
5.0	10.0±3.0**	0.60±0.04**	0.30±0.05

Results are analysed using Dunnett test; n=10; Value = mean±standard deviation.

Negative control = Untreated SD rats.

Positive control = SD rats orally treated with distilled water only (vehicle-treated control group).

AST: Aspartate aminotransferase; ALT: Alanine aminotransferase; ALP: Alkaline phosphatase; TC: Total cholesterol TAG: Triacylglycerol.

Determination of the serum levels of alanine aminotransferase (ALT) and aspartate aminotransferase (AST) are the most commonly used parameters of indicating hepatocellular injury. ALT is present in the highest concentrations in the liver and only small amount are found in the heart, skeletal muscle cells and red blood cells. The level of ALT in the circulation is markedly increased in hepatitis and from other acute liver damage. AST is found in many tissues including heart, muscle, kidney, brain and lung and also in the liver. When an organ such as heart or liver in injured, AST is released into the bloodstream. The elevation of the AST level in the blood is directly related to the extent of the tissue damage such as acute myocardial infarction and hepatic necrosis. Therefore, ALT is a more specific indicator for liver diseases compared to AST. The values of serum AST and ALT obtained from both treatment groups were within the normal range for the control group. No treatment-related changes were observed in any of the treatment groups for the measurement of liver weight and macroscopic examination *i.e.*, colour and texture changes of the organ. These results did not demonstrate any adverse liver effects.

Table 12.2: Effect of Oral Administration of *O. stamineus* Leaf Extract on Relative Organ Weight in Young Female SD Rats

Dose of O. stamineus (g/kg body weight)	Relative Organ Weight (g/100 g body weight)				
	Liver	Heart	Kidney	Lung	Spleen
Negative control	2.62±0.06	0.32±0.01	0.46±0.01	0.50±0.03	0.31±0.01
Positive control	2.61±0.10	0.30±0.02	0.46±0.02	0.51±0.03	0.32±0.01
0.5	2.63±0.08	0.31±0.02	0.47±0.01	0.52±0.02	0.31±0.01
1.0	2.63±0.12	0.33±0.01	0.46±0.02	0.54±0.02	0.32±0.01
3.0	2.65±0.12	0.31±0.00	0.49±0.02	0.53±0.02	0.32±0.01
5.0	2.67±0.10	0.32±0.02	0.46±0.03	0.51±0.01	0.32±0.01

Results are analysed using Dunnett test; n=5, value = mean±standard deviation.

Negative control = Untreated SD rats.

Positive control = SD rats treated with distilled water only (vehicle-treated control group).

Table 12.3: Body Weight, Water Intake and Food Consumption After Fourteen Days Recovery Period

Dose of O.stamineus (g/kg body weight)	Body Weight (g)		Water Intake (ml/rat/day)		Food Consumption (g/rat/day)	
	7th day	14th day	7th day	14th day	7th day	14th day
Negative control	106.3±2.0	116.3±1.8	11.0±0.2	14.0±0.3	8.2±1.0	11.6±0.8
Positive control	104.4±1.8	114.7±2.1	10.4±0.6	13.0±0.4	7.9±1.2	12.0±1.0
0.5	108.9±2.3	116.8±1.8	10.8±0.8	12.5±0.6	7.5±1.3	11.4±0.9
1.0	107.7±1.5	115.3±2.5	10.0±0.2	13.4±0.1	8.2±0.4	10.3±0.6
3.0	108.9±1.2	116.5±1.0	11.2±0.2	14.2±0.2	8.3±0.3	12.0±0.5
5.0	107.3±2.5	115.8±2.1	10.8±0.6	15.0±0.4	9.2±0.5	11.6±0.5

Results are analysed using Dunnett test; n=5, value = mean±standard deviation.

Negative control = Untreated SD rats.

Positive control = SD rats orally fed with distilled water only (vehicle-treated control group).

Renal damage has often been associated with the markedly increase in serum markers, known as urea and creatinine (Jahangir and Sultana, 2007). In this study, young female SD rats treated with 5 g/kg of methanol extract of *O. stamineus* had serum urea and creatinine significantly lower than the control group but these were not considered to be toxicologically significant. This observation indicated that kidney function is preserved by oral administration of *O. stamineus*. Hydroalcohol extract of *O. stamineus* has been tested for their diuretic activities in rats and it revealed that they led to an increase in urine flow and urinary sodium excretion (Beaux *et al.*, 1999).

One of the most striking results of the present study is the improvement of the lipid profile in response to *O. stamineus* extract treatment. As seen in Table 12.2, the serum total cholesterol level tended to be lower in the 5 g/kg treatment group than in the control group. Our previous study indicates that methanol extract of *O. stamineus* exhibited antioxidant activity (Chin *et al.*, 2008). This finding is in the agreement with other reports that the antioxidative effect had the added benefit of hypocholesterolemic effect (Zern and Fernandez, 2005; Sano *et al.*, 2004). The active compounds and mechanisms underlying the hypocholesterolemic effect of methanol extract of *O. stamineus*, however, remain unclear. Dietary foods enriched with polyphenols and catechins would accentuate to the improvement of lipid profile by increasing the LDL-receptor expression in a human hepatocytes cell line in culture (Pal *et al.*, 2003; Bursill *et al.*, 2001). Lipid metabolism usually maintains an elegant balance between its synthesis and degradation. Hence, further studies are necessary to examine the effect of *O. stamineus* extract on 3-hydroxyl-3-methylglutaryl (HMG-CoA) reductase, key regulatory enzyme in the hepatic production of cholesterol and the concentrations of circulating lipoproteins such as high density lipoprotein (HDL), low density lipoprotein (LDL) and very low density lipoprotein (VLDL).

Table 12.4: Relative Organ Weight after Fourteen Days Recovery Period

Dose of O. stamineus (g/kg body weight)	*Relative Organ Weight (g/100 g body weight)*				
	Liver	*Heart*	*Kidney*	*Lung*	*Spleen*
Negative control	2.61±0.02	0.32±0.01	0.47±0.02	0.50±0.03	0.30±0.01
Positive control	2.62±0.03	0.32±0.01	0.46±0.01	0.50±0.02	0.31±0.01
0.5	2.61±0.01	0.30±0.01	0.46±0.01	0.51±0.03	0.29±0.01
1.0	2.63±0.03	0.32±0.01	0.47±0.01	0.49±0.01	0.31±0.01
3.0	2.62±0.02	0.31±0.01	0.46±0.02	0.51±0.03	0.30±0.01
5.0	2.63±0.01	0.32±0.01	0.48±0.02	0.50±0.02	0.31±0.00

Results are analysed by using Dunnett test; n=5; value = mean±standard deviation.

Negative control = Untreated SD rats.

Positive control = SD rats orally fed with distilled water only (vehicle-treated control group).

According to OECD (2001d), the female redents are generally preferred over the male rodents due to the literature surveys of conventional LD_{50} tests that the females are slightly more sentitive to chemicals than males. It is generally accepted that toxicity varies with species/strain, age and gender (Cohen *et al.*, 1998). The available data from acute oral toxicity study reveals no evidence of toxicity of methanol extract of *O. stamineus* in SD female rats. Based on the chemical classification mentioned by Ecobichon (1995), methanol extract of *O. stamineus* was considered as "practically non toxic". LD_{50} could not be determined in this study due to the no lethality incident was observed. We suggested that the oral LD_{50} and No Observable Adverse Effect Level (NOAEL) for the methanol extract of *O. stamineus* were to be greater than 5 g/kg under the present experimentation condition.

Conclusion

Oral administration with methanol leaf extract of *O. stamineus* up to 500 mg/kg had no significant effect on the activity of aminopyrine-N-demethylase in female SD rat hepatocytes. The available data obtained from acute toxicity study demonstrated that methanol leaf extract of *O. stamineus* reveals no any adverse effects in SD rats. These findings could be compromise the safe use of this plant for medical purposes.

Acknowledgements

Authors would like to thank Prof Zhari Ismail for his generous gift of methanol extract of *O. stamineus*. Authors would like to thank the financial support of the Intensified Research in Priority Areas (IRPA) grant from the Malaysian Ministry of Science, Technology and Environmental.

References

Akowuah, G.A., Zhari, I., Norhayati, I., Sadikun, A., and Khamsah, S.M. (2004). Sinensitin, eupatorin, 3′-hydroxy-5,6,7,4′-tetramethoxyflavone and rosmarinic acid contents and antioxidative effect of *Orthosiphon stamineus* from Malaysia. *Food Chemistry*, 82: 559-566.

Beaux, D., Fleurentin, J., and Mortier, F. (1999). Effect of extracts of *Orthosiphon stamineus*, Benth, *Hieracium pilosell*, L., *Sambucus niagra* L. and *Arctostaphylos uva-ursi* (L.) Spreng. in rats. *Phytotherapy Research: PTR*, 13: 222-225.

Bursill, C., Roach, P.D., Bottema, C.D., and Pal, S. (2001). Green tea upregulates the low-density lipoprotein receptor through the sterol-regulated element binding protein in HepG2 liver cells. *Journal Agriculture Food Chemistry*, 49: 5639-5645.

Chan, P.K. and Hayes, A.W. (1994). Acute Toxicity and Eye Irritancy. *In:* Principles and Methods of Toxicology, Ed. By Hayes, A.W., Raven Press Ltd, New York, pp.579-647.

Chin, J.H., Akowuah, G.A., Hussin, A., Ismail, Z., Fei, Y.M. and Ismail, S. (2008). Toxicity and *In vivo* antioxidant effect of *Orthosiphon stamineus* leaf extracts in rats. *In*: Recent progress in medicinal plants, Vol. 21, Ed. By Singh, V.K., and Govil, J.N., Studium Press LLC, USA, pp.137-146.

Cohen, S.D., Hoivik, D.J. and Khairallah, E.A. (1998). Acetaminophen-induced hepatotoxicity. *In:* Toxicology of the liver, Ed. By Plaa, G.L. and Hewitt, W.R., Taylor and Francis, USA, pp.159-165.

Ecobichon, D.J. (1995). Acute Toxicity Studies. *In:* The Basic of Toxicity Testing, Ed. By Hollinger, M.A., CRC Press, Baca Raton, pp.35-58.

Gibson, G.G. and Skett, P. (1994). Introduction to drug metabolism. Blackie Academic and Professional, London.

Guengerich, F.P. (1996). *In vitro* techniques for studying drug metabolism. *Journal of Pharmakinetics and Biopharmaceutics*, 24: 521-533.

Havsteen, B. (1983). Commentary: flavonoids, a class of natural products of high pharmacological potency. *Biochemical Pharmacology*, 32: 1141-1148.

Hodgson, E. and Goldstein, J.A. (2001). Metabolism of Toxicants: Phase I Reactions and Pharmacogenetics. *In:* Introduction to Biochemical Toxicology, Ed. By Hodgson, E., and Smart, R.C., Wiley-Interscience, New York, pp.67-96.

Hussin, A.H., and Skett, P. (1988). Lack of effect of insulin in hepatocytes isolated from streptozotocin-diabetic male rats. *Biochemical Pharmacology*, 37 (9), 1683-1686.

Indubala, J. and Ng, L.T. (2000). Herbs: The green pharmacy of Malaysia. Vinpress Sdn. Bhd, Kuala Lumpur.

Jahangir, T., and Sultana, S. (2007). Perillyl alcohol protects against Fe-NTA-induced nephrotoxicity and early tumor promotional events in rat experimental model. *eCAM*, 4(4): 439-445.

Kamataki, T. (1993) Metabolism of Xenobiotics. *In:* Cytochrome P-450, Ed. By Omura, T., Ishimura, Y., and Fujii-Kuriyama, Y., Kodansha Ltd, Tokyo, pp.141-162.

Levine, B.S. (1995). Animal Clinical Pathology. *In*: CRC Handbook of Toxicology, Ed. By Derelanko, M.J., and Hollinger, M.A. CRC Press, USA, pp.517-539.

Loon, Y.H., Wong, J.W., Yap, S.P., and Yuen, K.H. (2004). Determination of flavonoids from *Orthosiphon stamineus* in plasma using a simple HPLC method with ultraviolet detection. *Journal of Chromatography B*, 816(1-2): 161-166.

Nash, T. (1953). The colorimetric estimation of formaldehyde by means of the Hantzsch reaction. *Biochemical Journal*, 55: 416-421.

OECD (Organization for Economic Cooperation and Development). (2001d) OECD Test Guideline 401: acute oral toxicity–fixed dose method. Organization for Economic Cooperation and Development, Paris.

Pal, S., Ho, N., and Santos, C. (2003). Red wine polyphenolics increase LDL receptor expression and activity and suppress the secretion of apoB100 from human HepG2 cells. *Journal of Nutrition*, 133: 700-706.

Rajesh, M.G., and Latha, M.S. (2004). Protective activity of *Glycyrrhiza glabra* Linn. on carbon-tetrachloride-induced peroxidative damage. *Indian Journal of Pharmacology*, 36: 284-287.

Saad, B., Dakwar, S., Said, O., Abu-Hijleh, G., Al Battah, F., Kmeel, A., and Aziazeh, H. (2006). Evaluation of medicinal plant hepatotoxicity in co-cultures of hepatocytes and monocytes. *eCAM*, 3(1): 93-98.

Sano, J., Inami, S., Seimiya, K., Ohba, T., Sakai, S., Takano, T., and Mizuno, K. (2004). Effects of green tea intake on the development of coronary artery disease. *Circulation Journal*, 68: 665-670.

Tezuka, Y., Stampoulis, P., Banskota, A.H., Awale, S., Tran, K.Q., Saiki, I., and Kadota, S. (2000). Constituents of the Vietnamese medicinal plant *Orthosiphon stamineus*. *Chemical and Pharmaceutical Bulletin*, 48: 1711-1719.

Timbrell, J. (2000). Principles of biochemical toxicology. Taylor and Francis Ltd, London.

Wiart, C. (2002). *Orthosiphon stamineus* Benth. *In:* Medicinal Plants of Southeast Asia, Ed. By Wong, F.K, Prentice Hall, Kuala Lumpur, pp.265-266.

Zern, T.L., and Fernandez, M.L. (2005). Cardioprotective effects of dietary polyphenols. *Journal of Nutrition*, 135: 2291-2294.

Zou, L., Harkey, M.R., and Henderson, G.L. (2002). Effects of herbal components on cDNA-expressed cytochrome P450 enzyme catalytic activity. *Life Sciences*, 71: 1579-1589.

Medicinal Plants: Phytochemistry, Pharmacology and Therapeutics, Vol. 1 *Pages 238–257*
Editors: **V.K. Gupta, G.D. Singh, Surjeet Singh and A. Kaul**
Published by: **DAYA PUBLISHING HOUSE, NEW DELHI**

Chapter 13

Capsicum Genus: Ethnobotany, Chemistry and Pharmacology Studies of the Pepper

Roosevelt H. Leal and Valdir F. Veiga Junior*
Departamento de Química, Universidade Federal do Amazonas
Av. Gal. Rodrigo Octávio Jordao, Japiim
69077-000–Manaus, AM-Brazil

ABSTRACT

Capsicum genus has a widespread use, ranging from medical and warlike ends to cooking. Being the most cultivated genus its use is known from the most ancient times. There are pain-inducing and sweet varieties; pain being attributed to a group of substances, the capsaicinoids. This paper presents a vision on *Capsicum* chemistry, biology and ethnopharmacology literature.

Keywords: *Capsicum, Pepper, Ethnobotany, Chemistry, Pharmacology, Capsaicin.*

Introduction

The species of the *Capsicum* genus are the most cultivated peppers worldwide, its use ranging from cooking to medical and warlike ends. The characteristic that gets more attention is the pungency in their fruits, varying from high pungency fruits to no pungency ones (bell peppers and sweet peppers).

* Corresponding Author: E-mail: valdirveiga@ufam.edu.br.

This characteristic feeling, commonly know as burning, is measured by the Scoville scale; some values found in ripe fruits are for instance between 15,000 and 300,000 (Gibbs and O'Garro, 2004). The fruits have varied shapes, colors and chemical compositions and are valued for their color, smell and pungency (Contreras-Padilla and Yahia, 1998). Besides their pungent components, known as capsaicinoids, other chemical constituents found are carotenoids, flavonoids and glycosides. The peppers and the products obtained from them are used since times immemorial in foods and in popular medicine. After finding use by ancient civilizations of the Americas, cultivation quickly spread worldwide, integrating medicinal arsenals of millenarian cultures in the East. Their popular uses are today even more numerous, and countless studies prove and reveal new therapeutic actions. Their pharmacological application is mainly related to neurology and the other biological activities such as antioxidants, antitumorals and antimicrobials. The genetic diversity of the peppers cultivated around of the world in their domesticated forms and mainly the diversity of the species in their origin centers, in their semi-domesticated and wild forms. The highest importance in improvement of cultivated plants, translated the possibility of transfer of important qualities, as resistance to diseases, tastes and flavors (Barbosa *et al.*, 2002; Noda *et al.*, 2003).

Botanical Aspects and Ethnopharmacology

Capsicum genus (Solanaceae) comprehends more than 200 varieties (Contreras-Padilla and Yahia, 1998). Several species that compose this genus are found in domesticated, semi-domesticated and wild forms (Reifschneider *et al.*, 2000) with several colours and forms. The five main species of the genus are: *C. annuum* (jalapeño and bell peppers), *C. frutescens* (tabasco), *C. chinense* (Habanero), *C. baccatum* (Aji) and *C. pubescens* (Rocoto and Manzano) (Pino, 2007). Their forms are prolonged, oval or round. The coloration of their ripe fruits can be red, orange, yellow and even black. Some botanical characteristics of three of the main cultivated species are: *C. annuum* has white, robust flowers with diameter between 1.4-1.8cm; *C. frutescens* has light green flowers, varying from white to greenish; its corolla has no stains and the lobes are positioned back after the anthesis *C. chinense* is a species that comes with two to five flowers per knot; the pedicel usually is found in the pendent form and the corolla can vary from white to white-greenish, with petals that have no points or marks (Barbosa *et al.*, 2002).

The use for the *Capsicum* species is extremely diversified: the fruits are used in human feeding, in the composition of medicines and in warlike industry in the form of pepper spray; they are also used in the treatment of domestic animal illnesses, as repellent of plagues and in indigenous rituals (Barbosa *et al.*, 2002; Wagner, 2003; Prasad *et al.*, 2006a; Mtambo *et al.*, 1999).

In human feeding, peppers and bell peppers are an important source of nutrients as carotenoids, phenols, vitamin C, folates, standing out for the abundance of these compounds (Howard *et al.*, 2000; Deepa *et al.*, 2007; Philips *et al.*, 2006). Concentrations of vitamin C vary among the pepper species, from 46 to 245mg/100g, values comparable to those of the guava (200mg/100g) and superior to those of the orange (60mg/100g) (Silva, 2006; Gnayfeed, 2001). The fruits of the different species of the *Capsicum* genus, the peppers, are consumed in natural form or processed as seasonings, pickles and currants. Paprika that is constituted by powdered dried pepper and oil-resin, which is the extract free of solvents used by the food industry to provide or to reinforce the intensity of foodstuff colors (Pieroni *et al.*, 2004).

In Asia, *C. frutescens* is used by populations in India to treat typhus, intermittent fevers, dropsy, gout, dyspepsia, cholera, rubefacient and stomach ache (Ching and Mohamed, 2001). *C. annuum* is used as an acid stimulant, rubefacient, and to treat scarlatina, hoarseness, dyspepsia, yellow fever, and diarrhoea (Ching and Mohamed, 2001). Other uses attributed to *Capsicum* (chilli) are to treat urinary symptoms, tonsillitis, snake-bite, diphtheria, tonic to loss of appetite, flatulence, to reduce swellings, lumbago, rheumatism, and gout. In Assam, (Northeast India) its use was observed in the fight against scabies (the crushed form is applied directly on the skin) (Dasgupta and Fowler, 1997; Saikia, 2006). In West Indies, chillies were used to relieve the sinking feeling in the epigastrium felt by drunkards and delirium tremens (Dasgupta and Fowler, 1997). In Turkey (Central Anatolia), hot red pepper fruits (*C. annuum*) are cooked in milk and ingested to relieve stomach ache (Sezik, 2001). In Asian countries like Korea, the spicy pepper is present in a quite significant way in the diet.

In England, chilli have been used in the treatment of various diseases, *e.g.*: dyspepsia, tympanitis, palsy, dropsies, for healing ulcers of the fauces, as a gargle for pharyngitis, linament for paralytic limbs, chronic gout, rheumatism, bronchial catarrh, chronic bronchitis (Dasgupta and Fowler, 1997). In Central Italy, its use as antirheumatic and antiotitis was performed using *C. annuum* macerate in olive oil form (Pieroni, 2004). Still in Italy (Castelmezzano, Pietrapertosa), *C. annuum* fruits were used as an aromatic in foods and as antihypertensive; the seeds were used in medicinal rituals, in massages and as antirheumatic (Pieroni, 2004). *C. annuum* in Uzbekistan is popularly used for poor digestion, chronic vomiting, lingual paralysis and in Russia for neuralgia, radiculitis and myositis treatment (Shakhidoyatov and Sagdullaev, 2001).

In the American continent, the use given by the Amerindians was to preserve foods from contamination of pathogenic mushrooms and bacteria (Reifschneider, 2000). Berg and Silva (1988) report that in indigenous and non indigenous communities of Roraima (Brazil) chilli pepper (*C. frutescens* L.) is used to combat the "pano branco" ("white cloth") skin affection. Barbosa *et al.* (2002) also report its use in the treatment of respiratory tract infections, ophthalmia (Yanomamis, Roraima, Brazil), malaria treatment (Wapichanas, Roraima, Brazil), and also at to indigenous rituals. In Southern Appalachia, United States, the fruit infusion from *C. annuum* L. var. *annuum* had its use mentioned to treat cold, influenza and to improve blood circulation (Cavender, 2006). In Latin America, chillies are reported to be used on children's gingers, a common practice by mothers who wish to deter them from the habit of sucking their thumbs (Dasgupta and Fowler, 1997). The Aztecs used it in cough treatment. Tarahumara Indians used them in bronchitis and throat irritation (Dasgupta and Fowler, 1997). Mayan inhabitants used chilli peppers (from several *Capsicum* species) in respiratory problems, complaints, earaches and sores. Huastec Mayan applied them on infected wounds and fresh burns, besides their use as flavouring components (Cichewicz and Thorpe, 1996; Molina-Torres *et al.*, 1999). In Jamaica, *C. frutescens* has popular use to treat diabetes mellitus (Tolan, *et al.*, 2004). In Northwest Argentina, *Capsicum annuum* L. dry fruits are crushed and the powder is placed on the wound to stop bleeding (Hilgert, 2001). In Colombia (Antioquia and Choco), the *C. frutescens* macerated ripe fruit is used to neutralize the hemorrhagic effect provoked by the snakebite of the *Bothrops atrox* species, whose effect can be verified *in vitro* (Otero *et al.*, 2000). In nowadays Mexico, peppers are above all an integral part of the national cultural identity.

In Africa, chilli peppers are applied as antiseptics, to enhance wound healing, and to fight parasitic infestations of the intestine (Dasgupta and Fowler, 1997). The aplication of *C. frutescens* in Tanzania in avian veterinary treatment of the Newcastle disease is reported too (Mtambo *et al.*, 1999). In Nigeria, Hausa people (ethnic group) uses *Capsicum* fruits as spice and leaf bundles (snack form) (Cook *et al.*, 2000). In Uganda, *C. frutescens* is used in the induction of labour during childbirth, being ingested (squeezing by hand, chewing leaves, seeds, fruits). In Faisalabad, Pakistan, *C. annuum* has veterinary use (systemic disorders of camel) where 250g are grated and drenched in 1L water.

Chemical Composition

The characteristic constituent phytochemicals of *Capsicum* genus are the xanthines derived from β-carotene called capsaicinoids (Figure 13.1), totaling around sixteen compounds. These alkaloids, the capsaicinoids (CAPS) according to their structure can be grouped in three classes of compounds (Schweiggert *et al.*, 2006): capsaicin analogues, which have insaturation and ramification in its alkyl chain (structures 1, 4, 5, 6, 13); dihydrocapsaicin analogues, saturated in its alkyl chain and possess ramification (structures 2, 3, 7, 8, 12); *N*-vanillyl-*n*-acylamide group analogues, which possess neither ramification nor insaturation (structures 9, 10, 11).

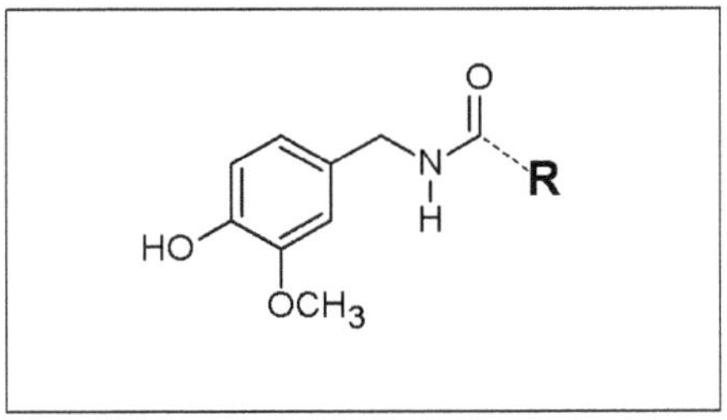

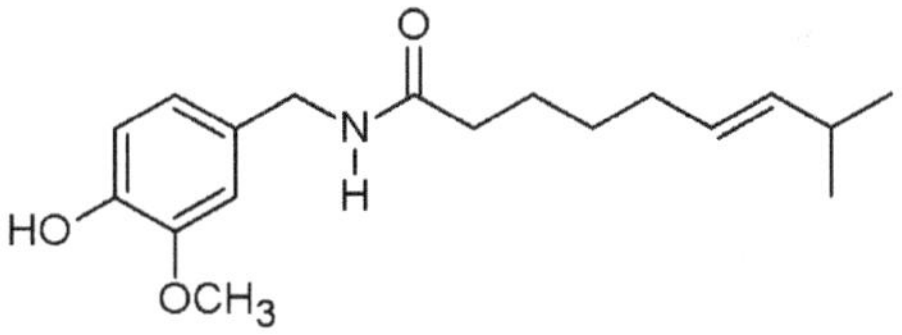

Compound	Structure
Capsaicin	(**1**)
Homocapsaicin I	(**5**): R = $(CH_2)_4CH{=}CH{-}CH_2CH{-}(CH_3)_2$
Homocapsaicin II	(**6**): R = $(CH_2)_4CH{=}CH{-}CH{-}(CH_3){-}CH_2{-}CH_3$
Norcapsaicin	(**4**): R = $(CH_2)_3CH{=}CH{-}CH{-}(CH_3)_2$
Nornorcapsaicin	(**13**): R = $(CH_2)_2CH{=}CH{-}CH{-}(CH_3)_2$

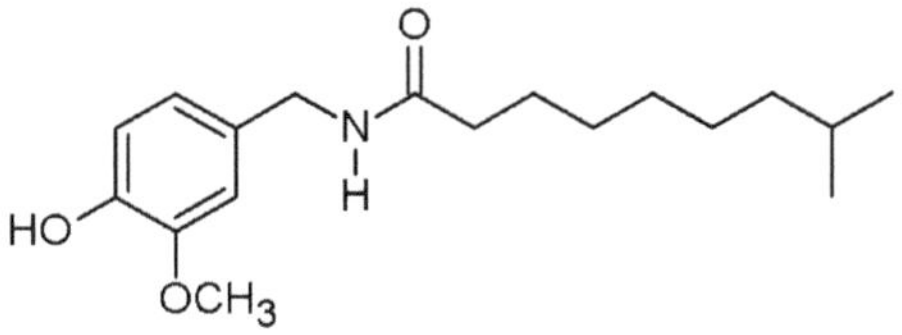

Compound	Structure
Dihydrocapsaicin	(**2**)
Homodihydrocapsaicin I	(**7**): R = $(CH_2)_7CH{-}(CH_3)_2$
Homodihydrocapsaicin II	(**8**): R = $(CH_2)_6CH{-}(CH_3){-}CH_2{-}CH_3$
Nordihydrocapsaicin	(**3**): R = $(CH_2)_5CH{-}(CH_3)_2$
Nornordihycapsaicin	(**12**): R = $(CH_2)_4CH{-}(CH_3)_2$

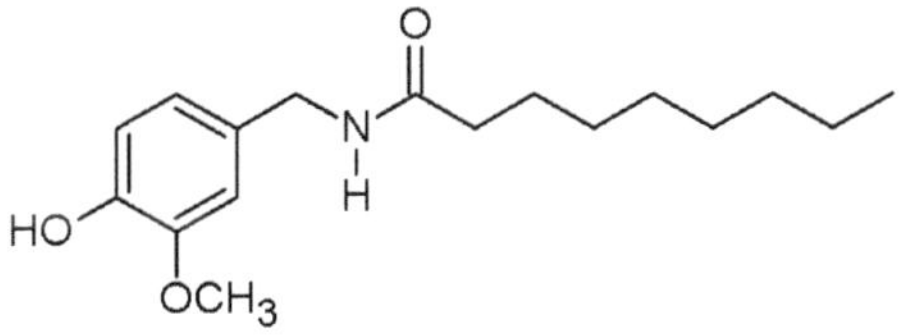

Compound	Structure
N-vanillyl-nonanamide	(**9**)
N-vanillyl-decanamide	(**11**): R = $(CH_2)_8CH_3$
N-vanillyl-octanamide	(**10**): R = $(CH_2)_6CH_3$

Figure 13.1: Chemistry, Structure of Capsaicinoids in the *Capsicum* Genus

The capsaicin biosynthesis occurs via the phenylpropanoid pathway; capsaicin is synthesized starting from the vanillylamine condensation with long chain fatty acids, which are synthesized from valine and vanillylamine originating from the mentioned pathway (Wagner, 2003; Titze *et al.*, 2002). Prasad *et al.* (2006b), studying the biosynthesis of capsaicin in the *C. frutescens*, relate that valine pathway is more crucial than phenylpropanoid pathway.

Besides fruits, CAPS are found in different plant organs like stem and leaves. The presence of CAPS in a plant is shown to be correlated with the flowering period and above all with the presence of fruits (Zewdie and Bosland, 2001) from which they would have their origin, being produced in glands located in their placenta. According to a recent report, capsaicinoids are not present in plants without fruits (Estrada *et al.*, 2002; Zewdie and Bosland, 2001) Environmental factors such as climate and soil, and other variables like cultural practices, crop and stockpiling and also genetic factors, influence incontestably on the qualitative and quantitative chemical composition in *Capsicum* genus.

Approaching qualitatively the proportion of capsaicinoids differs inside the *Capsicum* species and among them. There are studies in which capsaicin (1) is the major component (Garcés-Claver *et al.*, 2006; Poyrazoglu *et al.*, 2005) while in others it is dihydrocapsaicin (2) (Estrada *et al.*, 2002). Together, they account for 90 per cent of the pungent substances of *Capsicum* fruits (Garcés-Claver *et al.*, 2006). The nordihydrocapsaicin (3) is also reported (Schweiggert *et al.*, 2006; Poyrazoglu *et al.*, 2005; Sato *et al.*, 1999; Constant *et al.*, 1995) among the commonly observed pungent substances. Gibbs *et al.* (2004), studying *C. annuum, C. frutescens* and 28 other accessions of *C. chinense*, report that nordihydrocapsaicin was less abundant than capsaicin and homocapsaicin in all studied cultivars. Among minoritarian CAPS which have been found, several substances can be cited: norcapsaicin (4), nornorcapsaicin (13), homocapsaicin I (5), homocapsaicin II (6), nornordihydrocapsaicin (12), homodihydrocapsaicin I (7), homodihydrocapsaicin II (8), *N*-vanillyl-octanamide (10), *N*-vanillyl-decanamide (11) and *N*-vanillyl-nonanamide (9). This last one was previously known in synthetic form only, but was discovered occurring naturally and denominated nonivamide (9). There are also several isomers that occur as minoritarian constituents too (Constant and Cordell, 1996; Constant *et al.*, 1995; Schweiggert *et al.*, 2006; Luning *et al.*, 1995; Kopp and Jurenitsch, 1981; Paul Jr. *et al.*, 1975; Jurenitsch *et al.*, 1979). Studies demonstrate that quantitative variations of the chemical components can be found according to species and cultivars, geographical origin and part of the plant. Poyrazoglu *et al.* (2005) studied varieties of *C. annuum* and *C. frutescens* collected in different areas and observed for Mara variety the content of capsaicin (1), dihydrocapsaicin (2) and nordihydrocapsaicin (3) in the ranges: 0.81-1.42, 0.38-0.70 and 0.01-0.04 mg g^{-1}, respectively; to Süs, Cin and Isot the total content of capsaicinoids was 2.11, 4.70 and 0.55 mg g^{-1} respectively, and for their seeds 0.63, 1.70 and 1.60 mg g^{-1}. In another study, Choi *et al.* (2006) analyzing different varieties of peppers (*Capsicum*) found CAPS levels varying from 0.001 mg g^{-1} (PR Gang ja) to 0.12 mg g^{-1} (Chung yang). Homodihydrocapsaicin, as a general matter, was not found in the ripe fruits of 28 accessions of *C. chinense* nor in *C. annuum* and *C. frutescens.*

Capsaicin derivatives (Figure 13.2) have been object of several chemical and biological studies like 6'',7''-dihydro-5',5'''-dicapsaicin (14), isolated from *C. annuum* and (-)-capsaicinol (15) isolated from *C. frutescens*, both with similar antioxidant activity to capsaicin, without however having a pungent taste (Ochi *et al.*, 2003).

Other substances, isolated from non-pungent cultivars, like capsiate (16), dihydrocapsiate (17) have also been described to their antioxidant activities (Rosa *et al.*, 2002).

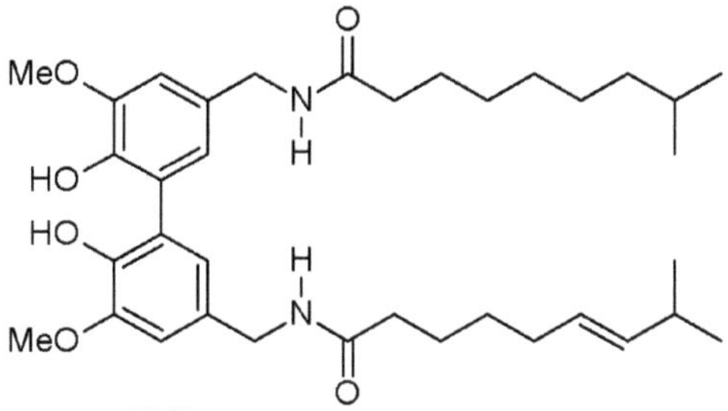

(14) 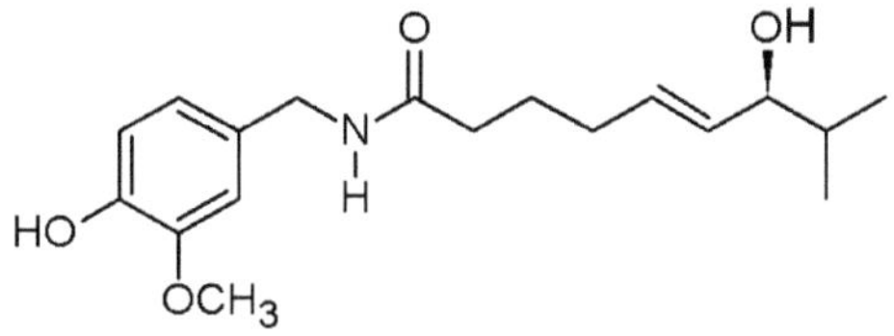 (15)

Figure 13.2: Chemistry Structure Derivatives of Capsaicin

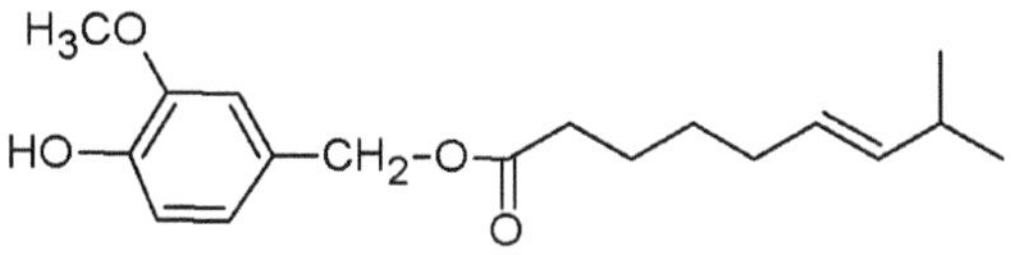

(16) 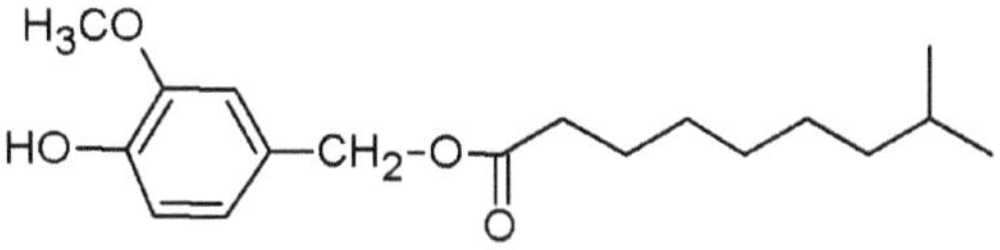 (17)

Figure 13.3: Substances Antioxidants Non-pungents Found in *Capsicum* Genus

In *C. annuum* cv. *"High Heat"*, *C. frutescens*, and *C. chinense* fruits the glucosides identified were: capsaicin-β-*D*-glucopyranoside and dihydrocapsaicin-β-*D*-glucopyranoside; Observing the correlation among the quantity of the capsaicinoids capsaicin and dihydrocapsaicin and the derived glucosides, it is noted that the glucosides are not detected in nonpunget cultivars of *C. annuum* L. (Higashiguchi *et al.*, 2006).

In polar fractions of fruits, leaves and branches of some *Capsicum annuum* varieties, it is possible to find acyclic diterpene glycosides of two classes: monomerics (capsianosides I-XI, XIII-XVII) and dimeric esters of those first ones (capsianosides A-G) (Yahara *et al.*, 1991; Izumitami *et al.*, 1990; Iorizzi *et al.*, 2002; Lee *et al.*, 2006; Song *et al.*, 2001; Lee *et al.*, 2008).

In *C. annuum* seeds and roots saponins, steroidal glycosides, deduced as glycosides furostanols, which are denominated capsicosides (A-D) are found (Yahara *et. al.*, 1994). Other substances found were proto-degalactotigonin and some oligoglycosides. In seeds of *C. annuum* L. var. *acuminatum* the capsicosides A, D, F, G and E (Figure 13.4), also 22-*O*-methylcapsicoside A (19) and 22-*O*-methylcapsicoside G (20) were described (Iorizzi *et al.*, 2002). Glycosides found in fruits of *C. anuum* L. var *acuminatum* are the capsoside A, capsoside B and the lignan glycoside icariside (Figure 13.4, 21) (Iorizzi *et al.*, 2001).

Besides fruits, the sesquiterpenes observed in the stems and roots of *C. annuum* (Figure 13.5) are canusesnols A-J(22-31) and nine more compounds reported are reported substances: capsidiol (32), *N-cis*-feruloyltyramine, *N-trans*-feruloyltyramine, *N-p-cis*-coumaroyltyramine, *N-p-trans*-coumaroyltyramine, lariciresinol, 13-hydroxycapsidiol, lubiminol, and drummondol (Kawaguchi *et al.*, 2004).

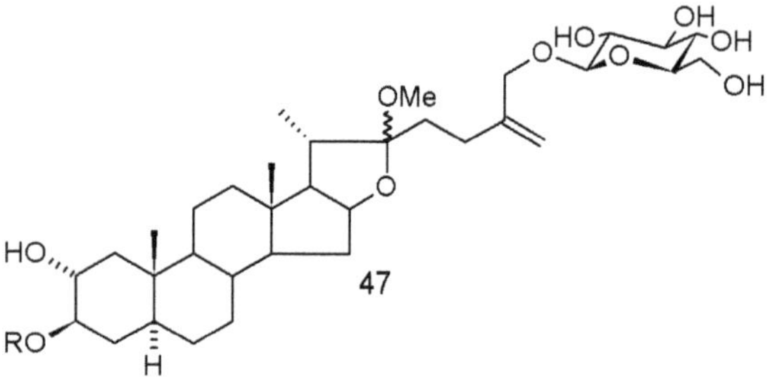

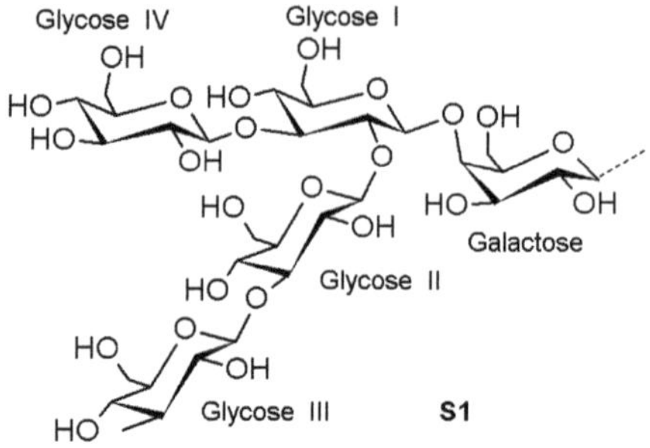

Capsicosideo E (**18**): R = S1

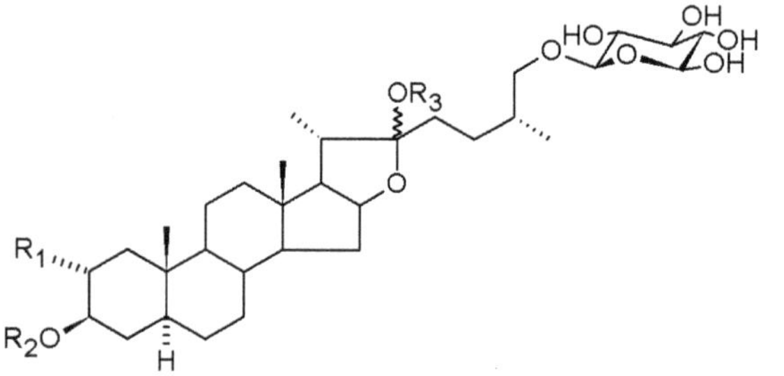

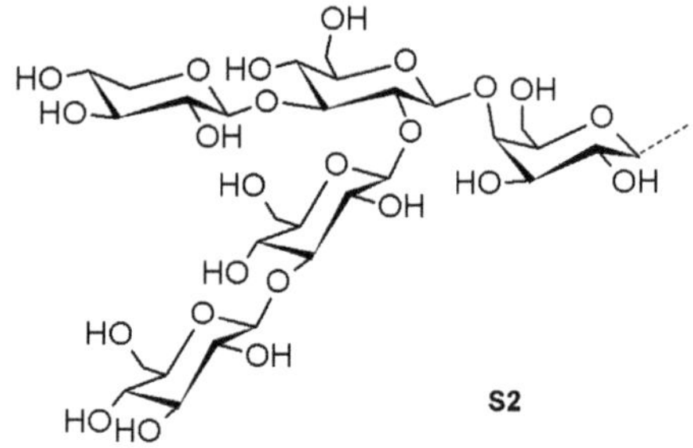

22-*O*-Methylcapsicoside A (**19**): R1 = OH, R2 = S1, R3 = Me

22-*O*-Methylcapsicoside G (**20**): R1 = H, R2 = S1, R3 = Me

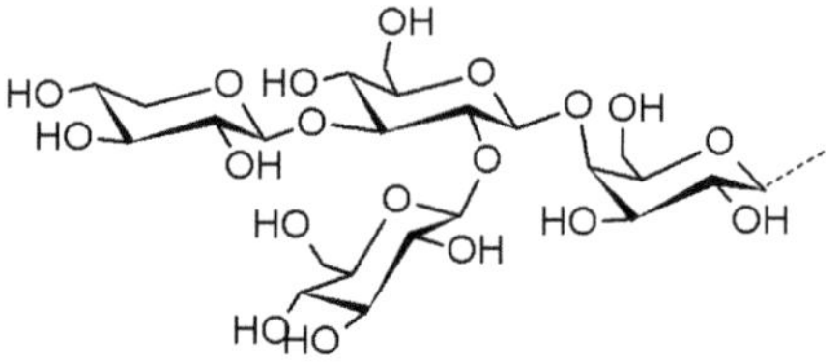

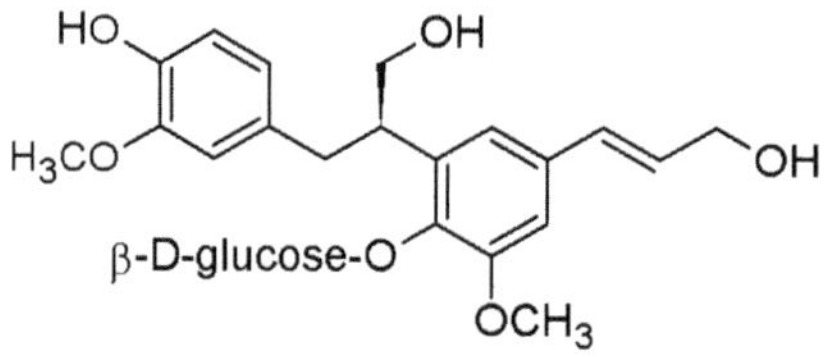

Icariside (**21**):

Figure 13.4: Chemistry Structure of Glycosides and Icariside

Among the main flavonoids found in *Capsicum* are the flavonoids aglycones, luteolin, apigenin (flavones) and quercetin. In their non-hydrolysed forms, flavonoids quercetin and luteolin are found in *Capsicum* as: quercetin 3-*O*-α-L-rhamnopyranoside-7-*O*-β-*D*-glucopyranoside, luteolin 6-*C*-β-*D*-glucopyranoside-8-*C*-α-L-arabinopyranoside, apigenin 6-*C*-β-D-glucopyranoside-8-*C*-α-*L*-arabinopyranoside known as schaftoside, lutoeolin 7-*O*-[2-(2-(β-*D*-apiofuranosyl)-β-*D*-glucopyranoside], quercetin 3-*O*-α-*L*-rhamnopyranoside and luteolin 7-*O*-[2-(β-*D*-apiofuranosyl)-4-(β-*D*-glucopyranosyl)-6-malonyl]-β-*D*-glucopyranoside (Materska *et al.*, 2003).

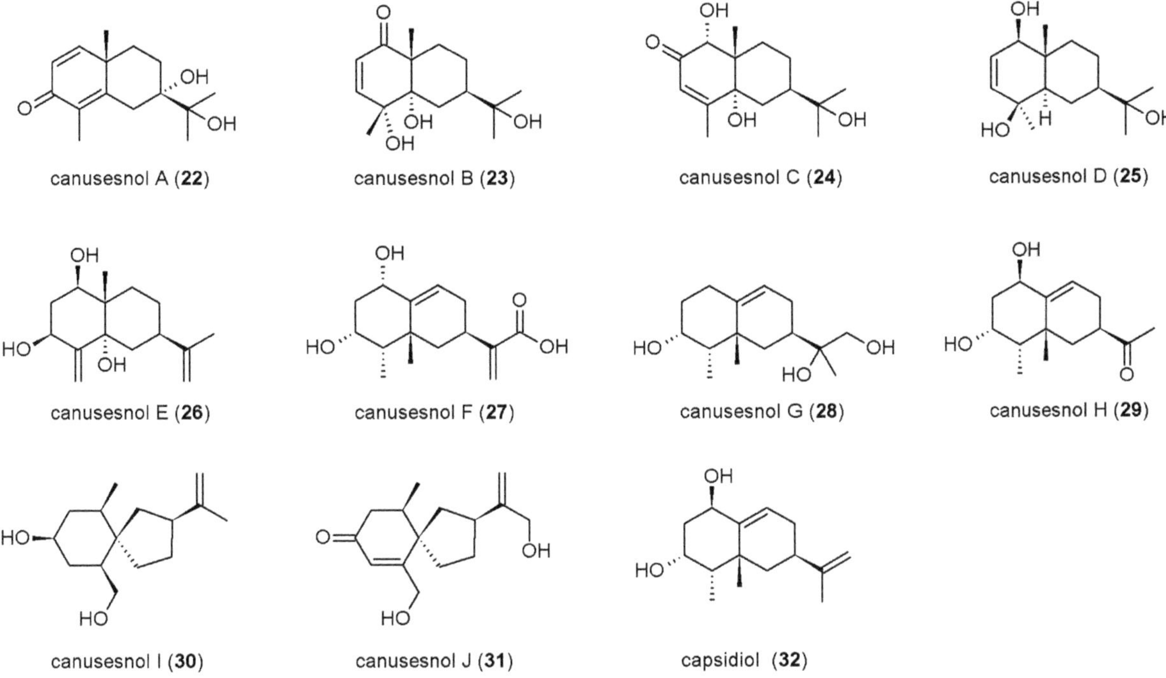

Figure 13.5: Chemistry Structure of Sesquiterpenes of the *Capsicum* Genus

Quantification of flavonoids in *Capsicum* species have been performed for quercetin and luteolin in some cultivars, the concentrations reported are: Banana Supreme (186.0 mg kg^{-1}), PI 357509 (86.0 mg kg^{-1}) and Rio Grande Gold (26.0 mg kg^{-1}) for quercetin and Fidel (37.0 mg kg^{-1}) and Banana Supreme (21.5 mg kg^{-1}) for luteolin. Miean and Mohamed (2001) observed in *C. frutescens* a concentration of 1.035,0 mg kg^{-1} for luteolin and 272.0 mg kg^{-1} for apigenin. Values found in *C. annuum* are: quercetin, 34.0 mg kg^{-1} and luteolin: 11.0 mg kg^{-1} (Sun *et al.*, 2007).

The colour determines the commercial value of the paprika oil-resin being usually associated to the sample quality: a great coloration capacity means a high quality (Mínguez-Mosquera and Pérez-Gálvez, 1998), which relates to the amount of carotenoids (Figure 13.6).

An important feature of *Capsicum* due to carotenoids is the vitamin concentration. Silva and Souza (2006) emphasize that Vitamin A concentration of green and red chilli peppers are considered one of the best sources of this vitamin about 10,500 and 11,000 IU respectively, close to the concentration of 13,000 IU found in carrot. The carotenoids contained in pepper species of *Capsicum* genus have antioxidant activity and the capacity to contribute significantly for the prevention of degenerative diseases like cancer (Etoh *et al.*, 2000). Some of these oxygenated carotenoids like capsanthin (33), capsorubin (34) and capsanthin 5,6-epoxi (35) are exclusive of *Capsicum* genus (Deepa *et al.*, 2007; Hornero-Méndez *et al.*, 2000).

The most common carotenoids in *Capsicum* species are: capsanthin (33), capsorubin (34), zeaxanthin (36), cucurbitaxanthin A (37), and β-carotene (38) (Deli and Tóth, 1997; Reifschneider, 2000; Mínguez-Mosquera and Hornero-Méndez, 1993; Deli *et al.*, 2001a; Hornero-Méndez *et al.*, 2000).

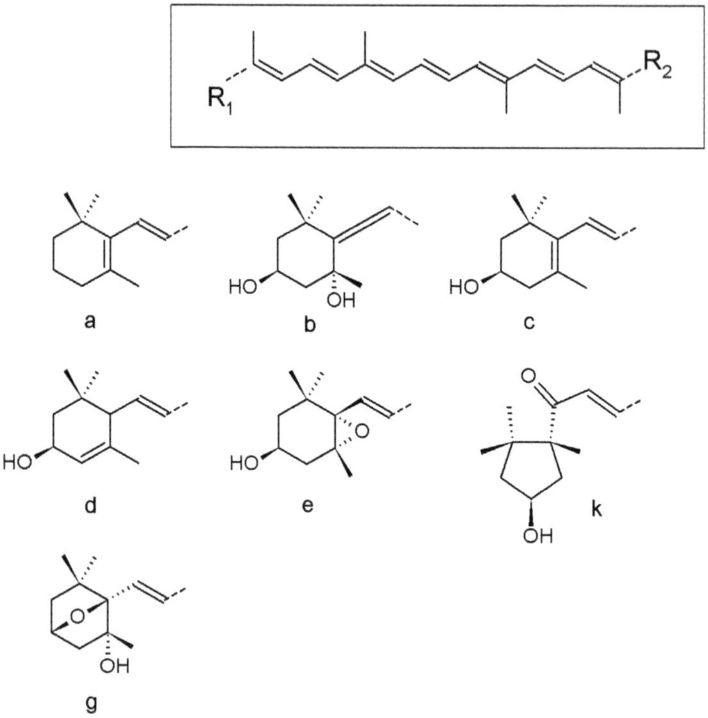

Capsanthin: (**33**): R_1= c, R_2 = f

Capsorubin: (**34**): R_1= R_2 = f

Capsanthin 5,6-epoxide: (**35**): R_1= e, R_2 = f

Zeaxanthin: (**36**): R_1= R_2 =c

Cucurbitaxanthin A: (**37**): R_1 = g, R_2 = c

β-carotene: (**38**): R_1 = R_2 = a

β-cryptoxanthin: (**39**): R_1 = c, R_2 = a

Lutein: (**40**): R_1 = c, R_2 = d

Neoxanthin: (**41**): R_1 = b, R_2 = e

Violaxanthin: (**42**): R_1 = R_2 = e

Cycloviolaxanthin: (**43**): R_1= R_2 = g

Capsanthin 3,6-epoxide: (**44**): R_1 = g, R_2 = f

Figure 13.6: Chemistry Structure of Carotenoids in the *Capsicum* Genus

Several other carotenoids are found as minor constituents in *Capsicum* fruits (Deli *et al.*, 1998; Maoka *et al.*, 2004; Hornero-Méndez *et al.*, 2000; Deli and Tóth, 1997; Reifschneider, 2000; Mínguez-Mosquera and Hornero-Méndez, 1993; Nagy *et al.*, 2007; Deli *et al.*, 2001b; Maoka *et al.*, 2001a).

Due to carotenoids type or concentration, only some varieties or cultivars possess potential for paprika or oil-resin production. In an assay that studied different cultivars focusing paprika production, it was observed that total carotenoid contents varied from 12,700mg kg^{-1} to 4,800mg kg^{-1} in dry weight (Hornero-Méndez *et al.*, 2002). Deli *et al.* (2001a) found in ripe fruits of *lycopersiciforme rubrum* variety 13.0g kg^{-1} in dry weight of carotenoids: capsanthin (37 per cent), zeaxanthin (8 per cent), cucurbitaxanthin A (7 per cent), capsorubin (3,2 per cent) and β-carotene (9 per cent). In another assay, the quantitative and qualitative carotenoid distribution was studied in the *Longum nigrum* variety, obtaining from ripe fruits a total carotenoid content of 32g kg^{-1} in dry weight (Deli *et al.*, 1992). In the two varieties, most used for paprika production, *Agridulce* and *Bola*, carotenoids can be found at 1,360mg kg^{-1} and 960mg kg^{-1} of the fresh weight (Mínguez-Mosquera and Hornero-Méndez, 1993).

Marin *et al.* (2004) in an assay with *C. annuum* cv. *vegasa*, observed that the total of carotenoid pigments increased 4 times for the ripe red fruits when compared to the immature fruits. It was also observed that immature green peppers contained an extremely high polyphenol content, while ripe red fruits had an extremely high pro-vitamin A content [β-carotene (38) and β-Cryptoxanthin (39)]. Great variation in carotenoid content, according to the maturation stage, can be observed through total carotenoids values found in the most used *C. annuum* cultivars in paprika production, *Agridulce* and *Bola*. Lutein (40) and neoxanthin (41) disappeared with maturation, while β-carotene and the violaxanthin (42) increased and other carotenoids appeared: zeaxanthin, capsanthin, capsorubin, β-cryptoxanthin, and cucurbitaxanthin A (capsolutein) appeared (Mínguez-Mosquera and Hornero-Méndez, 1994b). Some values for the total carotenoid content in relation to the fresh weight for these cultivars are respectively: green fruits 39.22 and 33.41 mg kg^{-1} and ripe fruits 1,359.98 and 961.80 mg kg^{-1}.

Breithaupt and Bamedi (2001) mention that carotenoids are found in alimentary plants in free form or as fatty acids esters. It was observed that during maturation there is a tendency to increment esterified forms and to reduce carotenoid free forms (Mínguez-Mosquera and Hornero-Méndez, 1994a).

Biological Activities

Capsaicinoids, the chemical substances present in the peppers and responsible for their pungency, CAPS, have a wide use in the pharmacology and neurology (Perucka and Oleszek, 2000).

Several human physiological processes are initiated by CAPS through mediation of chemical receivers; one of these processes is the endorfin liberation (Wagner, 2003). The CAPS, even when used in small levels in the diet, have been shown to be substances capable to increase the basal metabolism rate in humans. It is attributed to increment of the energy expense with fat burning, especially in those people with a high Body Mass Index and obese people, with consequent weight reduction, suppression of the corporal fat accumulation and decrease in the serum myocardial and aortic cholesterol levels, therefore being able to contribute in a diet therapy for obesity. In addition, the crude extract of *C. annuum* has been shown to have antidiabetic and antihypertension potential (Kwon *et al.*, 2007).

This activity is speacially observed at non-pungent capsaicinoids, as capsiate (16). Another compound, (-)-capsaicinol (15) also non-pungent, is reported to have the same thermogenesis and acceleration of the lipid metabolism properties (Inoue *et al.*, 2007; Kawabata *et al.*, 2006; Ohnuki *et al.*, 2001a; Ohnuki *et al.*, 2001b; Masuda and Nakatani, 1991; Westerterp-Plantenga *et al.*, 2006; Topuz and Ozdemir, 2007; Govindarajan and Sathyanarayana, 1991).

Capsaicin (1) decreases blood glucose levels, and is hypothesized that it can aid in lowering LDL even when consumed for a short period (Ching and Mohamed, 2001; Lee *et al.*, 2003). Topically used capsaicin is shown to be effective in the treatment of cutaneous allergy, and other uses in cutaneous disorders that involve pain and inflammation, urticary, psoriasis vulgaris. Other biological activities of capsaicin already reported are: anodyne effect, post-herpetic neuralgia, vasomotor rhinitis, hyperactive rhinopathy, cluster headaches, post-mastectomy pain, temporomandibular joint pain, osteoarthritis, rheumatoid arthritis, apocrine choromohydrosis; also provides relief in arthritis and respiratory ailments and neurological conditions like neurogenic pain, diabetic neuropathy, nostalgia paraesthetica, meralgia paraesthetica, antiinflammatory and pain in Guillain-Barré syndrome (Cordell and Araujo, 1993; Constant *et al.*, 1995; Davis *et al.*, 2007; Surh, 2002; Prasad *et al.*, 2006a; Iorizzi *et al.*, 2001; Dasgupta and Fowler, Surh, 2004 1997; Higashiguchi *et al.*, 2006). Use of capsaicin in the medical branch of neuro-urology is viewed as a breakthrough, given its use in the treatment of urinary incontinence (Dasgupta and Fowler, 1997); There is indication that the capsaicin is cardioprotective due to effects in platelet aggregation (Wang *et al.*, 1984). Activities such as antiangiogenic, antimetastatic, antitumoral, antiproliferative and chemoprotector are described to capsaicin; in this context the apoptosis study has been an area where several cellular lineages were researched; a conclusion for instance is that apoptosis in certain cellular types suggests that vanilloids (capsaicinoids) may be useful in prevention or treatment of skin cancers and other hyperproliferative skin disorders (Surh and Lee, 1996; Surh and Lee, 1996; Surh, 2004; Surh, 2002; Surh, 2005; Prasad *et al.*, 2006a; Kim *et al.*, 2006; Hail Jr. and Lotan, 2002).

Flavonoids present in *Capsicum* genus possess a wide spectrum of biological activities, such as antioxidation, antiinflammatory, antiplatelet, antiallergic and antithrobotic action. They also help to prevent diseases like cancer due to the inhibitory action of enzymes like lipoxygenase (Miean and Mohamed, 2001; Lee *et al.*, 1995). Quercetin had bioantimutagenic activity demonstrated; another substance also present in *Capsicum* with the same activity is 2,4-nonadienal (45) (Nakamura *et al.*, 1999; Hertog *et al.*, 1992).

Antioxidant Activity

The continued interest in the study and quantification of antioxidant constituents of fruits and vegetables is due to countless reports that associate the ingestion of antioxidant substances with the prevention of chronic and degenerative diseases. In the *Capsicum* genus, these studies have been very common since these species are rich in carotenoids, vitamins, provitamins, folates, polyphenols, and the capsaicinoids, that are exclusive to this genus.

The radical-scavenging and antioxidant activity has been verified for extracts obtained from *Capsicum* (Conforti *et al.*, 2006), as well as for the substances that are in these extracts (Conforti *et al.*, 2006; Matsufuji *et al.*, 1998). In terms of antioxidant activity, a compound that one can have as reference is α-tocoferol. Ching and Mohamed (2001) observed that red peppers contain a high amount of α-tocoferol, 29.07mg/100g, higher than bird pepper (*Capsicum frutescens*), with 16.84mg/100g; green pepper (15.39mg/100g) and the bell pepper (13.81mg/100g). Daood *et al.* (1996) reported a high content of α-tocoferol (40.5mg/100g) in red pepper too. The *in vivo* activity for capsaicin (1) was already reported as a potent antioxidant (Lee *et al.*, 2003), and many other CAPS, capsiate (16), dihydrocapsiate (17) and their analogues (Matsufuji *et al.*, 2004; Rosa *et al.*, 2002). Carotenoids as capsanthin (33), capsorubin (34), cicloviolaxantina (43) and capsanthin 3,6-epoxi (44), isolated from paprika (*Capsicum annuum*), inhibited oxidation of methyl linolate. The antioxidant activity followed the order: capsorubin (34) > capsanthin 3,6-epoxide (44) > capsanthin (33) > cicloviolaxantina (43) > β-carotene (18) (Maoka *et al.*, 2001b). Ochi *et al.* (2003) isolated for the first time, and have demonstrated in an assay using ADP/Fe^{2+}-induced liposomal lipid peroxidation, that 6″,7″-dihydro-5',5‴-dicapsaicin (14) possesses antioxidant activity comparable to capsaicin and is 25 times more potent than α-tocopherol. (-)-Capsaicinol (15) isolated from the fruits of *C. frutescens* possesses a higher antioxidative activity than α-tocoferol (Masuda and Nakatani, 1991). Icariside (21), a quite rare lignan glycoside, found in *C. annuum* L. var. *acuminatum*, showed an antioxidant potential in cultured cells (Iorizzi *et al.*, 2001).

Finally, it can be concluded from the results of several studies suggest that *Capsicum* extracts can act as *in vivo* antioxidants (Asai *et al.*, 1999). Flavonoids present in *Capsicum* like luteolin and quercetin contribute significantly to the pepper antioxidant potential (Lee *et al.*, 1995).

The concentrations of antioxidants in *Capsicum* fruits are affected by maturity stages. As the fruits ripen, an increment tendency in the vitamin C and carotenoids concentration is observed. On the other hand, a decline tendency can be observed in the capsaicin content, and in relation to the phenolic compounds, there can be still some variations when other factors are considered as the nature of the sample (fresh or dry) or the genotype (Marín *et al.*, 2004; Deepa *et al.*, 2007; Oboh and Rocha, 2008).

Several studies show that the concentration of a specific antioxidant can vary with the cultivar, the variety or the part of the *Capsicum* fruit. In *C. annuum*, for example, differences are found in the seeds (+-tocopherol) and in pericarp (α-tocopherol). There also are differences among cultivars for α-tocoferol, and differences not being found for the content of γ-tocopherol (Osuna-García *et. al.*, 1998). In some *C. annuum* varieties was observed that phenolic components were more abundant in ripe spicy peppers varieties than in sweet peppers varieties or in immature fruits; on the other hand the antioxidant activity was more pronounced in sweet varieties, standing out the ripe fruits of "Fushimi Amanaga" and "Wonder Bell" varieties (Saga and Sato, 2003). The coloration of the fruits seems to have certain relationship with the oxidant activity. Sun *et al.* (2007), studying 4 different colored (green, yellow, orange, and red) sweet bell peppers (*C. annuum*), found that the total phenolics content (folin-Ciocalteau method) for the fruit of red color was 4.2μmol and practically the half, 2.4μmol catechin equivalent/g fresh weight, in the fruits of green color. Variations in the antioxidants concentrations are also found when the part of the fruit is considered. In *C. pubescens*, it was observed that removing the seeds of this pepper reduces the antioxidant activity due to reduction of 50 per cent in total phenol content (Oboh and Rocha, 2007).

Antimicrobial Activity

Capsaicinoids show antimicrobial activity against several microorganisms *e.g. Bacilli, Clostridiae, Salmonellae, Helicobacter* (Cichewicz and Thorpe, 1996; Careaga *et al.*, 2003; Graham *et al.*, 1999). Capsaicin has been reported active against *Bacillus subtilis* (Molina-Torres *et al.*, 1999). Crude extracts of *C. annuum, C. baccatum, C. chinense, C. frutescens,* and *C. pubescens,* some of the main species of *Capsicum,* show activity against *Bacillus cereus, B. subtilis, Clostridium sporogenes, C. tetani, and Streptococcus pyogenes* (Cichewicz and Thorpe, 1996). The extract of *C. annuum* is also reported as bactericide against *Salmonella thyphimurium* and *Pseudomonas aeruginosa* (Careaga *et al.*, 2003). Other components besides capsaicin also had their activity demonstrated like capsidiol (32), which presents as bacteriostatic against the gastric pathogen *Helicobacter pylori*, associated to peptic ulceration, showing a MIC (minimum inhibitory concentration) of 200μg/mL. It can be considered very effective in an *in vitro* assay when compared with the commercial drug metronidazole (Marino *et al.*, 2006).

The glycosides furostanols, present in *C. annuum* L. var. *acuminatum* seeds show activity against yeast, as in the case of capsicoside E (18), 22-O-methylcapsicoside A (19) and 22-O-methylcapsicoside G (20) that exhibited activity against *Candida albicans*, a pathogenic yeast that causes cutaneous candidiasis. The activity against the yeasts is attributed to the oligosaccharide chain (S1, like S2, or S3 in other glycosides present in *Capsicum*) (Figure 13.3) combined with a *O*-methyl group in R_3 and the presence of hydroxyl group in position C-2 (Iorizzi *et al.*, 2002). A high level of fungicidal activity is observed against *Botrytis cinerea* in *Capsicum* species of different cultivars (WILSON *et al.*, 1997).

Besides the activities against the microorganisms mentioned above, the crude extract of *C. annuum* presents activity against *Schistosoma mansoni*, cause of schistosomosis (Molina-Torres *et al.*, 1999).

Flavonoids presence in *Capsicum*, like quercetin, provide antiviral activity in the sense that they inhibit the infectivity and/or replication of the viruses as the herpes simplex type, polio, parainfluenza type, syncytial viruses, and immunodeficiency virus (Lee *et al.*, 2005; Robbins, 2000).

Taking into account the resistance characters and productive capacity it was inferred that the *C. chinense* species is an important genetic resource as resistance source to *X. campestris* pv. *Vesicatoria* in the bell pepper improvement programs (Noda *et al.*, 2003).

Conclusion

The *Capsicum* genus is one of the most cultivated spices worldwide. The consumption and widespread use of these species in culinary and popular medicine turns them into an arsenal capable to fight important diseases like cancer and neurological diseases and promote prevention. The main factor that contributes to this effect is the unusual chemical composition that includes not only functional and nutritional molecules, like flavonoids, but other substances found in no other sources, like alkaloid capsaicin and other similar compounds, glycosides, and the exclusive carotenoids of *Capsicum* genus: capsanthin, capsorubin and capsanthin 5,6-epoxy.

Capsicum is a very interesting genus that requires more and more studies, since many of the research already accomplished was concentrated on the main cultivated and commercialized species: *C. annuum*. Many other *Capsicum* species are still object of few studies, and even ignored in many areas of the science.

Acknowledgements

Authors thanks to FAPEAM, CAPES and CNPq for financial support, and to Afonso R. L. Thury.

References

Asai, A., Nokagawa, K. and Miyazawa, T. (1999). Antioxidative Effects of Turmeric, Rosemary and *Capsicum* Extracts on Membrane Phospholipid Peroxidation and Liver Lipid Metabolism in Mice. *Biosci Biotechnol Biochem.*, 63: 2118-2122.

Barbosa, R.I., Luz, F.J.F., Nascimento Filho, H.R. and Maduro, C.B. (2002). Pimentas do Gênero *Capsicum* Cultivadas em Roraima, Amazônia Brasileira. I. Espécies Domesticadas. *Acta Amaz.*, 32: 132-177.

Berg, E.M. van den; Silva, M.H.L. (1988). ContribuiCão ao conhecimento da flora medicinal de Roraima. *Acta Amaz.*, 18: 23-35.

Breithaupt, D.E. and Bamedi, A. (2001). Carotenoid Esters in Vegetables and Fruits: A Screening with Emphasis on β-Cryptoxanthin Esters. *J Agr Food Chem.*, 54: 2064-2070.

Careaga, M., Fernández, E., Dorantes, L., Mota, L., Jaramillo, M.E. and Hernandez-Sanchez, H. (2003). Antibacterial activity of *Capsicum* extract against *Salmonella typhimurium* and *Pseudomonas aeruginosa* inoculated in raw beef meat. *Int J Food Microbiol.*, 83: 331-335.

Cavender, A. (2006). Folk medical uses of plant foods in southern Appalachia, United States. *J Ethnopharmacol.*, 108: 74-84.

Ching, L.S. and Mohamed, S. (2001). Alpha-Tocopherol Content in 62 Edible Tropical Plants. *J Agr Food Chem.*, 49: 3101-3105.

Cichewicz, R.H. and Thorpe, P.A. (1996). The antimicrobial properties of chile peppers (*Capsicum* species) and their uses in Mayan medicine. *J Ethnopharmacol.*, 52: 61-70.

Conforti, F., Statti, G.A. and Menichini, F. (2006). Chemical and biological variability of hot pepper fruits (*Capsicum annuum* var. *acuminatum L.*) in relation to maturity stage. *Food Chem.*, 102: 1096-1104.

Constant, H.L. and Cordell, G.A. (1996). Nonivamide, a Constituent of *Capsicum* oleoresin. *J Nat Prod.*, 59: 425-426.

Constant, H.L., Cordell, G.A., West, D.P. and Johnson, J.H. (1995). Separation and Quantification of Capsaicinoids Using Complexation Chromatography. *J Nat Prod.*, 58: 1925-1928.

Contreras-Padilla, M. and Yahia, E.M. (1998). Changes in Capsaicinoids during Development, Maturation, and Senescence of Chile Peppers and Relation with Peroxidase Activity. *J Agr Food Chem.*, 46: 2075-2079.

Cook, J.A., VanderJagt, D.J., Pastuszyn, A., Mounkaila, G., Glew, R.S., Millson, M. and Glew, R.H. (2000). Nutrient and Chemical Composition of 13 Wild Plant Foods of Niger. *J Food Comp Anal*, 13: 83-92.

Cordell, G.A. and Araujo, O.E. (1993). Capsaicin: identification, nomenclature, and pharmacotherapy. *An Pharmacother.*, 27: 330-336.

Daood, H.G., Vinkler, M., Markus, F., Hebshi, E.A. and Biacs, P.A. (1996). Antioxidant Vitamin Content of Spice Red Pepper (Paprika) as Affected by Technological and Varietal Factors. *Food Chem.*, 55: 365-372.

Dasgupta, P. and Fowler, C.J. (1997). Chillies: From Antiquity to Urology. British *J Urol.*, 80: 845-852.

Davis, C.B., Markey, C.E., Busch, M.A. and Busch, K.W. (2007). Determination of Capsaicinoids in Habanero Peppers by Chemometric Analysis of UV Spectral Data. *J Agr Food Chem.*, 55: 5925-5933.

Deepa, N., Kaur, C., George, B., Singh, B. and Kapoor, H.C. (2007). Antioxidant constituents in some sweet pepper (*Capsicum annuum L.*) genotypes during maturity. *LWT*, 40: 121-129.

Deli, J. and Tóth, G. (1997). Carotenoid composition of the fruits of *Capsicum annuum* Cv. *Bovet 4* during ripening. *Z Lebensm Unters Forsch.*, 205: 388-391.

Deli, J., Matus, Z. and Szabolcs, J. (1992). Carotenoid Composition in the Fruits of Black Paprika (*Capsicum annuum* Variety *longum nigrum*) during Ripening. *J Agr Food Chem.*, 40: 2072-2076.

Deli, J., Molnár, P., Matus, Z., Tóth, G., Steck, A. and Pfander, H. (1998). Isolation of Carotenoids with 3,5,6-Trihydroxy-5,6-dihydro–Beta-end Groups from Red Paprika (*Capsicum annuum*). *Helv Chim Acta.*, 81: 1233-1241.

Deli, J., Molnár, P., Matus, Z. and Tóth, G. (2001a). Carotenoid Composition in the Fruits of Red Paprika (*Capsicum annuum* var. *Lycopersiciforme rubrum*) during Ripening; Biosynthesis of Carotenoids in Red Paprika. *J Agr Food Chem.*, 49: 1517-1523.

Deli, J., Molnár, P., Matus, Z., Tóth, G.,Traber, B. and Pfander, H. (2001b). 'Prenigroxanthin' [(all-E,3R,3'S,6'S)-β,γ-carotene-3,3',6'-triol], a novel carotenoid from red paprika (*Capsicum annuum*). *Tetrahedron Lett.*, 42: 1395-1397.

Estrada, B., Bernal, M.A., Díaz, J., Pomar, F. and Merino, F. (2002). Capsaicinoids in Vegetative Organs of *Capsicum annuum L.* in Relation to Fruiting. *J Agr Food Chem.*, 50: 1188-1191.

Etoh, H., Utsunomiya, Y., Komori, A., Murakami, Y., Oshima, S. and Inakuma, T. (2000). Carotenoids in Human Blood Plasma after Ingesting Paprika Juice. *Biosci Biotechnol Biochem.*, 64: 1096-1098.

Garcés-Claver, A., Arnedo-Andrés, M.S., Abadía, J., Gil-Ortega, R. and Álvarez-Fernández, A. (2006). Determination of Capsaicin and Dihydrocapsaicin in *Capsicum* Fruits by Liquid Chromatography-Electrospray/Time-of-Flight Mass Spectrometry. *J Agr Food Chem.*, 54: 9303-9311.

Gibbs, H.A.A. and O'Garro, L.W. (2004). Capsaicin content of West Indies hot pepper cultivars using colorimetric and chromatographic techniques. *HortScienc.*, 39: 132-135.

Gnayfeed, M.H., Daood, H.G., Illés, V. and Biacs, P.A. (2001). Supercritical CO_2 and Subcritical Propane Extraction of Pungent Paprika and Quantification of Carotenoids, Tocopherols, and Capsaicinoids. *J Agr Food Chem.*, 49: 2761-2766.

Govindarajan, V.S. and Sathyanarayana, M.N. (1991). *Capsicum*–production, technology, chemistry and quality, part V. Impact on physiology, pharmacology, nutrition and metabolism; structure, pungency, pain and desensitisation sequences. *Food Sci Nutr.*, 29: 435-471.

Graham, D. Y., Anderson, S. Y. and Lang, T. (1999). Garlic or jalapeno peppers for treatment of *Helicobacter pylori* infection. *Am J Gastroenterol.*, 94: 1200-1202.

Hail Jr., N. and Lotan, R. (2002). Examining the Role of Mitochondrial Respiration in Vanilloid-Induced Apoptosis. *J Natl Cancer Inst.*, 94: 1281-1292.

Hertog, M.G.L., Hollman, P.C.H. and Katan, M.B. (1992). Content of Potentially Anticarcinogenic Flavonoids of 28 Vegetables and 9 Fruits Commonly Consumed in The Netherlands. *J Agr Food Chem.*, 40: 2379-2383.

Higashiguchi, F., Nakamura, H., Hayashi, H. and Kometani, T. (2006). Purification and Structure Determination of Glucosides of Capsaicin and Dihydrocapsaicin from Various *Capsicum* Fruits. *J Agr Food Chem.*, 54: 5948-5953.

Hilgert, N.I. (2001). Plants used in home medicine in the Zenta River basin, Northwest Argentina. *J Ethnopharmacol.*, 76: 11-34.

Hornero-Méndez, D., Costa-García, J. and Mínguez-Mosquera, M.I. (2002). Characterization of Carotenoid High-Producing *Capsicum annuum* Cultivars Selected for Paprika Production. *J Agr Food Chem.*, 50: 5711-5716.

Hornero-Méndez, D., de Guevara, R.G.-L. and Mínguez-Mosquera, M.I. (2000). Carotenoid Biosynthesis Changes in Five Red Pepper (*Capsicum annuum L.*) Cultivars during Ripening. Cultivar Selection for Breeding. *J Agr Food Chem.*, 48: 3857-3864.

Howard, L.R., Talcott, S.T., Brenes, C.H. and Villalon, B. (2000). Changes in Phytochemical and Antioxidant Activity of Selected Pepper Cultivars (*Capsicum* Species) As Influenced by Maturity. *J Agr Food Chem.*, 48: 1713-1720.

Inoue, N., Matsunaga, Y., Satoh, H. and Takahashi, M. (2007). Enhanced Energy Expendiutre and Fat Oxidation in Humans with High BMI Scores by the Ingestion of Novel and Non-Pungent Capsaicin Analogues (Capsinoids). *Biosci Biotechnol Biochem.*, 71: 380-389.

Iorizzi, M., Lanzotti, V., de Marino, S., Zollo, F., Blanco-Molina, M., Macho, A. and Muñoz, E. (2001). New Glycosides from *Capsicum annuum L.* Var. *acuminatum*. Isolation, Structure Determination, and Biological Activity. *J Agr Food Chem.*, 49: 2022-2029.

Iorizzi, M., Lanzotti, V., Ranalli, G., de Marino, S. and Zollo, F. (2002). Antimicrobial Furostanol Saponins from the Seeds of *Capsicum annuum L.* Var. *acuminatum*. *J Agr Food Chem.*, 50: 4310-4316.

Izumitani, Y., Yahara, S. and Nohara, T. (1990). Novel Acyclic Diterpene Glycosides, Capsianosides A-F and I-V from *Capsicum* Plants (Solanaceous Studies. XVI). *Chem Pharm Bull.*, 38: 1299-1307.

Jurenitsh, J., David, M., Heresch, F. and Kubelka, W. (1979). Detection and Identification of new Pungent Compounds in Fruits of *Capsicum*. *J Med Plant Res.*, 36: 61-67.

Kawabata, F., Inoue, N., Yazawa, S., Kawada, T., Inoue, K. and Fushiki, T. (2006). Effects of CH-19 Sweet, a Non-Pungent Cultivar of Red Pepper, in Decreasing the Body Weight and Suppressing

Body Fat Accumulation by Simpathetic Nerve Activation in Humans. *Biosci Biotechnol Biochem.*, 70: 2824-2835.

Kawaguchi, Y., Ochi, T., Takaishi, Y., Kawazoe, K. and Lee, K.-H. (2004). New Sesquiterpenes from *Capsicum annuum. J Nat Prod.*, 67: 1893-1896.

Kim, S., Lee, K.W., Park, J., Lee, H.J. and Hwang, I.-K. (2006). Effect of drying in antioxidant activity and changes of ascorbic acid and colour by different drying and storage in Korean red pepper (*Capsicum annuum L.*). *Int J Food Sci Technol.*, 41: 90-95.

Kopp, B. and Jurenitsch, J. (1981). Biosynthese der Capsaicinoide in *Capsicum annuum. L.* var. *annuum. J Med Plant Res.*, 43: 272-279.

Kwon, Y.-I., Apostolidis, E. and Shetty, K. (2007). Evaluation of pepper (*Capsicum Annuum*) for management of diabetes and hypertension. *J Food Biochem.*, 31: 370-385.

Lee, C.-Y.J., Kim, M., Yoon, S.-W. and Lee, C.-H. (2003). Short-term control of capsaicin on blood and oxidative stress of rats *in vivo. Phytother Res.*, 17: 454-458.

Lee, J.-H., Kiyota, N., Ikeda, T. and Nohara, T. (2006). Acyclic Diterpene Glycosides, Capsianosides VIII, IX, X, XIII, XV and XVI from the Fruits of Paprika *Capsicum annuum L.* var. *grossum* BAILEY and Jalapeño *Capsicum annuum L.* var. *annuum. Chem Pharm Bull.*, 54: 1365-1369.

Lee, J.-H., Kiyota, N., Ikeda, T. and Nohara, T. (2008). Three New Acyclic Diterpene Glycosides from the Aerial Parts of Paprika and Pimiento. *Chem Pharm Bull.*, 56: 582-584.

Lee, J.J., Crosby, K.M., Pike, L.M., Yoo, K.S. and Leskovar, D.I. (2005). Impact of genetic and environmental variation on development of flavonoids and carotenoids in pepper (*Capsicum* spp.). *Sci Hort.*, 106: 341-352.

Lee, Y., Howard, L.R. and Villalón, B. (1995). Flavonoid and Antioxidant Activity of Fresh Pepper (*Capsicum annuum*) Cultivars. *J Food Sci.*, 60: 473-476.

Luning, P.A., Ebbenhorst-Seller, T., Rijk, T. de and Roozen, J.P. (1995). Effect of hot-air drying on flavour compounds of bell peppers (*Capsicum annuum*). *J Sci Food Agricult.*, 68: 355-365.

Maoka, T., Akimoto, N., Fujiwara, Y. and Hashimoto, K. (2004). Structure of New Carotenoids with the 6-Oxo-K End Group from the Fruits of Paprika, *Capsicum annuum. J Nat Prod.*, 67: 115-117.

Maoka, T., Fujiwara, Y., Hashimoto, K. and Akimoto, N. (2001a). Capsanthone 3,6-Epoxide, a New Carotenoid from the Fruits of the Red Paprika *Capsicum annuum L.. J Agr Food Chem.*, 49: 3965-3968.

Maoka, T., Goto, Y., Isobe, K., Fujiwara, Y., Hashimoto, K. and Mochida, K. (2001a). Antioxidative Activity of Capsorubin and Related Compounds from Paprika (*Capsicum annuum*). *J Oil Sci.*, 50: 663-665.

Marín, A., Ferreres, F., Tomás-Barberán, F.A. and Gil, M.I. (2004). Characterization and Quantitation of Antioxidant Constituents of Sweet Pepper (*Capsicum annuum L.*). *J Agr Food Chem.*, 52: 3861-3869.

Marino, S. de, Borbone, N., Gala, F., Zollo, F., Fico, G., Pagiotti, R. and Iorizzi, M. (2006). New Constituents of Sweet *Capsicum annuum L.* Fruits and Evaluation of Their Biological Activity. *J Agr Food Chem.*, 54: 7508-7516.

Masuda, T. and Nakatani, N. (1991). Synthesis and Absolute Structure of (-)-Capsaicinol. *Agr Biol Chem.*, 55: 2337-2340.

Materska, M., Piacente, S., Stochmal, A., Pizza, C., Oleszek, W. and Perucka, I. (2003). Isolation and structure elucidation of flavonoid and phenolic acid glycosides from pericarp of hot pepper fruit *Capsicum Annuum L. Phytochemistry*, 63: 893-898.

Matsufuji, H., Chino, M. and Takeda, M. (2004). Effects of Paprika Pigments on Oxidation of Linoleic Acid Stored in the Dark or Exposed to Light. *J Agr Food Chem.*, 52: 3601-3605.

Matsufuji, H., Nakamura, H., Chino, M. and Takeda, M. (1998). Antioxidant Activity of Capsanthin and the Fatty Acid Esters in Paprika (*Capsicum annuum*). *J Agr Food Chem.*, 46: 3468-3472.

Miean, K.H. and Mohamed, S. (2001). Flavonoid (Myricetin, Quercetin, Kaempferol, Luteolin, and Apigenin) Content of Edible Tropical Plants. *J Agr Food Chem.*, 49: 3106-3112.

Mínguez-Mosquera, M.I. and Hornero-Méndez, D. (1993). Separation and Quantification of the Carotenoid Pigments in Red Peppers (*Capsicum annuum L.*), Paprika, and Oleoresin by Reversed-Phase HPLC. *J Agr Food Chem.*, 41: 1616-1620.

Mínguez-Mosquera, M.I. and Hornero-Méndez, D. (1994a). Changes in Carotenoid Esterification during the Fruit Ripening of *Capsicum annuum* Cv. *Bola*. *J Agr Food Chem.*, 42: 640-644.

Mínguez-Mosquera, M.I. and Hornero-Méndez, D. (1994b). Formation and Transformation of Pigments during the Fruit Ripening of *Capsicum annuum* Cv. *Bola* and *Agridulce*. *J Agr Food Chem.*, 42: 38-44.

Mínguez-Mosquera, M.I. and Pérez-Gálvez, A. (1998). Color Quality in Paprika Oleoresins. *J Agr Food Chem.*, 46: 5124-5127.

Mínguez-Mosquera, M.I., Pérez-Gálvez, A. and Garrido-Fernández, J. (2000). Carotenoid Content of the Varieties Jaranda and Jariza (*Capsicum annuum L.*) and Response during the Industrial Slow Drying and Grinding Steps in Paprika Processing. *J Agr Food Chem.*, 48: 2972-2976.

Molina-Torres, J., García-Chávez, A. and Ramírez-Chávez, E. (1999). Antimicrobial properties of alkamides present in flavouring plants traditionally used in Mesoamerica: affinin and capsaicin. *J Ethnopharmacol.*, 64: 241-248.

Mtambo, M.M.A., Mushi, E.J., Kinabo, L.D.B., Maeda-Machang'u, A., Mwamengele, G.L.M., Yongolo, M.G.S. and Temu, R.P.C. (1999). Evaluation of the efficacy of the crude extracts of *Capsicum frutescens*, Citrus lemon and *Opuntia vulgaris* against Newcastle disease in domestic fowl in Tanzania. *J Ethnopharmacol.*, 68: 55-61.

Nagy, V., Agoócs, A., Turcsi, E., Molnár, P., Szabó, Z. and Deli, J. (2007). Latoxanthin, a minor carotenoid isolated from the fruits of yellow paprika (*Capsicum annuum* var. *Lycopersiciforme flavum*). *Tetrahedron Lett.*, 48: 9012-9014.

Nakamura, Y., Suganuma, E., Matsuo, T., Okamoto, S., Sato, K., Ohtsuki, K. (1999). 2,4-Nonadienal and Benzaldehyde Bioantimutagens in Fushimi Sweet Pepper (Fushimi-Togarashi). *J Agr Food Chem.*, 47: 544-549.

Noda, H., Machado, F.M. and Martins, A.L.U. (2003). SeleCão de genótipos de pimentão resistentes a *Xanthomonas campestris* pv. *vesicatoria Doidge Dye.* sob condiCões naturais de infecCão. *Acta Amaz.*, 33: 371-380.

Oboh, G. and Rocha, J.B.T. (2007). Distribution and Antioxidant Activity of Polyphenols in Ripe and Unripe Tree Pepper (*Capsicum pubescens*). *J Food Biochem.*, 31: 456-473.

Oboh, G. and Rocha, J.B.T. (2008). Water extractable phytochemicals from *Capsicum pubescens* (tree pepper) inhibit lipid peroxidation induced by different pro-oxidant agents in brain: *in vitro*. *Eur Food Res Technol.*, 226: 707-713.

Ochi, T., Takaishi, Y., Kogure, K. and Yamauti, I. (2003). Antioxidant Activity of a New Capsaicin Derivative from *Capsicum annuum*. *J Nat Prod.*, 66: 1094-1096.

Ohnuki, K., Harmizu, S., Oki, K., Watanabe, T., Yazawa, S. and Fushiki, T. (2001a). Administration of Capsiate, a Non-Pungent Capsaicin Analog, Promotes Energy Metabolism and Suppresses Body Fat Accumulation in Mice. *Biosci Biotechnol Biochem.*, 65: 2735-2740.

Ohnuki, K., Niwa, S., Maeda, S., Inoue, N., Yazawa, S. and Fushiki, T. (2001b). CH-19 Sweet, a Non-Pungent Cultivar of Red Pepper, Increased Body Temperature and Oxygen Consumption in Humans. *Biosci Biotechnol Biochem.*, 65: 2033-2036.

Osuna-García, J.A., Wall, M.M. and Waddell, C.A. (1998). Endogenous Levels of Tocopherols and Ascorbic Acid during Fruit Ripening of New Mexican-Type Chile (*Capsicum annuum L.*) Cultivars. *J Agr Food Chem.*, 46: 5093-5096.

Paul Jr., T., Marlin, B. and Tesfaye, B. (1975). TLC Screening Techniques for the Qualitative Determination of Natural and Synthetic Capsaicinoids. *J Chromatogr Sci.*, 13: 577-579.

Perucka, I. and Oleszek, W. (2000). Extraction and determination of capsaicinoids in fruit of hot pepper *Capsicum annuum L.* by spectrophotometry and high-performance liquid chromatography. *Food Chem.*, 71: 287-291.

Phillips, K.M., Ruggio, D.M., Ashraf-Khorassani, M. and Haytowitz, D.B. (2006). Difference in Folate Content of Green and Red Sweet Peppers (*Capsicum annuum*) Determined by Liquid Chromatography-Mass Spectrometry. *J Agr Food Chem.*, 54: 9998-10002.

Pieroni, A., Quave, C.L. and Santoro, R.F. (2004). Folk pharmaceutical knowledge in the territory of the Dolomiti Lucane, inland southern Italy. *J Ethnopharmacol.*, 95: 373-384.

Pieroni, A., Quave, C.L., Villanelli, M.L., Mangino, P., Sabbatini, G., Santini, L., Boccetti, T., Profili, M., Ciccioli, T., Rampa, L.G., Antonini, G., Girolamini, C., Cecchi, M. and Tomasi, M. (2004). Ethnopharmacognostic survey on the natural ingredients used in folk cosmetics, cosmeceuticals and remedies for healing skin diseases in the inland Marches, Central-Eastern Italy. *J Ethnopharmacol.*, 91: 331-344.

Pino, J., González, M., Ceballos, L., Centurión-Yah, A.R., Trujillo-Aguirre, J., Latournerie-Moreno, L. and Sauri-Duch, E. (2007). Characterization of total capsaicinoids, colour and volatile compounds of Habanero chilli pepper (*Capsicum chinense Jack.*) cultivars grown in Yucatan. *Food Chem.*, 104: 1682-1686.

Poyrazoglu, E.S., Yemi, O., Kadakal, C. and Artük, N. (2005). Determination of capsaicinoid profile of different chilli peppers grown in Turkey. *J Sci Food Agr.*, 85: 1435-1438.

Prasad, B.C.N., Gururaj, H.B., Kumar, V., Giridhar, P., Parimalan, R., Sharma, A. and Ravishankar, G.A. (2006a). Influence of 8-methyl-nonenoic Acid on Capsaicin Biosynthesis in *In-Vivo* and *In-Vitro* Cell Cultures of *Capsicum* Spp.. *J Agr Food Chem.*, 54: 1854-1859.

Prasad, B.C.N., Gururaj, H.B., Kumar, V., Giridhar, P., Parimalan, R., Sharma, A. and Ravishankar, G.A. (2006b). Valine Pathway Is More Crucial than Phenyl Propanoid Pathway in Regulating Capsaicin Biosynthesis in *Capsicum frutescens Mill.* *J Agr Food Chem.*, 54: 6660-6666.

Reifschneider, F.J.B. (2000). *Capsicum*. Pimentas e pimentões do Brasil. Embrapa ComunicaCões para Transferência de Tecnologia/Embrapa HortaliCas, Brasília

Robbins, W. (2000). Clinical application of capsaicinoids. *Clin J Pain.*, 16: 86-89.

Rosa, A., Deiana, M., Casu, V., Paccagnini, S., Appendino, G., Ballero, M. and Dessí, M.A. (2002). Antioxidant Activity of Capsinoids. *J Agr Food Chem*, 50: 7396-7401.

Saga, K. and Sato, G. (2003). Varietal Differences in Phenolic, Flavonoid and Capsaicinoid Contents in Pepper Fruits (*Capsicum annuum L.*). *J Japan Soc Hort Sci.*, 72: 335-341.

Saikia, A.P., Ryakala, V.K., Sharma, P., Goswami, P. and Bora, U. (2006). Ethnobotany of medicinal plants used by Assamese people for various skin ailments and cosmetics. *J Ethnopharmacol.*, 106: 149-157.

Sato, K., Sasaki, S.S., Goda, Y., Yamada, T., Nunomura, O., Ishikawa, K. and Maitani, T. (1999). Direct Connection of Supercritical Fluid Extraction and Supercritical Fluid Chromatography as a Rapid Quantitative Method for Capsaicinoids in Placentas of *Capsicum*. *J Agr Food Chem.*, 47: 4665-4668.

Schweiggert, U., Carle, R. and Schiber, A. (2006). Characterization of major and minor capsaicinoids and related compounds in chili pods (*Capsicum frutescens L.*) by high-performance liquid chromatography/atmospheric pressure chemical ionization mass spectrometry. *Anal Chim Acta.*, 557: 236-244.

Sezik, E., Yesilada, E., Honda, G., Takaishi, Y., Takeda, Y. and Tanaka, T. (2001). Traditional medicine in Turkey X. Folk medicine in Central Anatolia. *J Ethnopharmacol.*, 75: 95-115.

Shakhidoyatov, R.Kh. and Sagdullaev, B.T. (2001). Capsaicine in *Capsicum annuum* Condensed Extract Determined by HPLC. *Chem Nat Comp.*, 37: 575-576.

Silva, E.C. da, Souza, R.J. de (2006). Cultura da pimenta. UFLA–Universidade Federal de Lavras http://www.editora.ufla.br/boletim/pdf/extensao/bol_68.pdf, Acessed: December 2006.

Song, W., Yahara, S., Maeda, Y., Yusa, K., Tanaka, Y. and Harada S. (2001). Enhanced Infection of an X4 Strain of HIV-1 Due to Capping and Colocalization of CD4 and CXCR4 Induced by Capsianoside G, a Diterpene Glycoside. *Biochem Biophys Res Commun.*, 283: 423-429.

Sun, T., Xu, Z., Wu, C.-T., Janes, M., Prinyawiwatkul, W. and No, H.K. (2007). Antioxidant Activities of Different Colored Sweet Bell Peppers (*Capsicum annuum L.*). *J Food Sci.*, 72: 98-102.

Surh, Y.-J. (2004). Cancer chemopreventive ingredients in Asian foods. *Environ Mutagen Res.*, 26: 219-220.

Surh, Y.-J. and Lee, S.S. (1995). Capsaicin, a double-edged sword: Toxicity, metabolism, and chemoprotective potential. *Life Sci.*, 56: 1845-1855.

Surh, Y.-J. and Lee, S.S. (1996). Capsaicin in Hot Chili Pepper: Carcinogen, Co-carcinogen or Anticarcinogen?. *Food Chem Toxic.*, 34: 313-316.

Thomas, B.V., Schreiber, A.A. and Weisskopf, C.P. (1988). Simple Method for Quantification of Capsaicinoids in Pepper Using Capillary Gas Chromatography. *J Agr Food Chem.*, 46: 2655-2663.

Titze, P., Seitz, E.M. and Petz, M. (2002). Pungency in Paprika (*Capsicum annuum*). 2. Heterogeneity of Capsaicinoid Content in Individual Fruits from One Plant. *J Agr Food Chem.*, 50: 1264-1266.

Tolan, Y., Ragoobirsingh, D., Morrison, E.Y.S.A. (2004). Isolation and purification of the hypoglycaemic principle present in *Capsicum frutescens*. *Phytother Res.*, 18: 95-96.

Topuz, A. and Ozdemir, F. (2007). Assessment of carotenoids, capsaicinoids and ascorbic acid composition of some selected pepper cultivars (*Capsicum annuum L.*) grown in Turkey. *J Food Comp Anal.*, 20: 596-602.

Wagner, C.M. (2003). Variabilidade e Base Genética da Pungência e de Caracteres do Fruto: ImplicaCões no Melhoramentode Uma PopulaCão de *Capsicum annuum* L. Tese de Doutorado–Escola Superior de Agricultura "Luiz de Queiroz"–Universidade de São Paulo.

Wang J.P., Hsu M.F. and Teng C.M. (1984). Antiplatelet effect of capsaicin. *Thromb Res.*, 31: 497-507.

Westerterp-Plantenga, M., Diepvens, K., Joosen, A.M.C.P., Bérubé-Parent, S. and Tremblay A. (2006). Metabolic effects of spices, teas, and caffeine. *Physiol Behav.*, 89: 85-91.

Yahara, S., Kobayashi, N., Izumitani, Y. and Nohara, T. (1991). New Acyclic Diterpene Glycosides, Capsianosides VI, G and H from the Leaves and Stems of *Capsicum annuum L. Chem Pharm Bull.*, 39: 3258-3260.

Yahara, S., Ura, T., Sakamoto, C. and Nohara, T. (1994). Steroidal Glycosides from *Capsicum annuum. Phytochemistry*, 37: 831-835.

Zewdie, Y. and Bosland, P.W. (2001). Capsaicinoid profiles are not good chemotaxonomic indicators for *Capsicum* species. *Biochem Syst Ecol.*, 29: 161-169.

Medicinal Plants: Phytochemistry, Pharmacology and Therapeutics, Vol. 1 *Pages* **258–296**
Editors: **V.K. Gupta, G.D. Singh, Surjeet Singh and A. Kaul**
Published by: **DAYA PUBLISHING HOUSE, NEW DELHI**

Chapter 14

Review of Plants Having Potential in the Management of Hyperlipidemia

T. D'souza and S.A. Mengi*
C.U. Shah College of Pharmacy, SNDT Women's University, Santacruz (West), Mumbai – 400 049, India

ABSTRACT

Throughout history humans have used plants as a remedy for various disease conditions. With the advent of modern synthetic molecules, plant medicine has often been relegated to the fringe of therapeutic modalities. However, it is increasingly being recognized that the current therapeutic options have several limitations especially in chronic disease conditions such as hyperlipidemia and atherosclerosis. Research is ongoing to discover newer drugs and several novel therapeutic targets are being explored. In this context there has been a renewed interest in plant research. Bioactives from plants such as garlic (*Allium sativum*), Guggul (*Commiphora mukul*), Soy (*Glycine max*), Citrus fruits and Psyllium (*Plantago ovata*) have demonstrated a potential in the treatment of hyperlipidemia. Further, the fact that today several plant bioactives have proved to act via known and well defined molecular pathways such as inhibition of microsomal triglyceride transfer protein (MTP), Acyl coenzyme A (CoA) : cholesterol acyl transferase (ACAT), Acyl coenzyme A (CoA) : diacylglycerol acyltransferase (DGAT) and Farnesoid X Receptors (FXR) has provided an added impetus to explore the untapped potential of medicinal plants. In the present review, the plant derived bioactives or natural products that have proved to have a potential in hyperlipidemia or whose molecular mechanism of action has been elucidated will be discussed, followed by an overview of the plants that have been investigated in this area in the past decade.

Keywords: *Citrus bioactives, Garlic, Guggul, Hyperlipidemia, Investigative plants, Novel targets, Polyphenols, Soy protein.*

---

* Corresponding Author: E-mail: sushmamengi@yahoo.co.in.

Introduction

While contagious diseases dominated the early centuries, followed by the increased incidence of various forms of cancer, today we are witnessing a dramatic increase in cardiovascular related mortality. Cardiovascular disease (CVD) has assumed epidemic proportion across the globe. One of the major contributory factors to cardiovascular disease is the growing menace of hyperlipidemia and the resulting coronary artery disease (CAD). Clinical studies have consistently demonstrated that lipid-lowering therapy can halt and even reverse the progression of atherosclerosis and reduce CVD events (Lipid Research Clinics Program, 1984; Blankenhorn *et al.*, 1993; Scandinavian Simvastatin Survival Study Group, 1994; Waters *et al.*, 1994; Levine *et al.*, 1995). Epidemiological studies have confirmed that hyperlipidemia has a central role in atherogenesis. It is of significance that studies have demonstrated that when total cholesterol levels were maintained below 160 mg/dl, CHD risk was markedly attenuated even in the presence of other risk factors (Grundy *et al.*, 1998). This can be attributed to the fact that lipid lowering actively opposes the events occurring right from the genesis of the atherosclerotic plaque to its rupture.

Although there are highly effective drugs available in this area of therapeutics, research is ongoing to discover drugs that overcome the limitations of the existing therapy. New drug discovery continues to be a challenge and successful outcomes are becoming increasingly rare. Indeed, in the area of hyperlipidemia, experts believe that the research pipeline is weak (Opar, 2007). Dramatic lifestyle changes in the past few decades and the high levels of stress in modern life often necessitate the concomitant use of several drugs, leading to adverse effects that then require further drug intervention. This cascade of subjecting the body to several drugs results in stress on vital organ systems. In this context there has been a renewed interest in plant research. Plants can be likened to experienced synthetic chemists producing a wide range of biologically active compounds. Of the large number of higher plants it is estimated that only around 6 per cent have been screened for biological activity and 15 per cent have been evaluated phytochemically (Lahlou, 2007). The recognition of the potential of plant derived drugs is amply reflected in recent publications of prominent scientific journals both debating and discussing the scope of plants in drug discovery (Balachandran and Govindarajan, 2007; Lahlou, 2007; Littleton, 2007; Mukherjee *et al.*, 2007). Further, the fact that today several plant bioactives have proved to act via known and well defined molecular pathways has provided an added impetus to explore the untapped potential of medicinal plants.

Lipid homeostasis is a complex process that is controlled mainly by events occurring at the intestine and the liver. Additionally, several nuclear receptors act as lipid sensors in these processes. Plant derived bioactives have proved to modulate various facets of lipid homeostasis at multiple levels. Further, plants are renowned for their potent antioxidant properties which contribute to the attenuation of atherosclerosis. An understanding of these factors requires a description of the events occurring at the intestine and liver and identification of the potential therapeutic targets.

Intestinal Absorption of Lipids

Dietary lipid comprises mainly of neutral fat or triglycerides, phospholipids, sterols like cholesterol, some minor lipids and fat-soluble vitamins. In order for the virtually insoluble lipids in the intestine to be absorbed, the large aggregates of dietary lipids need to be broken down into smaller droplets. The bile acids produced by the liver and secreted into the intestine are amphipathic molecules that effectively emulsify the dietary lipids into micelles resulting in the solubilization and transport of lipids in the aqueous environment of the intestine. The micelles are cylindrical in shape with the polar lipids arranged radially with their hydrophilic heads facing outward toward the aqueous phase (Figure

14.1A) (Hofmann, 1999). As the intestinal contents are mixed, micelles come in contact with the brush border of small intestinal enterocytes, and the lipids are taken up into the epithelial cells.

Absorption of Dietary Triglyceride by the Intestine

Dietary triglycerides (triacylglycerols) are hydrolyzed in the gut by the action of pancreatic lipase to fatty acids and monoacyl glycerol which are then absorbed separately by the intestine. In the enterocyte, the fatty acids and monoglycerides are re-esterified by the enzyme acyl-coenzyme A: diacylglycerol acyl transferase (DGAT) to form triglycerides (Figure 14.1B). Thus, pancreatic lipase inhibitors and DGAT inhibitors have a potential in the treatment of hypertriglyceridemia and obesity, wherein the absorption of dietary fats must be restricted (Shi and Burn, 2004; Chen and Farese, 2005).

Absorption of Cholesterol by the Intestine

Dietary cholesterol is mainly in the form of cholesteryl esters. In the intestine, these cholesteryl esters are acted upon by esterases, primarily secreted by the pancreatic exocrine glands. Intestinal cholesterol absorption is a multistep process that is regulated by the activity of several transporters and enzymes (Figure 14.1B). The cholesterol present in the micelles is taken up by the enterocytes via the Niemann-Pick C1 Like1 (NPC1L1) protein that is localized to the brush border of the jejunal enterocytes, which forms the interface between the intestinal lumen and the intracellular compartments (Altmann *et al.*, 2004). The cholesterol thus absorbed into the enterocyte is then re-esterified to cholesteryl esters by the enzyme Acyl coenzyme A:cholesterol acyltransferase (ACAT), a process that is essential to the incorporation of cholesterol into lipoprotein particles. A fraction of the cholesterol that enters into the enterocyte is pumped back out of the enterocyte into the intestinal lumen by the ATP-binding cassette (ABC) transporter complex ABCG5/G8 (Figure 14.1B) (Duan *et al.*, 2004). Thus modulation of the expression of NPC1L1, ACAT and ABCG5/G8 represents important new targets for cholesterol absorption inhibition.

Formation and Secretion of the Chylomicron on Particle by the Intestine

The triglycerides and cholesteryl esters formed in the enterocyte by the action of DGAT and ACAT respectively, are essentially insoluble in water and hence cannot be secreted or transported in the aqueous blood or lymph as free molecules. Microsomal triglyceride transfer protein (MTP) is responsible for the systematic addition of these triglycerides and cholesteryl esters to phospholipids and a protein moiety, Apolipoprotein B48 (ApoB48) to form a lipid and protein (lipoprotein) complex known as chylomicron (Figure 14.1C). MTP is a protein localized within the endoplasmic reticulum (ER) of the cells found in the intestine as well as the liver and is essential to the process of secretion of the atherogenic Apo-B containing lipoproteins by both the intestine as well as the liver (Swift *et al.*, 2003; Hussain *et al.*, 2003).Thus inhibitors of MTP are being investigated as a viable therapeutic option in the management of hyperlipidemia.

In the capillaries of the adipose tissue and muscle, the triglycerides of the chylomicrons are hydrolyzed by the enzyme lipoprotein lipase (Lpl) that is bound to the luminal surface of the endothelial cells. The liberated fatty acids cross the endothelium and enter the underlying adipocytes or muscle cells where they are either esterified again to triglycerides for storage or oxidized to provide energy. The triglyceride depleted chylomicron remnant is taken up by the liver via the LDL receptor or the LDL receptor related protein (LRP). The chylomicron particle then undergoes digestion in the lysosomes to release free cholesterol in the hepatocytes.

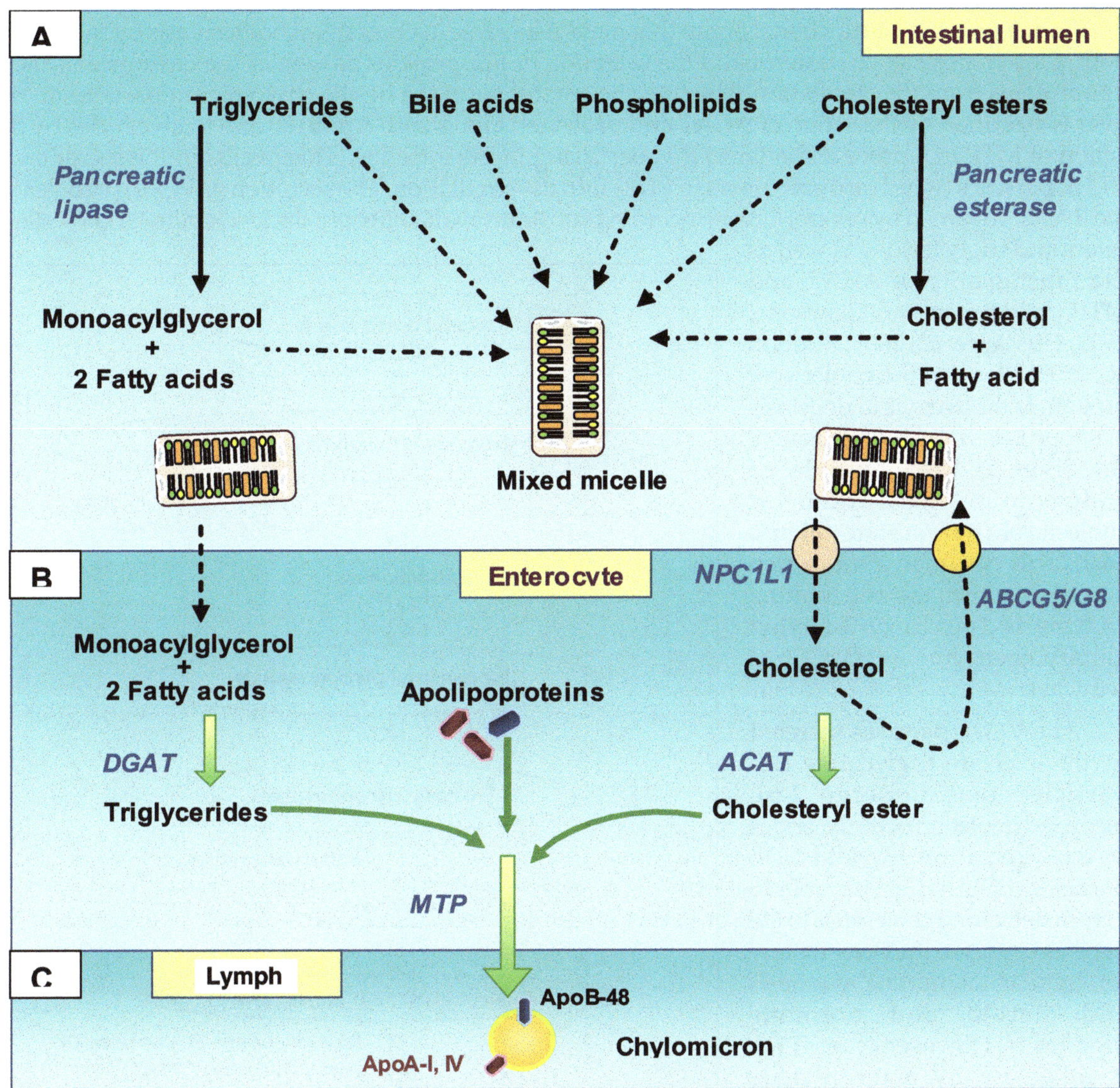

Figure 14.1: Intestinal Absorption of Lipids

(A) Solubilization of dietary lipids via interaction with bile acids to form mixed micelles.

(B) In the enterocytes, the monoacylglycerols and fatty acids are re esterified by the action of DGAT to form triglycerides while cholesterol is converted to cholesterol esters by the action of ACAT. Some of the unesterified cholesterol returns to the intestinal lumen via the ABCG5/G8 efflux transporter complex.

(C) Chylomicron particles are formed by the packaging of triglycerides, cholesteryl esters and apolipoproteins in a process mediated by MTP and secreted into the lymph.

Role of the Liver in Lipid Homeostasis

The liver is a multifunctional organ that plays a key role in cholesterol homeostasis by mediating both, the synthesis of cholesterol and the secretion of lipoproteins as well as the clearance of these lipoproteins from the circulation. The free cholesterol supplied by the chylomicron particles to the liver is esterified by the action of ACAT and packaged along with ApoB100 and triglycerides by the action of MTP in a process similar to that occurring in the intestine. This results in the secretion of VLDL particles (which are precursors to LDL) into the circulation. The secretion of VLDL particles by the liver is governed by several factors including substrate availability *viz.* the availability of cholesteryl esters and triglycerides as well as the functionality of ACAT and MTP (Sniderman and Cianflone, 1993; Hussain *et al.*, 2003; Rudel *et al.*, 2005). Besides the cholesterol brought to the liver via endocytosis of lipoproteins from the circulation, the liver is also capable of endogenous biosynthesis of cholesterol from acetate (Figure 14.2). This occurs in a multi step process in which the rate limiting enzyme is 3-hydroxy 3-methyl glutaryl coenzyme A (HMGCoA) reductase.

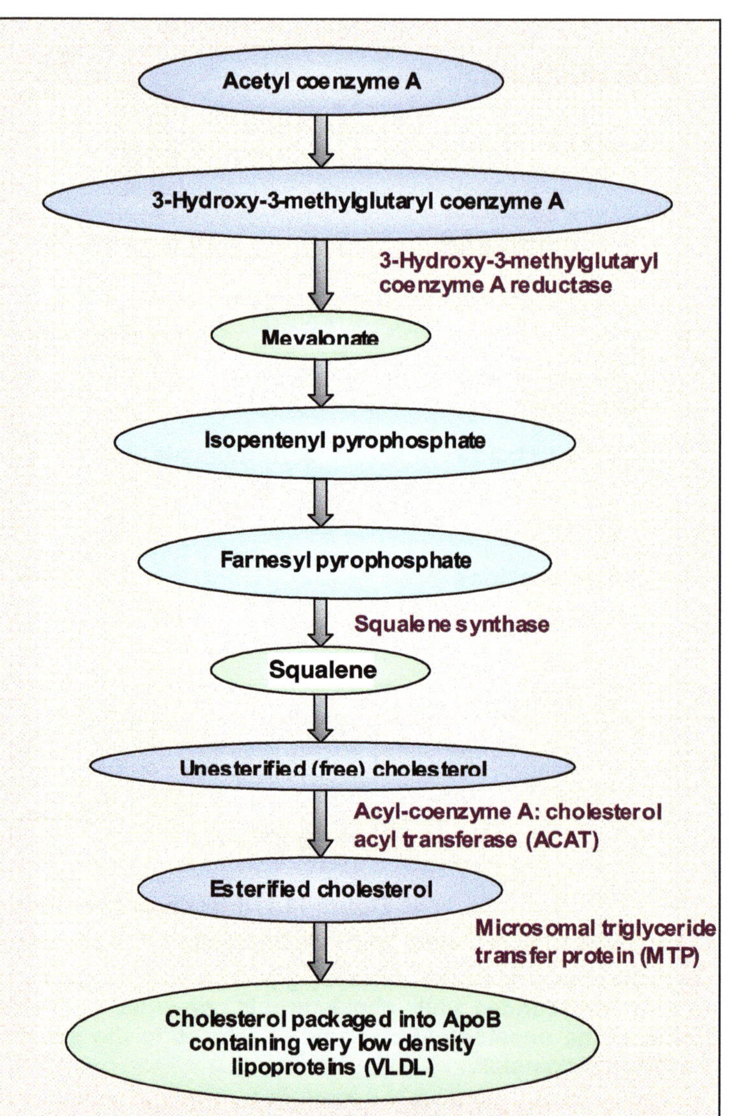

Figure 14.2: Endogenous Biosynthesis of Cholesterol by the Liver

The VLDL particles secreted by the liver are triglyceride rich particles that undergo LpL mediated depletion of triglycerides in the circulation to yield LDL particles. LDL has a vital role to play in delivering cholesterol to the various tissues of the body mainly for cellular membrane synthesis and steroid and hormone production. However, excess LDL is taken up by macrophages present in the subendothelial region of the vasculature to form lipid engorged macrophages known as foam cells which is the hallmark of the atherosclerotic lesion.

The liver is the only organ capable of excreting cholesterol out of the body wherein nonpolar cholesterol is degraded by the action of the hepatic enzyme, cholesterol 7α-hydroxylase, to the polar, water soluble bile acids that are then secreted back into the intestine. Additionally, the regulation of hepatic LDL-receptor expression and cycling are part of a complex process that regulates the removal of cholesterol from the blood stream (Brown and Goldstein, 1986). Approximately 75 per cent of the circulating LDL is removed by the liver in this fashion. This accounts for the tremendous success of the pharmacological modulation (upregulation) of the LDL-receptor.

Further, the liver also plays an important role in reverse cholesterol transport. HDL particles perform the important function of transferring excess cholesterol from the vasculature and other cells back to the liver in the process termed as reverse cholesterol transport (Figure 14.3). The cholesteryl esters picked up by the HDL particle is presented to the liver via either a direct or an indirect pathway.

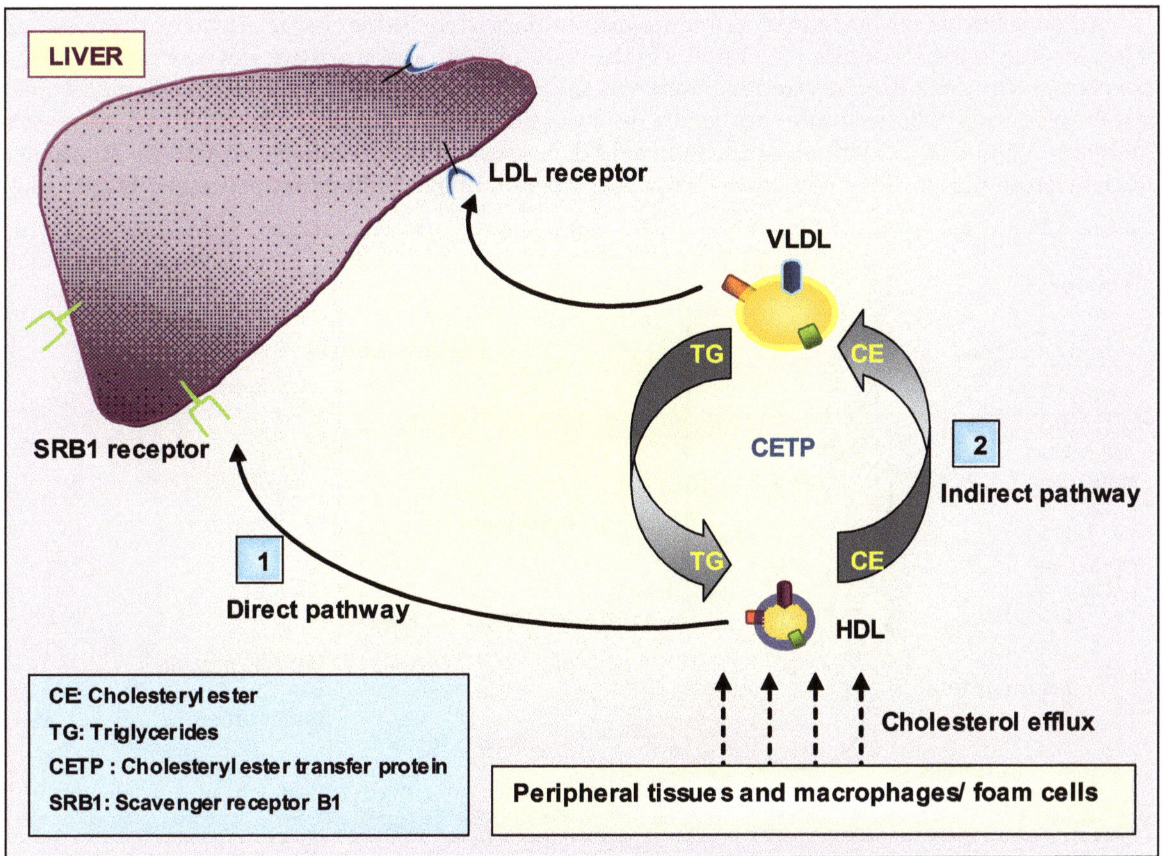

Figure 14.3: Transport of Cholesteryl Esters from the Peripheral Tissues and Macrophages to the Liver

HDL particle picks up cholesterol from the peripheral tissues and macrophages/foam cells. This cholesterol can be transported to the liver via two mechanisms:

(1) The Indirect pathway: this involves CETP mediated transfer of cholesteryl esters from HDL to Apolipoprotein B containing lipoproteins such as VLDL and their subsequent uptake by the LDL receptors of the liver.

(2) The Direct pathway: the HDL particle directly transfers its cholesteryl esters to the liver via interaction with the SRB1 receptors.

Cholesteryl ester transfer protein (CETP) mediates the exchange of cholesterol from the HDL particle to LDL and triglyceride rich lipoproteins (TRLs) *i.e.* The apoB containing lipoproteins. These particles are taken up by the liver via the LDL receptor. The direct pathway involves the selective uptake of cholesteryl esters by the liver via the SR-B1 receptors without endocytosis or breakdown of the HDL particle (Trigatti *et al.*, 2003). The core of the HDL particle is effectively depleted of cholesteryl esters and then released into the circulation for further interaction with the lipid laden macrophages (foam cells). Thus, the liver serves as an acceptor of cholesterol carried by the HDL particles, improving the functionality of the reverse cholesterol transport process. The cholesterol thus delivered to the liver becomes available for conversion to bile acids and excretion into the intestine.

Role of Oxidized Lipoproteins in Atherosclerosis

Atherosclerosis can be defined as a complex multifactorial disease characterized by the presence of lesions due to the accumulation of lipids in the walls of large and small arteries accompanied by a loss of elasticity of the affected arteries (Singh *et al.*, 2002). Several research workers have demonstrated that the oxidation of lipids, more specifically the oxidation of LDL, plays a central role in these events (Witztum, 1994). The oxidative modification of LDL has several ramifications and actively stimulates atherosclerotic plaque development and rupture by promoting inflammatory processes (Figure 14.4)

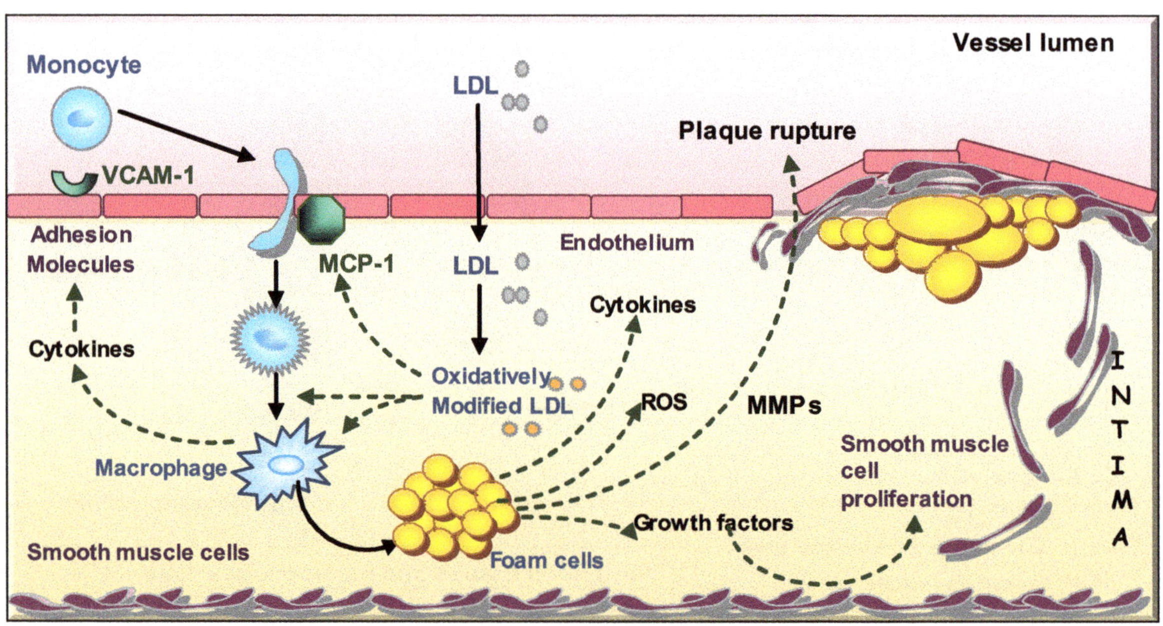

Figure 14.4: Schematic Representation of the Activating Effect of LDL Infiltration and Oxidative Modification on Inflammation in the Artery

Oxidatively modified LDL aids in the recruitment of monocytes into the subendothelial space (intima) by stimulating the endothelial cells to express adhesion molecules such as VCAM-1 and chemoattractants such as MCP-1. It is also readily taken up by the macrophages to form the lipid laden foam cells that release a variety of proinflammatory mediators such as cytokines, ROS, MMPs and growth factors.

VCAM: Vascular cell adhesion molecule-1, MCP: Monocyte chemoattractant protein, ROS: Reactive oxygen species, MMPs: Matrix metalloproteinases.

(Libby, 2002). It has been proposed that inhibiting this process could significantly attenuate the atherogenecity of the lipids and hence antihyperlipidemic agents possessing antioxidant activity is considered desirable.

Nuclear Receptors Acting as Sensors in Lipid Homeostasis

The homeostatic mechanisms that regulate lipid metabolism require cellular sensors that can monitor and coordinate the enzymatic cascades and events involved in lipid synthesis and catabolism. Nuclear receptors are transcription factors that are present in abundance in the various metabolic organ systems and have the capacity to regulate genes involved in lipid and energy metabolism directly in response to varying nutrient availability. Nuclear receptors playing a prominent role in lipid metabolism and atherosclerosis include the Peroxisome proliferator activated receptors (fatty acid sensor), the Farnesoid X receptor (bile acid sensor) and the Liver X receptor (sterol sensor) (Figure 14.5) (Shulman and Mangelsdorf, 2005). Screening of compounds as ligands for these receptors has gained tremendous momentum over the past two decades. The potential for obtaining such compounds from plants has been recognized by studies indicating that Guggulipid, a plant derived antihyperlipidemic compound, mediates its effect via the farnesoid X receptor (Urizar *et al.*, 2002).

Plants with Potential in the Management of Hyperlipidemia

Plants have served as a source of medicinal agents for thousands of years and have the distinct advantage of having been used empirically in the treatment of a wide variety of disease conditions. However, the demands of modern medicine (and rightly so) requires the evaluation of these plant bioactives using scientific methodologies and assays in order to gauge their potential in the management of the disease. In pursuit of this objective, several plant derived extracts and bioactives have been subjected to extensive preclinical and clinical studies. In the arena of hyperlipidemia, some of these plant bioactives have consistently demonstrated a potential to be used as therapeutic agents. Moreover, studies elucidating their mechanism of action have provided further proof of concept. These findings though, have not been without exception and controversies. In the following section an update will be provided on the status of these bioactives so as to be able to gauge their future potential.

Garlic: Bulbs of *Allium sativum*

Garlic and its preparations have been used by people of diverse cultures for thousands of years and are mentioned in several texts of traditional medicine as having an application in the treatment of cardiovascular disorders. The historical perspective of the therapeutic use of garlic and its scientific evaluation has been extensively reviewed (Rahman, 2001; Banerjee and Maulik, 2002). The most extensively studied preparation of garlic is the raw garlic homogenate or its aqueous extract, presumably because this is the commonest way garlic is consumed. Garlic oil, dried garlic powder (*Kwai*) and aged garlic extract (*Kyolic*) are other popular garlic preparations that have been investigated for therapeutic efficacy. Aged garlic extract (AGE) is prepared by soaking sliced raw garlic in aqueous ethanol solution for up to 20 months at room temperature a procedure that renders the garlic free of the odorous sulfur principles. The procedure is mentioned in the United States Pharmacopoeia/National Formulary monograph under Garlic Fluid Extract (Macan *et al.*, 2006).

Garlic is one of the most well studied plant products in the treatment of hyperlipidemia (Yeh and Liu, 2001, Thompson *et al.*, 2006). In preclinical studies, long term (2-9 months) feeding of garlic and garlic preparations (2 per cent garlic powder in diet) to rabbits fed a high-cholesterol diet resulted in a statistically significant reduction in atherosclerotic lesions. The chronic effects (> 4 weeks) of garlic (1-4 per cent in diet) and garlic protein on lipid metabolism in rats revealed a reduction in serum

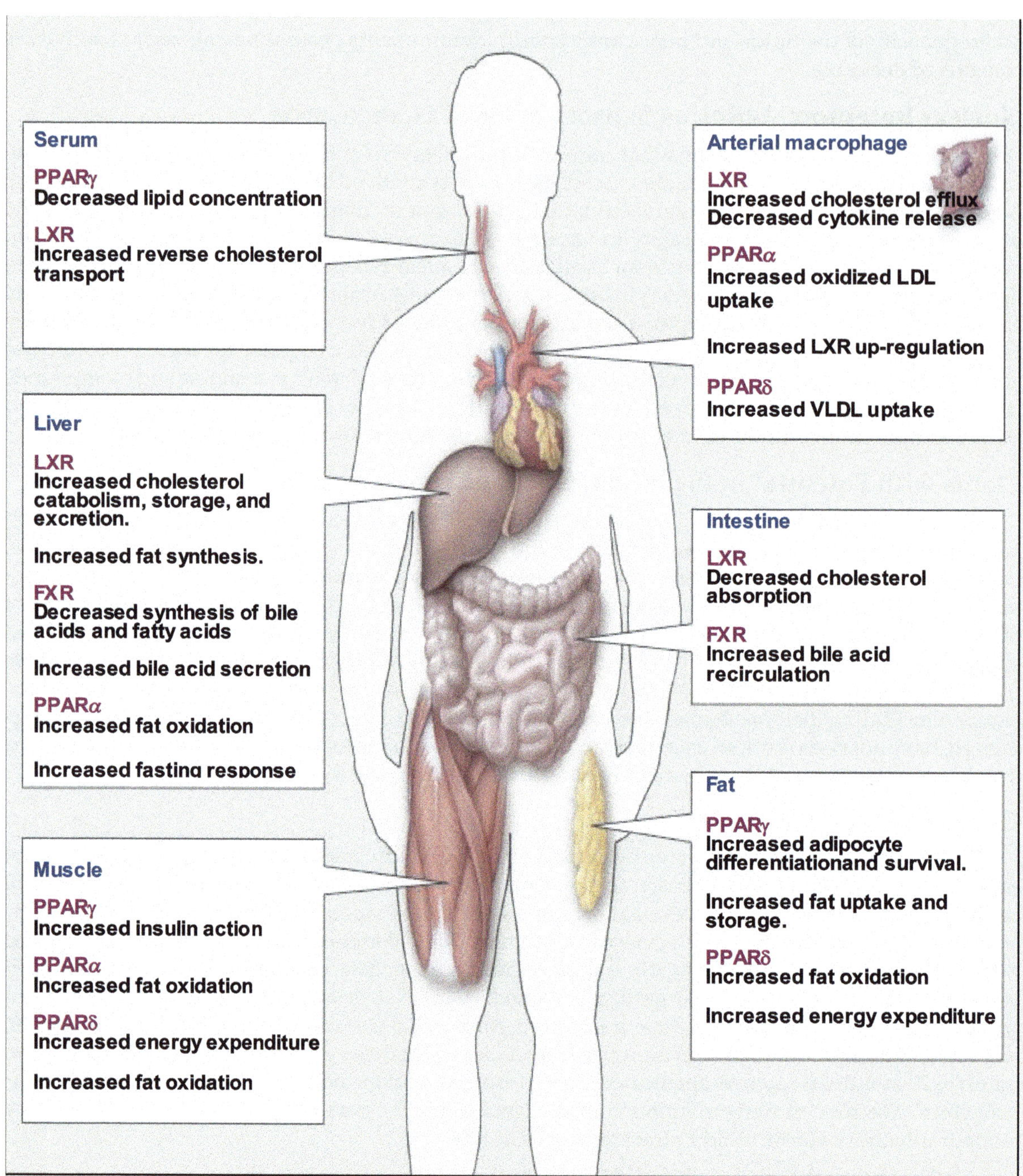

Figure 14.5: Regulation of Cholesterol and Lipid Handling in Metabolic Organ Systems by Nuclear Receptors
(Reproduced from Shulman and Mangelsdorf, 2005)

cholesterol, triglyceride and LDL cholesterol. Total lipid content and cholesterol levels in the liver were also decreased indicating that inhibition of the enzyme HMGCoA reductase could be one of the mechanisms of action. An excellent review of these studies has been compiled by Banerjee and Maulik (2002). Studies also indicate that garlic can attenuate hypercholesterolemia induced vascular alterations and prevent LDL oxidation, a process known to play a central role in atherogenesis (Slowing *et al.*, 2001; Lau, 2006). Moreover, since hypercholesterolemic patients are also often prescribed anticoagulants for associated complications and garlic has been alleged to predispose to platelet dysfunction, studies have been conducted to investigate the interaction of the aged garlic extract (AGE/Kyolic garlic), a popular garlic preparation and warfarin. The results of the study concluded that there was no synergistic effect and AGE can be safely administered with warfarin (Macan *et al.*, 2006).

The complex nature of the components of garlic as well as the tendency of some of these components to degrade depending on the method of preparation has made it a challenge to assign the therapeutic effects of the various preparations to any one chemical constituent (Amagase, 2006). The chemistry of the Allium species is highly complex, predominantly comprising of sulfur-containing compounds that are responsible for the characteristic flavor of garlic. S-allyl-L-cysteine sulfoxides (alliin), g-glutamyl-S-allyl-L-cysteines and (1)-S-(trans-1-propenyl)-L-cysteine sulfoxide are some of the abundantly present sulfur compounds. These sulfoxides are converted into thiosulfinates such as allicin (purported to be the active component) by the action of the enzyme alliinase when raw garlic is cut or crushed. Additionally, garlic also contains several volatile as well as water soluble organosulfur compounds. S-methyl cysteine sulfoxide obtained from another Allium species *viz. Allium cepa* (Onion) also significantly ameliorated the hyperlipidemic condition in rats maintained on a high cholesterol diet (Kumari and Augusti, 2007). Additionally, a variety of components including nonsulfur compounds such as steroidal saponins are believed to contribute to the therapeutic efficacy of garlic (Amagase, 2006).

Among the several mechanisms of action that have been proposed for garlic, it is interesting to note that both *in vitro* as well as *in vivo* studies indicate that inhibition of microsomal triglyceride transfer protein (MTP), is one of the mechanisms of action (Lin *et al.*, 2002). MTP is responsible for the packaging of triglycerides and cholesteryl esters with apolipoprotein B in the intestine and the liver to form chylomicrons and VLDL particles respectively. While MTP is the therapeutic target of several new synthetic molecules in the research pipeline, a notable hurdle in developing MTP inhibitors is that this effect in the liver leads to accumulation of fat (steatosis) as these agents block the assembly of VLDL but not the substrate (triglyceride and cholesteryl ester) accumulation in the liver (Burnett and Watts, 2007). Hence, it is encouraging to note that while *in vitro* studies indicate that fresh garlic decreases mRNA expression of MTP in both hepatic (HepG2) as well as intestinal (Caco-2) cell lines, *in vivo* studies in rats indicate that this effect is restricted to the intestine leading to increased excretion of fat (Lin *et al.*, 2002).

While garlic seems to be one of the most promising plant-derived anti hyperlipidemic agents, there are also studies which have reported the various forms and constituents of garlic to be ineffective in hyperlipidemia (Espirito Santo *et al.*, 2004). The results of clinical trials also demonstrate a dichotomy with respect to efficacy. While the majority of the clinical trials demonstrated a favorable effect on lipid profile, a meta-analysis of randomized clinical trials have indicated that while garlic was superior to the placebo, its effect was modest and its clinical efficacy doubtful (Stevinson *et al.*, 2000). This observation has been countered by arguments that the cholesterol lowering activity of garlic is mainly due to allicin (which is formed from alliin by the action of the enzyme alliinase) when raw garlic is cut or crushed. On the other hand the clinical studies employed dried garlic/commercial preparations such as tablets that presume that a biologically significant amount of allicin is formed after consumption (Lawson, 2001).

This highlights the need for uniformity in the preparation and standardization of the various garlic preparations. Thus, while a plethora of evidence points to the therapeutic potential and health benefits of garlic consumption, the challenge lies in the development of a standardized and stable preparation that retains the therapeutic efficacy and safety.

Guggul: Gum resin of *Commiphora mukul*

Guggul is an extract from the resin of the myrrh tree *Commiphora mukul*. The medicinal use of guggul dates back to 600 BC, when it was used for obesity, atherosclerosis, and various inflammatory conditions. The plant sterols E- and Z-guggulsterone are believed to be the bioactive compounds. An ethyl acetate extract of this resin termed as guggulipid has been found to lower LDL cholesterol and triglyceride levels in clinical studies (Gopal *et al.*, 1986). Guggulipid as a treatment has been developed mainly by research groups working in India. In the 1980s several clinical trials attested to the beneficial effects of guggulipid on the lipid profile (Agarwal *et al.*, 1986; Gopal *et al.*, 1986; Nityanand *et al.*, 1989). It received regulatory approval in India in 1987 for use as a lipid-lowering drug and has been feted as an example of successful translation of knowledge from traditional systems of medicine (Ayurveda) to modern clinical practice.

Research on guggul received an additional boost by findings that indicated its mechanism of action to be via the farnesoid X receptors (FXR). A brief digression to highlight the role of FXR in lipid homeostasis is of order. The biosynthesis of bile acids from cholesterol by the action of the enzyme cholesterol 7α hydroxylase (CYP7A1) is the most significant pathway for the elimination of cholesterol from the body. FXR is referred to as a bile acid sensor and its activation by bile acids leads to suppression of bile acid synthesis by CYP7A1, increased biliary excretion, detoxification of bile acids and decreased import back into the hepatocytes (Figure 14.6) (Claudel *et al.*, 2005). On the other hand, CYP7A1 expression becomes derepressed by antagonism of FXR. This leads to increased conversion of cholesterol to bile acids and subsequent upregulation of the LDL receptor with increased clearance of LDL from the plasma.

In 2002 studies demonstrated that guggulsterones strongly inhibit FXR activation by chenodeoxycholic acid (CDCA) which is the most potent of the bile acid agonist ligands by directly competing for the FXR ligand binding domain (Urizar *et al.*, 2002). Simultaneously, other cell based assays confirmed that guggulsterones antagonize the bile acid receptor (Wu *et al.*, 2002). Further, guggulsterone treatment decreased hepatic cholesterol in wild-type mice fed a high-cholesterol diet but was not effective in FXR-null mice indicating that its mechanism of action was FXR antagonism (Urizar *et al.*, 2002). Subsequent studies however, have revealed that guggulipid also activates FXR controlled targets such as the bile salt export pump (BSEP), with a predominance of transactivation rather than antagonism of FXR, thereby indicating that it may be acting as a partial agonist to FXR (Cui *et al.*, 2003; Deng *et al.*, 2007).

Although its effect on FXR provides a rational and valid basis to the lipid lowering effects seen in the earlier clinical trials, in 2003, results of a double-blind, randomized clinical trial of guggulipid in an American population on a typical western diet, failed to demonstrate a beneficial effect on lipid profile. The investigators of the trial have suggested that guggulipid may have different lipid effects in different populations. A positive finding of the study was that guggulipid produced a marginal decrease in cardiovascular surrogate markers such as Lp(a) and CRP which have a role in the inflammatory component of atherosclerosis (Szapary *et al.*, 2003). Considering all the evidence in

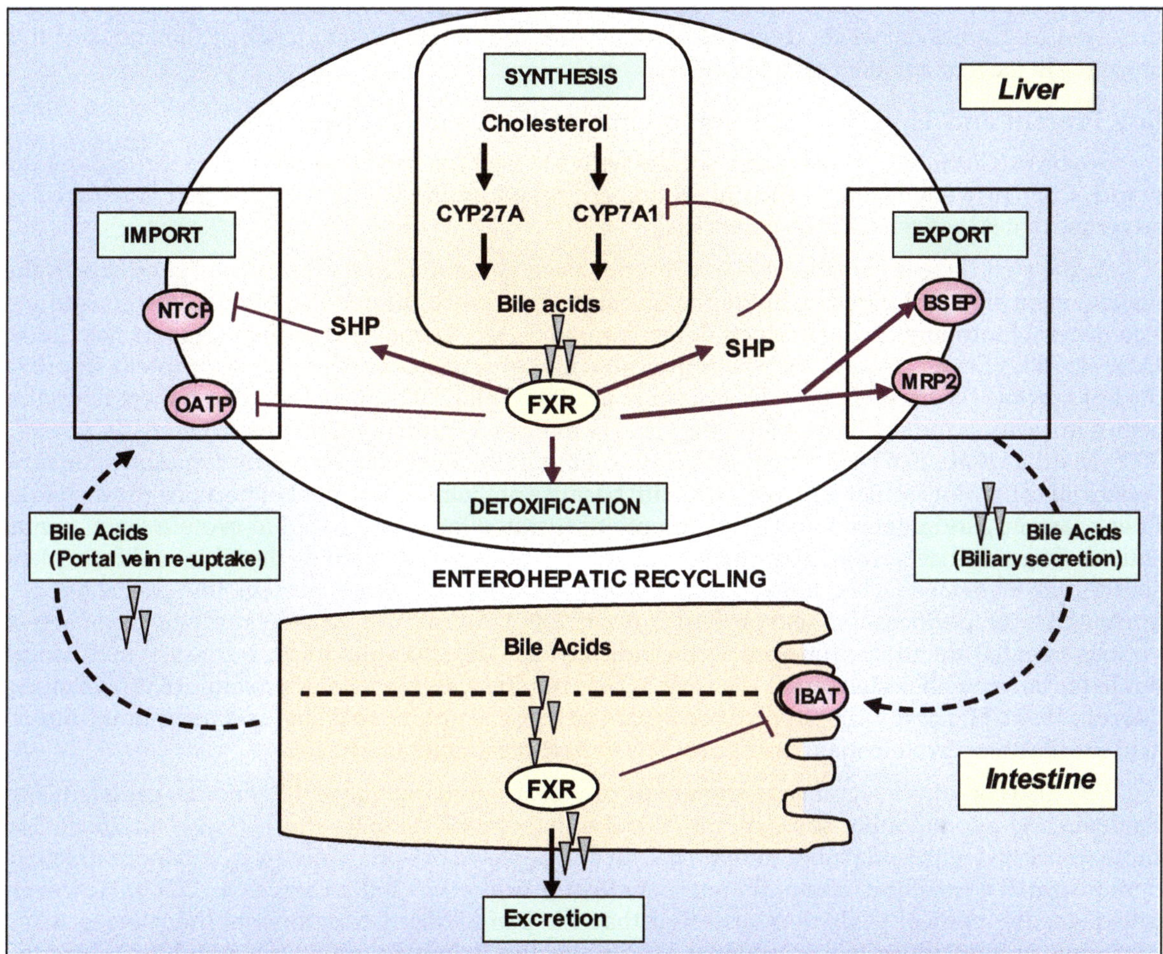

Figure 14.6: Role of FXR in the Regulation of Bile Acids Synthesis, Transport and Detoxification (Adapted from Claudel *et al.*, 2005)

Cholesterol 7α-hydroxylase (CYP7A1) is the rate controlling enzyme of one of the pathways by which the liver converts cholesterol to bile acids. Activation of FXR by ligands/bile acids induces the expression of the atypical nuclear receptor small heterodimer partner (SHP). SHP represses CYP7A1 gene transcription thereby inhibiting bile acid synthesis. FXR also induces the expression of transporters such as the bile salt export pump (BSEP) and multidrug resistance-associated protein 2 (MRP-2) that enable the hepatocytes to secrete the synthesized bile acids into the bile canaliculi. On the other hand it inhibits the expression of the intestinal bile acid transporter (IBAT) which is responsible for the uptake of the bile acids from the lumen of the ileum back into the enterocytes. Further, FXR inhibits the reuptake of bile acids from the portal vein by inhibiting the expression of bile acid import transporters such as Na^+ taurocholate cotransporting polypeptide (NTCP) and organic anion transporter polypeptides (OATPs).

totality, we can conclude that guggulipid is a plant bioactive with considerable potential. However, detailed clinical studies on a wider and more diverse population using guggulipid as well as guggul prepared by traditional methods could possibly provide conclusive evidence of the status of this bioactive in the management of hyplipidemia.

Soy Protein and Isoflavones: Components of Soybean, *Glycine max*

Soybean (*Glycine max*) is a legume species native to East Asia and now cultivated throughout the world. Currently soy is one of the only foods approved by the US FDA (1999) that is allowed to advertise that it lowers cardiovascular risk.

In the past decade considerable interest has been generated in the use of soy products in the management of hyperlipidemia. Epidemiological studies have indicated that populations consuming a considerable amount of soy products demonstrated better plasma lipid profiles (Nagata *et al.*, 1998; Ho *et al.*, 2000). Several clinical trials have indicated that soy components, mainly soy protein, improve the lipid profile (Wong *et al.*, 1998; Desroches *et al.*, 2004; Taku *et al.*, 2007). In contrast, there have also been clinical trials indicating that this effect is very marginal and cannot be substantiated (Sacks *et al.*, 2006; Matthan *et al.*, 2007). However, these investigators also agree that many soy products should be beneficial to cardiovascular and overall health because of their high content of polyunsaturated fats, fiber, vitamins, and minerals and low content of saturated fat as compared to protein from animal sources. In general, when dietary protein from animal sources is replaced by that obtained from plant sources, a beneficial effect on lipid profile is observed. In the case of soy protein, this effect has been attributed to its specific amino acid profile (Erdman, 2000). Animal experiments studying the effects of various essential amino acids on lipid profile indicate that while the amino acids lysine and methionine tended to be hypercholesterolemic, the amino acid arginine was hypocholesterolemic (Kurowska and Carroll, 1994). Hence it has been proposed that the higher arginine to lysine and methionine amino acid profile of soy protein may contribute to its hypocholesterolemic effects.

Soy also contains a significant amount of phytoestrogens *viz.* the isoflavonoids, genistein and daidzein and two saponins, soyasaponin A and B that contribute to its effects (Lee *et al.*, 2005). Soy protein enriched with isoflavones compared with that depleted of isoflavones eg. by ethanol extraction, demonstrated a greater cholesterol lowering effect (Lucas *et al.*, 2001; Taku *et al.*, 2007). However, unexpectedly, clinical trials demonstrated that the isoflavonoid components themselves when consumed without its protein component were ineffective in lowering cholesterol and thus currently soy protein but not isoflavone pills have been recommended (Hodgson *et al.*, 1998).

The mechanism of action of the cholesterol lowering activity of soy has been proposed to have several components (Figure 14.7). Studies have indicated that soy protein enhances the conversion of cholesterol to bile acids by the liver resulting in upregulation of LDL-C receptor and subsequent increase in clearance of LDL from the plasma. It has also been proposed that soy could increase thyroid hormones that modulate lipid metabolism (Potter, 1995).

Polyphenolic Plant Bioactives

Polyphenols are phytochemicals found in abundance in several legumes, berries, fruits such as grapes, apple and pear and vegetables such as broccoli, parsley, cabbage and celery. Additionally, polyphenols are also present in red wine, chocolate, green tea and olive oil.

In recent years the polyphenols have become the focus of much attention due to their potent antioxidant properties and possible health benefits in diseases ranging from cancer to coronary artery disease. The polyphenol class of compounds include flavonoids such as flavanols, flavones,

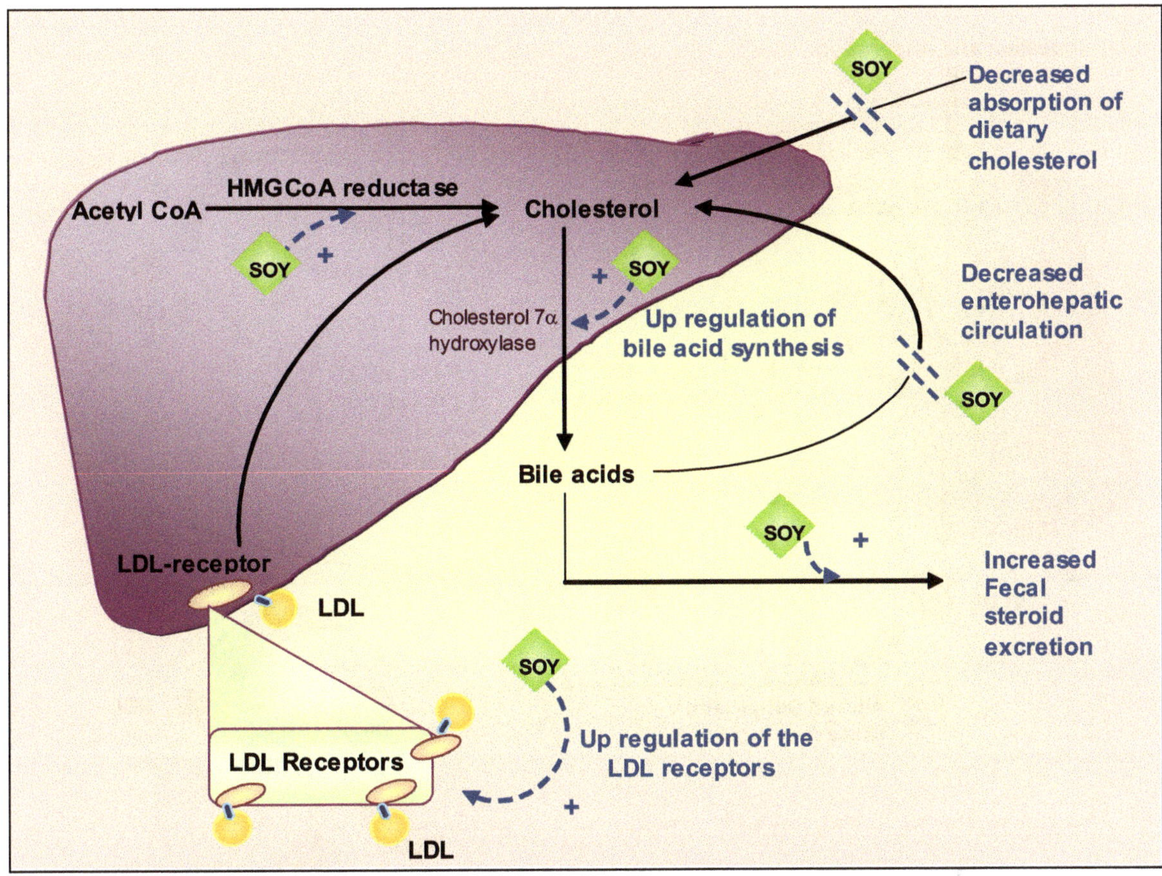

Figure 14.7: The Mechanism of Action of the Cholesterol Lowering Activity of Soy (Adapted from Potter, 1995)

Soy increases the conversion of cholesterol to bile acids. Consequently, hepatic cholesterol metabolism shifts to provide cholesterol for enhanced bile acid synthesis. As a result cholesterol biosynthesis as well as low density lipoprotein (LDL) receptor activity is increased. The net result is increased clearance of LDL from the plasma. Additionally, the uptake of bile acids and cholesterol from the intestine to the liver is also decreased.

isoflavones, anthocyanidins and proanthocyanidins, tannins such as theaflavins and gallic and ellagic acid esters as well as coumarins and stilbenes.

Some of the polyphenols that have been investigated for their effect on hyperlipidemia and atherosclerosis include polyphenols isolated from grapes, red wine, tea, citrus fruits, apple and soy. Studies have indicated that several factors contribute to the lipid lowering effects of the polyphenols (Figure 14.8) (Zern and Fernandez, 2005).

Resveratrol

Resveratrol, a stilbene polyphenol is perhaps the most well known therapeutically active polyphenol. While it is often mentioned exclusively in context of *Vitis vinifera* (grape) species, it was

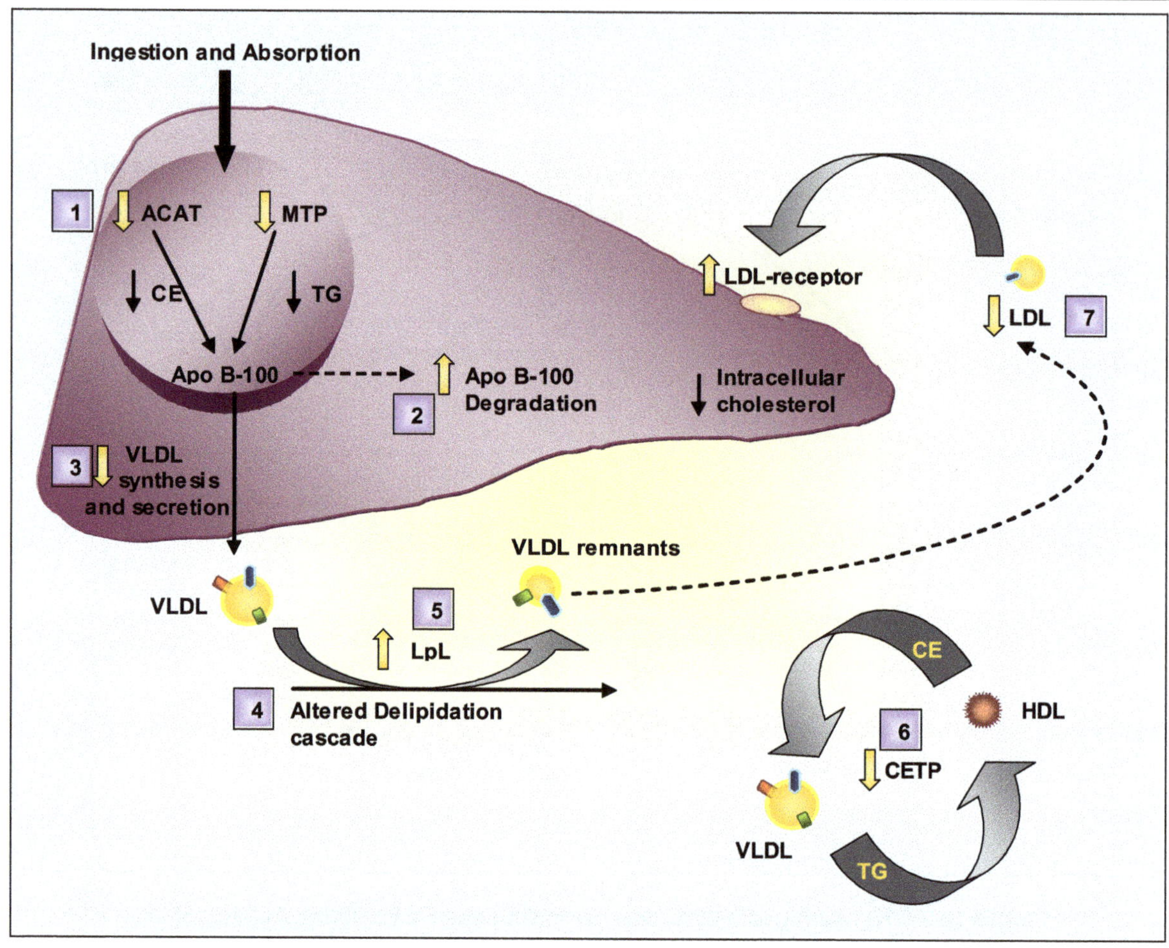

Figure 14.8: Pathways Contributing to the Lipid Lowering Effect of the Polyphenols (Adapted from Zern and Fernandez, 2005)

(1) Polyphenols decrease both MTP and ACAT activity involved in lipid assembly for VLDL secretion. (2) Without sufficient lipid components, the degradation of apo B-100 is increased. (3) The significant decrease in substrate availability results in a decrease in both VLDL synthesis and secretion. (4) The delipidation cascade is further altered due to the decrease in VLDL particles in circulation. (5) Alterations to the VLDL particle, including significant decreases in apo E, may induce an increase in LPL activity, and therefore, decrease plasma TG and VLDL concentrations. (6) CETP activity may also be affected by the decrease in VLDL substrate. (7) The VLDL decrease yields a significant decrease in LDL concentrations. Due to the significant alteration in hepatic cholesterol concentrations, the LDL receptor may be upregulated to maintain hepatic cholesterol homeostasis.

first isolated from the roots of white hellebore (*Veratrum grandiflorum*) in 1940, and later, in 1963, from the roots of *Polygonum cuspidatum*, a plant used in Oriental medicine (Baur and Sinclair, 2006). In the early 1990s resveratrol shot into prominence as the compound responsible for the cardioprotective effects of red wine (the French paradox).

Resveratrol has a multi pronged effect, addressing several aspects of atherosclerosis *viz.* decreased platelet aggregation, vasorelaxation, decreased expression of adhesion molecules and cytokines, reduced lipid peroxidation and improved serum cholesterol and triglyceride concentrations (Zern and Fernandez, 2005; Baur and Sinclair, 2006). Additionally, the protective effect of red wine has also been attributed to other phenolic compounds such as gallic acid, catechin and quercetin.

Tea Polyphenols

The leaves of the tea plant *Camellia sinensis* are a rich source of polyphenols like catechins eg. (-)-epigallocatechin-3-gallate (EGCG), (-)-epigallocatechin (EGC), (-)-epicatechin-3-gallate (ECG), (-)-epicatechin (EC), (+)-gallocatechin, and (+)-catechin as well as flavonoids such as theaflavins and thearubigins. Several studies indicate that these polyphenols reduce intestinal absorption of cholesterol possibly by interfering with micelle formation and solubility. Additionally, they are also known to upregulate the LDL receptor (Bays and Stein, 2003).

Naringenin and Hesperetin

The citrus fruits contain a diverse range of flavonoids including numerous flavanone and flavone O–and C-glycosides and methoxylated flavones. Naringenin and hesperetin belong to the class of flavonoids called flavanones. They are found in abundance as the glycosides naringin and hesperidin in grapefruit and oranges, respectively. These glycosides are hydrolyzed by intestinal bacteria to their active forms, naringenin and hesperetin.

It has been hypothesized that the hypocholesterolemic effect of the citrus juices are due to their flavonoid components. The mechanism of action of both naringenin and hesperetin is similar to the general mechanism proposed for polyphenols *viz.* mediating a decrease in the availability of lipids for assembly of apoB-containing lipoproteins, by reducing the activities of ACAT2 and MTP as well as promoting the expression of the LDL receptor (Wilcox *et al.*, 2001).

Dietary Fiber

Epidemiological studies have provided evidence that a high intake of dietary fiber may reduce the relative risk of coronary heart disease. This has prompted the US FDA to allow manufacturers to claim reduced CHD risk with high fiber products such as whole oat foods.

Dietary fiber generally implies non digestible carbohydrate components of plant parts. They are classified into two different types: soluble dietary fibers such as pectins, gums, β-glucans, starches and other storage polysaccharides and insoluble dietary fibers *viz.* cellulose and lignins. The soluble fibers are generally present in high levels in oats, barley, nuts, fruits, beans and vegetables while whole grains and cereals are a major food source of insoluble fiber. An excellent comprehensive review of the various types of dietary fiber, their sources and functions has been compiled by Tungland and Meyer (2002).

The soluble and insoluble fibers have very different influences on normal gut physiology and disease processes. Dietary insoluble fiber such as cellulose provides bulk, gentle laxation and ease of elimination. Due to its high affinity for water, cellulose increases stool weight, decreases transit time and intraluminal pressure (Tungland and Meyer, 2002).

Water soluble dietary fibers are known to effectively lower plasma cholesterol. The mechanism implicated is interference with bile acids absorption by biding and sequestering bile acids and reducing their reabsorption. This leads to increased diversion of cholesterol to bile acids in the liver, up regulation of lipoproteins receptors and decrease in plasma cholesterol.

However, many soluble fibers are extensively degraded by the colonic microflora and yet the bile acids are not fully absorbed. It has been demonstrated that the microflora in the colon has the capacity to ferment dietary fibers resulting in the production of short chain fatty acids such as acetate, propionate and butyrate which depress the solubility of the bile acids and their reabsorption.

Succinyl CoA that arises from propionate metabolism is known to stimulate the synthesis of bile acids via induction of cholesterol 7α hydroxylase. Propionate could also be an effective inhibitor of fatty acid synthesis and subsequent production of VLDL by the liver (Thomas *et al.*, 1983; Moundras *et al.*, 1994; Matheson *et al.*, 1995; Gerhardt and Gallo, 1998). Further, inulin oligofructans may also have a "prebiotic" effect and may stimulate useful colonic microflora, such as bifidobacteria which improve gut function and may also prevent bowel cancer (Loh *et al.*, 2006; Roberfroid, 2007).

Plant Derived Inhibitors of Pancreative Lipase and DGAT

In the recent years, obesity and its related disorders have become the focus of much research. Several prominent research workers have stressed the fact that obesity has reached epidemic proportions (Melnikova and Wages). Research into the mechanisms influencing the regulation of fat intake and absorption has gained momentum worldwide. Studies have demonstrated that as long as fat stays in the intestine, satiety is promoted. This satiety is mediated by the fat-stimulated peptide hormones, the best known being CCK (cholecystokinin). Hence, retarded fat digestion with prolonged time for delivery of fatty acids promotes satiety.

Pancreatic lipase (PL) is an exocrine enzyme of pancreatic juice that plays a key role in the hydrolysis of esters of glycerol and long-chain fatty acids, ultimately leading to the absorption of the fatty acids. Thus it is proposed that inhibition of pancreatic lipase reduces the efficiency of dietary fat absorption in the small intestine as well as promotes satiety. Further, researchers have recognized the potential of screening pancreatic lipase inhibitors from plant sources (Birari and Bhutani, 2007).

The bioactives of several plants used in traditional oriental medicine have demonstrated a significant inhibition of pancreatic lipase. These include chikusetsusaponins isolated from *Panax japonicus* rhizomes, triterpenoid saponins from *Acanthopanax senticosus* fruits and *Gypsophila oldhamiana* roots (Han *et al.*, 2005; Li *et al.*, 2007; Zheng *et al.*, 2007) Bioactives from the rhizomes of *Alpinia officinarum*, thylakoids isolated from chloroplast membranes and soy proteins have also demonstrated PL inhibitory activity (Gargouri *et al.*, 1984; Shin *et al.*, 2004; Albertsson *et al.*, 2007)

Acyl coenzyme A (CoA): diacylglycerol acyltransferase (DGAT) as discussed earlier is responsible for the re-esterification of the absorbed fatty acids and glycerol in the enterocyte and hepatocyte and is essential to the process of triglyceride formation. Flavonoids from *Sophora flavescens*, polyacetylenes from the roots of *Panax ginseng* and chalcone xanthohumols from *Humulus lupulus* are some of the bioactives that have demonstrated an inhibitory effect on DGAT which could have a beneficial effect in the management of obesity (Casaschi *et al.*, 2004; Chung *et al.*, 2004; Lee *et al.*, 2004).

General Trend in the Preclinical Screening of Plant Bioactives and Extracts as Antihyperlipidemics

In the area of research in medicinal plants having antihyperlipidemic potential, several *in vivo* as well as *in vitro* studies have been carried out. *In vivo* studies have generally involved the use of rats, rabbits and hamsters maintained on a high fat/cholesterol diet. Some studies have also been conducted on genetically altered animals such as ApoE knockout mice. With the incidence of obesity and the metabolic syndrome gaining ground in recent times, diabetic dyslipidemic animal models using

Table 14.1: Literature Survey of the Plants Investigated for Efficacy as Antihyperlipidemic Agents

Sl.No.	*Name of the Plant*	*Animal Model*	*Extract/Fraction*	*Parameters Measured*	*Reference*
1.	*Sophora flavescens*	Poloxamer 407-induced hyperlipidemic and cholesterol-fed rats	MeOH extract and 4 fractions	Total cholesterol (TC), triglycerides (TG), High density lipoprotein cholesterol (HDL-C), Low density lipoprotein cholesterol (LDL-C), Athero Index (A.I.)	Kim *et al.*, 2008
2.	*Cynodon dactylon*	Streptozotocin induced diabetic rats	Aqueous extract	Blood glucose, TC, TG, HDL-C, LDL-C	Singh *et al.*, 2007
3.	*Pueraria thunbergiana* (Flower)	✰ Trition WR1339-induced hyperlipidemic mice ✰ High fat diet induced hyperlipidemic mice	Kakkalide and irisolidone	TC, TG, epididymal fat pad weight.	Min and Kim, 2007
4.	*Ajuga iva* L. (whole plant)	Streptozotocin induced diabetic rats	Lyophilised aqueous extract	Blood glucose,TC, TG	El-Hilaly *et al.*, 2007
5.	*Momordica charantia* (Bitter gourd, karela; fruit)	✰ Alloxan induced diabetic rats ✰ Old obese rats	Fruit extract	Glycosylated haemoglobin, mean blood glucose, serum insulin, cholesterol, triglcerides, protein and glycogen content of liver. Serum LDL-C, HDL-C, VLDL-C, Histopathology of pancreas.	Fernandes *et al.*, 2007
6.	*Panax notoginseng* (root)	Sprague-Dawley male rats on a high-fat/high-cholesterol diet	*n*-butanol extract	Serum TC, TG, LDL-C, Hepatic TC, TG Express-level analysis of LXRalpha target genes and FXR target genes and LDLR mRNA level	Ji and Gong, 2007
7.	*Ulmus davidiana*	Triton WR-1339-induced mice	Glycoprotein	TC, TG, LDL-C Antioxidant assays: Thiobarbituric acid reactive species (TBARS), catalase and glutathione peroxidase (GPx), superoxide dismutase (SOD) activity and nitric oxide (NO) production	Ko *et al.*, 2007
8.	*Tribulus alatus* and *Tribulus terrestris* Comparative study	Diabetic rats	Alcoholic extract	Fasting glucose levels, glycosylated hemoglobin, TC, TG, LDL-C	El-Tantawy and Hassanin, 2007
9.	*Glycine max* L. (black soybean; seed coats)	High Fat Diet (16 per cent lard oil) induced hyperlipidemic rats	Anthocyanins	Body weight, adipose tissue weight, and serum lipids	Kwon *et al.*, 2007

Contd...

Table 14.1–Contd...

Sl.No.	Name of the Plant	Animal Model	Extract/Fraction	Parameters Measured	Reference
10.	Monascus-fermented red mold dioscorea (RMD)	High cholesterol diet-induced hyperlipidemic hamsters	Dietary inclusion	TC, TG, HDL-C LDL-C Total antioxidant status, catalase, SOD activity antilipid peroxidation.	Lee *et al.*, 2007
11.	*Cymbopogon citratus* (lemon grass; fresh leaves)	Normal male Wistar rats	Aqueous extract	Fasting glucose levels, Plasma TC, TG, HDL-C, LDL-C, VLDL-C Acute oral dose toxicity study.	Adeneye and Agbage, 2007
12.	*Eclipta prostrata* (leaves)	Atherogenic diet induced hyperlipidemic rats	Aqueous extract	TC, TG, HDL-C, total protein	Dhandapani, 2007
13.	*Panax ginseng* (red ginseng, steamed and dried root)	✰ Corn-oil-induced hyper-triglycemidemic mice ✰ Triton WR-1339-induced hyperlipidemic mice	Steamed and dried root (RG) and Bifidodoterium-fermented (FRG) Saponin and Polysaccha-ride fractions of RG and FRG	Serum TC, TG, postprandial blood glucose elevation	Trinh *et al.*, 2007
14.	*Pleurospermum kamtschaticum*	✰ Poloxamer-407 induced rats ✰ Triton WR-1339-induced rats ✰ 30 per cent corn oil diet induced rats ✰ High cholesterol diet induced rats	MeOH extract and its fractions Buddlejasaponin IV isolated from the BuOH fraction	Serum TC, TG, HDL-C, LDL-C Blood TBARS, hydroxy radical levels, SOD activity	Jung *et al.*, 2007
15.	*Telfairia occidentalis* (fluted pumpkin)	High cholesterol diet induced rats	Mixed in diet	Plasma TC, heart enlargement. Lipid peroxidation assay	Adaramoye *et al.*, 2007
16.	*Cichorium intybus*	Streptozotocin-induced diabetic rats	Ethanolic (80 per cent) extract	Glucose tolerance test, serum glucose, TC, TG, insulin levels, hepatic glucose-6-phosphatase activity	Pushparaj *et al.*, 2007
17.	*Nardostachys jatamansi*	Doxorubicin (15mg/kg) intoxicated rats resulting in myocardial injury.	Ethanolic extract	Serum and cardiac lipids (cholesterol, triglycerides, free fatty acids and phospholipids), Lipid metabolizing enzymes, Histopathology.	Subashini *et al.*, 2007

Contd...

Table 14.1–Contd...

Sl.No.	Name of the Plant	Animal Model	Extract/Fraction	Parameters Measured	Reference
18.	Cocoa product rich in dietary fiber naturally containing antioxidant polyphenols	Rats fed a high cholesterol diet	Cocoa product	Serum lipid profile, total antioxidant capacity, and malondialdehyde. Antioxidant enzymes: catalase, glutathione reductase (GR), glutathione peroxidase (GPx), and superoxide dismutase (SOD). Concentrations of glutathione and malondialdehyde in the liver.	Lecumberri *et al.*, 2007
19.	*Ananas comosus* L. (pineapple ; leaves)	☆ Fructose-fed mice ☆ High-fat diet fed mice ☆ Alloxan induced mice ☆ Triton WR-1339-induced hyperlipidemic mice	Ethanolic extract	Serum lipid profile, lipoprotein lipase (LPL), HMGCoA reductase activity, liver weight.	Xie *et al.*, 2007
20.	*Aronia melanocarpa* (Black chokeberry; fruit)	Streptozotocin-induced diabetic rats	Juice (rich in phenolic antioxidants *viz.* flavonoids from the anthocyanin subclass)	Plasma glucose, TC, TG, HDL-C, LDL-C	Valcheva-Kuzmanova *et al.*, 2007
21.	*Ajuga iva* L.	Rats fed a high cholesterol (1 per cent) diet	Aqueous extract	Plasma TC, TG, HDL-C, VLDL-C. TBARS, glutathione reductase, superoxide dismutase glutathione peroxidase activity in the liver, heart, kidney and adipose tissue.	Chenni *et al.*, 2007
22.	*Morus alba* L (Mulberry; leaves)	Triton WR-1339 induced hyperlipidemic mice	Total flavonoids	Serum TC, TG, HDL-C, LDL-C	Chen and Li, 2007
23.	*Cinnamonum zeylanicum* (cinnamon; bark)	Streptozotocin-induced diabetic rats	Cinnamaldehyde	Plasma glucose, glycosylated hemoglobin (HbA(1C), insulin Plasma enzymes: aspartate amino transferase (AST), alanine amino transferase (ALT), lactate dehydrogenase (LDH), alkaline phosphatase (AP), Serum TC, TG, HDL-C. Hepatic glycogen	Subash Babu *et al.*, 2007
24.	*Momordica charantia* (Bitter gourd/karela; fruit)	Alloxan-induced diabetic rats	Juice and alcoholic extract	Serum TC, TG, glucose, urea, creatinine, ALT, AST and AP	Abd El Sattar El Batran, 2006

Contd...

Table 14.1–Contd...

Sl.No.	Name of the Plant	Animal Model	Extract/Fraction	Parameters Measured	Reference
25.	*Diospyros kaki* (Persimmon; leaf)	Rats fed a high fat diet	Powdered whole leaf	Plasma TC, TG, HDL-C, A.I., leptin. Hepatic cholesterol and triglyceride. Hepatic lipid droplet accumulation Hepatic HMG-CoA and ACAT activities. Body weight and relative weight of interscapular brown adipose tissue, epididymal white adipocyte size. Fecal triglyceride, cholesterol and acidic sterol	Lee *et al.*, 2006
26.	*Lagenaria siceraria* (Bottle gourd; fruit)	✰ Triton-induced hyperlipidemic rats. ✰ Normocholesteremic rats.	Four different extracts: petroleum ether– (NOT EFFECTIVE), chloroform, alcoholic and aqueous extracts	Serum TC, TG, HDL-C	Ghule *et al.*, 2006
27.	*Opuntia ficus-indica* (Prickly pear cactus; fruit)	Triton WR-1339-induced mice	Isolated glycoprotein	Plasma TC, TG, HDL-C TBARS and NO levels Antioxidant enzymes:SOD, CAT and GPx	Oh and Lim, 2006
28.	*Withania coagulans* (fruits)	High fat diet induced hyperlipidemic rats	Aqueous extract	Serum TC, TG, HDL-C Histopathology of liver.	Hemalatha *et al.*, 2006
29.	*Ajuga iva* (whole plant)	Normal and streptozotocin (STZ) induced diabetic rats	Lyophilized aqueous extract	Lipid profile	El-Hilaly *et al.*, 2006
30.	*Morus alba* L. (mulberry; root bark)	Rats fed high fat (25 per cent coconut oil) high cholesterol (2 per cent) diet.	3 fractions obtained by column chromatography of the 70 per cent alcohol extract	Plasma TC, TG, HDL-C, LDL-C plasma and liver lipid peroxides and glutathione-S-transferase enzyme levels, serum paraoxonase enzyme level, LDL oxidation, LDL aggregation and LDL retention	El-Beshbishy, 2006
31.	*Scoparia dulcis* (sweet broomweed; whole plant)	Normal and streptozotocin (STZ) induced diabetic rats	Aqueous extract	Blood glucose, serum LDL-C, HDL-C, Athero Index Serum and tissue cholesterol, triglycerides, free fatty acids, phospholipids. Hepatic HMGCoA reductase activity	Pari and Latha, 2006
32.	*Allium porrum* L. (leek; bulbs)	Rabbits fed a high cholesterol diet	Hydroalcoholic extract	Plasma TC, TG, HDL-C, LDL-C.	Movahedian *et al.*, 2006

Contd...

Table 14.1–Contd...

Sl.No.	Name of the Plant	Animal Model	Extract/Fraction	Parameters Measured	Reference
33.	*Inula japonica* (flower)	Alloxan induced diabetic mice	Aqueous extract and Two fractions	Oral glucose tolerance test Plasma glucose and insulin levels Serum triglyceride levels	Shan *et al.*, 2006
34.	*Rhus verniciflua* stokes (fruit)	Triton WR-1339 induced hyperlipidemic mice.	Glycoprotein	Plasma TC, TG, HDL-C, LDL-C, HMG-CoA reductase TBARS, nitric oxide production Anti-oxidant enzymes: catalase (CAT), superoxide dismutase (SOD), and glutathione peroxidase (GPx)	Oh *et al.*, 2006
35.	*Hibiscus sabdariffa* (roselle; dried calyx)	Rats fed a high cholesterol diet	Aqueous extract	Serum TC, TG, HDL-C, LDL-C TBARS and conjugated dienes formed during LDL oxidation	Hirunpanich *et al.*, 2006
36.	*Gardenia jasminoides* (fructus)	✰ Corn oil feeding-induced triglyceridemic mice ✰ Triton WR-1339-induced hyperlipidemic mice ✰ Mice fed a high cholesterol diet ✰ Mice fed a high fat diet ✰ Mice fed a high carbohydrate diet	Crocetin and crocin obtained from the aqueous extract	Serum lipid profile Pancreatic lipase activity	Lee *et al.*, 2005
37.	*Clerodendron cole-brookianum* (leaves)	Ischemic-reperfusion injury in isolated rat hearts	Aqueous extract	Endogenous antioxidant enzyme activities (SOD, Catalase, GSH and GPx) Lipid peroxidation	Devi *et al.*, 2005
38.	*Eugenia jambolana* (Jamun; seed kernel)	Streptozotocin-induced diabetes in rats.	Ethanolic extract	Cholesterol, phospholipids, triglycerides and free fatty acids levels in the plasma, liver and kidney	Ravi *et al.*, 2005
39.	*Dolichos biflorus* Linn.	Rats fed a high fat diet.	Methanolic extract	Plasma TC, TG, LDL-C, HDL-C, tissue cholesterol	Muthu *et al.*, 2005
40.	*Melissa officinalis* (Lemon balm; leaves)	Rats fed a lipid diet containing 2 per cent cholesterol, 20 per cent sunflower oil and 0.5 per cent cholic acid added to normal chow Additionally 3 per cent ethanol was also administered daily.	Extract	Serum total cholesterol, total lipid, ALT, AST, ALP. Liver tissue glutathione and lipid peroxidation. Microscopic examination of the liver.	Bolkent *et al.*, 2005

Contd...

Table 14.1–Contd...

Sl.No.	Name of the Plant	Animal Model	Extract/Fraction	Parameters Measured	Reference
41.	*Boswellia serrata* (Frankincense, Salai guggal; oleoresin gum)	Rats fed a lipid diet (2.5 per cent cholesterol, 1 per cent cholic acid, 15.7 per cent saturated fat) Lipopolysaccharide induced nitric oxide (NO) production by macro-phages under *in vivo* and *in vitro* conditions.	Water-soluble fraction of the oleoresin gum	Serum lipid profile, blood urea, serum glutamate-pyruvate transaminase (SGPT) Transverse section of liver and kidneys.	Pandey *et al.*, 2005
42.	Dioscorea rhizome (yam; tuberous rhizomes)	Rabbits fed a lipid diet (0.5 per cent cholesterol and 10 per cent corn oil)	Powdered rhizome	Serum TC, TG. Lucigenin chemiluminescence, and luminol chemiluminescence. Antioxidant enzymes: superoxide dismutase and catalase Hepatic DNA 8-hydroxy-2'-deoxygua-nosine (8-OHdG), Aortic histopathology.	Chang *et al.*, 2005
43.	*Averrhoa bilimbi* (Bimbli; leaves)	High fat diet fed-streptozotocin-induced diabetic rats.	Semi-purified fractions of the 80 per cent ethanolic extract	Blood glucose, TC, TG, HDL-C. Liver TBARS Cytochrome P450 values.	Tan *et al.*, 2005
44.	*Capparis spinosa*	✰ Streptozotocin-induced diabetic rats. ✰ Normal rats.	Aqueous extract	Plasma TC, TG, body weight	Eddouks *et al.*, 2005
45.	*Iris germanica*	Rats fed high fat diet	Ethanolic extract	Serum TC, TG, HDL-C, total lipids.	Choudhary *et al.*, 2005
46.	*Malus domestica* (Apple; fruit)	Human Caco2/TC7 enterocytes	Procyanidins	Cholesteryl ester synthesis and Lipoprotein secretion.	Vidal *et al.*, 2005
47.	*Camellia sinensis*	Normal rats (tea; leaves)	Oolong, black, puerh, and green tea	Serum TC, TG, HDL-C, LDL-C Antioxidant enzyme SOD Body weight	Kuo *et al.*, 2005
48.	*Ananas comosus* (Pineapple; leaves)	Diabetic-dyslipidemic rats induced by alloxan and a high-fat/high-cholesterol diet.	Ethanolic extract	Oral glucose tolerance test Blood glucose, Postprandial TG Serum TC, TG, LDL-C, HDL-C Glycated albumin Lipid peroxidation products in the blood, brain, liver, kidneys	Xie *et al.*, 2005

Contd...

Table 14.1–Contd...

Sl.No.	Name of the Plant	Animal Model	Extract/Fraction	Parameters Measured	Reference
49.	*Lycium barbarum* (Chinese Wolfberry/ Himalayan Goji berry; fruit)	Alloxan-induced diabetic or hyperlipidemic rabbits	Water decoction, Crude polysaccharide extract Purified polysaccharide fraction	Blood glucose, serum TC, TG, HDL-C. Total antioxidant capacity: Trolox equivalent antioxidant capacity (TEAC) and Oxygen radical absorbance capacity (ORAC) assay.	Luo *et al.*, 2004
50.	*Nigella sativa* (Kalonji; seeds)	Normal rats	Petroleum ether extract	Plasma glucose, insulin, TC, TG, HDL-C. Response to insulin was evaluated in hepatocytes isolated from animals of all groups by Western blot analysis of phosphorylated MAPK p44/42erk and PKB.	Le *et al.*, 2004
51.	*Curcuma longa* (Turmeric; rhizome) Capsicum species (Chilli peppers; fruit) Allium sativum (Garlic; bulb)	Rats fed a high-fat (30 per cent) diet	Curcumin, Capsaicin and Garlic	Antioxidant status of red blood cells: Intracellular total thiols, glutathione, lipid peroxides content of erythrocytes. Hepatic antioxidant enzyme levels.	Kempaiah and Srinivasan, 2004
52.	*Coriandrum sativum*	Triton-induced hyperlipidemic rats		TC, TG	Lal *et al.*, 2004
53.	*Humulus lupulus* (Hops; female flowers)	Diabetic KK-Ay mice C57BL/6N mice fed a high fat diet	Isohumulones	Plasma glucose, triglyceride, and free fatty acid levels. Glucose tolerance and insulin resistance. Liver fatty acids oxidation Size and apoptosis of adipocytes	Yajima *et al.*, 2004
54.	*Momordica charantia* (Bitter gourd/melon, karela; fruit)	Golden Syrian hamsters fed diets supplemented with and without cholesterol.	Methanolic fraction	Food efficiency (weight gain/food intake) Serum TC, TG. Liver triglyceride and total cholesterol	Senanayake *et al.*, 2004
55.	*Coix lachrymajobi* (Adlay; seed)	High fat diet induced obesity (DIO) rats	Crude extract	Food intake, body weight, weights of epididymal and peritoneal fat. Microscopic examination of the size of the adipocytes of white adipose tissue (WAT) Leptin and TNF-alpha mRNA expressions in WAT Serum TC, TG, Leptin.	Kim *et al.*, 2004

Contd...

Table 14.1–Contd...

Sl.No.	Name of the Plant	Animal Model	Extract/Fraction	Parameters Measured	Reference
56.	*Nigella sativa* (Kalonji; seeds)	Primary cultured mouse hepatocytes	Diterpene alkaloids isolated from the methanolic extract: [nigellamines A3, A4, A5, and C]	Triglycerides	Morikawa *et al.*, 2004
57.	*Semecarpus anacardium* (Marking nut/Oriental cashew; nuts	✰ Rats fed an atherogenic diet ✰ Rat peritoneal macrophages cell culture	Fraction	Serum lipid profile. Liver and kidneys function tests. LPS induced NO production in cell culture	Tripathi and Pandey, 2004
58.	*Cocos nucifera* (Coconut; fruit)	Ethanol fed rats	Coconut kernel protein	Serum TC, TG, Athero index, LpL. HMG-CoA reductase, malic enzyme, glucose-6-phosphate dehydrogenase activity in the liver. Fecal excretion of neutral sterols and bile acids.	Mini and Rajamohan, 2004
59.	*Clerodendron colebrookianum* (leaves)	✰ Rats fed a High-fat diet ✰ Normal rats	Crude extract Methanolic extract Ethylacetate extract	Serum TC, TG, HDL-C, LDL-C.	Devi and Sharma, 2004
60.	*Argania spinosa* (seeds)	Meriones shawi rodents (Gerbillideae family) fed a high calorie and high cholesterol diet.	Argan oil	Serum TC, TG, HDL-C, LDL-C	Berrougui *et al.*, 2003
61.	*Alpinia officinarum* (Galangal; rhizome)	✰ Corn oil feeding-induced triglyceridemic mice. ✰ Triton WR-1339-induced hyperlipidemic mice. ✰ High cholesterol diet-induced hyperlipidemic mice. (NOT EFFECTIVE) ✰ Pancreatic lipase *in vitro* assay.	Ethyl acetate fraction of the aqueous extract and 3-Methyl ether galangin isolated from the ethylacetate fraction of the aqueous extract.	Serum TC, TG Pancreatic lipase activity	Shina *et al.*, 2003
62.	*Eugenia jambolana* (Jamun; seed kernel)	Alloxan-induced diabetic rabbits	Ethanol extract	Blood glucose, glycosylated haemoglobin (GHb), serum insulin level. Serum TC, LDL-C, HDL-C. Liver and muscle glycogen content Histopathological studies of liver, pancreas and aorta	Sharma *et al.*, 2003

Contd...

Table 14.1–Contd...

Sl.No.	Name of the Plant	Animal Model	Extract/Fraction	Parameters Measured	Reference
63.	*Opuntia ficus-indica* (Prickly pear cactus; fruit)	Patients with isolated heterozygous familial hypercholesterolemia (FH)	Dietary inclusion	Uptake of autologous (123)I-radiolabeled LDL by the liver	Palumbo *et al.*, 2003
64.	*Acorus calamus* (Sweet flag/Vekhand; rhizome)	Rats fed hyperlipidemic diet.	50 per cent Ethanolic extract. Aqueous extract Saponins	Serum TC, TG, HDL-C.	Parab and Mengi, 2002
65.	*Arachis hypogaea* (Peanut/groundnut)	✰ Alloxan induced diabetic rats ✰ Normal rats	Aqueous extract	Blood glucose, serum TC, TG, HDL-C, LDL-C.	Bilbis *et al.*, 2002
66.	*Emblica officinalis* (Gooseberry/Amla; fruit) and *Mangifera indica* (Mango; fruit)	Hyperlipidmeic rats	Flavonoids	Lipid levels in serum and tissues. HMG CoA reductase activity. LCAT activity.	Anila and Vijayalakshmi, 2002
67.	*Crataegus monogyna* (Hawthorn; dried fruits)	Rabbits fed a high cholesterol (1 per cent) diet	Fruit powder	Serum TC, TG, HMG CoA reductase, 7alpha-hydroxylase, intestinal acyl CoA:cholesterol acyltransferase activity.	Zhang *et al.*, 2002
68.	*Teucrium polium* (Felty Germander; aerial parts)	Hyperlipidmeic rats	Aqueous extract	Serum TC and TG *et al.*, 2001	Rasekh
69.	*Cocos nucifera* (Coconut; fruit)	Rats fed high fat, high cholesterol diet	Coconut protein	Serum TC, TG, HDL-C, LDL-C Hepatic cholesterogenesis Fecal excretion of bile acids Superoxide dismutase and Catalase activity and malondialdehyde content of the heart.	Salil and Rajamohan, 2001
70.	Dietary plant stanol esters derived from vegetable oil (sitostanol 65.7 per cent, campestanol 30.1 per cent) and from wood (sitostanol 87.6 per cent,campestanol 9.5 per cent)	ApoE*3-Leiden transgenic mice	Dietary plant stanol esters	Plasma TC, LDL-C, IDL-C, VLDL-C. Atherosclerotic lesion area. Adherence of monocytes to the vessel wall.	Volger *et al.*, 2001

Contd...

Table 14.1–Contd...

Sl.No.	Name of the Plant	Animal Model	Extract/Fraction	Parameters Measured	Reference
71.	*Momordica cymbalaria* (fruit)	Alloxan-induced diabetic rats	Fruit powder	Fasting blood glucose, Serum TC, TG. Hepatic glycogen level	Rao *et al.*, 1999
72.	*Salvadora persica* (Toothbrush tree/ Miswak; stem)	✰ Rats fed a hypercholesterolemic diet ✰ Triton induced hyperlipidemic rats	Lyophilized stem decoction	Serum TC,TG, HDL-C, LDL-C	Galati *et al.*, 1999
73.	*Terminalia arjuna* (Arjuna; bark), *Terminalia belerica* (Bibbhitaki; fruits), *Terminalia chebula* (Chebulic myrobalan/ Haritaki; fruits)	Rabbits fed cholesterol-enriched diet	Dietary inclusion	Plasma and tissue lipid components. Histopathological examination of the aorta.	Shaila *et al.*, 1998
74.	*Diospyros kaki* (Persimmon; leaf)	✰ Rats fed a high cholesterol (1 per cent) diet ✰ Normal rats	Dietary inclusion	Plasma TC, TG, HDL-C Liver TC Lipid peroxides	Gorinstein *et al.*, 1998
75.	*Cocos nucifera* (Coconut; fruit)	Normal rats	Hemicellulose component of coconut fiber	Serum TC, TG, HDL-C HMG CoA reductase activity Incorporation of labeled acetate into free cholesterol. Hepatic bile acids concentration Fecal sterols and bile acids excretion.	Sindhurani and Rajamohan, 1998

streptozotocin (an agent that damages the pancreatic β-cells) have also been employed. In the *in vivo* studies the plant bioactives have been mainly evaluated for their effect on lipid profile, total liver lipids, fecal neutral sterols and bile acids. Additionally, several antioxidant enzymes such as superoxide dismutase (SOD), catalase (CAT) and glutathione peroxidase (GSH) have also been estimated. Free radical scavenging and antilipid peroxidation assays have been performed by *in vitro* as well as *in vivo* methods.

Cell based assays using hepatic and intestinal cell lines have aided in the elucidation of the mechanism of action of some of the plant bioactives. For example, it was confirmed that apple procyanidins significantly decreased the lipoprotein synthesis and secretion by the intestine using human Caco-2/TC7 enterocytes apically supplied with complex lipid micelles (Vidal *et al.*, 2005), while the inhibitory effects of bioactives of garlic on triglyceride incorporation into VLDL was studied in cultured rat hepatocytes (Liu and Yeh, 2001). The current focus of research in antihyperlipidemic plant bioactives encompasses crude extracts as well as highly characterized fractions and isolated bioactives. The plants that have been investigated range from medicinal plants mentioned in the traditional systems of medicine to those used as spices and food products with purported health benefits. Table 14.1 represents a literature search (excluding topics discussed in earlier sections) of relevant preclinical research, investigating a range of plant bioactives that have demonstrated considerable potential in the management of hyperlipidemia, but have yet to be critically evaluated in clinical studies.

Conclusion and Summary

Knowledge of the mechanism of action involved in lipid homeostasis has expanded rapidly in the last two decades. Moreover, high throughput techniques have enabled the pharmaceutical industry to screen a large number of molecules at a faster rate. However, the expected increase in new drugs has not been forthcoming due to safety and efficacy issues. On the other hand the current times could be the proverbial golden opportunity for research workers in the area of plant bioactives for hyperlipidemia and the metabolic syndrome. With the knowledge of a wider variety of therapeutic targets as well as analytical techniques at their disposal, screening of medicinal plants to identify lead molecules or bioactive fractions could provide newer therapeutic options or supplement and enhance the existing therapies. Identification of the molecular targets and mechanism of action of several plant bioactives in hyperlipidemia has provided an added impetus to the interest in plant research. While plant bioactives have a tremendous potential in the management of hyperlipidemia, the challenge is to standardize these bioactives to ensure consistent efficacy and also to subject these bioactives to rigorous testing and trials on par with the evaluation of synthetic molecules.

References

Abd El Sattar El Batran, S., El-Gengaihi, S.E., and El Shabrawy, O.A. (2006). Some toxicological studies of *Momordica charantia* L. on albino rats in normal and alloxan diabetic rats. *Journal of Ethnopharmacology*,108 (2): 236-242.

Adaramoye, O.A., Achem, J., Akintayo, O.O., and Fafunso, M.A. (2007). Hypolipidemic effect of *Telfairia occidentalis* (fluted pumpkin) in rats fed a cholesterol-rich diet. *Journal of Medicinal Foods*, 10(2): 330-336.

Adeneye, A.A., and Agbaje, E.O. (2007). Hypoglycemic and hypolipidemic effects of fresh leaf aqueous extract of *Cymbopogon citratus* Stapf. in rats. *Journal of Ethnopharmacology*, 112(3): 440-444.

Agarwal, R.C., Singh, S.P., Saran, R.K., Das, S.K., Sinha, N., Asthana, O.P., Gupta, P.P., Nityanand, S., Dhawan, B.N., and Agarwal, S.S. (1986). Clinical trial of gugulipid—a new hypolipidemic agent of plant origin in primary hyperlipidemia. *Indian Journal of Medical Research*, 84: 626-634.

Albertsson, P.A., Köhnke, R., Emek, S.C., Mei, J., Rehfeld, J.F., Akerlund, H.E., and Erlanson-Albertsson, C. (2007). Chloroplast membranes retard fat digestion and induce satiety: effect of biological membranes on pancreatic lipase/co-lipase. *Biochemistry Journal*, 401(3): 727-733.

Altmann, S.W., Davis, H.R., Yao, X., Tetzloff, G., Iyer, S.P., Maguire, M., Golovko, A., Zeng, M., Wang, L., Murgolo, N., and Graziano, M.P. (2004). Niemann-Pick C1 Like 1 protein is critical for intestinal cholesterol absorption. *Science*, 303:1201-1204.

Amagase, H. (2006). Clarifying the real bioactive constituents of garlic. *Journal of Nutrition*, 136: 716S–725S.

Anila, L., and Vijayalakshmi, N.R. (2002). Flavonoids from *Emblica officinalis* and *Mangifera indica*-effectiveness for dyslipidemia. *Journal of Ethnopharmacology*, 79(1): 81-87.

Balachandran, P., and Govindarajan, R. (2007). Ayurvedic drug discovery. *Expert Opinion on Drug Discovery*, 2(12):1631-1652.

Banerjee, S.K., and Maulik, S.K. (2002) Effect of garlic on cardiovascular disorders: a review. *Nutrition Journal*, 1: 1-14.

Baur, J.A., and Sinclair, D.A. (2006). Therapeutic potential of resveratrol: the *in vivo* evidence. *Nature Reviews Drug Discovery*, 5: 493-506.

Bays, H., and Stein, E.A. (2003). Pharmacotherapy for dyslipidaemia–current therapies and future agents. *Expert Opinion on Pharmacotherapy*, 4(11): 1901-1938.

Berrougui, H., Ettaib, A., Herrera Gonzalez, M.D., Alvarez de Sotomayor, M., Bennani-Kabchi, N., and Hmamouchi, M. (2003). Hypolipidemic and hypocholesterolemic effect of argan oil (*Argania spinosa* L.) in Meriones shawi rats. *Journal of Ethnopharmacology*, 89(1): 15-8.

Bilbis, L.S., Shehu, R.A., and Abubakar, M.G. (2002). Hypoglycemic and hypolipidemic effects of aqueous extract of *Arachis hypogaea* in normal and alloxan-induced diabetic rats. *Phytomedicine*, 9(6): 553-555.

Birari, R.B., and Bhutani, K.K. (2007). Pancreatic lipase inhibitors from natural sources: unexplored potential. *Drug Discovery Today*, 12(19-20): 879-889.

Blankenhorn, D.H., Azen, S.P., Kramsch, D.M., Mack, W.J., Cashin-Hemphill, L., Hodis, H.N., DeBoer, L.W., Mahrer, P.R., Masteller, M.J., Vailas, L.I., Alaupovic, P., and Hirsch, L.J. (1993). Coronary angiographic changes with lovastatin therapy: the Monitored Atherosclerosis Regression Study (MARS). *Annals of Internal Medicine*, 119(10): 969-976.

Bolkent, S., Yanardag, R., Karabulut-Bulan, O., and Yesilyaprak, B. (2005). Protective role of *Melissa officinalis* L. extract on liver of hyperlipidemic rats: a morphological and biochemical study. *Journal of Ethnopharmacology*, 99(3): 391-8.

Brown, M.S., and Goldstein, J.L. (1986). A receptor-mediated pathway for cholesterol homeostasis. *Science*, 232: 34-47.

Burnett, J.R., and Watts, G.F. (2007). MTP inhibition as a treatment for dyslipidemias: time to deliver or empty promises. *Expert Opinion on Therapeutic Targets*, 11(2): 181-189.

Casaschi, A., Maiyoh, G.K., Rubio, B.K., Li, R.W., Adeli, K., and Theriault, A.G. (2004). The chalcone xanthohumol inhibits triglyceride and apolipoprotein B secretion in HepG2 cells. *Journal of Nutrition,* 134: 1340–1346.

Chang, W.C., Yu, Y.M., Wu, C.H., Tseng, Y.H., and Wu, K.Y. (2005). Reduction of oxidative stress and atherosclerosis in hyperlipidemic rabbits by Dioscorea rhizome. *Canadian Journal of Physiology and Pharmacology,* 83(5): 423-430.

Chen, J., and Li, X. (2007). Hypolipidemic effect of flavonoids from mulberry leaves in triton WR-1339 induced hyperlipidemic mice. *Asia Pacific Journal of Clinical Nutrition,* 16(1): 290-294.

Chenni, A., Yahia, D.A., Boukortt, F.O., Prost, J., Lacaille-Dubois, M.A., and Bouchenak, M. (2007). Effect of aqueous extract of *Ajuga iva* supplementation on plasma lipid profile and tissue antioxidant status in rats fed a high-cholesterol diet. *Journal of Ethnopharmacology,* 109(2): 207-213.

Choudhary, M.I., Naheed, S., Jalil, S., Alam, J.M., and Atta-ur-Rahman. (2005). Effects of ethanolic extract of *Iris germanica* on lipid profile of rats fed on a high-fat diet. *Journal of Ethnopharmacology,* 98(1-2): 217-220.

Chung, M.Y., Rho, M.C., Ko, J.S., Ryu, S.Y., Jeune, K.H., Kim, K., Lee, H.S., and Kim, Y.K. (2004). *In vitro* inhibition of diacylglycerol acyltransferase by prenylflavonoids from *Sophora flavescens. Planta Medica,* 70: 258–260.

Claudel, T., Staels, B., and Kuipers, F. (2005). The Farnesoid X Receptor: A molecular link between bile acids and lipid and glucose metabolism. *Arteriosclerosis Thrombosis and Vascular Biology,* 25: 2020-2030.

Cui, J., Huang, L., Zhao, A., Lew, J.L., Yu, J., Sahoo, S., Meinke, P.T., Royo, I., Pelaez, F., and Wright, S.D. (2003). Guggulsterone is a farnesoid X receptor antagonist in coactivator association assays but acts to enhance transcription of bile salt export pump. *Journal of Biological Chemistry,* 278: 10214–10220.

Deng, R., Yang, D., Radke, A., Yang, J., and Yan, B. (2007). The hypolipidemic agent guggulsterone regulates the expression of human bile salt export pump: dominance of transactivation over Farsenoid X Receptor-mediated antagonism. *Journal of Pharmacology and Experimental Therapeutics,* 320(3):1153-1162.

Desroches, S., Mauger, J.F., Ausman, L.M., Lichtenstein, A.H., and Lamarche, B. (2004). Soy protein favorably affects LDL size independently of isoflavones in hypercholesterolemic men and women. *Journal of Nutrition,* 134: 574–579.

Devi, R., Banerjee, S.K., Sood, S., Dinda, A.K., and Maulik, S.K. (2005). Extract from *Clerodendron colebrookianum* Walp protects rat heart against oxidative stress induced by ischemic-reperfusion injury (IRI). *Life Sciences,* 77(24): 2999-3009.

Devi, R., and Sharma, D.K. (2004). Hypolipidemic effect of different extracts of *Clerodendron colebrookianum* Walp in normal and high-fat diet fed rats. *Journal of Ethnopharmacology,* 90(1): 63-68.

Dhandapani, R. (2007). Hypolipidemic activity of *Eclipta prostrata* (L.) L. leaf extract in atherogenic diet induced hyperlipidemic rats. *Indian Journal of Experimenal Biology,* 45(7): 617-619.

Duan, L.P., Wang, H.H., and Wang, D.Q. (2004). Cholesterol absorption is mainly regulated by the jejunal and ileal ATP-binding cassette sterol efflux transporters Abcg5 and Abcg8 in mice. *Journal of Lipid Research,* 45:1312–1323.

Eddouks, M., Lemhadri, A., and Michel, J.B. (2005). Hypolipidemic activity of aqueous extract of *Capparis spinosa* L. in normal and diabetic rats. *Journal of Ethnopharmacology,* 98(3): 345-350.

El-Beshbishy, H.A., Singab, A.N., Sinkkonen, J., and Pihlaja, K. (2006). Hypolipidemic and antioxidant effects of *Morus alba* L. (Egyptian mulberry) root bark fractions supplementation in cholesterol-fed rats. *Life Sciences,* 78(23): 2724-2733.

El-Hilaly, J., Tahraoui, A., Israili, Z.H., and Lyoussi, B. (2007). Acute hypoglycemic, hypocholesterolemic and hypotriglyceridemic effects of continuous intravenous infusion of a lyophilised aqueous extract of *Ajuga iva* L. Schreber whole plant in streptozotocin-induced diabetic rats. *Pakistan Jouranl of Pharmaceutical Sciences,* 20(4): 261-268.

El-Hilaly, J., Tahraoui, A., Israili, Z.H., and Lyoussi, B. (2006). Hypolipidemic effects of acute and sub-chronic administration of an aqueous extract of *Ajuga iva* L. whole plant in normal and diabetic rats. *Journal of Ethnopharmacology,* 105(3): 441-448.

El-Tantawy, W.H., and Hassanin, L.A. (2007). Hypoglycemic and hypolipidemic effects of alcoholic extract of *Tribulus alatus* in streptozotocin-induced diabetic rats: a comparative study with *T. terrestris* (Caltrop). *Indian Journal of Experimental Biology,* 45(9):785-790.

Erdman, J.W. (2000). AHA Science Advisory: soy protein and cardiovascular disease: a statement for healthcare professionals from the Nutrition. Committee of the AHA. *Circulation,* 102: 2555–2559.

Espirito Santo, M.S., Vlijmen, B.J.M., Buytenhek, R., Duyvenvoorde, W., Havekes, L.M., Arnault, I., Auger, J., and Princen, H.M.G. (2004). Well-characterized garlic-derived materials are not hypolipidemic in ApoE*3-leiden transgenic Mice. *Journal of Nutrition,* 134: 1500–1503.

Fernandes, N.P., Lagishetty, C.V., Panda, V.S., and Naik, S.R. (2007). An experimental evaluation of the antidiabetic and antilipidemic properties of a standardized *Momordica charantia* fruit extract. *BMC Complementary and Alternative Medicine,* 7: 29.

Galati, E.M., Monforte, M.T., Forestieri, A.M., Miceli, N., Bader, A., and Trovato, A. (1999). *Salvadora persica* L.: hypolipidemic activity on experimental hypercholesterolemia in rat. *Phytomedicine,* 6(3): 181-185.

Gargouri, Y., Julien, R., Pieroni, G., Verger, R., and Sarda, L. (1984). Studies on the inhibition of pancreatic and microbial lipases by soybean proteins. *Journal of Lipid Research,* 25(11): 1214-1221.

Gerhardt, A.L., and Gallo, N.B. (1998). Full-fat rice bran and oat bran similarly reduce hypercholesterolemia in humans. *Journal of Nutrition,* 128: 865–869.

Ghule, B.V., Ghante, M.H., Saoji, A.N., and Yeole, P.G. (2006). Hypolipidemic and antihyperlipidemic effects of *Lagenaria siceraria* (Mol.) fruit extracts. *Indian Journal of Experimental Biology,* 44(11): 905-909.

Gopal, K., Saran, R.K., Nityanand, S., Gupta, P.P., Hasan, M., Das, S.K., Sinha, N., and Agarwal, S.S. (1986). Clinical trial of ethyl acetate extract of gum gugulu (gugulipid) in primary hyperlipidemia. *Journal of the Association of the Physicians of India,* 34(4): 249-251.

Gorinstein, S., Bartnikowska, E., Kulasek, G., Zemser, M., and Trakhtenberg, S. (1998). Dietary persimmon improves lipid metabolism in rats fed diets containing cholesterol. *Journal of Nutrition*, 128(11): 2023-2027.

Grundy, S.M., Balady, G.J., Criqui, M.H., Fletcher, G., Greenland, P., Hiratzka, L.F., Houston-Miller, N., Kris-Etherton, P., Krumholz, H.M., LaRosa, J., Ockene, I.S., Pearson, T.A., Reed, J., Washington, R., and Smith, S.C. (1998). Primary prevention of coronary heart disease: guidance from Framingham: a statement for healthcare professionals from the AHA Task Force on risk reduction. American Heart Association. *Circulation*, 97(18):1876-1887.

Han, L.K., Zheng, Y.N., Yoshikawa, M., Okuda, H., and Kimura, Y. (2005). Antiobesity effects of chikusetsusaponins isolated from *Panax japonicus* rhizomes. *BMC Complementary and Alternative Medicine*, 5: 9.

Hemalatha, S., Wahi, A.K., Singh, P.N., and Chansouria, J.P. (2006). Hypolipidemic activity of aqueous extract of *Withania coagulans* Dunal in albino rats. *Phytotherapy Research*, 20(7): 614-617.

Hirunpanich, V., Utaipat, A., Morales, N.P., Bunyapraphatsara, N., Sato, H., Herunsale, A., and Suthisisang, C. (2006). Hypocholesterolemic and antioxidant effects of aqueous extracts from the dried calyx of *Hibiscus sabdariffa* L. in hypercholesterolemic rats. *Journal of Ethnopharmacology*, 103(2): 252-260.

Ho, S.C., Woo, J., Leung, S.S., Sham, A.L., Lam, T.H., and Janus, E.D. (2000). Intake of soy products is associated with better plasma lipid profiles in the Hong Kong Chinese population. *Journal of Nutrition*, 130: 2590–2593.

Hodgson, J.M., Puddey, I.B., Beilin, L.J., Mori, T.A., and Croft, K.D. (1998). Supplementation with isoflavonoid phytoestrogens does not alter serum lipid concentrations: a randomized controlled trial in humans *Journal of Nutrition*, 128: 728–732.

Hussain, M.M., Shi, J., and Dreizen, P. (2003). Microsomal triglyceride transfer protein and its role in apoB-lipoprotein assembly. (2003). *Journal of Lipid Research*, 44: 22–32.

Ji, W., and Gong, B.Q. (2007). Hypolipidemic effects and mechanisms of *Panax notoginseng* on lipid profile in hyperlipidemic rats. *Journal of Ethnopharmacology*, 113(2): 318-324.

Jung, H.J., Nam, J.H., Park, H.J., Lee, K.T., Park, K.K., Kim, W.B., and Choi, J. (2007). The MeOH extract of *Pleurospermum kamtschaticum* and its active component buddlejasaponin (IV) inhibits intrinsic and extrinsic hyperlipidemia and hypercholesterolemia in the rat. *Journal of Ethnopharmacology*, 112(2): 255-261.

Kempaiah, R.K., and Srinivasan, K. (2004). Influence of dietary curcumin, capsaicin and garlic on the antioxidant status of red blood cells and the liver in high-fat-fed rats. *Annals of Nutrition and Metabolism*, 48(5): 314-320.

Kim, H.Y., Jeong, M., Jung, H.J., Jung, Y.J., Yokozawa, T., and Choi, J.S. (2008). Hypolipidemic effects of *Sophora flavescens* and its constituents in poloxamer 407-induced hyperlipidemic and cholesterol-fed rats. *Biological and Pharmaceutical Bulletin*, 31(1): 73-78.

Kim, S.O., Yun, S.J., Jung, B., Lee, E.H., Hahm, D.H., Shim, I., and Lee, H.J. (2004). Hypolipidemic effects of crude extract of adlay seed (*Coix lachrymajobi* var. mayuen) in obesity rat fed high fat diet: relations of TNF-alpha and leptin mRNA expressions and serum lipid levels. *Life Sciences*, 75(11):1391-1404.

Ko, J.H., Lee, S.J., and Lim, K.T. (2007). Hypolipidemic effect and antioxidant activity of glycoprotein isolated from *Ulmus davidiana* Nakai in Triton WR-1339-treated mouse. *Cell Biochemistry and Function*, 25(5): 495-500.

Kumari, K., and Augusti, K.T. (2007). Lipid lowering effect of S-methyl cysteine sulfoxide from *Allium cepa* Linn in high cholesterol diet fed rats. *Journal of Ethnopharmacology*, 109(3): 367-371.

Kuo, K.L., Weng, M.S., Chiang, C.T., Tsai, Y.J., Lin-Shiau, S.Y., and Lin, J.K. (2005). Comparative studies on the hypolipidemic and growth suppressive effects of oolong, black, pu-erh, and green tea leaves in rats. *Journal of Agriculture and Food Chemistry*, 53(2): 480-489.

Kurowska, E.M., and Carroll, K.K. (1994). Hypercholesterolemic responses in rabbits to selected groups of dietary essential amino acids. *Journal of Nutrition*, 124: 364-370.

Kwon, S.H., Ahn, I.S., Kim, S.O., Kong, C.S., Chung, H.Y., Do, M.S., and Park, K.Y. (2007). Antiobesity and hypolipidemic effects of black soybean anthocyanins. *Journal of Medicinal Food*, 10(3): 552-556.

Lahlou, M. (2007). Screening of natural products for drug discovery. *Expert Opinion on Drug Discovery*, 2(5): 697-705.

Lal, A.A., Kumar, T., Murthy, P.B., and Pillai, K.S. (2004). Hypolipidemic effect of *Coriandrum sativum* L. in triton-induced hyperlipidemic rats. *Indian Journal of Experimental Biology*, 42(9): 909-912.

Lau, B.H.S. (2006). Suppression of LDL oxidation by garlic compounds is a possible mechanism of cardiovascular health benefit. *Journal of Nutrition*, 136: 765S–768S.

Lawson, L.D. (2001). Garlic for total cholesterol reduction. *Annals of Internal Medicine*, 135(1): 65.

Le, P.M., Benhaddou-Andaloussi, A., Elimadi, A., Settaf, A., Cherrah, Y., and Haddad, P.S. The petroleum ether extract of *Nigella sativa* exerts lipid-lowering and insulin-sensitizing actions in the rat. *Journal of Ethnopharmacology*, 94(2-3): 251-259.

Lecumberri, E., Goya, L., Mateos, R., Alía, M., Ramos, S., Izquierdo-Pulido, M., and Bravo, L. (2007). A diet rich in dietary fiber from cocoa improves lipid profile and reduces malondialdehyde in hypercholesterolemic rats. *Nutrition*, 23(4): 332-341.

Lee, C.L., Hung, H.K., Wang, J.J., and Pan, T.M. (2007). Red mold dioscorea has greater hypolipidemic and antiatherosclerotic effect than traditional red mold rice and unfermented dioscorea in hamsters. *Journal of Agriculture and Food Chemistry*, 55(17): 7162-7169.

Lee, I.A., Lee, J.H., Baek, N.I., and Kim, D.H. (2005). Antihyperlipidemic effect of crocin isolated from the fructus of *Gardenia jasminoides* and its metabolite Crocetin. *Biological and Pharmaceutical Bulletin*, 28(11): 2106-2110.

Lee, J.S., Lee, M.K., Ha, T.Y., Bok, S.H., Park, H.M., Jeong, K.S., Woo, M.N., Do, G.M., Yeo, J.Y., and Choi, M.S. (2006). Supplementation of whole persimmon leaf improves lipid profiles and suppresses body weight gain in rats fed high-fat diet. *Food and Chemical Toxicology*, 44(11): 1875-1883.

Lee, S.O., Simons, A.L., Murphy, P.A., and Hendrich, S. (2005). Soyasaponins lowered plasma cholesterol and increased fecal bile acids in female golden Syrian hamsters. *Experimental Biology and Medicine*, 230(7): 472-478.

Lee, S.W., Kim, K., Rho, M.C., Chung, M.Y., Kim, Y.H., Lee, S., Lee, H.S., and Kim, Y.K. (2004). New Polyacetylenes, DGAT inhibitors from the roots of *Panax ginseng*. *Planta Medica*, 70: 197–200.

Levine, G.N., Keaney, J.F., and Vita, J.A. (1995). Cholesterol reduction in cardiovascular disease: clinical benefits and possible mechanisms. *New England Journal of Medicine*, 332: 512-521.

Li, F., Li, W., Fu, H., Zhang, Q., and Koike, K. (2007). Pancreatic lipase-inhibiting triterpenoid saponins from fruits of *Acanthopanax senticosus*. *Chemical and Pharmaceutical Bulletin*, 55(7): 1087-1089.

Libby, P. (2002). Inflammation in atherosclerosis. *Nature*, 420: 868–874.

Lin, M.C., Wang, E.J., Lee, C., Chin, K.T., Liu, D., Chiu, J.F., and Kung, H.F. (2002). Garlic inhibits microsomal triglyceride transfer protein gene expression in human liver and intestinal cell lines and in rat intestine. *Journal of Nutrition*, 132: 1165–1168.

Lipid Research Clinics Program. (1984). The Lipid research Clinics Primary Trial results. I. Reduction in incidence of coronary heart disease. *Journal of the American Medical Association*, 251: 351-364.

Littleton, J. (2007). The future of plant drug discovery. *Expert Opinion on Drug Discovery*, 2(5): 673-683.

Loh, G., Eberhard, M., Brunner, R.M., Hennig, U., Kuhla, S., Kleessen, B., and Metges, C.C. (2006). Inulin alters the intestinal microbiota and short-chain fatty acids concentrations in growing pigs regardless of their basal diet. *Journal of Nutrition*, 136: 1198–1202.

Lucas, E.A., Khalil, D.A., Daggy, B.P., and Arjmandi, B.H. (2001). Ethanol-extracted soy protein isolate does not modulate serum cholesterol in golden syrian hamsters: a model of postmenopausal hypercholesterolemia. *Journal of Nutrition*, 131: 211–214.

Luo, Q., Cai, Y., Yan, J., Sun, M., and Corke, H. (2004). Hypoglycemic and hypolipidemic effects and antioxidant activity of fruit extracts from *Lycium barbarum*. *Life Sciences*, 76(2):137-149.

Macan, H., Uykimpang, R., Alconcel, M., Takasu, J., Razon, R., Amagase, H., and Niihara, Y. (2006). Aged garlic extract may be safe for patients on warfarin therapy. *Journal of Nutrition*, 136: 793S–795S.

Matheson, H.B., Colon, I.S., and Story, J.A. (1995). Cholesterol 7α-hydroxylase activity is increased by dietary modification with psyllium hydrocolloid, pectin, cholesterol and cholestyramine in rats. *Journal of Nutrition*, 125: 454-458.

Matthan, N.R., Jalbert, S.M., Ausman, L.M., Kuvin, J.T., Karas, R.H., and Lichtenstein, A.H. (2007). Effect of soy protein from differently processed products on cardiovascular disease risk factors and vascular endothelial function in hypercholesterolemic subjects. *American Journal of Clinical Nutrition*, 85: 960–966.

Melnikova, I., and Wages, D. (2006). Antiobesity therapies. *Nature Reviews Drug Discovery*, 5:369-370.

Min, S.W., and Kim, D.H. (2007). Kakkalide and irisolidone: HMG-CoA reductase inhibitors isolated from the flower of *Pueraria thunbergiana*. *Biological and Pharmaceutical Bulletin*, 30(10): 1965-1968.

Mini, S., and Rajamohan, T. (2004). Influence of coconut kernel protein on lipid metabolism in alcohol fed rats. *Indian Journal of Experimental Biology*, 42(1): 53-7.

Morikawa, T., Xu, F., Ninomiya, K., Matsuda, H., and Yoshikawa, M. (2004). Nigellamines A3, A4, A5, and C, new dolabellane-type diterpene alkaloids, with lipid metabolism-promoting activities from the Egyptian medicinal food black cumin. *Chemical and Pharmaceutical Bulletin*, 52(4): 494-497.

Moundras, C., Behr, S.R., Demigne, C., Mazur, A., and Remesy, C. (1994). Fermentable polysaccharides that enhance fecal bile acid excretion lower plasma cholesterol and apolipoprotein E-rich HDL in rats. *Journal of Nutrition,* 124: 2179-2188.

Movahedian, A., Sadeghi, H., Ghannadi, A., Gharavi, M., and Azarpajooh, S. (2006). Hypolipidemic activity of *Allium porrum* L. in cholesterol-fed rabbits. *Journal of Medicinal Food,* 9(1): 98-101.

Mukherjee, P.K., Rai, S., Kumar, V., Mukherjee, K., Hylands, P.J., and Hider, R.C. (2007). Plants of Indian origin in drug discovery. *Expert Opinion on Drug Discovery,* 2(5): 633-657.

Muthu, A.K., Sethupathy, S., Manavalan, R., and Karar, P.K. (2005). Hypolipidemic effect of methanolic extract of *Dolichos biflorus* Linn. in high fat diet fed rats. *Indian Journal of Experimental Biology,* 43(6): 522-525.

Nagata, C., Takatsuka, N., Kurisu, Y., and Shimizu, H. (1998). Decreased serum total cholesterol concentration is associated with high intake of soy products in Japanese men and women. *Journal of Nutrition,* 128: 209–213.

Nityanand, S., Srivastava, J.S., and Asthana, O.P. (1989). Clinical trials with gugulipid. A new hypolipidaemic agent. *Journal of Association of Physicians of India,* 37(5): 323-328.

Oh, P.S., Lee, S.J., and Lim, K.T. (2006). Hypolipidemic and antioxidative effects of the plant glycoprotein (36 kDa) from *Rhus verniciflua* stokes fruit in Triton WR-1339-induced hyperlipidemic mice. *Bioscience, Biotechnology and Biochemistry,* 70(2): 447-456.

Oh, P.S., and Lim, K.T. (2006). Glycoprotein (90 kDa) isolated from *Opuntia ficus-indica* var. saboten MAKINO lowers plasma lipid level through scavenging of intracellular radicals in Triton WR-1339-induced mice. *Biological and Pharmaceutical Bulletin,* 29(7): 1391-1396.

Opar, A. (2007). Where now for new drugs for atherosclerosis? *Nature Reviews Drug Discovery,* 6: 334-335.

Palumbo, B., Efthimiou, Y., Stamatopoulos, J., Oguogho, A., Budinsky, A., Palumbo, R., and Sinzinger, H. (2003). Prickly pear induces upregulation of liver LDL binding in familial heterozygous hypercholesterolemia. *Nuclear Medicine Review Central and Eastern Europe,* 6(1): 35-39.

Pandey, R.S., Singh, B.K., and Tripathi, Y.B. (2005). Extract of gum resins of *Boswellia serrata* L. inhibits lipopolysaccharide induced nitric oxide production in rat macrophages along with hypolipidemic property. *Indian Journal of Experimental Biology,* 43(6): 509-516.

Parab, R.S., and Mengi, S.A. (2002). Hypolipidemic activity of *Acorus calamus* L. in rats. *Fitoterapia,* 73(6): 451-455.

Pari, L., and Latha, M. (2006). Antihyperlipidemic effect of *Scoparia dulcis* (sweet broomweed) in streptozotocin diabetic rats. *Journal of Medicinal Food,* 9(1): 102-107.

Potter, S.M. (1995). Overview of proposed mechanisms for the hypocholesterolemic effect of soy. *Journal of Nutrition,* 125(Suppl): 606S–611S.

Pushparaj, P.N., Low, H.K., Manikandan, J., Tan, B.K., and Tan, C.H. (2007). Antidiabetic effects of *Cichorium intybus* in streptozotocin-induced diabetic rats. *Journal of Ethnopharmacology,* 111(2): 430-434.

Rahman, K. Historical perspective on garlic and cardiovascular disease. *Journal of Nutrition,* 131: 977S–979S.

Rao, B.K., Kesavulu, M.M., Giri, R., and Appa Rao, C. (1999). Antidiabetic and hypolipidemic effects of *Momordica cymbalaria* Hook. fruit powder in alloxan-diabetic rats. *Journal of Ethnopharmacology*, 67(1): 103-109.

Rasekh, H.R., Khoshnood-Mansourkhani, M.J., and Kamalinejad, M. (2001). Hypolipidemic effects of *Teucrium polium* in rats. *Fitoterapia*, 72(8): 937-939.

Ravi, K., Rajasekaran, S., and Subramanian, S. (2005). Antihyperlipidemic effect of *Eugenia jambolana* seed kernel on streptozotocin-induced diabetes in rats. *Food and Chemical Toxicology*, 43(9):1433-1439.

Roberfroid, M. (2007). Prebiotics: The concept revisited. *Journal of Nutrition*, 137: 830S–837S.

Rudel, L.L., Lee, R.G., and Parini, P. (2005). ACAT2 is a target for treatment of coronary heart disease associated with hypercholesterolemia. *Arteriosclerosis Thrombosis and Vascular Biology*, 25: 1112-1118.

Sacks, F.M., Lichtenstein, A., Van Horn, L., Harris, W., Kris-Etherton, P., and Winston, M. (2006). Soy Protein, Isoflavones, and Cardiovascular Health: An American Heart Association Science Advisory for Professionals from the Nutrition Committee. *Circulation*, 113: 1034-1044.

Salil, G., and Rajamohan, T. (2001). Hypolipidemic and antiperoxidative effect of coconut protein in hypercholesterolemic rats. *Indian Journal of Experimental Biology*, 39(10):1028-1034.

Scandinavian Simvastatin Survival Study Group. (1994). Randomised trial of cholesterol lowering in 4444 patients with coronary heart disease: the Scandinavian Simvastatin Survival Study (4). *Lancet*, 344: 1383-1389.

Senanayake, G.V., Maruyama, M., Sakono, M., Fukuda, N., Morishita, T., Yukizaki, C., Kawano, M., and Ohta, H. (2004). The effects of bitter melon (*Momordica charantia*) extracts on serum and liver lipid parameters in hamsters fed cholesterol-free and cholesterol-enriched diets. *Journal of Nutritional Science and Vitaminology*, 50(4): 253-257.

Shaila, H.P., Udupa, S.L., and Udupa, A.L. (1998). Hypolipidemic activity of three indigenous drugs in experimentally induced atherosclerosis. *International Journal of Cardiology*, 67(2):119-124.

Shan, J.J., Yang, M., and Ren, J.W. (2006). Antidiabetic and hypolipidemic effects of aqueous-extract from the flower of *Inula japonica* in alloxan-induced diabetic mice. *Biological and Pharmaceutical Bulletin*, 29(3): 455-459.

Sharma, S.B., Nasir, A., Prabhu, K.M., Murthy, P.S., and Dev, G. (2003). Hypoglycaemic and hypolipidemic effect of ethanolic extract of seeds of *Eugenia jambolana* in alloxan-induced diabetic rabbits. *Journal of Ethnopharmacology*, 85(2-3): 201-206.

Shi, Y., and Burn, P. (2004). Lipid metabolic enzymes: Emerging drug targets for the treatment of obesity. *Nature Reviews Drug Discovery*, 3: 695-710.

Shin, J.E., Han, M.J., Song, M.C., Baek, N.I., and Kim, D.H. (2004). 5-Hydroxy-7-(49-hydroxy-39-methoxyphenyl)-1-phenyl-3-heptanone: a pancreatic lipase inhibitor isolated from *Alpinia officinarum*. *Biological and Pharmaceutical Bulletin*, 27(1): 138-140.

Shin, J.E., Joo Han, M., and Kim, D.H. (2003). 3-Methylethergalangin isolated from *Alpinia officinarum* inhibits pancreatic lipase. *Biological and Pharmaceutical Bulletin*, 26(6): 854-857.

Shulman, A.I., and Mangelsdorf, D.J. (2005). Retinoid X Receptor heterodimers in the metabolic syndrome. *New England Journal of Medicine*, 353: 604-615.

Sindhurani, J.A., and Rajamohan, T. (1998). Hypolipidemic effect of hemicellulose component of coconut fiber. *Indian Journal of Experimental Biology*, 36(8): 786-789.

Singh, R.B., Mengi, S.A., Xu, Y.J., Arneja, A.S., and Dhalla, N.S. (2002). Pathogenesis of atherosclerosis: a multifunctional process. *Experimental and Clinical Cardiology*, 26(1): 1-9.

Singh, S.K., Kesari, A.N., Gupta, R.K., Jaiswal, D., and Watal, G. (2007). Assessment of antidiabetic potential of *Cynodon dactylon* extract in streptozotocin diabetic rats. *Journal of Ethnopharmacology*, 114(2): 174-179.

Slowing, K., Ganado, P., Sanz, M., Ruiz, E., and Tejerina, T. (2001). Study of garlic extracts and fractions on cholesterol plasma levels and vascular reactivity in cholesterol-fed rats. *Journal of Nutrition*, 131: 994S–999S.

Sniderman, A.D., and Cianflone, K. (1993). Substrate delivery as a determinant of hepatic apoB secretion. *Arteriosclerosis Thrombosis and Vascular Biology*, 13: 629-636.

Stevinson, C., Pittler, M.H., and Ernst, E. (2000). Garlic for treating hypercholesterolemia: a meta-analysis of randomized clinical trials. *Annals of Internal Medicine*, 133: 420-429.

Subash Babu, P., Prabuseenivasan, S., and Ignacimuthu, S. (2007). Cinnamaldehyde—a potential antidiabetic agent. *Phytomedicine*, 14(1): 15-22.

Subashini, R., Ragavendran, B., Gnanapragasam, A., Yogeeta, S.K., and Devaki, T. (2007). Biochemical study on the protective potential of *Nardostachys jatamansi* extract on lipid profile and lipid metabolizing enzymes in doxorubicin intoxicated rats. *Pharmazie*, 62(5): 382-387.

Swift, L.L., Zhu, M.Y., Kakkad, B., Jovanovska, A., Neely, M.D., Valyi-Nagy, K., Roberts, R.L., Ong, D.E., and Jerome, W.G. (2003). Subcellular localization of microsomal triglyceride transfer protein. *Journal of Lipid Research*, 44: 1841–1849.

Szapary, P.O., Wolfe, M.L., Bloedon, L.T., Cucchiara, A.J., DerMarderosian, A.H., Cirigliano, M.D., and Rader, D.H. (2003). Guggulipid for the treatment of hypercholesterolemia a randomized controlled trial. *Journal of the American Medical Association*, 290: 765-772.

Taku, K., Umegaki, K., Sato, Y., Taki, Y., Endoh, K., and Watanabe, S. (2007). Soy isoflavones lower serum total and LDL cholesterol in humans: a meta-analysis of 11 randomized controlled trials. *American Journal of Clinical Nutrition*, 85: 1148–1156.

Tan, B.K., Tan, C.H., and Pushparaj, P.N. (2005). Antidiabetic activity of the semi-purified fractions of *Averrhoa bilimbi* in high fat diet fed-streptozotocin-induced diabetic rats. *Life Sciences*, 76(24): 2827-2839.

Thomas, M., Leelamma, S., and Kurup, P.A. (1983). Effect of blackgram fiber (*Phaseolus mungo*) on hepatic hydroxymethylglutaryl-CoA reductase activity, cholesterogenesis and cholesterol degradation in rats. *Journal of Nutrition*, 113: 1104-1108.

Thomson, M., Al-Qattan, K.K., Bordia, T., and Ali, M. (2006). Including garlic in the diet may help lower blood glucose, cholesterol, and triglycerides. *Journal of Nutrition*, 136: 800S–802S.

Trigatti, B.L., Krieger, M., and Rigotti, A. (2003). Influence of the HDL receptor SR-BI on lipoprotein metabolism and atherosclerosis. *Arteriosclerosis Thrombosis and Vascular Biology*, 23:1732-1738.

Trinh, H.T., Han, S.J., Kim, S.W., Lee, Y.C., and Kim, D.H. (2007). Bifidus fermentation increases hypolipidemic and hypoglycemic effects of red ginseng. *Journal of Microbiology and Biotechnology*, 17(7):1127-1133.

Tripathi, Y.B., and Pandey, R.S. (2004). *Semecarpus anacardium* L, nuts inhibit lipopolysaccharide induced NO production in rat macrophages along with its hypolipidemic property. *Indian Journal of Experimental Biology*, 42(4): 432-436.

Tungland, B.C., and Meyer, P.D. (2002). Dietary fibre and human health. *Comprehensive Reviews in Food Science and Food Safety*, 3: 78-92.

Urizar, N.L., Liverman, A.B., Dodds, D.T., Silva, F.V., Ordentlich, P., Yan,Y., Gonzalez, F.J., Heyman, R.A., Mangelsdorf, D.J., and Moore, D.D. (2002). A natural product that lowers cholesterol as an antagonist ligand for FXR. *Science*, 296:1703-1706.

Valcheva-Kuzmanova, S., Kuzmanov, K., Tancheva, S., and Belcheva, A. (2007). Hypoglycemic and hypolipidemic effects of *Aronia melanocarpa* fruit juice in streptozotocin-induced diabetic rats. *Methods and Findings in Experimental and Clinical Pharmacology*, 29(2):101-105.

Vidal, R., Hernandez-Vallejo, S., Pauquai, T., Texier, O., Rousset, M., Chambaz, J., Demignot, S., and Lacorte, J.M. (2005). Apple procyanidins decrease cholesterol esterification and lipoprotein secretion in Caco-2/TC7 enterocytes. *Journal of Lipid Research*, 46(2): 258-268.

Volger, O.L., Mensink, R.P., Plat, J., Hornstra, G., Havekes, L.M., and Princen, H.M. (2001). Dietary vegetable oil and wood derived plant stanol esters reduce atherosclerotic lesion size and severity in apoE*3-Leiden transgenic mice. *Atherosclerosis*, 157(2): 375-381.

Waters, D., Higginson, L., Gladstone, P., Kimball, B., May, M.L., Boccuzzi, S.J., Lesperance, J., and the CCAIT Study Group. (1994). Effects of monotherapy with an HMG-CoA reductase inhibitor on progression of coronary atherosclerosis as assessed by serial quantitative arteriography. The Canadian Coronary Atherosclerosis Intervention Trial. *Circulation*, 89: 959-968.

Wilcox, L.J., Borradaile, N.M., Dreu, L.E., and Huff, M.W. (2001). Secretion of hepatocyte apoB is inhibited by the flavonoids, naringenin and hesperetin, via reduced activity and expression of ACAT2 and MTP. *Journal of Lipid Research*, 42: 725–734.

Witztum, J.L. (1994). The oxidation hypothesis of atherosclerosis. *Lancet*, 344: 793-795.

Wong, W.W., Smith, E.O.B., Stuff, J.E., Hachey, D.L., Heird, W.C., and Pownell, H.J. (1998). Cholesterol-lowering effect of soy protein in normocholesterolemic and hypercholesterolemic men. *American Journal of Clinical Nutrition*, 68(suppl):1385S–1389S.

Wu, J., Xia, C., Meier, J., Li, S., Hu, X., and Lala, D.S. The hypolipidemic natural product guggulsterone acts as an antagonist of the bile acids receptor *Molecular Endocrinology*, 16(7):1590–1597.

Xie, W., Wang, W., Su, H., Xing, D., Cai, G., and Du, L. (2007). Hypolipidemic mechanisms of *Ananas comosus* L. leaves in mice: different from fibrates but similar to statins. *Journal of Pharmacological Sciences*, 103(3): 267-274.

Xie, W., Xing, D., Sun, H., Wang, W., Ding, Y., and Du, L. (2005). The effects of *Ananas comosus* L. leaves on diabetic-dyslipidemic rats induced by alloxan and a high-fat/high-cholesterol diet. *American Journal of Chinese Medicine*, 33(1): 95-105.

Yajima, H., Ikeshima, E., Shiraki, M., Kanaya, T., Fujiwara, D., Odai, H., Tsuboyama-Kasaoka, N., Ezaki, O., Oikawa, S., and Kondo, K. (2004). Isohumulones, bitter acids derived from hops, activate both peroxisome proliferator-activated receptor alpha and gamma and reduce insulin resistance. *Journal of Biological Chemistry*, 279(32): 33456-33462.

Yeh, Y., and Liu, L. (2001). Cholesterol-lowering effect of garlic extracts and organosulfur compounds: human and animal studies. *Journal of Nutrition,* 131: 989S–993S.

Zern, T.L., and Fernandez, M.L. (2005). Cardioprotective effects of dietary polyphenols. *Journal of Nutrition,* 135: 2291–2294.

Zhang, Z., Ho, W.K., Huang, Y., James, A.E., Lam, L.W., and Chen, Z.Y. (2002). Hawthorn fruit is hypolipidemic in rabbits fed a high cholesterol diet. *Journal of Nutrition,* 132(1): 5-10.

Zheng, Q., Li, W., Han, L., and Koike, K. (2007). Pancreatic lipase-inhibiting triterpenoid saponins from *Gypsophila oldhamiana. Chemical and Pharmaceutical Bulletin,* 55(4): 646-650.

Medicinal Plants: Phytochemistry, Pharmacology and Therapeutics, Vol. 1 *Pages* **297–314**
Editors: **V.K. Gupta, G.D. Singh, Surjeet Singh and A. Kaul**
Published by: **DAYA PUBLISHING HOUSE, NEW DELHI**

Chapter 15

A Review on Phytochemistry and Pharmacology of *Alangium* Sp.

Papiya Bigoniya*, Alok Shukla and C.S. Singh
Radharaman College of Pharmacy, Fatehpur Dopra, Ratibad, Bhopal – 462 002, M.P., India

ABSTRACT

Alangium is a deciduous rambling shrub or small tree, distributed over the plains and foothills throughout the India. The root, root-bark, leaves, fruits and seeds of this genus have been used in indigenous Indian systems of medicine for a long time. The root is laxative and anthelmintic. The root bark is bitter purgative, anthelmintic, astringent, pungent, having emetic property, useful in fever and skin diseases and also prescribed for biliousness and colic. The leaves are used as poultice in rheumatic pains. The fruits are astringents and are reputed in the indigenous system of medicine for laxative, tonic and refrigerant properties and are useful in emaciation and haemorrhages. The seeds are reputed for their cooling and tonic property and also used in treatment of haemorrhage. The plant is used as an antidote to snake poison. The bark is used as an antipyretic, in insanity, epilepsy, jaundice, hepatitis and asthma.

An alkaloid deoxytubulosine was isolated from the flowers, which reportedly showed a strong binding with DNA.The fruits were found to contain alkaloids like-cephaeline, N-methylcephaeline (alamarckine), deoxytubulosine alangiside and sterol. The seeds were reported to contain several alkaloids having various structural skeletons including benzopyridoquinolozine skeleton. These were characterized as alamarckine, emetin, cephaeline and psychotrin,

* Corresponding Author: E-mail: p_bigoniya2@hotmail.com; Phone: 91-0755-2477941, 91-0755-2896218, 09827011258.

alangamide, venoterpine, salsoline, isocephaeline, alangimarine, alamarine, alangimaridine and alamaridine. The seeds were reported to contain betulinic acid considered to be sterol named alangol or alengol. The leaves are reported to contain saponins, alkaloids, sterol and terpenoids.

Keywords: *Alangiaceae, Alangium, Alanine, Antimicrobial, Cytotoxicity, Deoxytubulosine.*

Introduction

Plant and plant products are being used as a source of medicine since long. According to World Health Organization (WHO) more than 80 per cent of the world's population, mostly in a poor and developing countries depend on traditional plant-based medicines for their primary healthcare needs (WHO, 1993). Medicinal plants are the nature's gift to human being to make disease free healthy life. It plays a vital role to preserve our health. India is one of the most medico-culturally diverse countries in the world where the medicinal plant sector is part of a time-honored tradition that is respected even today. The utility of plants as therapeutic agents in traditional medicine system is still prevalent today. For example, the middle eastern civilization developed the Greco-Arabic system of medicine (Unani system of medicine), which is practiced in Indian sub continent. Similarly, the Chinese race developed the Chinese system of medicine largely based on it unique system of theories including the concept of Yen and Yang; the idea of Wv, Xing (the five elements), the theory of influence imparted from nature. The Ayurveda and Sidha system of medicines were contributed by Indians. All these systems procure more than 80 per cent of their medicaments from plants (Gupta *et al.*, 2007). The earliest mention use of the plants in medicine is found in the Rig-Veda, which was written between 4500 and 1600 BC. During British period due to Western culture our traditional art of natural healing has nearly disappeared. Now it is reappearing due to realization of its importance in curing diseases with very few side effects. Owing to the global trend towards improved 'quality of life', there is considerable evidence of an increase in demand for medicinal plant (Kotnis, 2004). Medicinal plants, which form the backbone of traditional medicine, have been subjected for very intense pharmacological studies in the last few decades. This has been brought about by the acknowledgement of the value of medicinal plants as potential sources of new compounds of therapeutic value and as sources of lead compounds in the drug development. There arises a need therefore to screen medicinal plants for bioactive compounds as a basis for further pharmacological studies. Plants are considered to be promising source of medicine in the traditional health care system. The efficacy and safety of herbal medicine have turned the major pharmaceutical population towards medicinal plant's research.

Alangium Genus

Alangium is a genus of shrubs or small trees. The leaves of this genus are alternate, petiolate, oblong, quite entire, 3-nerved from the base, persistant where as the flowers are white subsilky, hermaphrodite, in axillary fascicles, embracteate, shortly pedicelled and articulated with the pedicelled. Calyx-tube turbinate, often sulcate, larege limb, 5-10 toothed or truncate. Petals are 5-10 in number, linear–oblong, revolute and valvate. Stamens are usually 2-4 times as many as petals, filaments are filiform or flattened with more or less villous along with long anthers. Cushioned-shaped disk having depression in centre, lobed or crenulate. Ovary is 1-celled, ovule solitary in each cell, pendulous, style narrowly clavate or filiform, stigma clavate or capitate, many lobed and the lobes are conduplicate. Berry crowned with the calyx–limb. Seeds are oblong, with thin testa, albumen usuallly fleshy, foliaceousm cotyledons and elongate, cylindric, thick radicle (Kirtikar and Basu, 2006).

Alangium alpinum (C.B.Clarke) W.W.Sm. and Cave
Alangium barbatum (R. Br.) Baill.
Alangium chinense (Lour.) Harms
Alangium faberi Oliv.
Alangium grisolleoides Capuron
Alangium javanicum (Blume) Wangerin
Alangium kurzii Craib
Alangium kwangsiense Melch.
Alangium longiflorum Merr.
Alangium platanifolium (Siebold and Zucc.) Harms
Alangium salviifolium (L.f.) Wangerin
Alangium villosum (Blume) Wangerin
Alangium vitiense (A.Gray) Baill. ex Harms

Alangium salviifolium (Linn.f.) Wang

Alangiaceae includes 1 genera and approximately 17 species. Plants of Alangiaceae family are tropical and subtropical trees or shrubs and sometimes spiny. Leaves are alternate, simple. Flowers are hermaphrodite, in axillary cymes with articulated pedicles. Calyx having 4-10 teeths which are turncate. Petals are mostly linear, valvate, 4-10 in number and sometimes coherent at base. Stamens the same number as and alternate with the petals or 2-4 times as many, free or slightly connate at the base, more or less villous inside, 2 celled anthers, linear and lengthwise opening. Disk is cushion like with inferior ovary, 1-2 celled, simple style, clavate or 2-3 lobed, ovule solitary, pendulus with 2 integuments. Fruit is a drupe crowened by the sepals and 1–seeded. Seeds with the embryo are near about equal to the endosperm (Kirtikar and Basu, 2006).

Synonym(S)

Alangium lamarckii Thw., *Grewia salvifolium* Linn.f.

Vernacular Name

Alangium salviifolium is commonly called akhaul, akol akola, anedhera, dhera in hindi; ankola, ankota, bodha, dirghakilaka, ghalanta, kankarola, lambakarna in sanskrit; akarkanta, angkula, ankoda, dhalakura in Bengali; ankol, ankoli, ankul in Marathi; adigolam, alangi, alinjil, eralingil in Tamil; ankola in Urdu; ankulo, baghonokhiya in Uriya and mulanninchil in ceylon (Kirtikar and Basu, 2006).

Geographical Distribution

Alangium salviifolium is a shrub or small tree distributed over the plains, foothills throughout the greater part of India, Sri Lanka, China, Malaya and Phillipines. It is also abundant in tropical and subtropical regions from Africa east to Australia and Fiji.

Taxonomical Classification

Kingdom:	Plantae
Subkingdom:	Viridaeplantae
Phylum:	Magnoliophyta
Subphylum:	Spermatophytina
Infraphylum:	Angiospermae
Class:	Magnoliopsida
Subclass:	Cornidae
Superorder:	Cornanae
Order:	Cornales
Family:	Alangiaceae
Genus:	Alangium
Specific epithet:	Salviifolium *Alangium salviifolium*
Botanical name:	*Alangium salviifolium*

Botanical Description

A small thorny decuduous tree/shrub with more less spinescent branches which grows up to height of 5-10 meters. Bark light coloured and young parts pubescent. Leaves variable 7.5-12.5 by 2.5-5.7 cm narrowly oblong or ovate–lanceolate, more or less acuminate, subobtuse, entire, glabrous above, pubescent on the nerves and prominently reticulately veined beneath, base rounded or acute, petioles 6-13 mm long, densely pubescent. Flowers few, in axillary fascicles, pedicles 3-6 mm long, densely pubescent, jointed at the top. Calyx turbinate 3 mm long, densely silky pubescent, teeth triangular, 0.85 mm long. Petals 5-10 (usually 6), densely pubescent outside, 1.3-2 cm long and about 5 mm wide, narrowly linear, reflected. Stamens numerous (more than 20), nearly as long as petals, filaments hairy at base. Style as long as the stamens, stigma very large. Fruit when young ovoid or ellipsoid, becoming nearly globular when ripe 1.3-2 cm diameter. Crowned by the persistant calix limb, finely pubescent, not or obscurely ribbed, purplish red, endocarp bony, albumen freshly outside, friable inside, not at all ruminate, cotyledons foliaceous, flat not crumpled (Kirtikar and Basu, 2006).

Ethnopharmacological Uses

The root is acrid, bitter, slightly pungent, oily, sharp, heating, anthelmintic, alterative, cures erysipelas, biliousness, inflammations, snake-bites and fish-poison. The juice is emetic, alexipharmic, cures kapha, vata, pain, inflammations, biliousness, diseases of blood, rat–bite, hydrophobia, lumbago, dysentery, diarrhoea, anthelmintic. The seeds have taste and flavour, cooling, aphrodisiac, indigestible, tonic, laxative, cure burning sensations. Consumption of seed causes biliousness, erysipelas, kaph and loss of appetite.

The root bark is used in piles. The stem is good in vomiting and diarrhoea. The fruit is sweet, laxative, expectorant, anthelmintic, alexiteric useful in inflammation, diseases of the blood and burning of the body. In native practice, the root-bark is used as anthelmintic and purgative. In Bombay, the leaves are used as a poultice to relieve rheumatic pains.

It has proved itself an efficient and safe emetic in doses of fifty grains; in smaller doses it is nauseant and febrifuge. The bark is very bitter and its repute in skin diseases is not without foundation. It is a good substitute for Ipecacuanha and proves useful in relieving pyrexia. Doses as a nauseant, diuretic and febrifuge: 6-10 grains of root bark; as an alternative: 2-5 grains. It is given in leprosy and syphilis. The natives consider it to be alexiteric, especially in cases of bites from rabid animals.

The Mundas of Chota Nagpur use the root as a purgative in dyspepsia and in gout. In the Salem district, 40 grains of powered bark is made into a bolus and given in cases of cobra poisoning. Both the bark and the root are prescribed as antidotes to snake-venom (Charaka, Sharangdharasambhita, Bhavaprakasha). The root and the bark are equally useless in the symptomatic treatment of snake bite (Kirtikar and Basu, 2006; Nadkarni, 2002).

Phytochemistry

The root bark was reported to yield ceryl alcohol and a light brown wax. The wax was found to be composed of non-saponifiable matter, myristic, palmitic, oleic, linoleic acids and resin acids. Myricyl alcohol, stigmasterol and β-sitosterol were also detected. The investigation of root bark were showed presence of different alkaloids identified as alangine (mp 80-82°), alangine (mp 205-208°), alangine A, alangine B, alanginine, akharkantine, ankoline, lamarkine along with five alkaloids bases designated as B1 to B5 (Chopra and Chauhan, 1934; Basu *et al.*, 1950; Basu and Gode, 1957). The structure of alangine A was established as 3-anisyl-2-piperidyl-*n*-propanol (Bhakuni *et al.*, 1960). Alkaloids marckine, marckidine, tubulosine (mp 257°), cephaeline (mp 102°), psychotrine and alangicine were isolated from root bark (Pakrashi and Ali, 1967). From root and stem bark emetine, cephaeline, psychotrine (mp121°), N-methylcephaeline and deoxytubulosine were isolated (Budzikiewicz *et al.*, 1964; Pakrashi, 1966). The root also contained alkaloids tubulosine and isotubulosine (Desai *et al.*, 1966; Shoeb *et al.*, 1975).

The stem bark was reported to contain lamarckinine (mp 265°). A new alkaloid demethylcephaeline–along with cephaeline, psychotrine, tubulosine and demethylpsychotrine were isolated from stem bark (Achari and Pakrashi, 1970). New benzoquinolizidine alkaloid–alancine and isoalamarine were also isolated and characterized from stem bark (Chattopadhyay *et al.*, 1984; Pakrashi *et al.*, 1980). The total non alkaloidal extract of the stem bark contained β-sitosterol, stigmasterol and a viscous oil.

In a preliminary study the leaves revealed presence of alkaloids and saponins on the other hand absence of tannins (Joshi and Sabnis, 1989). The leaves were found to contain a new phenolic alkaloid ankorine (mp 174°), campesterol, episterol and two unidentified triterpenoids (Dasgupta and Sharma, 1966). Presence of deoxytubulosine, alangimarckine (mp 184°) and choline chloride were reported by Dasgupta, (1965, 1966). A new sterol stigmasta-5, 22, 25-trien-3β-ol and a monoterpenoid lactum–alangiside was isolated and structure elucidated by Kapil *et al.* (1971) and Shoeb *et al.* (1975). Achari *et al.* (1974) reported isolation of N-benzoyl-L-phenylalaninol (mp 169°). Structures of new D, E-cis fused neohopane derivatives–alangidiol and isoalangidiol were established and isolated from leaves (Achari *et al.*, 1975). β-amyrin acetate, triacontanol and β-sitosterol were isolated from leaves. Five new alkaloids–isoalangimarine, isoalamarine, alangimarinone, dihydroalamarine and dihydroisoalamarine were isolated along with alangimarine, alamarine and alangimaridine. Structures of (+) 9-demethylpsychotrine and bharatamine were established by synthesis. A new alkaloid alamaridine was isolated and its stereo structure was established and confirmed by synthesis. Deacetylipecoside synthase, the enzyme catalyzing the condensation of dopamine and secologanin to form the (R)-epimer of deacetylipecoside had been purified and partially characterized by De-Eknamkulw *et al.* (2000).

The seeds revealed the presence of sterol, tannins, sugar, colouring matters and cellulose (Bhargava and Dutt, 1942). Seeds were reported to contain several alkaloids with various structural skeleton including benzoquinolizine or benzopyridoquinolozine nucleus characterized as alamarckine, emetin, cephaeline and psychotrin (Budzipiewicz *et al.*, 1964). Betulinic acid, earlier recogzined to be a sterol called alangol or alengol betulinaldehyde, betulin, lupeol, hydroxylactone A of betulinic acid, deoxybetulonic acid and β-sitosterol were reported in seeds (Lakshminarasimhaiah *et al.*, 1942; Pakrashi *et al.*, 1968). Isolation and structural elucidation of new phenolic alkaloid–alangamide (mp-213°), novel alkaloids–alangimarine, alamarine, alangimaridine venoterpine, salsoline, isocephaeline, deoxytubulosine, demethyltubulosine, cephaeline, psychotrine, and ankorine were done on seeds (Achari *et al.*, 1980). New isomeric alkaloids 10–demethylprotoemetinol and 9–demethylprotoemetinol were isolated from seeds (Ali *et al.*, 1982). Stereospecific synthesis of ankorine, alangicine, alangimarckine, desmethylpsychotrine, demethyltubulosine and 10-demethylprotoemetinol was reviewed by Fujii, (1983). Isolation and structure determination of new protoberberine alkaloid called bharatamine (mp-182°) from seeds. Alamaridine isoalangamarine, alangimerinone, dihydroisoalamarine were isolated from seeds (Bhattacharya *et al.*, 1986; 1988). Presences of a terpene, laciniliene were reported by Mukhopadhyaya *et al.* (1987). Bhattacharjya *et al.* (1988) reported the synthesis of 5–epialamaridine, isoalamaridine and its 5–epimer.

Alkaloids like cephaeline, N-methylcephaeline, deoxytubulosine, alangiside and a sterol were isolated from fruits (Salgar and Merchant, 1964; 1966; Battersby *et al.*, 1965; 1966; Desai *et al.*, 1966; Shoeb *et al.*, 1975). Synthesis of bharatamine, 3-O-demethyl-2-O-methylalangiside along with isolation and characterization of alangiside from dried fruits were reported. From the water soluble fraction of the dried fruits, four tetrahydroisoquinoline–monoterpene glycosides, 6-O–methyl-N-deacetyliso-ipecosidic acid, 7-O-methyl-N-deacetylisoipecosidic acid, 6, 7-di-O-methyl-N-deacetylisoipecosidic acid, 6''-O-α-D–glucopyranosyl-6-O methyl-N-deacetylisoipecosidic acid and an iridoid glycoside, 6'-O–α-D-glucopyranosylloganic acid were isolated, together with six known compounds (Itoh *et al.*, 2001).

Two new alangium alkaloids, 1', 2'-dehydrotubulosine and alangine were isolated from the dried fruits along with tubulosine, isotubulosine, deoxytubulosine, cephaeline, isocephaeline, psychotrine, neocephaeline, protoemetine, protoemetinol, salsoline, alangiside and 10-O-demethylcephaeline, 2'-N-(1''-deoxy-1''-beta-D-fructopyranosyl) cephaeline (Itoh *et al.*, 2000).

The flowers were reported to contain an alkaloid deoxytubulosine. Anjum *et al.* (2002) reported isolation of 1-methyl-1H-pyrimidine-2, 4-dione and 3-O-β-D-glucopyranosyl-(24β)-etylcholesta–5, 22, 25–triene from flowers.

Pharmacological Activity

Antimicrobial

The alcoholic and aqueous extracts of the plant were tested for antibacterial activity. The alcoholic extract was active against *Staphylococcus aureus* and *Escherichia coli* whereas the aqueous extract showed activity only against *Escherichia coli* (George and Pandalai, 1949). The root bark extracts revealed antitubercular activity against mycobacterial strains *M. phlei* and M-607 and antifungal activity against *Helminthosporium sativum* (Bhatnagar *et al.*, 1961). The 80 per cent ethanolic extract of the root revealed antibacterial activity against *Escherichia coli, Pseudomonas aeruginosa, Bacillus subtilis* and *staphylococcus aureus*. The extract was active at a concentration of 25 mg/ml against the first two bacteria while it was active against the other two at a concentration of 12.5 mg/ml. The extract also revealed antifungal activity against *Aspergillus niger* and *Candida albicans*. The aqueous root extract of the plant also showed *in-vitro* antibacterial activity against *Pseudomonas aeruginosa, Bacillus megaterium, Shigella dysenteriae, Vibrio cholerae* and *Staphylococcus aureus* in decreasing order (Gond and Shankhapal, 1998).

The lyophilized powder extract (4.59 per cent) of pulverized wood was tested for its inhibitory effect by agar disc diffusion test. The extract gave inhibitory zone diameters of 25.23 and 14.78 mm against isolates of dermatophytes and *Candida albicans* respectively. Ketoconazole, used as a reference antifungal agent, had inhibitory zone diameters of 33.15 and 27.93 mm against dermatophytes and *C. albicans*, respectively. There was no significant difference between the extract and ketoconazole in their inhibition against dermatophytes ($p > 0.01$), but their difference was significant against *C. albicans* ($p < 0.01$). Using Buehler's method, different amounts of extract (3, 6 and 9 mg/inch^2 gauze pad) were

Figure 15.1: Chemical Constituents of *Alangium* sp.

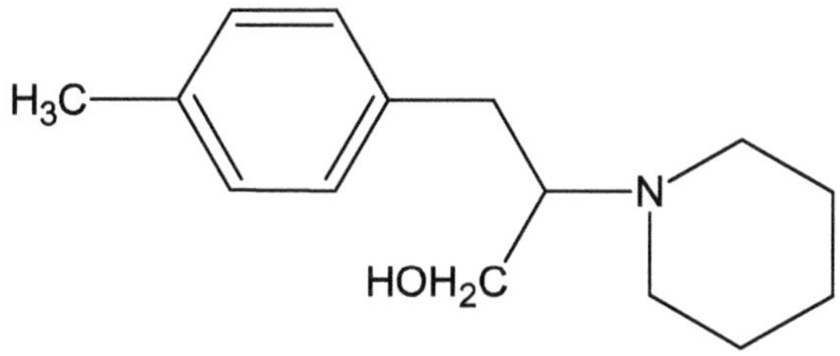

Alangine

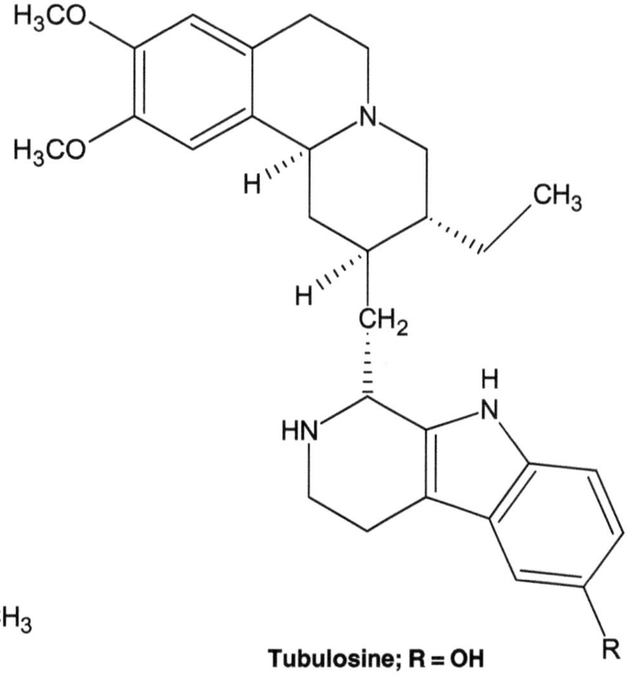

Tubulosine; R = OH
Isotubulosine (3' epimer); R = OH
Deoxytubulosine; R = H

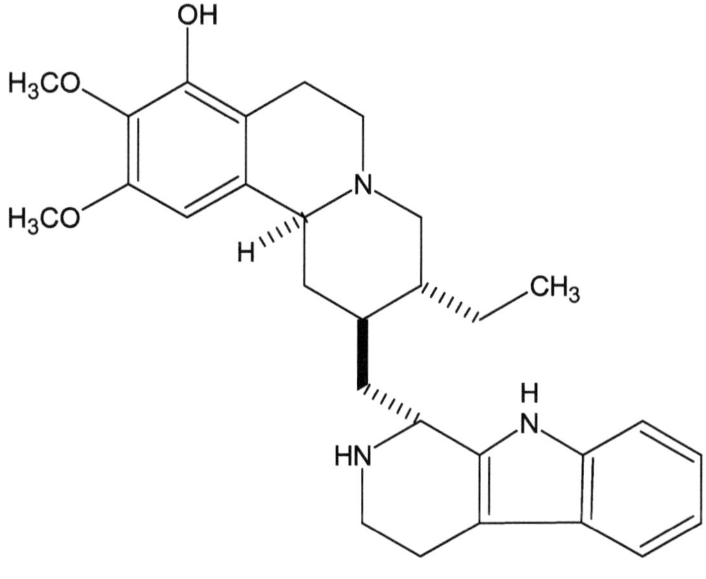

Alangimarckine

Contd...

Figure 15.1–Contd...

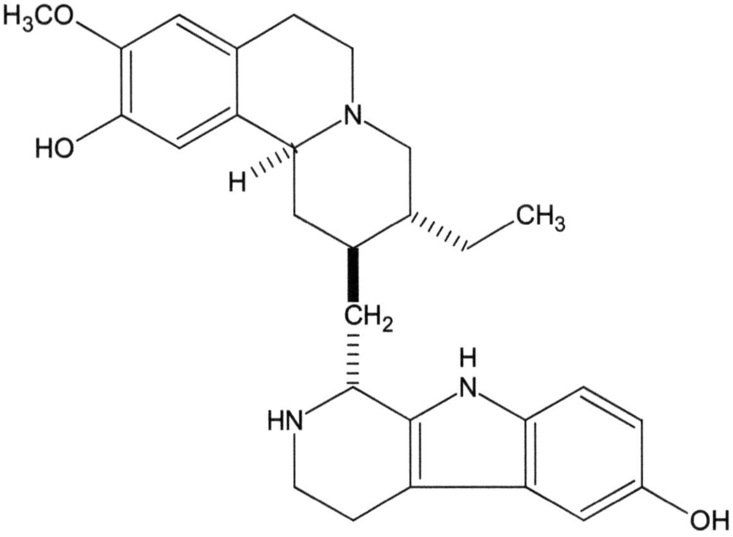

Demethyltubulosine

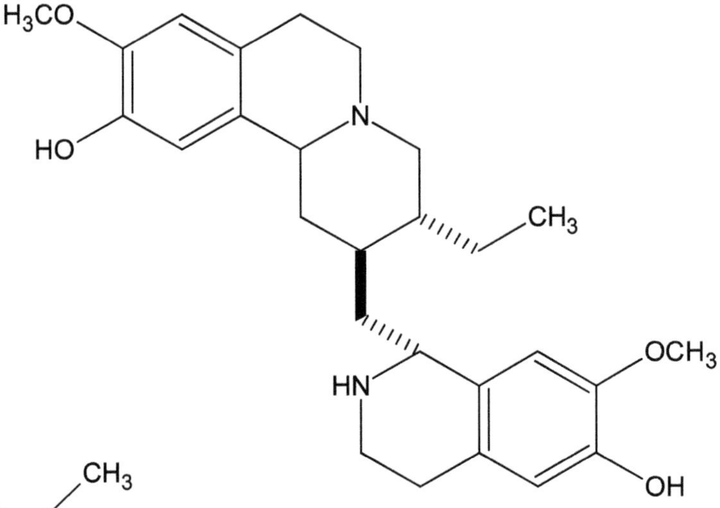

Demethylcephaeline

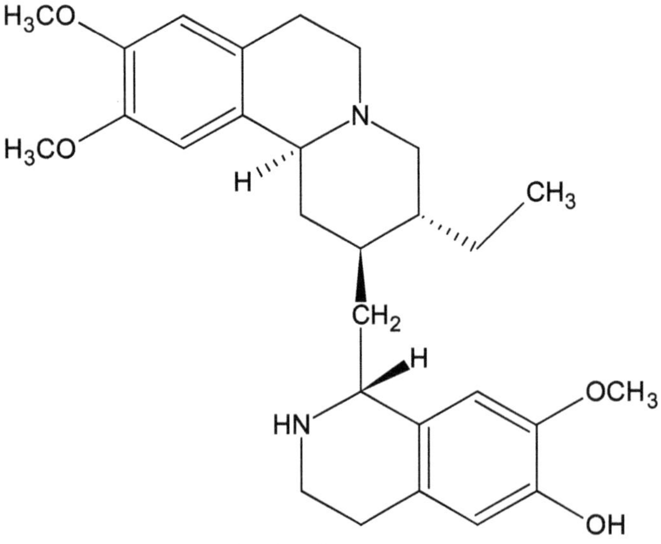

Cephaeline

Contd...

Figure 15.1–Contd...

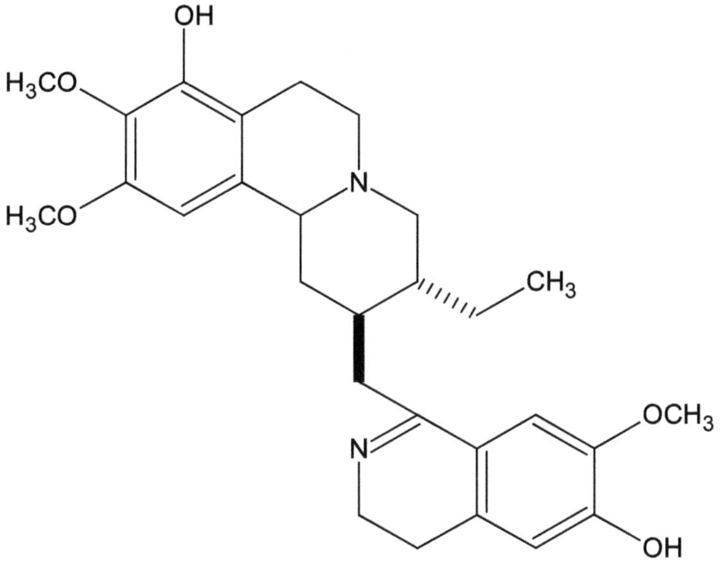

Alangicine

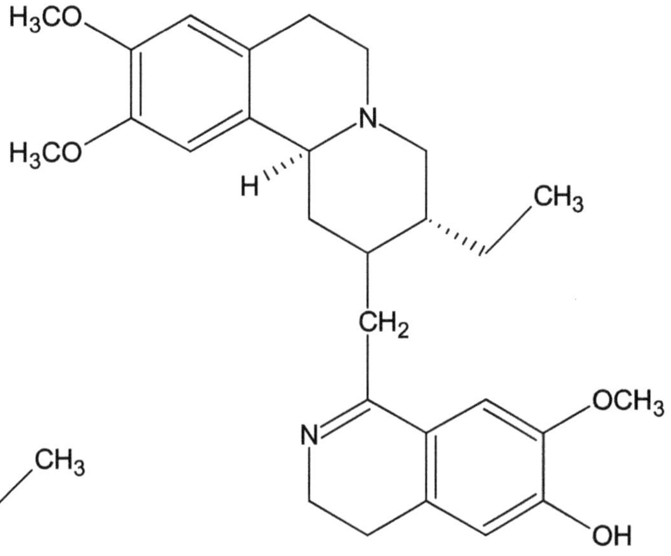

Demethylphychotrine

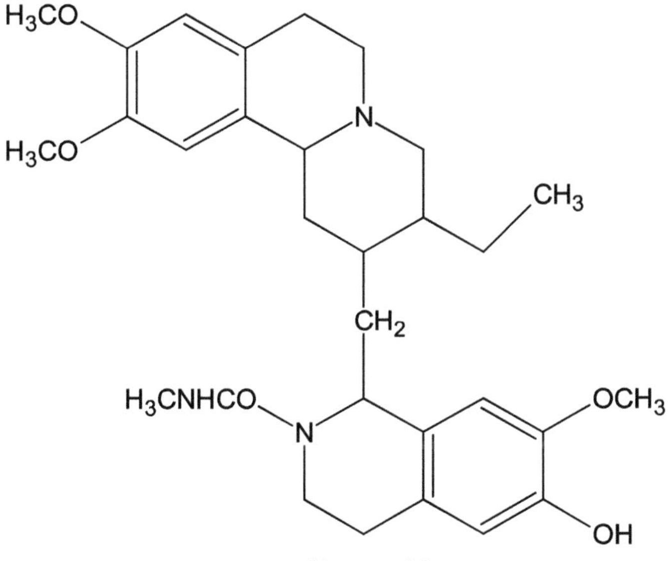

Alangamide

Contd...

Figure 15.1–Contd...

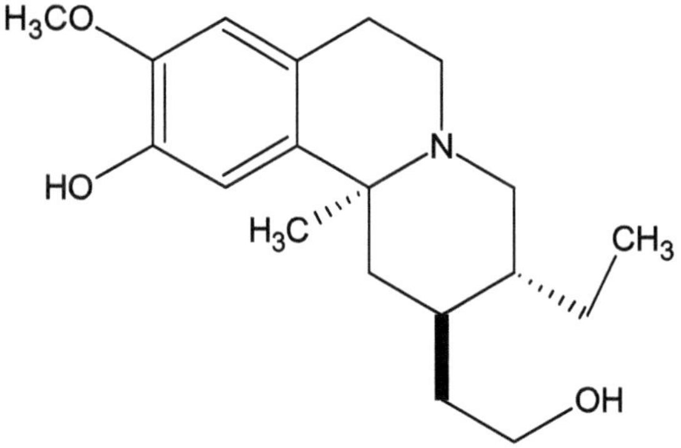

H_3CO, HO, H_3C, N, CH_3, OH

10–Demethylprotoementinol

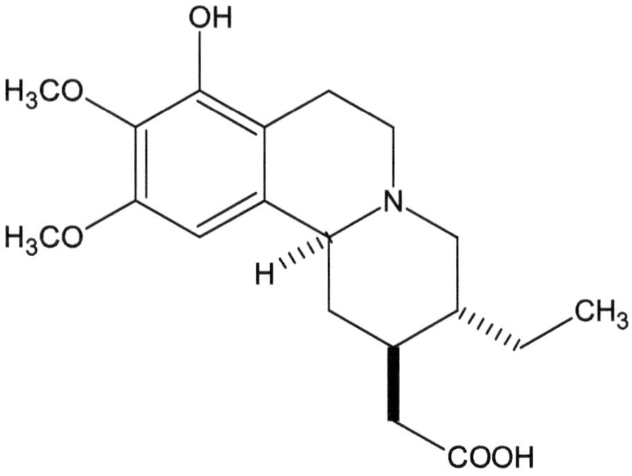

OH, H_3CO, H_3CO, N, H, CH_3, COOH

Alancine

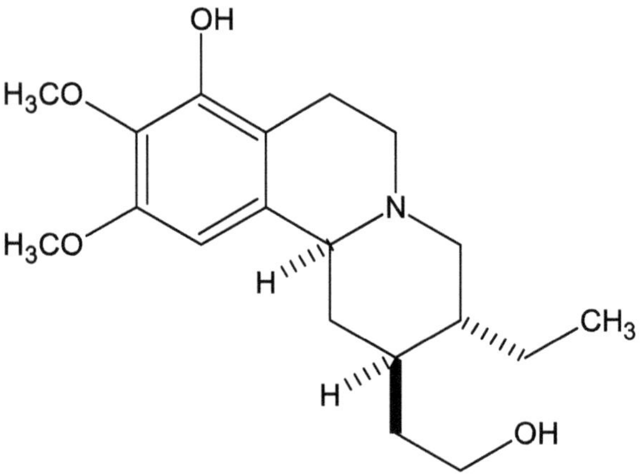

OH, H_3CO, H_3CO, N, H, H, CH_3, OH

Ankorine

R'O, R"O, N, O, N, R

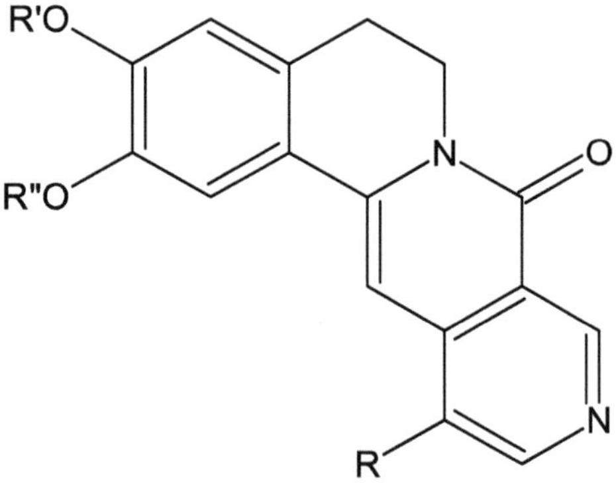

Isoalangimarine
R = CH=CH R' = H, R" = CH3
Isoalamarine
R = CH(OH)CH_3, R '= H, R" = CH_3
Alangimarinon
R = AC, R' = CH_3, R" = H

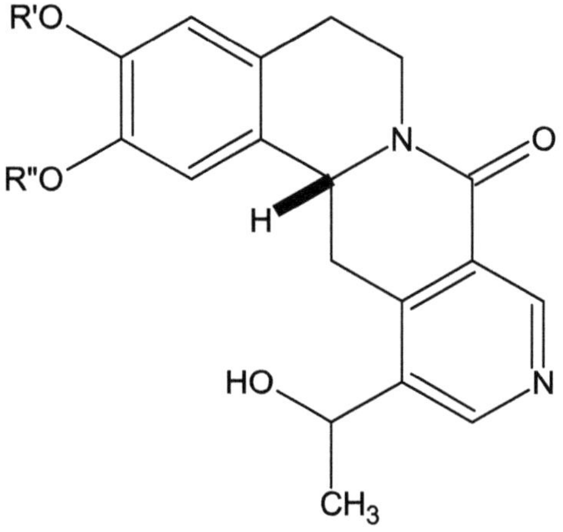

R'O, R"O, N, O, H, HO, N, CH_3

Dihydroalamarine
R"= H, R'= CH_3
Dihydroisoalamarine
R"= CH_3, R'=H

Contd...

Figure 15.1–Contd...

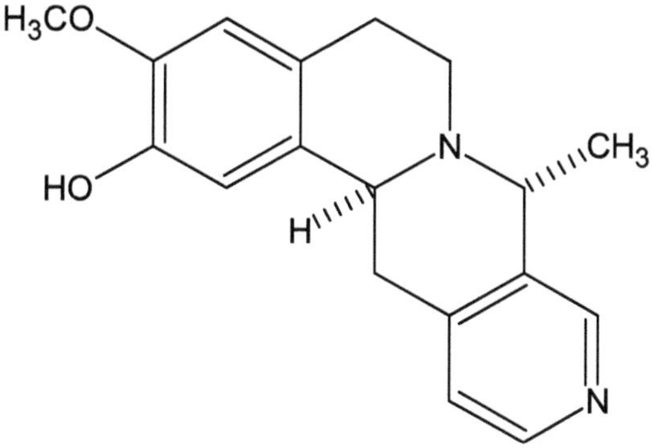

Alamaridine

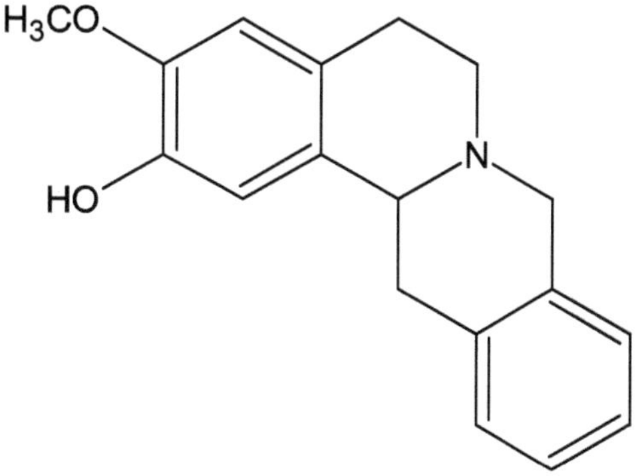

Bharatamine

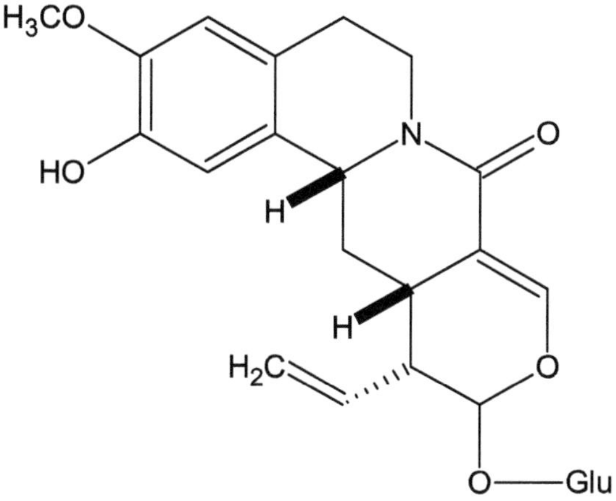

Alangiside

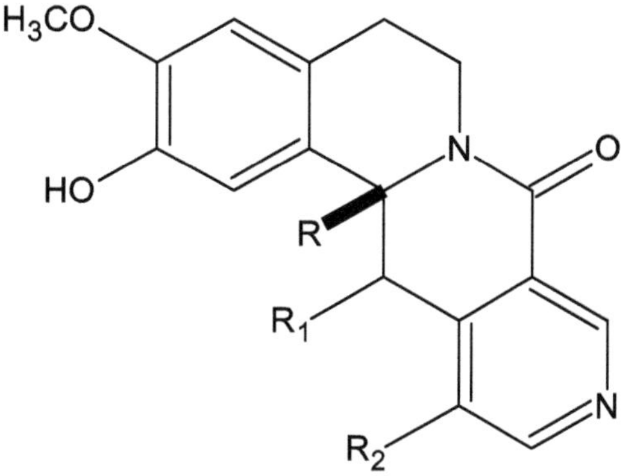

Alangimarine
R, R_1 = Δ, R_2 = CH=CH$_2$
Alamarine
R, R_1 = Δ, R_2 = CH(CH$_3$)OH
Alangimaridine
R,R_1= H, R_2 = CH=CH$_2$

tested in five male New Zealand white rabbits. All tested amounts of extract did not induce dermatitis among those rabbits within 1 week. The results demonstrated the inhibitory effect of *Alangium salviifolium* subsp *hexapetalum* against fungi without any local toxicity (Wuthi-udomlert *et al.*, 2002).

1-Methyl-1H-pyrimidine-2, 4-dione and 3-O-beta-D-glucopyranosyl-(24beta)-ethylcholesta-5, 22, 25-triene, isolated from the flowers showed remarkable antibacterial activities against a number of Gram-positive and Gram-negative bacterial species (Anjum *et al.*, 2002).

The methanol extract of flowers showed a wide spectrum of antibacterial activity against both gram-positive and gram-negative bacteria (Mossaddik *et al.*, 2000).

Antiinflammatory Activity

The total alkaloidal fraction of leaves were administered in a dose of 10 mg/100 g bw per day using formalin–induced arthritis model and betamethasone as standard for study of antiinflammatory activity. Remarkable increase in inflammatory reaction was observed during the first five days and extract reduced foot volume from the 11th day onwards in formalin-induced model. The results revealed that the drug was toxic and 66.7 per cent of rats died during treatment. After the administration of the drug a reduction in the food intake and faecal output of rats was observed (Gupta and Tandon, 2004).

Anthelmintic

The root bark extract showed anthelmintic activity only against poultry ascarids, but had no effect against bursate worms of sheep and hook worms of dog (Dubey and Gupta, 1968).

Cardiovascular Activity

An amorphous yellow alkaloid AL60 from stem bark showed biphasic action on blood pressure on intact cats. At low dose it caused a transient fall in blood pressure followed by a prolonged rise, where as in higher doses (0.4-1.6 mg/kg), it exerted hypotensive activity only. In contrast, spinal cats showed only a brief high pressure with improvement in cardio dynamic activity which was independent of doses. Animals treated with the dibenamine with or without prior administration of tetraethylammonium chloride showed that the alkaloid exhibited a sustained and prolonged hypotension. Remarkable vasodepression was recorded in atropinized, vagotomized, carotid occluded and hypertensive animals. In intact cats, AL60 in low dose induced a positive inotropic effect in cardiac muscle but in higher doses it depressed the heart. At higher and lower doses the total alkaloid isolated from the seeds exerted a sustained and prolonged hypo and hypertensive effect in intact cats respectively where as in spinal preparations the total alkaloids at the same dose level showed insignificant responses. Hypotensive activity was observed in atropinized, vagotomized, carotid occluded and tetraethylammonium chloride treated animals. The total alkaloids inhibited or reversed the pressor response of adrenaline in the preparations. It partially antagonized the vasodepressor effect of histamine (Dutta and Pakrashi, 1962b, 1963).

The hypotensive effect was not affected by pretreatment with 1 mg/kg of atropine sulphate where as pentolinium tartarate pretreated dogs reduced the hypertensive action of the alkaloids. The alkaloid also had anticholinesterase activity on dog's blood (Sanyal *et al.*, 1965).

The quaternary base salt isolated from air-dried powder leaves produced increasing fall in carotid blood pressure of anaesthetized dogs. The hypotension produced by 2 mg/kg of the drug was found to be nearly identical with those of 2µg/kg of acetylcholine chloride and 2 mg/kg of choline chloride. The effect was not altered by prior incubation with blood nor by pretreatment of the animal with eserine. Pretreatment with atropine 1 mg/kg however not only block the hypotensive effect of the drug but also caused a rise in the carotid blood pressure with the same dose. This property of the drug was identical with that of choline chloride. Acetylcholine did not cause any rise in the carotid blood pressure when its equipotent dose was repeated after atropinization. The base increased the tone and amplitude of contraction of isolated illeum of rabbit (Sanyal *et al.*, 1966).

Effect on Smooth Muscles

The stem bark alkaloid exerted spasmodic and spasmolytic effects in smooth muscle in low and higher doses respectively Extract produced spasmolytic action in guinea pig ileum. The total alkaloidal fraction of the leaves exhibited a non-specific antispasmodic effect on rat and rabbit ileum. A biphasic action on rabbit ileum, rat uterus and relaxant action on rat ileum was observed. Increases in rhythmic movements were observed at lower concentrations but at higher concentration a decrease in rhythmic movements and relaxation was observed. The quarternary base isolated from leaves had same spasmodic potency as that of choline chloride but much less than that of acetylcholine. 1μg/ml of atropine sulphate completely blocked the spasmodic effect of the base. It produced slow developing spasmodic contraction of the rectus abdominis muscle of the frog. The spasm produced by 0.2 mg/ml of the drug was same with that of 2 μg/ml of acetylcholine and 0.2 mg/ml of choline. This spasmodic effect of the drug could be blocked by pretreating the tissue with 50 μg/ml of tubocurarine chloride (Dutta and Pakrashi, 1960, 1962a, 1962b, 1963; Sanyal *et al.*, 1966).

Cytotoxicity

Thymidylate synthase is a key target enzyme in chemotherapy. The biological activity of the beta-carboline-benzoquinolizidine alkaloid deoxytubulosine demonstrated to exhibit potent cytotoxicity and inhibited the cell growth of *L. leichmannii* and thymidylate synthase activity at IC_{50} value 40 μMol. The deoxytubulosine concentrations more than 80 μMol resulted in a total loss of the thymidylate synthase activity, suggesting that the beta-carboline-benzoquinolizidine alkaloid had a promising potential as antitumor agent. The deoxytubulosine binding to thymidylate synthase appeared to be irreversible and tight through a possible covalent linkage. Inhibition kinetics showed that thymidylate synthase has a Ki value of 7×10^{-6} Mol for deoxytubulosine and that the inhibition is a simple linear "noncompetitive" type (Rao *et al.*,, 1998).

Beta-carboline-benzoquinolizidine plant alkaloid deoxytubulosine was evaluated and assessed for its biochemical and biological activity employing the biomarker dihydrofolate reductase purified from *Lactobacillus leichmannii*, a key target in cancer chemotherapy. Deoxytubulosine was demonstrated to exhibit potent cytotoxicity. The alkaloid potently inhibited the cell growth of *L. leichmannii* and the cellular enzyme activity of dihydrofolate reductase at IC_{50} value 40 and 30 μMol for the cell growth and enzyme inhibitions, respectively. Deoxytubulosine concentrations more than 75 μMol resulted in a total loss of the dihydrofolate reductase activity suggesting that the beta-carboline-benzoquinolizidine alkaloid had potential antitumor agent. It also had potential antimicrobial activity. Deoxytubulosine binding to dihydrofolate reductase appeared to be slow and reversible. Inhibition kinetics revealed that dihydrofolate reductase had a Ki value of 5×10^{-6} Mol for deoxytubulosine and enzyme inhibition is a simple linear 'non-competitive' type (Rao and Venkatachalam, 1999).

Deoxytubulosine inhibited the thymidylate synthatase a key target enzyme purified from *Latobacillus leichannii*. Cytotoxicity studies showed that cell growth of *L. leichmannii* was inhibited at IC_{50} value 40-45 μMol, the concentrations more than 80-90 μMol resulted in complete loss of the enzyme activity. Ki values of the enzyme calculated for deoxytubulosine were 7×10^{-6} Mol. These are typed as 'non-competitive' inhibitors of thymidylate synthatase. Alkaloids inhibited the elevated thymidylate synthatase activity of leukocytes in cancer patients with clinically diagnosed chronic myelocytic leukemia, acute lymphocytic leukemia and metastatic solid tumours in a dose of IC_{50} value 50 μMol. (Rao *et al.*, 1999).

Biological evaluation of alkaloids showed that compound (-)-10-O-demethylisocephaeline and 10-O-demethylcephaeline exhibited potent cytotoxic activity against human lung carcinoma (A 549) and breast adenocarcinoma (MCF-7) with $ED_{(50)}$ values of 0.013 and 0.062 μMol respectively. The stereoisomer 1st compound was less potent than 2nd and related compounds with different hydroxyl/methoxy substitution patterns were also less potent or inactive (Sakurai *et al.*, 2006).

Miscellaneous

The alkaloidal fraction did not show any analgesic, anticonvulsant or diuretic action in rats. The 50 per cent ethanolic extract of leaves exhibited hypoglycaemic activity in rats, antiprotozoal activity against *Entamoeba histolytica* and antispasmodic activity in isolated guinea pig ileum. The minimum toxic dose of the extract was found to be 1000 mg/kg bw orally in mice. The extract was devoid of antibacterial, antifungal, anthelmintic, antiviral and antispirochaetal activities and effects on respiration, CVS and CNS in experimental animals (Sanyal *et al.*, 1965; Dhar *et al.*, 1968).

Alangimarckine showed hypoglycaemic effect with sodium retention with little effect on blood pressure, but independent of the dose. The alkaloid produced a moderate cytostatic activity *in vitro* (Merchant and Salgar, 1975).

The flowers also contained deoxytubulosine, a potent antiplatelet aggregation component which has a strong binding with DNA. Petroleum ether, ethyl acetate, chloroform, methanol and aqueous extracts of powdered stem bark did not show any significant CNS activity in mice but showed abortifacient activity when given during the first 8th day of pregnancy. Petroleum ether and ethyl acetate have some antiimplantation action. The extract also caused resorption of some implantation sites (Murugan *et al.*, 2000).

Conclusion and Discussion

In the present review we have made an attempt to congregate the taxonomical, botanical, ethnopharmacological, phytochemical and pharmacological information on *Alangium salviifolium*, a medicinal herb used in the Indian system of medicine. Literature Survey revealed the presence of alkaloids, saponins, monoterpenoids, sterols, tannins, sugars, colouring matter, cellulose, tetrahydroisoquinoline-monoterpene glycoside and iridoid glycoside in different parts of this plant. Research on alkaloids of beta-carboline-benzoquinolizidine basic structure has gained a special attention in recent times. Several phytoconstituent in the plant have shown promising cardiovascular, antiinflammatory, antimicrobial, antiplatelet, anticonvulsant, antipyretic, antidiabetic, abortifacient, anthelmintic, and antispasmodic activity etc. The cytotoxic activity of beta-carboline-benzoquinolizidine group alkaloid deoxytubulosine is definite, but most of the alkaloids are too toxic to be clinically used. Investigation of natural products to isolate more potent and structural modification of the known compounds to retain its parent activity are still the best possible ways to develop safe and effective anticancer drugs.

Cardiac disease claims several million deaths every year on a global basis which is mainly due to change in life style of human being. In spite of the fact that clinically used cardiovascular drug, digitoxin is originally derived from plants, further search for isolation and identification of new cardioactive drugs from natural sources are extremely limited. Ethnopharmacological approach in the search for new cardiovascular compounds from plants appears to be helpful compared to the random screening approach. However a promising phytopharmacological basis is needed to use phytoactive constituent as templates for designing new derivatives with improved cardioactive properties. Alkaloid AL60 has demonstrated a promising cardiovascular activity by producing biphasic action on blood pressure. At low dose it caused a transient fall in blood pressure followed by a prolonged rise, where as in higher doses it exerted hypotensive activity only (Pakrashi and Achari, 1970). Therefore, these alkaloids offer a promising source for the development of new cardiovascular agents. Total alkaloidal fraction of plant has been screened for antiinflammatory activity but having less efficacy, where as alcoholic, aqueous and lyophilized powder extract would be worthwhile in serving as a tool for microbial control. It also finds immense utility in abdominal problems, rheumatic pain, snake biting, haemorrhage, skin diseases and liver disfunctioning. This review will definitely help the researchers as well as practitioners dealing with this plant to know its nature and proper uses. Taking great concern of the useful benefits of the plant, it can be advocated as a potent medicinal plant for general population. Effects should be directed towards formulation development with the phytoactive constituents or with enriched fractions of *Alangium salviifolium* to get herbal remedies for anticancer and cardiovascular diseases. Approach for formulation development and clinical studies have not been done so far. More patient oriented clinical studies should be carried out to explore the practical medicinal values of this plant which can also help in exploitation of its economical potential by marketing herbal formulation.

Acknowledgements

The authors are grateful to the CDRI, Lucknow and NISCAIR, New Delhi, India for providing library facilities.

References

Achari, B., Ali, E., Ghosh, D., Sinha, R.R., and Pakrashi, S.C. (1980). Studies on Indian medicinal plants. Part 56. further investigations on the alkaloids of *Alangium lamarckii. Planta Medica (suppl)*, 40: 5-7.

Achari, B., Pal, A. and Pakrashi, S.C. (1974). Studies on Indian medicinal plants: Part XXXI. N-Benzoyl-L-phenylalaninol from *Alangium lamarckii. Indian Journal of Chemistry*, 12: 1218-19.

Achari, B., Pal, A. and Pakrashi, S.C. (1975). Studies on Indian medicinal plants: Part XXXVI. New D: E-*Cis*-fused neohopane derivatives from *Alangium lamarckii. Tetrahedron Letter*, 48: 4275-78.

Ali, E., Sinha, R.R., Achari, B. and Pakrashi, S.C. (1982). Demethylproteometinols from *Alangium lamarckii. Heterocycles*, 19: 2301-04

Anjum, A., Ekramul, H.M., Mukhlesur, R.M. and Sarker, S.D. (2002). Antibacterial compounds from the flowers of *Alangium salviifolium. Fitoterapia*, 73(6): 526-28.

Basu, N.K. and Gode, K.D. (1957). Studies on the alkaloids of *Alangium lamarcki* Thw. *Journal of Indian Chemical Society*, 34: 629–39.

Basu, N.K., Nair, N.S. and Bhattacharya, N.N. (1950). Chemical investigation of *Alangium lamarcki* Thw. *Indian Journal of Pharmacy*, 12: 98-9.

Battersby, A.R., Merchant, J.R., Ruveda, E.A. and Salgar, S.S. (1965). Structure, synthesis and stereochemistry of deoxytubulosine. *Chemical Communication*, 14: 315-17.

Bhakuni, D.S., Dhar, M.M. and Dhar, M.L. (1960). Structure of alangine-A, an alkaloid from *Alangium lamarcki* Thwaits. *Journal of Science and Industrial Research*, 19B: 8-10.

Bhargava, P.N. and Dutt, S. (1942). Chemical examination of the seeds of *Alangium lamarckii* Thw. Isolation of alangol. *Proceeding of the Indiana Acadmy of Science*, 16A: 328-31.

Bhatnagar, S.S., Santapau, H., Desa, J.D.H., Maniar, A.C.,Ghadially, N.C., Solomon, M.J., Yellore, S. and Rao, T.N.S. (1961). Biological activity of Indian medicinal plants. Part I. Antibacterial, antitubercular and antifungal action. *The Indian Journal of Medical Research*, 49: 799-13.

Bhattacharjya, A., Mukhopadhyay, R., Sinha, R.R., Ali, E. and Pakrash, S.C. (1988). Studies on Indian medicinal plants: part 91-structure and synthesis of alamaridine, a novel 5-methylbenzopyrioquinolizine alkaloid from *Alangium lamarckii. Tetrahedron*, 44(12): 3477-88.

Bhattacharjya, A., Mukhopadhyay, R. and Pakrashi, S.C. (1986). Structure and synthesis of alamaridine, a novel benzopyroquinolizine alkaloid from *Alangium lamarckii. Tetrhedron*, 27: 1215-16.

Budzikiewicz, H., Pakrashi, S.C. and Vorbruggen, H. (1964). Isolation of emetin, cephaeline, and psychotrin from *Alangium lamarckii* and their identification with alamarckine and N–methylcephaeline. *Tetrahedron*, 20: 399-408.

Chattopadhyay, S.K., Slatkin, D.J., Schiff, P.L.Jr. and Ray, A.B. (1984). Alancine, a new benzoquinolizidine alkaloid from *Alangium lamarckii. Heterocycles*, 22: 1965-68.

Chopra, R.N. and Chowhan, J.S. (1934). *Alangium lamarckii*: Its chemistry and pharmacological action. *Indian Journal of Medical Reserch*, 21: 507-12.

Dasgupta, B. (1966). Chemical investigations of *Alangium lamarckii* II. Isolation of choline from the leaves. *Experientia*, 22: 287-88.

Dasgupta, B. and Sharma, S. (1966). Chemical investigations of *Alangium lamarckii*. III. Isolation of steroids and terpenoids from the leaves. *Experientia*, 22: 647-51.

De-Eknamkul, W., Suttipanta, N. And Kutchan, T.M. (2000). Purification and characterization of deacetylipecoside synthase from *Alangium lamarckii* Thw. *Phytochemistry*, 55(2): 177-81.

Desai, P.D., Ganguly, A.K., Govindachari, T.R., Joshi, B.S., Kamat, V.N., Manmade, A.H., Mohamed, P.A., Nagle, S.K., Nayak, R.H., Saksena, A.K., Sathe, S.S. and Viswanathan, N. (1966). Chemical investigation of some Indian plants. Part II. *Indian Journal of Chemistry*, 4:457-59.

Dhar, M.L., Dhar, M.M., Dhawan, B.N. and Ray, C. (1968).Screening of Indian plants for biological activity. Part I. *Indian Journal of Experimental Biology*, 6: 232-47.

Dubey, M.P. and Gupta, I. (1968). Some studies on the anthelmintic activity of *Alangium lamarckii* Thwaites-(Hindi-akol) root bark. *Indian Journal of Physiology and Pharmacology*, 12: 25-31.

Dutta, A.K. and Pakrashi, S.C. (1962 a). Studies on cardiovascular drugs. Part IV. Effect of the new alkaloid from the stem bark of *Alangium lamarckii* Thw. on cardiovascular system and smooth muscles. *Annals of Biochemistry and Experimental Medicine*, 22: 129-46.

Dutta, A.K. and Pakrashi, S.C. (1962b). Studies on Cardiovascular drugs. Part III. Preliminary studies on the total alkaloids from the seeds of *Alangium lamarckii* Thw. *Annals of Biochemistry and Experimental Medicine*, 22: 23-24.

Dutta, A.K. and Pakrashi, S.C. (1963). Studies on cardiovascular drugs. Part V. Pharmacological investigation of the total alkaloids from the seeds of *Alangium lamarckii* Thw. *Annals of Biochemistry and Experimental Medicine*, 23: 285-98.

Dutta, A.K. and Pakrashi, S.C., 1960. Studies on cardiovascular drugs. Part I. Preliminary pharmacological investigation of a new alkaloid from *Alangium salviifolium* Thw. *Annals of Biochemistry and Experimental Medicine*, 20: 279-80.

Fujii, T. (1983). Structure and synthesis of benzoquinolizidine alkaloids isolated from *Alangium lamarckii. Yakugaku Zasshi*, 103(3): 257-72.

George, M. and Pandalai, K.M. (1949). Investigation of plant antibiotics. Part IV. Further search for antibiotic substances in Indian medicinal plants. *The Indian Journal of Medical Research*, 37: 169-81.

Gond, G.S. and Sankhapal, K.V. (1998). Antimicrobial activity of some tribal plants. *Indian Drugs*, 35: 778-79.

Gupta, A.K. and Tandon, (2004). Reviews on Indian Medicinal Plants, Vol. I, Indian Council of Medical Research, New Delhi, pp.432-38.

Gupta, B., Srivastava, R.S. and Goyal, R. (2007). Plant review therapeutic uses of *Euphorbia thymifolia*: A Review, *Pharmacognosy Reviews*, 1(2): 299.

Itoh, A., Ikuta, Y., Tanahashi, T. and Nagakura, N. (2000). Two alangium alkaloids from *Alangium lamarckii*. *Journal of Natural Product*, 63(5): 723-25.

Itoh, A., Tanahashi, T., Tabata, M., Shikata, M., Kakite, M., Nagai, M. and Nagakura, N. (2001). Tetrahydroisoquinoline-monoterpene and iridoid glycosides from *Alangium lamarckii*. *Phytochemistry*, 56(6): 623.

Joshi, N.C. and Sabnis, S.D. (1989). A phytochemical study of South Gujarat Forests plants with special reference to the medicinal and of ethnobotanical interest. *Bulletin of Medical and Ethnobotanical Research* 10: 61-82.

Kapil, R.S., Shoeb, A. and Popli, S.P. (1971). Alangiside: A monoterpenoid lactum. *Journal of the Chemical Society. Chemical Communication*, 904-05.

Kirtikar, K.R. and Basu, B.D. (2006). Indian Medicinal Plants. Vol. II, 4th reprint Ed., Jayyed Press, Delhi, pp.1237-39.

Kotnis, M.S., Patel, P., Menon, S.N. and Sane, R.T. (2004). Renoprotective effect of *Hemisdesmus indicus*, a herbal drug used in gentomicin-induced renal toxicity. *Nephrology (carlton)*, 3: 142-52.

Lakshminarasimhaiah, A., Manjunath, B.L. and Nagaraj, B.S. (1942). *Journal of Mysore University*, 3B: 113.

Merchant, J.R. and Salgar, S.S. (1975). Some further data on the alkaloids deoxytubulosine and alangimarckine. *Indian Journal of Chemistry*, 13: 100-01.

Mosaddik, M.A., Kabir, K.E. and Hassan P.(2000). Antibacterial activity of *Alangium salviifolium* flowers. *Fitoterapia*, 71(4): 447-49.

Mukhopadhyay, R., Ghosh Dastidar, P.P., Ali, E. and Pakrashi, S.C. (1987). Studies on Indian medicinal plants 87. Lacinilene C–a rare sesquiterpene from *Alangium lamarckii*. *Journal of Natural Product*, 50: 1185.

Murugan, V., Shareef, H., Sharma, R., G.V.S., Ramanathan, M. and Suresh, B. (2000). Antifertility activity of the stem bark of *Alangium salviifolium* (Linn.f.) Wang in wistar female rats. *Indian Journal of Pharmacology*, 32: 388-89.

Nadkarni, K.M. (2002). Indian Materia Medica, Vol. I, reprint Ed., Popular Prakashan, pp 58-60.

Pakrashi, S. C., Bhattacharjya, J., Mookerjee, S., Samatan, T. B. and Vorbrüggen, H. (1968). Studies on Indian medicinal plants-XVIII, the non-alkaloidal constituents from the seeds of *Alangium lamarckii* Thw. *Phytochemistry*, 7(3): 461-66.

Pakrashi, S.C. (1966). Chemical investigation of root bark and stem bark of *Alangium lamarcki* Thwaites–A correction. *Current Science*, 35: 468-69.

Pakrashi, S.C. and Achari, B. (1970). Demethylcephaeline, a new alkaloid from *Alangium lamarckii*.Characterization of AL60, the hypotensive principal from the stem bark. *Experientia*, 26: 933-34.

Pakrashi, S.C. and Ali, E. (1967). Newer alkaloids From *Alangium lamarckii* Thw. *Tetrahedron Letter*, 23: 2143-46.

Rao, K.N. and Venkatachalam, S.R. (1999). Dihydrofolate reductase and cell growth activity inhibition by the beta-carboline-benzoquinolizidine plant alkaloid deoxytubulosine from *Alangium lamarckii*: Its potential as an antimicrobial and anticancer agent. *Bioorganic and Medical Chemistry*, 7(6): 1105-10.

Rao, K.N., Bhattacharya, R.K. and Veankatachalam, S.R. (1999). Inhibition of thymidylate synthase by pergularinine, tylophorinidine and deoxytubulosine. *Indian Journal of Biochemistry and Biophysics*, 36(6): 442-48.

Rao, K.N., Bhattacharya, R.K. and Venkatachalam, S.R. (1998) Thymidylate synthase activity and the cell growth are inhibited by the beta-carboline-benzoquinolizidine alkaloid deoxytubulosine. *Journal of Biochemical and Molecular Toxicology*, 12(3): 167-73.

Sakurai, N., Nakagawa-Goto, K., Ito, J., Sakurai, Y., Nakanishi, Y., Bastow, K.F., Cragg, G. and Lee, K.H. (2006). Cytotoxic Alangium alkaloids from *Alangium longifolium*. *Phytochemistry*, 67(9): 894-97.

Sanyal, A.K., Dasgupta, B. and Das, P.K.(1965). Studies of *Alangium lamarckii*, Thw. I. Pharmacological studies of the total alkaloidal extract of the leaves. *The Indian Journal of Medical Research*, 53(11), 1055-61.

Sanyal, A.K., Dasgupta, B., Gambhir, S.S. and Das, P.K. (1966). Studies on *Alangium lamarckii*, Thw. II. Chemical and pharmacological studies with a quaternary base from the leaves. *The Indian Journal of Medical Research*, 54(11): 1060-63.

Shoeb, A., Raj, K., Kapil, R.S. and Popli, S.P.(1975). Alangiside, the monoterpenoid alkaloidal glycoside from *Alangium lamarckii* Thw. *Journal of the Chemical Society*, 13: 1245-48.

WHO, IUCN and WWF, Guidelines on the conservation of medicinal plants, (IUCN Gland Switzerland), (1993).

Wuthi-udomlert, M., Prathanturarug, S. and Wongkrajang, Y. (2002). Antifungal activity and local toxicity study of *Alangium salviifolium* subsp hexapetalum. *Southeast Asian Journal of Tropical Medicine and Public Health*, 33(3): 152-54.

Medicinal Plants: Phytochemistry, Pharmacology and Therapeutics, Vol. 1 *Pages* ***315–329***
Editors: **V.K. Gupta, G.D. Singh, Surjeet Singh and A. Kaul**
Published by: **DAYA PUBLISHING HOUSE, NEW DELHI**

Chapter 16

An Overview of the Ayurvedic Medicinal Plant *Phyllanthus amarus* for its Botanical, Phytochemical and Biological Explorations

P. Koul*, S. Singh, R. Sharma and V. K. Gupta
Indian Institute of Integrative Medicine (CSIR),
Canal Road, Jammu – 180 001, J&K State, India

ABSTRACT

Since pre-historic days attempts are being made to find out suitable drugs from natural source for the treatment of diseases because synthetic medicines cause various inevitable side effects. Recently, much importance has been imparted to develop the formulations from the plant source which are mostly free from toxic actions. The plant families are the rich source of organic compounds, many of which are well known for their therapeutic properties. *Phyllanthus amarus* (Euphorbiaceae) is an annual herb, which is reported to contain lignans, alkaloids, flavonoids, galloatnoids, glycosides and alkaloids. It is commonly called Bhumi-amala. The plant species is distributed throughout the hotter parts of India. It grows well under tropical conditions, however rarely survives under dry or very low temperature conditions although water logging does not show any lethal effects. The plant grows abundantly throughout India up to 700msl altitude. The plants are propagated through seeds. Since the active constituents of *P. amarus* are concentrated more in the leaves, production of higher leaf mass is desired for the extraction. Plant bears highest number of leaves during September and this time suitable for harvesting.

* Corresponding Author: E-mail: pkoul@iiim.res.in.

The therapeutic effects has been acknowledged as antiviral, antiparasitic, antimalarial, antimicrobial, anticancer, antidiabetic, antihypercholesterolemic, cellular protective and wound-healing properties. It also acts on kidney stones and Uric Acid. It protects liver and detoxifies the toxicity and for treating hepatitis B virus.

***Keywords**: Phyllanthus, Hepatoprotective, Antiviral, Anticancer, Antidiabetic.*

Introduction

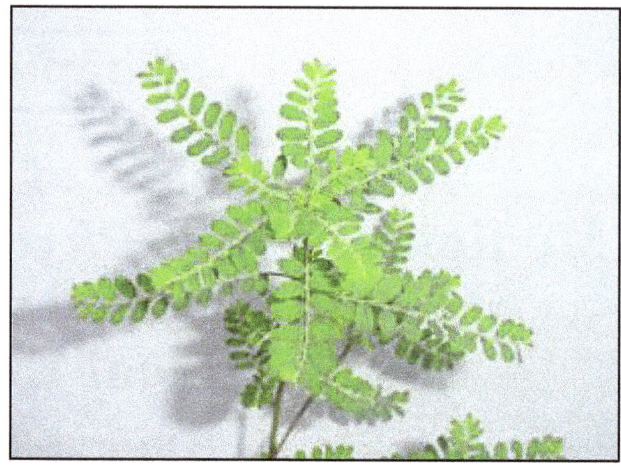

Phyllanthus amarus belongs to family Euphorbiaceae. Commanly in Hindi it is called Jaramla, Jangli amli, Bhuinanvalah, Bhonyabali, Sada-hasurmani and Bhumi-amala and in Sanskrit it is named as Bahuphala, Mahidhatrika, Bhumyamalaki, Bhupatra. The synonyms of *Phyllanthus amarus* are *Phyllanthus niruri* L. *Phyllanthus fraternus* and *Phyllanthus nanus.* The plant species is distributed throughout the hotter parts of India, in upper Gangetic plain, Bundelkhand, Assam, Bengal, Bihar, Orissa, Punjab, Deccan, Konkan and South Indian states. It is common in Central and Southern India extending to Sri Lanka. The plant grows abundantly throughout India up to 700msl altitude. Whole plant is used as the crude drug. A number of other species of *Phyllanthus* are found mixed in the commercial samples or used as substitutes. Among these *Phyllanthus urinaria* L. is used more commonly. This species has large leaves and reddish fruits (on ripening). The commercial samples originating from south India have been found to be a mixture of *P. amarus. hyllanthus debilis* willd and *P. simplex* Retz. are also reported to be used as substitute/adulterant to *P. amarus.* It grows well under tropical conditions, however rarely survives under dry or very low temperature conditions although water logging does not show any lethal effects.

The plants are propagated through seeds. About 1kg seeds are sufficient for seedlings for transplanting in one hectare of land. For raising the seedlings, the seeds are sown in well prepared nursery beds. Well decomposed farm yard manure should be mixed with top layer of the soil while preparing the beds. Being minute, the seeds are mixed with dry soil or sand to allow uniform distribution of seeds on the nursery bed. Later a thin layer of soil is spread to cover the nursery beds. Appropriate moisture is maintained in the beds till the seeds have germinated. In north Indian plains, the month of April-May was found very well for sowing for higher rate of germination of seeds and good herb yield. Approximately 15-30 days old seedlings, which are about 10 cm tall, are transplanted in the field at horizontal and vertical spacing of 15 cm each. Proper irrigation just after transplanting ensures establishment of seedlings. The crop raised by transplanting of seedlings gives improved yield of herbage. The medicinal plants have to be grown without chemical fertilizers and use of pesticides. Organic manures like Farm Yard Manure (FYM), Vermi-Compost, and Green Manure etc. may be used as per requirement of the species. To prevent diseases, bio-pesticides could be prepared (either single or mixture) from Neem (kernel, seeds and leaves), Chitrakmool, Dhatura, Cow's urine etc. Plants are harvested when the rainy season is over, when they are still green and herbaceous. Since the active constituents of *P. amarus* are concentrated more in the leaves, production of higher leaf mass is desired for the extraction. Plant bears highest number of leaves during September and this time is suitable for harvesting.

Chemistry

The main active constituents of *P. amarus* are lignans (phyllanthin, hypophyllanthin, nirurin etc), flavonoids (quercetin, quercetrin, rutin etc), terpens, alkaloids etc. The leaves are the rich source of phyllanthin a diarylbutane and hypophyllanthin an aryltetrahydronaphthalene type of lignin. Enantiomer of norsecurinine, 4–methoxy securinine, 4–methoxy-norsecurinine, nirphyllin and phyllnirurin, phyllantheol, phyllathenol, nirphyllin and phyllnirurin,3,7,11,15,19,23-hexamethyl–2Z, 6Z, 10Z. 14E, 18E, 22E-tetracosahexen-1 ol, tricontanol, phthalic acid bis-ester (phyllester) with β-sitosterol, dotriacontanoic acid and a rare sterol 24-isopropylcholesterol (aerial parts); lintetralin, niranthin, nirtetralin, phyllanthin, hypophyllanthin, phyltetralin, vitamin C (leaves); phyllochrysine alkaloids (leaves, stem); lupa 20 (29)-ene-3-ol, 3,5,7-trihydroxyflavonal-4′-0-α-L(-)–rhamnopyranoside,5,3′,4′-trihydroxy flavanone-7-0-α-L(-)-rhamnopyranoside, nirurin[5,6,7,4′-tetrahydroxy 8-(3-methylbut-2-aryl)flavones-5-0-rutinoside], phyllanterpenyl ester, pentacosanyl ester, heptacosanoic acid, phyllanthusone, phyllanthosterol, phyllanthosecosteryl ester, phyllanthostigmasterol and fraternusterol (root); estradiol (bark,root); ricinoleic, linoleic and linolenic acid (seed oil); corilagin, ellagic acid, gallic acid, geraniin an angiotensin converting enzyme inhibitor, and the flavonoids-FG_1 and FG_2 (plant).

Root

(-)-Epi-gallocatechin-3-O-gallate, Lupeol, Lupeol acetate, Nor-securinine, Phyllanthine.

Root Culture

(+)-Catechin, (+)-Gallocatechin, (-)-Epi-catechin, (-)–Epi-Catechin-3-gallate, (-) Epi-gallocatechin, Gallic acid.

Leaf

4-Hydroxy-lintetralin, 2,3-dimethoxy-iso-lintetralin, Ascorbic acid 0.41 per cent, Asteragalin,β sitosterol, Hydroxy niranthin, Iso-quercitrin, Linnanthin, Lintetralin, Niranthin, Nirtetralin, Phyllanthine, Phyllochrysine, Phyltetralin, Quercetin, Quercitrin, Rutin.

Leaf Ethanolic Extract

(-)-Limonene 4.5 per cent, Cymene 11 per cent.

Plant

(-)-Nor-serurinine, 4-Hydroxy-sesamin, Corilagin, Ellagic acid, Estradiol, Geranin 0.23 per cent, Hinokinin, Iso-lintetralin, Nirtetralin, Nirurine, Nirurinetin, Phyllanthus, Phyltetralin 14 per cent, Quercetin, Repandusinic acid 0.12 per cent, Rutin, Trans-phytol.

Seed Oil

Linoleic acid 21 per cent, Linolenic acid 51.4 per cent, Ricinoleic acid 1.2 per cent.Aerial: 24-Isopropyl cholesterol, Dotriacontanoic acid, Nirphyllin, Nirurine, Phyllanthenone, phyllantheol, phyllester, Phyllnirurin, phylltetrin, Triacontan-1-al, Triancontan-1-ol.

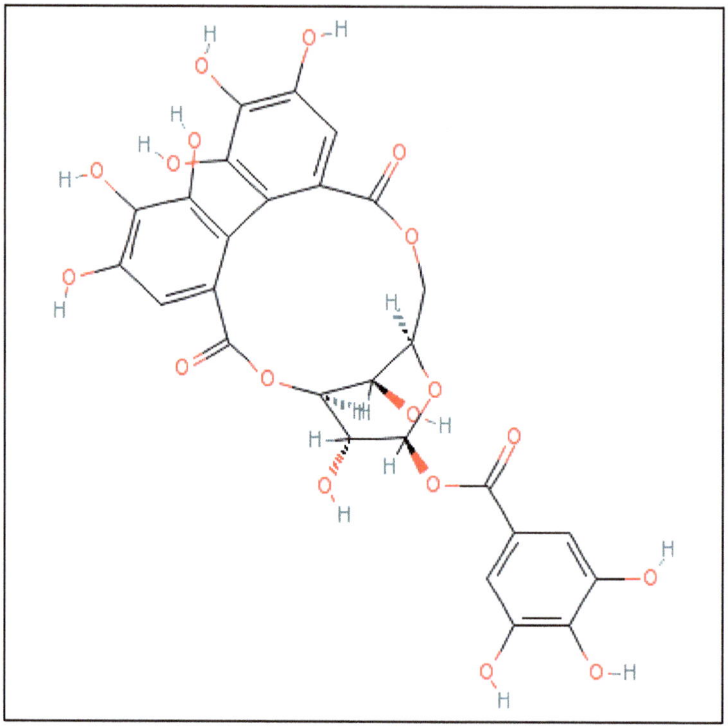

Corilagin

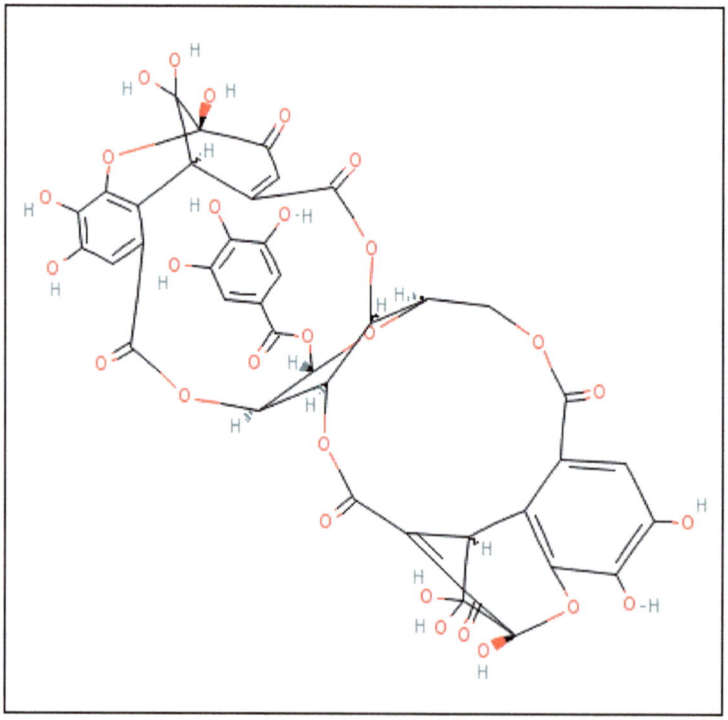

Amariin

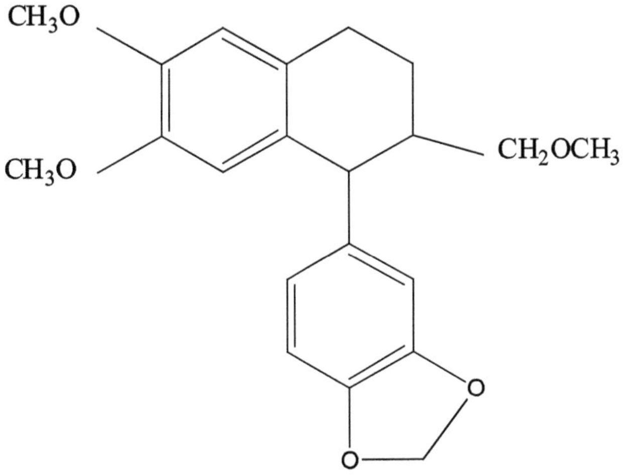

Lintetralin

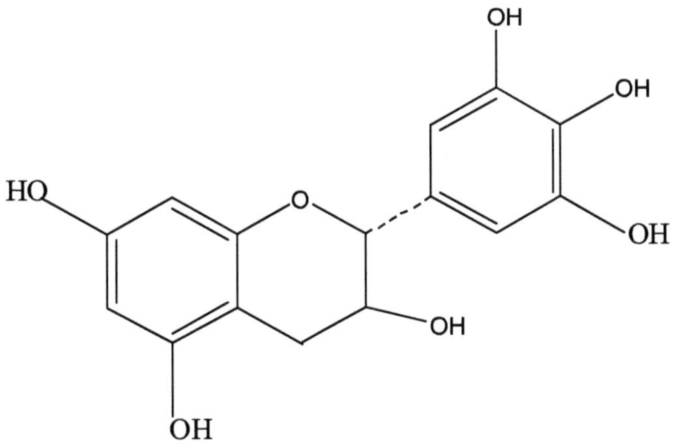

Gallocatecin

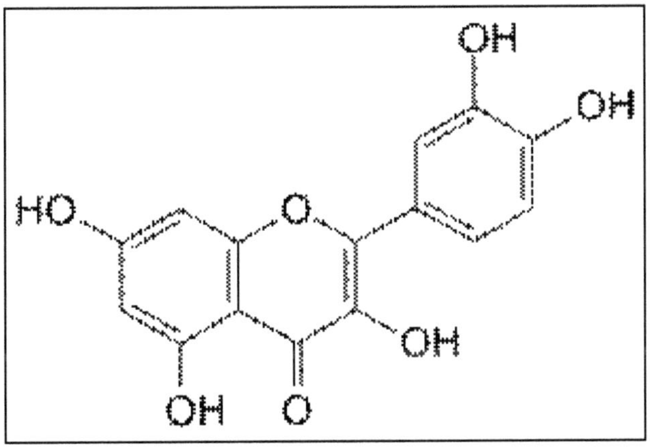

Quercetin

Chemical Markers for Authentication and Identification

The secondary metabolites present in *P. amarus* are alkaloids, flavanoids, hydrolysable tannins and major lignans. Phyllanthin (bitter constituent) and hypophyllanthin (non-bitter compound) are

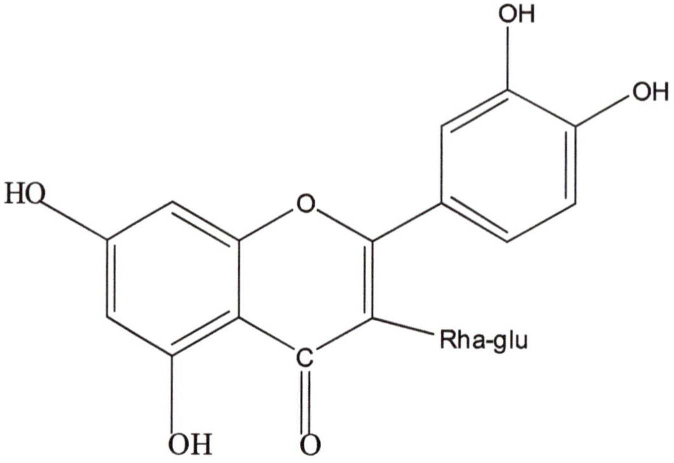

Rutin

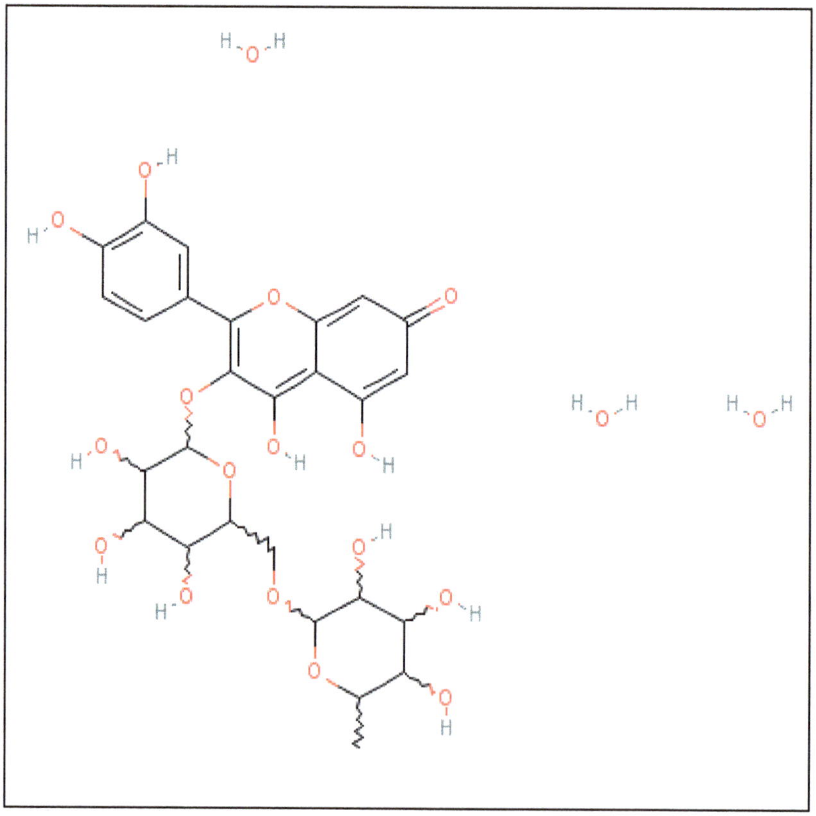

Geraniin

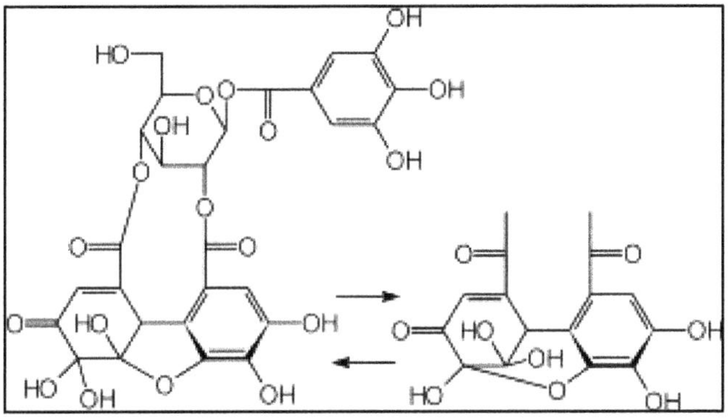

Furosin

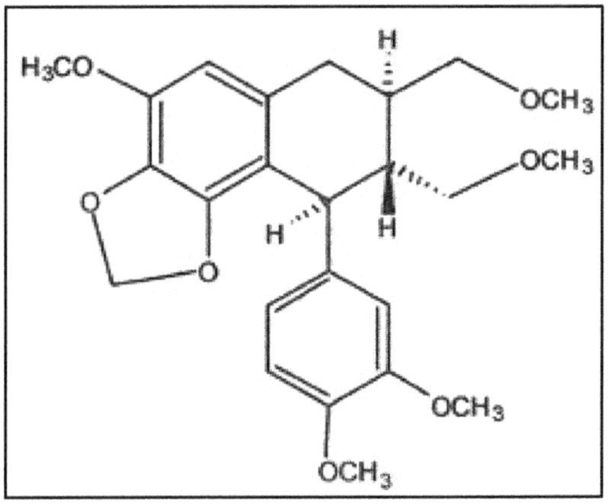

Phyllanthusiin

isolated from the leaves. From the roots rutin, querecetin were isolated. Lintetralin was also isolated from the plant. Amariin, a novel hydrolysable tannin together with geraniin, furosin, phyllanthusin have been isolated from the polar fraction. Several chemical investigations have been conducted where the structures of most of these phytochemicals were determined by UV, IR, Mass and NMR spectroscopy. Houghton *et al.* (1996) isolated securinega type alkaloids by Column Chromatography (CC) and preparative Thin Layer Chromatography (TLC). This group did qualitative analysis by using TLC, and spots were detected by UV radiation (254 nm and 365 nm). The unknown compounds were determined by means of UV, IR, mass and NMR spectroscopy (Foo, 1992, 1993, 1995).

The extracts (50 per cent methanol in water, 99 per cent methanol and 50 per cent methanol in chloroform) were analyzed by thin layer chromatography based upon the presence of secondary metabolites. *P. amarus* material was air dried under shade for two weeks at 40°C. The dried plant material was ground with a Wiley Mill grinder to 2 mm or smaller particle size. Plant material and solvent were agitated with a laboratory rotator at 30 rpm for three days at room temperature, *i.e.* 18-23°C. The supernatant was filtered with Whatman filter paper No. 4 and concentrated with blown air to 1ml. The concentrated liquid extracts were stored at 4°C (May, 2002) until TLC analysis (Rugutt, 1996).

Extraction Method Development

In order to determine the extraction rate, 10 g of ground plant material of *P. amarus* was extracted with 100 ml (1:10, w/v) of the following solvents: A, 50 per cent methanol in D.D. water; B, 99 per cent methanol; or C, 50 per cent methanol in chloroform. All solvents used were HPLC grade from Fisher Scientific Chemicals. Plant material and solvent were agitated with an orbital shaker at 115 rpm for three days at room temperature, *i.e.* 18-23°C. The supernatant was drained and the residue was rinsed with 100 ml extraction solvent A, B, or C for 24 hours. The pooled extracts were filtered through Whatman No. 4 filter paper and concentrated at 60 °C using a rotary evaporator. The weight of the powders of *P. amarus was* recorded (Vitanyi *et al.*, 1997).

Phytochemical Analysis of Crude Extracts by Using TLC Method

Thin layer chromatography (TLC) was employed in this study to analyze the compounds present in the crude plant extracts of the solvents 50 per cent methanol in D.D. water, 99 per cent methanol and

50 per cent methanol in chloroform. Normal phase silica gel GF precoated TLC (scored 10×20 cm) plates; 250 microns (Analtech, Uniplate No. 02521) were used. The solvent extracts (three per plate) were applied as separate spots to a TLC plate about 1.3 cm from the edge (spotting line), using 20 µl capillary tubes (microcaps disposable pipettes, Drummond Scientific Company). The mobile phase, chloroform/methanol= 9:1; 95:5; 98:2 (v/v), for each crude extract from *P. amarus* was chosen by trial and error. For the powder extracts of *P. amarus*, mobile phases with different polarities had to be used, namely, chloroform/methanol= 5:5; 7:3; 9:1 and chloroform/methanol= 9:1; 95:5, respectively. All TLC separations were performed at room temperature, *i.e.* 18-23°C. After sample application of 3 µl for *P. amarus*, the plates were placed vertically into a solvent vapor saturated TLC chamber. Three mobile phases were respectively used: chloroform/methanol= 9:1; 95:5; 98:2 (volume ratio). The spotting line was about 0.5 cm from the developing solution. After the mobile phase had moved about 80 per cent from the spotting line, the plate was removed from the developing chamber and dried in a fume hood (Houghton, 1996, Wagner and Bladt, 1996).

Phytochemical Analysis of Powder Extracts by Using TLC Method

Extraction solvent B (absolute methanol) was used to produce powder for bio-assay analysis, because this solvent had a good extraction rate for *P. amarus*. The TLC fingerprint of the produced *P. amarus* powders was compared with those of the crude solvent extracts. Twenty-five milligrams of crude powder from methanol extract (B) of *P. amarus* were dissolved in two solvents of different polarities: 1 ml methanoldeionized and distilled water (1); 1 ml absolute methanol (2). The mixture to be analyzed (3 µl *P. amarus)* was spotted near the bottom of the plate (1.3 cm). The mobile phases in which the *P. amarus* plates were placed are: $CHCl_3$/MeOH = 5:5;7:3; 9:1. The eluted spots were visualized at UV 254 nm and spraying with 10 per cent ethanolic phosphomolybdic acid reagent. The secondary metabolites present in extracts of *P. amarus* fractions eluted from *P. amarus* extract with mobile phase that can be detected with UV-254 nm are: alkaloids; flavonoids; and lignans. Phosphomolybdic acid (PMA) is a general reagent that detects a large variety of organic compounds, in this case phenols and indole derivatives. The use of mobile phase chloroform/methanol= 9:1 gave a separation that is not equally spread over the plate. The two last compounds were still not completely separated. Mobile phase chloroform/methanol= 98:2 is less polar, so the less polar compounds were eluted and the more polar compounds did not travel along with the mobile phase (Fernand, 1998).

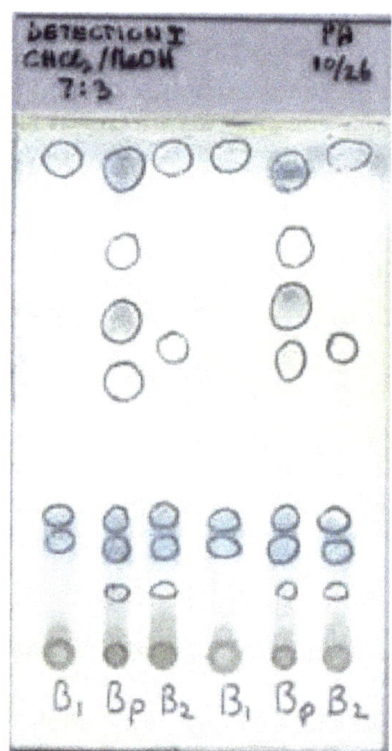

Fractions eluted from *P. amarus* extract with mobile phase

$CHCl_3$/MeOH= 7:3 and detected by UV-254 nm and PMA reagent

B1= Powder extract dissolved in 50% MeOH in H_2O

Bp= *P. amarus* crude extract

B2= Powder extract dissolved in 99%MeOH.

Phyllanthin and hypophyllanthin are estimated using C_{18} µ Bondapak (30 cm X 3.9mm) column by UV detection at 280 nm. The mobile phase consists of methanol : water (30:34) at the flow rate of 1.8 ml/min (Handa, 1999).

Bioactivity

Phyllanthus amarus is a small herb indigenous to Amazon Basin. It is well known for its medicinal properties and widely used by Ayurveda. It is reported to contain lignans, alkaloids, flavonoids, galloatnoids, glycosides and alkaloids. It possesses antiviral, antiparasitic, antimalarial, antimicrobial, anticancerous, antidiabetic and anticholesterol agents. It acts on kidney stones and Uric Acid. It protects liver and detoxifies the toxicity. It has cellular protective and wound-healing properties also. Further activity guided phytochemical phytoanalytical studies may indicate to development of novel agents to be used in various disorders.

Pharmacological Studies

Hepatoprotective Activity

In search of the effective and standardized hepatoprotective combination therapy, silymarin and standardized extract of *Phyllanthus amarus* has been evaluated against CCl_4-induced hepatotoxicity in rats. Eight groups of rats were used. The animals of group A served as normal and were given only vehicle. The animals of group B served as toxin control and were administered with CCl_4 (50 per cent solution of CCl_4 in liquid paraffin, 2 ml/kg b.w., intraperitoneally). The animals of groups C–H received silymarin (100 mg/kg b.w.), *Phyllanthus amarus* aqueous extract (100 mg/kg b.w.), *Phyllanthus amarus* ethanolic extract (100 mg/kg b.w.), silymarin (50 mg/kg b.w.)+*P. amarus* aq. ext. (50 mg/kg b.w.), silymarin (50 mg/kg b.w.) + *P. amarus* eth. ext. (50 mg/kg b.w.) and marketed formulation (M.F.) 5 ml/ kg b.w. for 6 days orally as well as CCl_4 (2 ml/kg b.w.) on 4th day intraperitoneally. The test materials were found effective as hepatoprotective as evidenced by plasma and liver biochemical parameters. The combination of silymarin and *Phyllanthus amarus* showed synergistic effect for hepatoprotection and silymarin with ethanolic extract of *P. amarus* showed better activity due to the higher concentration of phyllanthin in ethanolic extract in comparison to aqueous extract of *P. amarus* as estimated by HPLC. Moreover, *P. amarus* leaf extract could protect the liver against ethanol-induced oxidative damage by possibly reducing the rate of lipid peroxidation and increasing the antioxidant defence mechanism in rats (Yadav *et al.*, 2008).

Hepatitis B Surface Antigen Inactivation

Water extract of dried entire plant at a concentration of 0.2 mg/ml was active on hepatitis virus vs reaction of woodchuck hepatitis surface antigen with hepatitis B (Human) antibody. At a concentration of 0.63 mg/ml the extract was active on hepatitis B virus vs reaction of hepatitis B surface antigen with hepatitis B antibody. Both water and methanol extracts of the dried whole plant, at variable concentrations were active. Water extract of dried leaves, was active against hepatitis B surface antigen inactivation was assayed. IC_{50} 650 mg/ml. water extract was active. IC_{50} 1.2 mcg/ml. Water extract of dried leaves, was active. Hepatitis B surface antigen inactivation was assayed. IC_{50} 3.30 mcg/ml. Chloroform extract and water extract of dried leaves, stem, and also of dried roots, at a concentration of 2.0 per cent were active (Lee *et al.*, 1996).

Antiviral Activity

The pure isolates of *Phyllanthus amarus viz.*, Niranthrin, nirtetralin, geraniin suppressed effectively both HbSAg and HBeAg expression with the highest inhibition at 74.3 per cent, 45.3 per cent, 33.9 per cent, 68.1 per cent, and 52.3 per cent,46.6 per cent respectively (Yang *et al.*, 2007). It down-regulates HBV mRNA transcription by a specific mechanism involving interactions between HBV enhancer I and C/EBP transcription factors (Ott *et al.*, 1997). The aqueous, butanol and alcoholic extracts of *Phyllatnthus amarus* were prescribed for the treatment of chronic hepatitis B virus infection at the doses of 25,50, and 200 mg/kg body weight (Niu *et al.*, 1990). A clinical study was carried out for the eradication of hepatitis B virus with this plant extract. This species were collected from Central Thailand. Sixtyfive adult symptomatic chronic carriers were treated. Thirty four received *Phyllanthus amarus* extract at a dose 600mg per day for 30 days and thirty one received placebo in identical capsules, at day 30 the conversion rate of HbsAg was 6 per cent in the experimental group. A further 30 days treatment were given to 20 subjects in the *Phyllanthus amarus* group and twenty placebo recipients given *Phyllanthus amarus* 1,200 mg per day for 30 days. The study indicated that the whole plant extract except root had a minimal effect to eradicate HBsAg (Grewal, 2003). Another clinical study on chronic carrier of hepatitis B virus was encouraging and recommended continued evaluation of this plant. In this preliminary study, carriers of hepatitis B virus were treated with *Phyllanthus amarus* for 30 days. Fifty nine percent subjects had lost hepatitis B surface antigen when tested 15-20 days after the end of the treatment compared with only 4 per cent placebo treated controls (Handa, 1999).

Antibacterial Activity

Water extract of fresh whole plant at a concentration of 10 per cent on agar plate was inactive on *Neisseria gonorrhea*. Saline extract of leaves, at a concentration of 10 per cent on agar plate was active on *Pasteurella pestis* and *Staphylococcus aureus*, and inactive on *Escherichia coli*. Chloroform extract of dried leaves, at a concentration of 1.0 g/ml on agar plate was inactive on *Bacillus subtilis, Escherichia coli, Pseudomonas aeruginosa and staphylococcus aureus*. Methanol extract was active on *Staphylococcus aureus*, but inactive on *Bacillus subtilis, Escherichia coli,* and *Pseudomonas aeruginosa* (Kloucek *et al.*, 2005).

Anticancer and Cytoprotective Activity

Numerous studies were documented that treatment with *Phyllanthus amarus* enhanced the life span of animals with liver cancer (Rajeshkumar *et al.*, 2000).When the aqueous extract of *Phyllanthus amarus* was administered to cancer bearing mice it lowered the tumor incidents, level of carcinogen-metabolizing enzymes, levels of liver cancer markers dose dependently (Kumar *et al.*, 2005). It is also established that extracts of *Phyllanthus amarus* have prevented or inhibited the cells from mutation with the existence of chemical agents those are known to create cellular mutation and breaking down of DNA strands and finally leads to the formation of cancerous cells (Hari Kumar, 2006).These experimental data indicated that *Phyllanthus amarus* possesses the ability to inhibit the unusual enzymatic pathways peculiar to cancer cells proliferation and growth rather than a direct toxic effect of killing the different types of cancer cells. The extract of *Phyllanthus amarus* has been administered orally (750mg/kg and 250mg/kg body weight) in the radiation (6Gy) induced BALB/c mice for its protective activity against carcinogenesis. The WBC count, bone marrow cellularity and α-esterase activity increased significantly as compared to only radiation–exposed mice. The antioxidant enzymes such as superoxided dismutase (SOD), Catalase (CAT), Glutahione-S-transferase (GST), gluthaione peroxidase (GPX), and glutathione reductase, both in blood and tissue, which were reduced by radiation induced (Kumar and Kuttan, 2004). The life span of hepatocellular carcinoma induced by N-nitrosodiethylamine (NDEA) bearing rats increased significantly after treatment with the aqueous extract of *Phyllanthus amarus* (150mg/kg body weight). Likewise the increased glutahione and GST content in NDEA+ *Phyllanthus amarus* treated group were also controlled (Rajeshkumar and Kuttan, 2000). N-methyl N′-nitro-N-nitrosoguanidene (MNNG) induced stomach cancer in Wistar rats was significantly inhibited by the administration of *Phyllanthus amarus* extracts; it also reduced the incidence of gastric neoplasms in rats (44 per cent) as well as their numbers. The elevated enzymes levels in the stomach were also found to reduce by *Phyllanthus amarus* treatment (Raphael *et al.*, 2006).

Antiinflammatory Activity

Phyllanthus amarus is a herbal medicine traditionally applied in the treatment of viral hepatitis. On investigation, *P. amarus* for antiinflammatory activity *in vitro* against different models *viz.*, rat

Kupffer cells (KC), in RAW264.7 macrophages, in human whole blood, and in mice showed significant protection of the elevated inflammation related biomarkers such as iNOS, COX-2 TNF-alpha and NF-kappa B. cells were stimulated with lipopolysaccharide (LPS) in the presence or absence of *P. amarus* extracts (hexane, aqueous ethanol), mice were treated with galactosamine/LPS as a model for acute toxic hepatitis. Nitrite was measured by Griess assay, prostaglandin (PGE-2) by radioimmunoassay, and cytokines by enzyme-linked immunosorbent assay. iNOS and COX-2 were determined by Western blot, activation of NF-kappaB by EMSA. Results of aqueous ethanol and hexane extracts showed an inhibition of LPS-induced production of NO and PGE(2) in KC and in RAW264.7. The extracts also attenuated the LPS-induced secretion of tumor necrosis factor (TNF-alpha) in RAW264.7 as well as in human whole blood. Both extracts reduced expression of iNOS and COX-2 and inhibited activation of NF-kappa B. *P. amarus* inhibited induction of interleukin (IL)-1beta, IL-10, and interferon-gamma in human whole blood and reduced TNF-alpha production *in vivo*. These results show that standardized extracts of *P. amarus* inhibit the induction of iNOS, COX-2, and TNF-alpha. Therefore, *P. amarus* has the antiinflammatory potential both by *in vitro* and *in vivo* systems (Kiemer *et al.*, 2003).

Antispasmodic and Analgesic Activity

Researchers proved *P. amarus* as antispasmodic including uterine relaxant effect and finally it is concluded that "smooth muscle relaxation within the urinary or biliary tract probably facilitates the expulsion of kidney or bladder calculi" (Nadkarni, 1982).The pain-relieving effects of PA were also performed against six different laboratory-induced pain models *viz.*, acetic acid induced writhing, formalin-induced pedal edema, tail flick response to radiant heat, hot plate method etc. The hydrolysable tannin geraniin of *P. amarus* was seven times more potent as a pain reliever than aspirin or acetaminophen; it is also effective for its antiulcerous properties and to protect the gastrointestinal tract.

Antidiabetic, Antioxidant and Anticholesterol Activity

The Methanolic extract of *Phyllanthus amarus* was administered 200mg/kg and 1000mg/kg body weight in alloxan induced diabetic rats and found to normalize the elevated blood sugar by 6 per cent and 18.7 per cent respectively. The antioxidant potentiality of the extract was also established by inhibiting the lipid peroxidation, scavenge hydroxyl and superoxide radicals *in vitro* (Raphael *et al.*, 2002).The antidiabetic activity of the aqueous extracts of leaf and seed of the plant was studied at oral dose of 150, 300 and 600 mg/kg body weight. The experiment showed dependent decrement of the fasting plasma glucose level and cholesterol content and reduction of body weights in treated mice in a dose-dependent manner (Adeneye *et al.*, 2006).

Immunomodulatory Activity

Aqueous decoction of the leaf and seeds of *Phyllanthus amarus* is used as blood-forming remedy and immunobooster in immunocompromised patients particularly HIV/AIDS and tuberculous patients. In one of the study, haematopoietic and immunomodulatory activities of the aqueous extract of *Phyllanthus amarus*, were investigated in normal and cyclophosphamide (CYCLO)-treated, young adult, male Swiss albino mice for 14 days. Results of the study showed *P. amarus* to induce significant ($P<0.05$, $P<0.01$, $P<0.001$) elevation in packed cell volume (PCV) and total leucocytes count dose-dependently in normal and attenuated leucopaenia and anaemia in cyclophosphamide (CYCLO)-treated mice. The data, thus, generated has a positive correlation with its folkloric use. In the near future, the plant may constitute a new source of haematopoietic and immuomodulatory drug (Adeneye and Arogundade, 2007).

Antidiarrheal Activity

Fifty per cent aqueous ethanol extract of dried aerial parts at a concentration of 300 mg/kg was inactive for antidiarrheal activity on both guinea pig and rabbit ileums vs. *E. coli*-Inte Rotoxin-induced diarrhea (Adeneye *et al.*, 2006).

Antifungal Activity

Petroleum ether extract of whole plant showed antifungal activity against *Helminthosporium sativa*. The leaf extract showed antifungal activity against *Alternaria alternate*, while it had no activity against *Curvalaria lunata* (Abad *et al.*, 2007).

Miscellaneous Activities

Phyllanthus amarus was also evaluated for the following activities such as Nematocidal activity wherein it showed positive response against *Toxacara canis* at 1 mg ml concentration, *Molluscicidal activity;* petroleum ether extract at a concentration of 25.0 ppm was active on *Biomphalaria pfeifferi* and *Bulinus truncates*, Cytotoxic activity; water extract of dried whole plant at a concentration of 50.0 ug/ml was active against woodchuck hepatitis virus DNA polymerase. At this dose it showed an inhibition of 25 per cent. Both methanol and water extracts, at variable dosages were also active; 50 per cent Ethanol/water extract of a commercial sample of the whole plant, administered intravenously at variable dosages to dogs showed positive chronotropic effect; *P amarus* (aqueous extract) showed chromosome aberration protective effect at 685mg/kg p.o. in lead nitrate and aluminum sulphate induced damage to the bone marrow chromosomes (Raphael *et al.*, 2002).

Clinical Studies Status

P. amarus has been used since ages as a drug. Several clinical studies have been conducted with different extracts of different parts of this plant and also with the pure isolates also. Few of the studies have been coded for the reference (Premila, 2006).

In Infective Hepatitis

A study at the Indian Institute of Research in Yoga and allied Sciences, Tirupati has been conducted on 160 children (1-12years of age) which claimes to be effective in the treatment of infective hepatitis. Out of 160 children, 101 cases were cured and 59 cases dropped out. In majority of cases, disappearance of jaundice, hepatitis tenderness and bile salts and pigments from urine was observed in 2nd week.

In a preliminary study, carriers of hepatitis B virus were treated with a preparation of *Phyllanthus amarus.* 59 per cent treated patients had lost hepatitis B surface antigen when tested 15-20 days after the end of the treatment compared with only 4 per cent of the placebo treated controls. In no case did the surface antigen return. Clinical observation revealed few or no toxic effect.

In another clinical trial *P. amarus* was administered to 30 asymptomatic carriers of Hepatitis B surface antigen (HbsAg) in a dosage of 250-2500mg thrice daily for 4 to 8 weeks. None of the 30 subjects cleared HbsAg. *P. amarus* was well tolerated, with no clinical side effects or changes in the organ profiles for safety evaluation. It was concluded that *P. amarus* was not effective in clearing HbsAg in asymptomatic carriers of the antigen.

A study was made to know whether the powder of *P. amarus* plant favorably influenced the duration of disease in patients with acute virus B hepatitis when compared to placebo. The powder of the plant was given in capsule form and an antacid powder in similar capsule was used as placebo. Persons with encephalopathy, pre existing medical conditions or serum bilirubin above 350 iu/1 were excluded from the study. The analysis showed that *P. amarus* powders did not significantly reduce the duration of jaundice in persons with virus B hepatitis.

A clinical trial was conducted on 25 patients of jaundice. The patients were given 1gm of *P.amarus* in tablet form thrice daily for 8 days and 500mg TDS for next 8 days. Complete relief was observed in 22 patients (88 per cent) and partial relief in 2(8 per cent) patients. The time required for clinical improvement was 2-7 days.

Toxicity

Aqueous extract of fresh leaves and roots is found to be nontoxic in 2 g/kg., p.o. in acute toxicity studies. Clinical trials conducted so far have not revealed any toxic effects for the species. Since the drug is known to possess contraceptive properties in mice, it may be avoided during pregnancy. Hypophyllanthin and phyllanthin are toxic to fish and frog.

Clinical Usage in Formulations

The plant species is used in the preparation of various formulations like Chyavanprasha, Citraka Haritaki, Madhuyashtiaddi Taila, Pippalyddi Ghrita, Satavari guda, Laghuvishagarbha taila, Shwasahara kashaya. These formulations have been used for different diseases.

Conclusion

Phyllanthus amarus (Euphorbiaceae) is an annual herb which is reported to contain lignans, alkaloids, flavonoids, galloatnoids, glycosides and alkaloids. The pharmacological evaluation mentioned in this review establish the therapeutic value of this herb. The therapeutic effects has been acknowledged as antiviral, antiparasitic, antimalarial, antimicrobial, anticancer, antidiabetic, antihypercholesterolemic, cellular protective and wound-healing properties. It also acts on kidney stones and Uric Acid. It protects liver and detoxifies the toxicity and for treating hepatitis B virus. Thus activity guided phytochemical and phytoanalytical may lead to the development of novel agents for various disorders from *Phyllanthu amarus* alone or in combination with other important medicinal plants. The available literature regarding the chemical compositions and pharmacological activities appear to be very impressive and explains the utility of this herb as medicine.

References

Abad, M.J., Ansuategui, M. and Bermejo, P. (2007). Active antifungal substances from natural sources. ARKIVOC, 7: 116-145.

Adeneye, A.A. Amole, and Adeneye, O.O., A. K. (2006). Hypoglycemic and hypocholesterolemic activity of the aqueous leaf and seed extract of *Phyllanthus amarus. Fototerapia,* 77 (7-8): 511-514.

Adeneye, A.A. and Arogundade, M. O. (2007). Immuno-Stimulatory and Haematopoietic Activities of the Leaf and Seed Aqueous Extract of *Phyllanthus Amarus* in Normal and Cyclophosphamide-Treated Mice. *Nigerian Journal of Health and Biomedical Sciences,* 6 (2): 53-57.

Fernand, V. E. (1998). Initial characterization of crude extracts from *Phyllanthus amarus* Schum. and Thonn. and *Quassia amara* L. using normal phase thin layer chromatography. *Thesis Master of Science.* B.S., University of Suriname, South American.

Foo, L.Y. (1993). Amarulone, a novel cyclic hydrolysable tannin from *Phyllanthus amarus. Natural Product Letters,* 3: 45-52.

Foo, L.Y. (1995). Amariinic acid and related ellangitannins from *Phyllanthus amarus*. *Phytochemistry*, 39: 217-224.

Foo, L.Y., and Wong, H. (1992). Phyllanthusiin-D, an unusual hydrolysable tannin from *Phyllanthus amarus*. *Phytochemistry*, 31(2): 711-713.

Grewal, R.C. (2003). *Medicinal plants* (Reprint). Campus Books International, New Delhi: pp.297-304.

Handa, S.S. (1999). *Indian herbal Pharmacopoeia* Vol.-II. RRL Jammu and IDMA Mumbai:pp 85-92.

Hari Kumar, K. B. and Kuttan R. (2006). Inhibition of drug metabolizing enzymes (cytochrome P450) in vitro as well as in vivo by *Phyllanthus amarus* Schum and Thonn. *Biol. Pharm. Bull.*, 29(7): 1310-1313.

Houghton, P. J., Woldemariam, T. Z., O'Shea, S. and Thyagarajan, S.P. (1996). Two securinega-type alkaloids from *Phyllanthus amarus*. *Phytochemistry*, 43: 715-717.

Kiemer, A. K., Hartung, T., Huber, C. and Vollmar, A.M. (2003). *Phyllanthus amarus* has antiinflammatory potential by inhibition of iNOS, COX-2 and cytokines via the NF-kappaB pathway. *Hepatol.*, 38(3): 289-297.

Kloucek, P., Polesny, Z., Svobodova, B., Vlkova, E. and Kokoska, L. (2005). Antibacterial screening of some Peruvian medicinal plants used in Caller?a District. Journal of Ethnopharmacology, 99: 309–312

Kumar, K.B. and Kuttan, R. (2004). Protective effect of an extract of Phyllanthus amarus against radiation-induced damage in mice. J Radiat Res., 45(1): 133-139.

Kumar, K.B. and Kuttan, R. (2005). Chemoprotective activity of an extract of *Phyllanthus amarus* against cyclophosphamide induced toxicity in mice. *Phytomedicine*, 12(6-7): 494-500.

Lee, C.D., Otte, M., Thyagrajan, S.P., Shafritz, D. A., Burk, R.D. and Gupta, S. (1996). *Phyllanthus amarus* down-regulates hepatitis B virus mRNA transcription and replication. *European Journal of Clinical investigation*, 26: 1069-1078.

Nadkarni, N.K. (1982). *Indian Materia Medica*. Popular prakashen, Bombay. Vol.-1: pp.948.

Niu, J.Z., Wang, Y Y., Qiao, M., Goawans, E., Edwards, P., Thyagarajan, S.P., Gust, I. and Locarmini, S. (1990). *J. Med. Virol.*, 32 (4): 212-8.

Ott, M., Thyagarajan, S. P. and Gupta, S. (1997). *Phyllanthus amarus* suppresses hepatitisB virus by interrupting interaction between HBV enhancer I and cellular transcription factors. *Eur J,Clin Invest.*, 7(11): 908-915.

Premila, M.S. (2006). Hepatoprotective agents. In: Ayurvedic herbs–A clinical guide to the healing plants of traditional Indian medicine. Health and Fitness, Hawarth Press. 61-83.

Rajesh kumar, N. V. and Kuttan, R. (2000). *Phyllanthus amarus* extract administration increases the life span of rats with hepatocellular carcinoma. *J Ethnopharmacol.*, 73(1-2): 215-219.

Raphael, K. R., Ajith, T.A., Joseph, S. and Kuttan, R. (2002). AntiMutagenic Activity of *Phyllanthus amarus* Schum and Thonn *In Vitro* as Well as *In Vivo*. *Teratogenesis, Carcinogenesis, and Mutagenesis*, 22: 285–291.

Raphael, K.R., Sabu, M. and Kuttan, R. (2002). Hypoglycemic effect of methanol extract of *Phyllanthus amarus* Schum. and Thonn. on alloxan induced diabetes mellitus in rats and its relation with antioxidant potential. *Indian J Exp Biol.* 40(8): 905-909.

Raphael, K.R., Sabu, M., Kumar, K.H. and Kuttan, R. (2006). Inhibition of N-Methyl N'–nitro-N-nitrosoguanidine (MNNG) induced gastric carcinogenesis by *Phyllanthus amarus* extract. *Asian Pac J Cancer Prev.,* 7(2): 299-302.

Rugutt, J.K. (1996). *Control of African Striga species by natural productsfrom native plants.* Dissertation Louisiana State University, USA. pp.226.

Vitányi, G., Bihátsi-Karsai, E., Lefler, J. and Lelik, L (1997). Application of high performance liquid chromatography/mass spectrometry with thermospray ionization to the detection of quassinoids extracted from *Quassia amara* L. *Rapid Communications in Mass Spectrometry,* 11: 691-693.

Wagner, H. and Bladt, S. (1996). *Plant Drug Analysis: A Thin Layer Chromatography Atlas* (Second edition). Springer-Verlag Berlin Heidelberg New York Tokyo. pp.384.

Yadav, N.P., Pal, A., Shanker, K., Bawankule, D.U., Darokar, M.P. and Khanuja, S.P. (2008). Synergistic effect of silymarin and standardized extract of *Phyllanthus amarus* against CCl_4-induced hepatotoxicity in Rattus norvegicus. *Phytomedicine,* 15(12): 1053-61.

Yang, C.M., Cheng, H.Y., Lin, T.C., Chiang, L.C. and Lin, C.C. (2007). The *in vitro* activity of geraniin and 1, 3, 4, 6-tetra-O-galloyl-beta-D-glucose isolated from *Phyllanthus urinaria* against herpes simplex virus type 1 and type 2 infection. *Journal of Ethnopharmacology,* 110(3): 555-558

Medicinal Plants: Phytochemistry, Pharmacology and Therapeutics, Vol. 1 *Pages 330–337*
Editors: **V.K. Gupta, G.D. Singh, Surjeet Singh and A. Kaul**
Published by: **DAYA PUBLISHING HOUSE, NEW DELHI**

Chapter 17

In vitro Antisickling Activity of Anthocyanins Extracts from *Morinda lucida* Benth (Rubiaceae)

P.T. Mpiana[1]*, V. Mudogo[1], K.N. Ngbolua[2], D.S.T. Tshibangu[1] and E.K. Atibu[1]
[1]Département de Chimie, [2]Département de Biologie, Faculté des Sciences B.P. 190, Université de Kinshasa, Kinshasa XI, R.D. Congo

ABSTRACT

In the present work, anthocyanins extracts from a Congolese plant *Morinda lucida* were evaluated for their antisickling activity using microscopic technique. The red blood cells (RBCs) were observed to change from the sickled shape to normal biconcave cells in the presence of 2 per cent sodium metabisulfite. The treated SS RBCs demonstrated a remarkable similarity to normal blood values (Radius =3.3±0.3mm).The minimal concentration of normalization (MCN) of sickle cell erythrocytes was 0.195 µg/mL. The antisickling activity was found to be dose dependent. Anthocyanins extracts was found to be responsible of the inhibition of the sickling process, thus, justifying the claims of the traditional medical practitioners and suggesting a possible correlation between the chemical composition of this plant and its use in traditional medicine.

Keywords: *Morinda lucida, Sodium metabisulfite, Antisickling activity, Anthocyanins extracts.*

* Corresponding Author: E-mail: ptmpiana@yahoo.fr.

Introduction

Several reports indicate that pharmacological agents that inhibit haemoglobin S (HbS) gelation could be used in the control of the sickling process of red blood cells (RBCs), which is a major pathological event of the sickle cell disease (SCD) (Iwu *et al.*, 1988; Nwaoguikpe *et al.*, 2005).

Sickling of RBCs occur as a result of polymerization of deoxygenated HbS molecules, so that, they become stacked linearly. Clinical symptoms occur in homozygote individuals and develop from at about 6 months old. There is a chronic haemolytic anaemia and recurrent painful vasocclusive crises because of the sickled RBCs blocking small vessels. This leads to tissue ischemia and infarction, mostly affecting the liver, spleen, lungs, brain and retina. These crises may be precipitated by infection, cold, exercise, dehydration and pregnancy (Parveen and Michael, 1999).

Many investigations have been carried out on the role of phenolics such as benzoic acid derivatives and divanilloyl quinic acids in the management of SCD (Elujoba and Sofowora, 1977b, Adesanya and Sofowora, 1983; Osoba *et al.*, 1989; Akojie and Fung, 1992; Ouatara *et al.*, 2004) and the importance of the plant materials in the maintenance of health is well established (Neuwinger, 2000; Cordeiro *et al.*, 2004; Elujoba *et al.*, 2005a, Ekeke *et al.*, 1997).

These phytochemical compounds have been found to reduce the *in vitro* sickling of RBCs.

Different species of plants from tropical Africa region are very rich sources of phenolics. Because of the antisickling effects of certain phenolics such as anthocyanins (Mpiana *et al.*, 2007a, Mpiana *et al.*, 2007b), we were prompted to investigate the antisickling potency of a Congolese plant *Morinda lucida* Benth., which is a medical plant widely used by traditional medical practitioner in Democratic Republic of Congo (DRC) to cure the SCD.

The plant *Morinda lucida* Benth. belongs to the family of Rubiaceae. It is commonly known as Nsiki (Bas Congo), Mukakadi or Mutebenolozi (Bandundu), Endombe or Kolomboka (Equateur), Mundundama (Kasai-Occidental), Kakate (Kasai-Oriental), isuku (Katanga) in the specified Congolese languages.

It is a small tree, approximately 15m (50ft) high, widely distributed in Tropical Africa. It has been found in DRC, Republic of Congo, Benin, Ivory Coast, Nigeria, Central African Republic, Senegal, Togo, Sao Tomé et Principé.

The plant has been reported to have varying traditional medicinal uses (Kerharo, 1974). It has been shown to have antibacterial (Bokolo *et al.*, 2006), antitrypanocidal, and antimalarial (Azuzu and Chineme, 1990) activities. Anthocyanins are powerful free radical scavengers (Kahkonen *et al.*, 2003a). They also show antioxidant activity in lipid environments (Satué-Gracia *et al.*, 1997).

The antisickling activity of anthocyanins extracted from this plant is evaluated *in vitro* on *SS* blood using Emmel's test in the presence of Sodium metabisulfite (Courtejoie and Hartaing, 1992). This activity is expressed as the normalization of sickled cells. The minimal concentration of normalization (MCN) of sickle cell erythrocytes will be determined.

Materials and Methods

Plant Material

The leaves of *Morinda lucida* Benth were collected from plants growing in Kinshasa, DRC and were authenticated by Mr. B.L. Nlandu of the INERA (Institut National d'Etudes et Recherches

Agronomiques). Voucher specimen is on deposit at the INERA Herbarium of the Faculty of Science (Université de Kinshasa).

Extraction

The dried and powdered plant material (leaves, 10 g) was repeatedly extracted by cold percolation with 95 per cent ethanol (EtOH) and water (100 ml x 1) for 48 hrs. Fractions were filtered and concentrated to dryness under reduced pressure using a rotary evaporator. Extraction of anthocyanins was then done using 100 g of dried powdered plant material with distillated water and diethyl ether following an established protocol as previously reported (Mpiana *et al.*, 2007a, Mpiana *et al.*, 2007c).

Biological Material

The sodium citrate suspension of blood samples used to evaluate the antisickling activity of the plant extracts in this study were taken from known sickle cell adolescent patients attending the "Centre de Médecine Mixte et d'Anémie *SS*" and "Centre Hospitalier Monkole", both located in Kinshasa area, DRC. None of the patients had been transfused recently with Hb AA blood. All antisickling experiments were carried out with freshly collected blood. In order to confirm their *SS* nature, the above-mentioned blood samples were first characterized by haemoglobin electrophoresis on cellulose acetate gel at pH 8.5. They were found to be *SS* blood and were then stored at±4° C in a refrigerator.

Antisickling Assay

In order to evaluate the antisickling activity of our plant extract samples, an *in vitro* antisickling assay was performed, in which the 2 per cent sodium metabisulfite pre-treated blood sample is put in contact with plants extracts at different concentrations, according to Emmel's test procedure as previously reported (Mpiana *et al.*, 2007a; Mpiana *et al.*, 2007b; Mpiana *et al.*, 2007c; Mpiana *et al.*, 2007d).

The RBCs were analysed by measuring various parameters including the area, perimeter, and the radius of each RBC using a computer assisted image analysis system (Motic Images 2000, version 1.3) and statistical data analysis were processed using Microcal Origin 6.1 package software. The graph was obtained by computer simulation using the same software. The *in vitro* bioassay was performed in triplicate and the number of observed erythrocytes was determined using Thomas' cell. All results presented in this study are mean±S.D

Results and Discussion

Two extracts from a plant used in Congolese traditional medicine were tested for their sickling reversal activities. Both aqueous and EtOH extracts of *Morinda Lucida* have shown a sickling reversal activity, thus, justifying the claims of the traditional medical practitioners and suggesting a possible correlation between the chemical composition of this plant and its use in traditional medicine. *Morinda Lucida* EtOH extract was found to exhibit the highest antisickling activity. The phytochemical screening revealed the presence of anthocyanins, tannins, alkaloids and steroids.

Figures 17.1 and 17.2 illustrate the morphology of *SS* blood erythrocytes (control) and that of *SS* blood erythrocytes in the presence of *Morinda lucida* EtOH extract.

As it can be seen from the images, the normalization of erythrocytes of *SS* blood sample treated with *Morinda lucida* extract indicates the influence of the extract on the sickliness of cells.

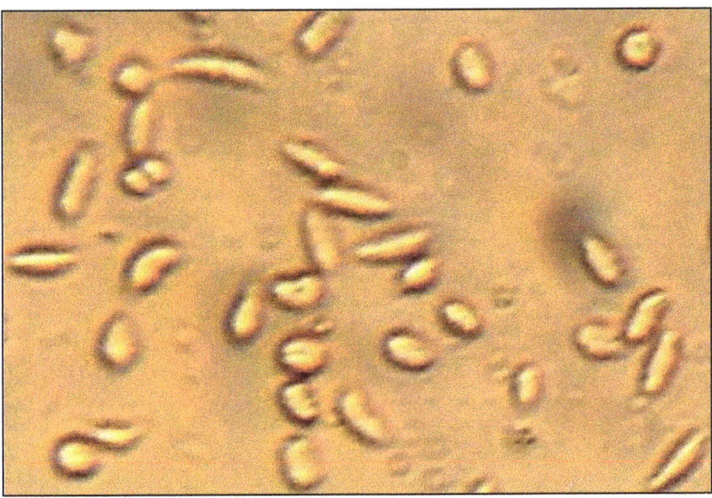

Figure 17.1: Morphology of Drepanocytes of Untreated SS Blood (Control) (X500)

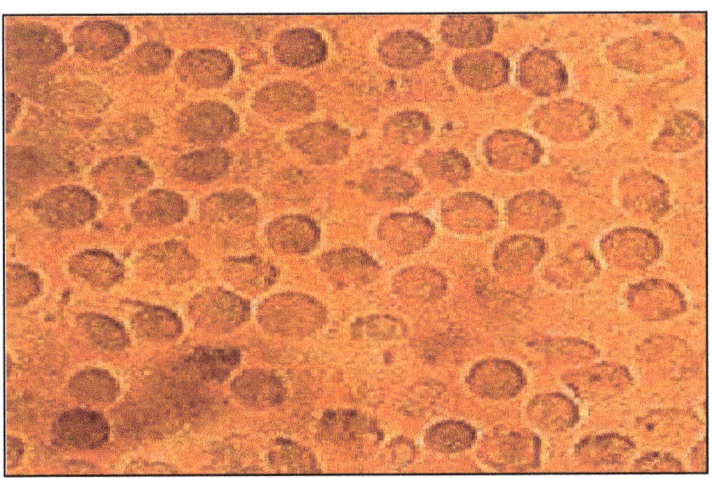

Figure 17.2: Morphology of Drepanocytes of Treated with 39.06 µg/ml of ElOH Extract of *Morinda lucida* (X500)

Figure 17.3 shows the dose dependent antisickling activity of anthocyanins extract of *Morinda lucida*.

Figure 17.3 shows the normalization of sickled cells with the anthocyanins extracts concentration. This normalization increases with the extract concentration and reach a maximum and constant value at 0.195 µg/mL (MCN). This corresponds to a normalization rate of 74 per cent. So, the antisickling activity of *Morinda lucida* anthocyanins extracts is dose dependent.

Figure 17.4 illustrates the morphology of *SS* blood erythrocytes treated with alkaloids (left) or anthocyanins extracts (right) of *Morinda lucida*.

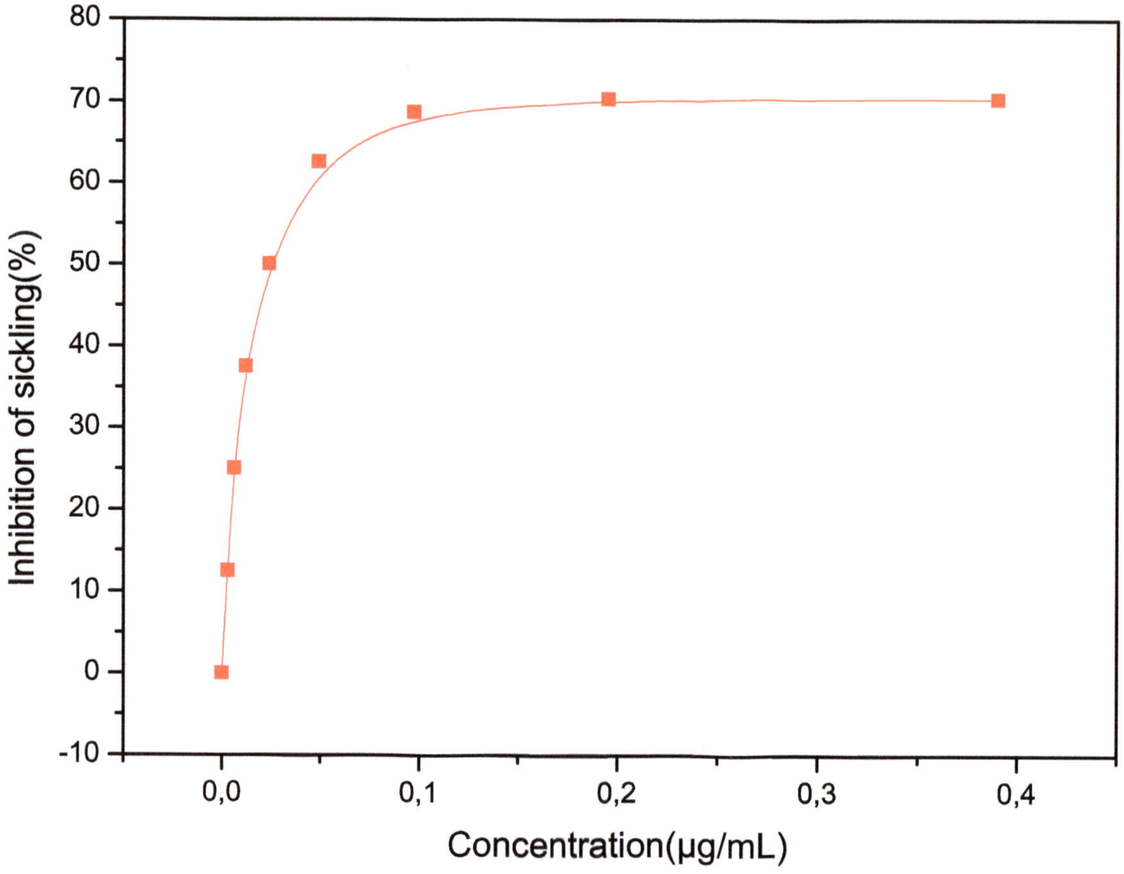

80
70
60
50
40
30
20
10
0
-10

Inhibition of sickling(%)

0,0 0,1 0,2 0,3 0,4

Concentration(μg/mL)

Figure 17.3: Concentration-Dependent Antisickling Effect of Anthocyanins Extracts of *Morinda lucida*

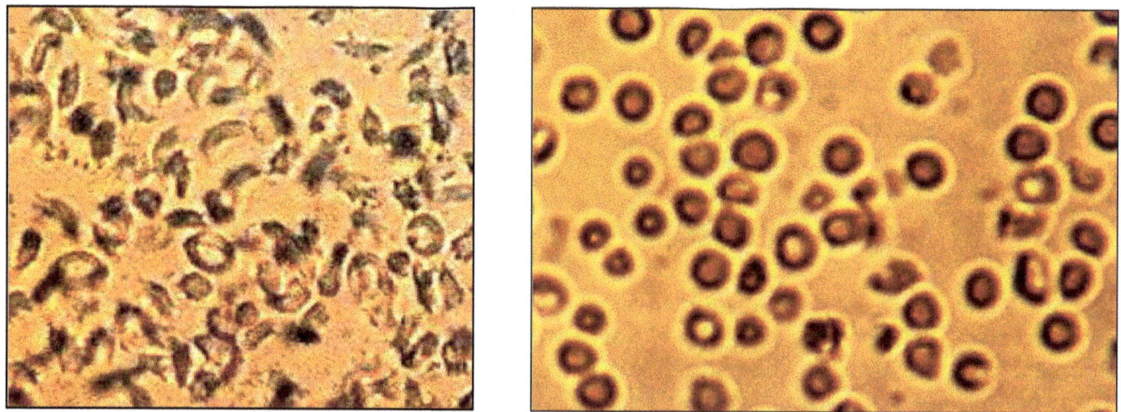

Figure 17.4: Morphology of SS Blood Erythrocytes Treated with 0.195 μg/mL of Either Alkaloids (left) or Anthocyanins Extracts (right) of *Morinda lucida* (X500)

These morphological *SS* blood cells were observed in hypoxic conditions, *i.e.* after deoxygenation of haemoglobin. As it can be seen from the above images, a normalization of erythrocytes of *SS* blood sample treated with EtOH extract (Figure 17.2) and anthocyanins extracts (Figure 17.4, right) of *Morinda lucida* indicates the influence of the extract on the sickliness of RBCs while Alkaloids extracts (Figure 17.4, left) has not shown any activity.

The computer program used in this study did not give the average radius for the erythrocytes (Table 17.1), because sickled cells of untreated *SS* blood is not circular. The average radius appeared after treatment of *SS* blood cells with *Morinda lucida* anthocyanins extracts, indicating the re-appearance of the normal and classical biconcave form of RBCs.

Statistical treatments according to Student's t-test (Tomassone, 1993), applied with a probability threshold of both 0.01 and 0.05 for 20 degrees of freedom (dof), enabled the determination of a significant difference between the average values of both the perimeter and the surface of the untreated and treated erythrocytes on the images, thus confirming the modification of the RBCs form in the presence of anthocyanins extract. Indeed, the RBCs were observed to change from the sickled shape to normal biconcave cells. These values were in agreement with previously reported values (Mpiana *et al.*, 2007a; Mpiana *et al.*, 2007b). The treated SS RBCs demonstrated a remarkable similarity to normal blood values.

Table 17.1: Average Values of Radius, Perimeter and Surface of Erythrocytes Before and After Treatment with Anthocyanins Extracts (ACE) of *Morinda lucida*

Measured Parameters	*Untreated SS RBCs*	*SS RBCs (+ACE)*
Radius (μm)	-	3.3±0.3
Perimeter (μm)	32.9±1.5	19.5±1.2
Surface (μm²)	20.3±1.0	32.8±1.8

Therefore, from the above results; anthocyanins might be potential antisickling drug candidate for sickle cell patients.

Anthocyanins have been shown to act as powerful antioxidants helping to protect the cells from free radicals. There is considerable current interest in the possible health effects of anthocyanins in humans owing to their reported positive effects on blood vessel walls (Kahkonen *et al.*, 2003a, Kahkonen *et al.*, 2003b, Mian *et al.*, 1977; Wang *et al.*, 1997). The antioxidant activity of anthocyanins is mainly due to their redox properties, which allow them to act as reducing agents, hydrogen donators, and singulet oxygen quenchers. In addition, they have a metal chelation potential.

Our results in this study suggest that the effectiveness of the antisickling activity of *Morinda lucinda* Benth. leaves extract is related to the anthocyanins, and the observed bioactivity may be probably due to the anthocyanins behaviour consisting in a non covalent binding reaction to proteins (Charpentier *et al.*, 1998; Wagner *et al.*,1983). The curve of the concentration-dependent antisickling effects of anthocyanins extracts of *Morinda lucida Benth.* is similar to that of *Ocimum basilicum* L. and *Alchornea cordifolia*. However, the MCN value of *Morinda lucida* Benth. (0.195μg/mL) is less than that of *Ocimum basilicum* L. (13μg/ml) and more than that of *Alchornea cordifolia* (0.097μg/mL) (Mpiana *et al.*, 2007a, Mpiana *et al.*, 2007b).

The ability of the anthocyanins extracts, in this study, to reverse the pathological events leading to sickling of RBCs under low oxygen tension may represent a rational explanation for the use of this plant in managing sickle cell disease by Congolese traditional medical practitioners.

Further studies, involving the structure-antisickling activity relationship of anthocyanins from *Morinda lucida* Benth. and other Congolese plants using a combination of chromatographic and spectroscopic techniques are in progress.

Acknowledgements

The authors are indebted to Third World Academy of Science (TWAS) (Grant No. 07-077 LDC/ CHE/AF/AC-UNESCO FR-3 144 804) for providing financial assistance.

References

Adesanya, S.A., Sofowora, A. (1983).Biological standardisation of Zanthoxylum roots for antisickling activity. *Planta Med.*, 48:27–33.

Akojie, F.O. and Fung, L.W.(1992). Antisickling Activity of Hydroxybenzoic Acids in *Cajanus cajan. Planta Med.*, 58(4): 317-320.

Azuzu and Chineme C.N. (1990). Effects of *Morinda lucida* leaf extract on *Trypanosoma brucei-brucei* infection in mice. *Journal of Ethno pharmacology*, 30 (3): 307-313.

Bokolo,M.K., Tshibangu, D.S.T., Shetonde, O.M. and Mbala, M.B.(2006). *In vitro* antibacterial activity of flavonoïdes of *Morinda lucida Benth* leaves. *Ann. Fac. Sci.*, 1:29-32.

Charpentier, B., Hamon, F.L., Harlay, A., Huardar, A. and Ridoux, L.(1998). Guide du préparateur en pharmacie, Masson, Paris.

Cordeiro, J.V. and Oniyangi, O.(2004). Phytomedicine (medicines derived from plants) for sickle cell disease. *The Cochrane Database of Systematic Reviews*, Issue 3, Art.No.: CD004448.pub2.

Elujoba, A.A., Odeleye, O.M., Ogunyemi, C.M.(2005).Traditional Medicine Development for Medical and Dental Primary Health care Delivery System in Africa. *Afr.J.Trad.CAM.*, 2 (1): 46–61.

Elujoba, A.A., Sofowora E.(1977). Detection and estimation of total acid in the antisickling fraction of *Fagara* species. *Planta Med.*, 32: 54–59.

Iwu, M.N., Igboko, A.O., Onwubiko, H. and Ndu, U.E.(1988). Effects of *Cajanus cajan* on gelation and oxygen affinity of sickle cell Hemoglobin. *J. Ethnopharm.*, 20:99-104.

Kahkonen,M.P., Heinamaki, J. and Heinonen, M.(2003). Antioxidant activity of anthocyanins and their aglycons. *J. Agric Food Chem.*, 52: 628–633.

Kahkonen, M.P., Heinamaki, J. and Heinonen, M.(2003). Berry anthocyanins: isolation, identification and antioxidant activities. *J. Agric Food Chem.*, 83: 1403–1411.

Kerharo, J.(1974). La pharmacopée Sénégalaise traditionnelle, Plantes médicinales et toxiques. Ed. Vigot. France.

Mian,E., Curri,S.B., Lietti,A. and Borbardelli,E.(1977). Anthocyanosides and the walls of microvessels: further aspects of the mechanism of action of their protective effect in syndromes due to abnormal capillary fragility. *Minerva Med.*, 68: 3565–3581.

Mpiana, P.T., Mudogo, V., Ngbolua, K.N, Tshibangu, D.S.T, Shetonde, O.M., and Mbala B.M.(2007). *In vitro* Antisickling Activity of Anthocyanins From *Ocimum basilicum L.* (Lamiaceae). *Int. J. Pharmacol.*, 3 (4): 371-374.

Mpiana, P.T., Mudogo, V., Tshibangu, D.S.T., Ngbolua, K.N, Shetonde, O.M., Mangwala P.K. and Mavakala, B.K.(2007).*In vitro* Antisickling Activity of Anthocyanins Extracts of a Congolese Plant: *Alchornea cordifolia M.Arg.*. *Journal of Medical Sciences*, 7(7):1182-1186.

Mpiana, P.T., Tshibangu, D.S.T., Shetonde, O.M. and Ngbolua, K.N.(2007). *In vitro* antidrepanocytary activity (antisickle cell anaemia) of some Congolese plants. *Phytomedicine*, 14: *192-195.*

Mpiana, P.T., Mudogo, V., Tshibangu, D.S.T., Shetonde, O.M., Ngbolua, K.N. and Mbala, M.B.(2007). Antisickling activity of some congolese plants, In: Drug discovery from African flora, The 12th Symposium of the Natural Product Research Network for Eastern and Central Africa, Hotel Africana, July 22-26, Kampala, Uganda, P.45.

Neuwinger, M.D.(2000). African Traditional Medicine. Medpharm Scientific Publisher. Stuttgart, 590p.

Nwaoguikpe R.N., Uwakwe A.A.(2005). The antisickling effect of dried fish (tilapia) and dried prawn (Astacus red). *J. Appl. Sci. Environ. Mgt.*, 9 (3): 115-119.

Osoba,O., Adesanya, S., Durosimi, M.(1989). Effect of *Zanthoxylum xanthoyloides* and some substituted benzoic acids on glucose-6-phosphate and 6-phosphogluconate deshydrogenases in Hb SS red blood cells, *Journal of Ethnopharmacology*, 27: 177-183.

Ouattara, B., Angenot, L.,Guissou, P., Fondu, P., Dubois, J., Frederich, M., Jansen, O., van Heugen, J.-C., Wauters, J.-N., Tits, M.(2004). LC/MS/NMR analysis of isomeric divanilloylquinic acids from the root bark of *Fagara zanthoxyloides* Lam. *Phytochemistry*, 65 : 1145–1151.

Parveen and Michael C.(1999). Sickle syndrome in clinical Medicine (4th Ed.) W.B. Saunders. London.pp 337-379.

Satué–Gracia, M.T., Heinonen, M. and Frankel, E.N.(1997). Anthocyanins as antioxidants on human low–density lipoprotein and lecithin–liposome systems. *J. Agric Food Chem.*, 45: 3362–3367.

Tomassone, R., Dervin, C., Masson, J.P.(1993). Biométrie: modélisation des phénomènes biologiques, Masson, Paris.

Wagner, H., Bladt, S. and Zgainski, E.M.(1985). Plant drug analysis. Springer–Verlag, Berlin.

Wang,H., Cao,G. and Prior, R.L.(1997).Oxygen radical absorbing capacity of anthocyanins. *J.Agric Food Chem.*, 45: 304–309.

Medicinal Plants: Phytochemistry, Pharmacology and Therapeutics, Vol. 1 *Pages 338–353*
Editors: **V.K. Gupta, G.D. Singh, Surjeet Singh and A. Kaul**
Published by: **DAYA PUBLISHING HOUSE, NEW DELHI**

Chapter 18

Studies on the Phenolic Compound Profiles and Antioxidant Activity in Fruit Portions of Marx Red Bartlett and Starkrimson Pear Cultivars

Z. Chikwambi* and M. Muchuweti
Department of Biochemistry, Faculty of Science,
University of Zimbabwe, Harare, Zimbabwe

ABSTRACT

Plant secondary metabolites, for example phenolic compounds and DNA polymorphisms constitute biochemical markers, used in the evaluation of germplasm for different purposes. In this study, an evaluation of the phenolic content, HPLC phenolic profiles, 1, 1–Diphenyl–2–picryl hydrazyl (DPPH•) scavenging activity, and β-carotene-linoleic acid antioxidant activity, in common pear (*Pyrus communis* L.) cultivars Starkrimson, Marx red Bartlett (MRB), Clapp's favourite and their reverted spots was done. The distribution of the phenolic content in pear fruit showed compartmentalization of the secondary metabolites, with higher content in the peel than the pulp. Clapp's favourite had the highest total phenolic content while MRB mutant A had the least. The HPLC profiles however showed variations in composition, quantities and distribution of phenolic compounds in peel and pulp before and after acid hydrolysis. DPPH• free radical scavenging activity of the methanolic extracts from the peel and pulp showed positive correlation with total phenolic content. The β-carotene-linoleic acid antioxidant activity did not show a direct relationship with total phenolic content. Presence or absence of secondary

* Corresponding Author: E-mail: muchuweti@medic.uz.ac.zw; Phone: 00263 (0) 4 308047; Fax: 00263 4 308046.

metabolites alone can not be used as a marker in pear breeding but would require complementing with genetic information. The results show some of the challenges in finding markers linked to color of the peel among different pear cultivars, which have a high degree of similarity to one another.

Keywords: *Pyrus communis L., Starkrimson, Clapp's favourite, Marx red Bartlett, Antioxidant activity, Scavenging activity, Phenolic compounds.*

Introduction

Common pear (*Pyrus communis* L.) is a deciduous pome fruit of the Rasaceae family, subfamily Maloideae. Pears thrive best in temperate climates and have a higher chilling requirement than apple, confining their production to the coolest areas with more than 400 chilling hours (Rehm and Espig, 1991; Rice *et al.*, 1986). In Zimbabwe production is mainly in the eastern highlands.

The ultimate objective of the production, handling and distribution of fresh fruits and vegetables is to satisfy consumer's requirements (Escarpa and Gonzalez, 2001). In general the attractiveness of fruits and vegetables to consumers is determined by sensory quality attributes such as colour, astringency, bitterness and aroma and to different aspects of fruits including health benefits (Macheix *et al.*, 1990; Mozetic *et al.*, 2002; Kuti, 2004; Barberan and Espin, 2001). Flavonoids and hydroxycinnamic acid derivatives, secondary metabolites, contribute largely to both fruit colour and through fruit consumption, to human health (Hamauzu, 2006; Mozetic *et al.*, 2002).

There is considerable evidence for the role of antioxidant constituents of fruits and vegetables in the maintenance of health and disease prevention (Veberic *et al.*, 2005; Cao *et al.*, 1998; Goh *et al.*, 2003). Recent studies have shown that the majority of the antioxidative and possible anticarcinogenic activity of fruits and vegetables may originate from the flavonoids and other phenolic compounds (Vallejo *et al.*, 2003; Yang *et al.*, 2001). The term phenolic antioxidant refers to both simple phenolic acids and flavonoids (Harborne, 1998). They are products of secondary plant metabolism and are ubiquitous natural components of plants (Becker *et al.*, 2004), whose evolution, accumulation, content and composition in fruit tissues is invaluable in breeding for improved functional fruits.

Consumption of different pear cultivars contributes to different antioxidant phenolics levels in the diets (Veberic *et al.*, 2005). Characterization of major phenolic families involved is invaluable to the informed recommendation of particular diets and markets with an optimal knowledge of the contents and activity of these natural antioxidants (Chun *et al.*, 2005; Rooyen and Bower, 2003; Miller, 1998).

Colour differences were noted in 2004-2005 season, on the fruits of Starkrimson (red) and Marx red Bartlett (red) common pear trees at Nyanga Experiment Station. New green coloured pear bud mutants were identified on these trees. In this study phenolic compound HPLC profiles, free radicals scavenging activity, and antioxidant activity of the of the phenolic compounds in the wild types and their bud mutants were evaluated and used to discriminate between wild type pear cultivars and their bud mutants with different peel colour. The chemical composition and activities constitute a biochemical marker, which can be used in finger printing cultivars for proper referencing of the germplasm.

Materials and Methods

Pear Samples

The pears investigated in the study are described in Table 18.1. The fruit samples were harvested ripe from Rhodes Inyanga Experiment Station, February 2006. The collected fruits samples were stored at –20 °C and analysed at the University of Zimbabwe's Department of Biochemistry, in February to May 2006. Peel and pulp portions of the fruit were used as fresh samples.

Table 18.1: Pears Investigated in the Study

Origin	*Cultivar*	*Fruit Colour*	*Average Fruit Mass (g)*
South Africa	Starkrimson	Deep red	268
NES, Zimbabwe	Starkrimson mutant	Green with red blush	270
South Africa	Clapp's Favourite	Green with red blush	265
South Africa	Marx red Bartlett	Light red	272
NES, Zimbabwe	Marx red Bartlett mutant A	Green with red blush	204
NES, Zimbabwe	Marx red Bartlett mutant B	Green with red blush	323

NES: Nyanga Experiment Station.

Chemicals

Ethylenediaminetetraacetic acid (EDTA); 1, 1–Diphenyl–2–picryl hydrazyl (DPPH?); Polyoxyethylene sorbitan monopalmitate (Tween 80); Ethanol; lead acetate-water (1:10,v/v), methanol-water (1:1, v/v), butanol, acetic acid, Folin-Ciocalteu reagent, acetic acid, acetonitrile, vanillic, caffeic acid, p-coumaric acid, protocatechuic acid, ferulic acid, p-hydroxybenzaldehyde, p-hydroxybenzoic acid, (Sigma H 5882: Sigma Co., St Louis, 2004) All the other solvents/chemicals used were of analytical grade and purchased from Sigma Aldrich.

Extraction for Total Phenolics

Total phenolic compounds were extracted from the peel and pulp as described by Makkar (1999). The peel, or pulp sample (2 g) was extracted with 50 per cent aqueous methanol (10 ml). The cell walls were broken by sornicating for 10 min followed by centrifugation at 3, 000 rpm for 10 min. Supernatant was transferred into sample bottles for analysis.

Determination of Total Phenolic Content using Folin-Ciocalteu Method

Total phenolic compounds were determined following the method by Makkar (1999). To a sample (20 ml), distilled water (2.98 ml) was added to make up to 3 ml followed by 1N Folin C. reagent (500 ml) and sodium carbonate (500 ml). After 40 min at room temperature absorbance at 725 nm was read on a Spectronic 20 Genesys Tm spectrophotometer against a blank that contained methanol instead of sample. Total phenolics were expressed in terms of Gallic Acid Equivalent (GAE).

Extraction and hydrolysis for HPLC

Total phenolic compounds were extracted from the peel, and pulp. The peel and pulp sample (2 g) was sornicated for 10 min and hydrolysed with 2 M HCL in boiling water bath for 30 min followed by extraction with 50 per cent aqueous methanol (5 ml). The hydrolysates were centrifuged at 3 000 rpm for 10 min. The supernatant was filtered through and transferred into sample bottles for analysis.

Chromatographic Conditions in HPLC

A Shimadzu HPLC with a SCL-6B Shimadzu systems controller, C-R AX Shimadzu chromatopac, Shimadzu SPD-10 AV UV-Vis detector fitted with a Dynamax 60 A C18 column was used for analysis of phenolic compounds. The amount of sample injected was 5 µl and the flow rate was 1 ml/min. Two mobile phases were employed for elution, water-acetic acid (98:2, v/v, A) and water-acetonitrile-acetic acid (78:20:2, v/v/v, B). The gradient profile used is shown in Table 18.2. Detection was carried out at 280 nm.

Table 18.2: Time Programme for HPLC Analysis of Phenolic Compounds

Time (Minutes)	*Per cent Solvent A*	*Per cent Solvent B*
0	100	0
55	20	80
70	10	90
75	10	90
80	100	0
85	Stop	Stop

Free Radical Scavenging Activity with 2, 2–Diphenyl–1–picrylhydrazyl (DPPH•)

DPPH• (0.001 g) was dissolved into absolute alcohol (100 ml). To DPPH• (3 ml) the extract (20 ml) was added and mixed. The discoloring of DPPH? was monitored by taking absorbance readings at 517 nm at 30°C in a spectrophotometer at an interval of 15 min. Alcohol was used as a blank while ascorbic acid (50 mg/ml) was used as control. Scavenging activity was calculated as: [Absorbance at time n (t_n)/absorbance at time zero (t_o)]

Antioxidant Activity Using β-carotene-linoleic Acid Model System

β-Carotene (2 mg) was dissolved in 10 ml chloroform. One ml of the b-carotene solution was pipetted into a 100 ml round-bottom flask and evaporated using a rotavapor at 40°C for 10 min. Tween 80 (400 ml), linoleic acid (40 ml) as well as distilled water (100 ml) were added to the 100 ml flask containing β-carotene. The contents were vigorously shaken to form an emulsion. A blank devoid of β-carotene was used to zero the machine. Absorbance was read at 470 nm at an interval of 15 min for 120 min.

Results

Determination of Total Phenolic Compounds in *Pyrus communis* L. (Common Pear)

Secondary metabolites, for example phenolic compounds, are important in determining the nutritional value of a fruit as well as the adaptability of the plant to environmental factors. These factors assist the breeders in identifying the write germplasm in their programs. It is invaluable then to quantify and qualify these compounds for proper reference of the germplasm.

The reaction of phenolic compounds with the Folin and Ciocalteu's phenol reagent was measured at 725 nm to give the amount of phenolic compounds in 50 per cent methanol extracts. The phenolic content was determined by reference to a standard gallic acid curve.

The green coloured Clapp's favourite peel had the highest total phenolics (1.541 mg GAE/g); while Starkrimson peel had the least. The amount of total phenolics in Clapp's favourite peel extracts (Table 18.3) is more than double that of wild type Starkrimson peel. It can be observed that green coloured fruits have peel extracts containing higher total phenolics compared to the red coloured Starkrimson fruit peels. The pulp extracts of Starkrimson (0.065 mg GAE/g) had the highest total phenolics, while those of Clapp's favourite (0.014 mg GAE/g) had the least.

Table 18.3: Total Phenolics Content in Mature Common Pear Fruit Peel and Pulp 50 per cent Methanolic Extracts (mg GAE/g fresh weight) of Clapp's Favourite Origin. The uncertainties shown are standard deviations for at least three measurements.

Cultivar	*Fruit Portion*	*Mean Concentration mg GAE/g of Fruit Weight*
Starkrimson wild type	peel	0.561±0.004
Starkrimson mutant	peel	0.966±0.005
Clapp's Favourite	peel	1.541±0.006
Starkrimson wild type	pulp	0.065±0.003
Starkrimson mutant	pulp	0.051±0.004
Clapp's Favourite	pulp	0.014±0.004

Table 18.4 shows the total phenolics content of the wild type Marx red Bartlett peel to be the highest (1.389 mg GAE/g), while mutant A had the least (0.420 mg GAE/g). The peel extract total phenolics content of mutant A is about twice less than that of mutant B and almost three times less than that of the wild type. Mutant B pulp had the highest total phenolics content with about twice the content in wild type Marx red Bartlett and mutant A pulps. The quantities of total phenolics in the wild type and mutant A are almost the same with total phenolics of 0.014 mg GAE/g.

Table 18.4: Total Phenolics Content in Mature Common Pear Fruit Peel and Pulp 50 per cent Methanolic Extracts (mg GAE/g fresh weight) of Marx Red Bartlett Origin. The uncertainties shown are standard deviations for at least three measurements.

Cultivar	*Fruit Portion*	*Mean Concentration mg GAE/g of Fruit Weight*
Marx red Bartlett wild type	peel	1.389±0.004
Marx red Bartlett mutant A	peel	0.420±0.003
Marx red Bartlett mutant B	peel	0.948±0.005
Marx red Bartlett wild type	pulp	0.014±0.001
Marx red Bartlett mutant A	pulp	0.014±0.004
Marx red Bartlett mutant B	pulp	0.029±0.004

Phenolic Profiles

HPLC Phenolic Profiles of Fruit Portions of Clapp's Favorite Origin

The relative content of flavonoids and phenolic acids among the pears studied varied considerably, as shown in Figure 18.1. Certain similarities were observed within cultivars. In the members of the Clapp's favourite origin, that is wild type Starkrimson and its mutant, eight phenolic compounds (gallic acid, protochatechuic acid, p-hydroxybenzoic acid, p–hydroxybenzaldehyde, vanilic acid,

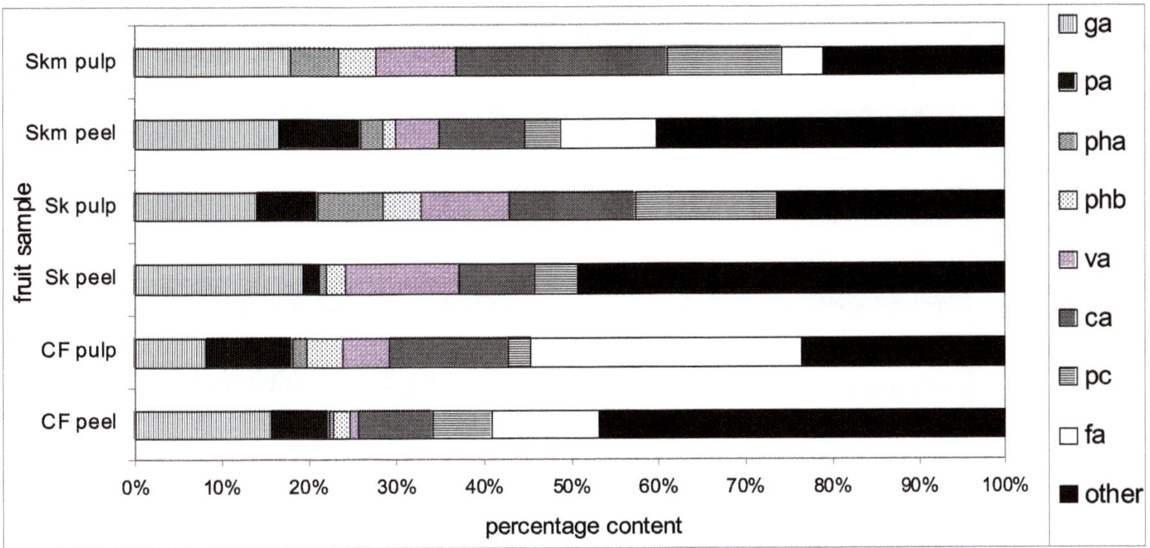

Figure 18.1: The Proportion of Simple Phenolic Compounds in Pear Fruits of Clapp's Favourite Origin (peel and pulp), Hydrolysed with 2 M HCl for 30 min and Extracted with 50 per cent Methanol (v/v), as Assessed by HPLC, Detection at 280 nm. The following compounds were identified: va, ca, pc, pa, fa, pha, phb, ga representing, vanillic, caffeic acid, p-coumaric acid, protocatechuic acid, ferulic acid, p-hydroxybenzaldehyde, p-hydroxybenzoic acid, gallic acid respectively. Skw, Starkrimson wild type; Skm, Starkrimson mutant; CF, Clapp's favourite.

p-coumaric acid, caffeic acid and ferulic acid) were identified, but varied in percentage distributions. In Clapp's favourite peel, the main phenolic compound was gallic acid while ferulic acid was the main compound in the pulp. The peels of Starkrimson wild type and its mutant had gallic acid as the major compound, while the pulps had ferulic acid and caffeic acid respectively, as the major compounds. Unlike Starkrimson wild type and Clapp's favourite, the pulp of the mutant of Starkrimson did not have protochatechuic acid in its profile, or couldn't be resolved.

Phenolic Profiles of Fruit Portions of Marx Red Bartlett Origin

There were major differences in phenolic compound profiles of wild type Marx Red Bartlett and its mutants, A and B. Gallic acid was identified in wild type Marx Red Bartlett peel, mutant A pulp and peel, and mutant B pulp, and was the major compound in mutant A pulp and mutant B pulp, but could not be identified in mutant B peel and wild type Marx Red Bartlett pulp. In mutant A and mutant B peels caffeic acid was the major compound. The peel of mutant B had vanillic acid as the major compound.

Scavenging Effect on 2, 2-diphenyl-1-picrylhydrazyl (DPPH)

The recent interest in phenolic acids has stemmed from their potential protective role, through ingestion of fruits and vegetables, against oxidative damage from diseases (coronary heart disease, stroke, and cancers). Phenolic compounds are essential for the growth and reproduction of plants, and are produced as a response for defending injured plants against pathogens. The importance of antioxidant activities of phenolic compounds and their possible usage in processed foods as a natural antioxidant has reached a new high in recent years.

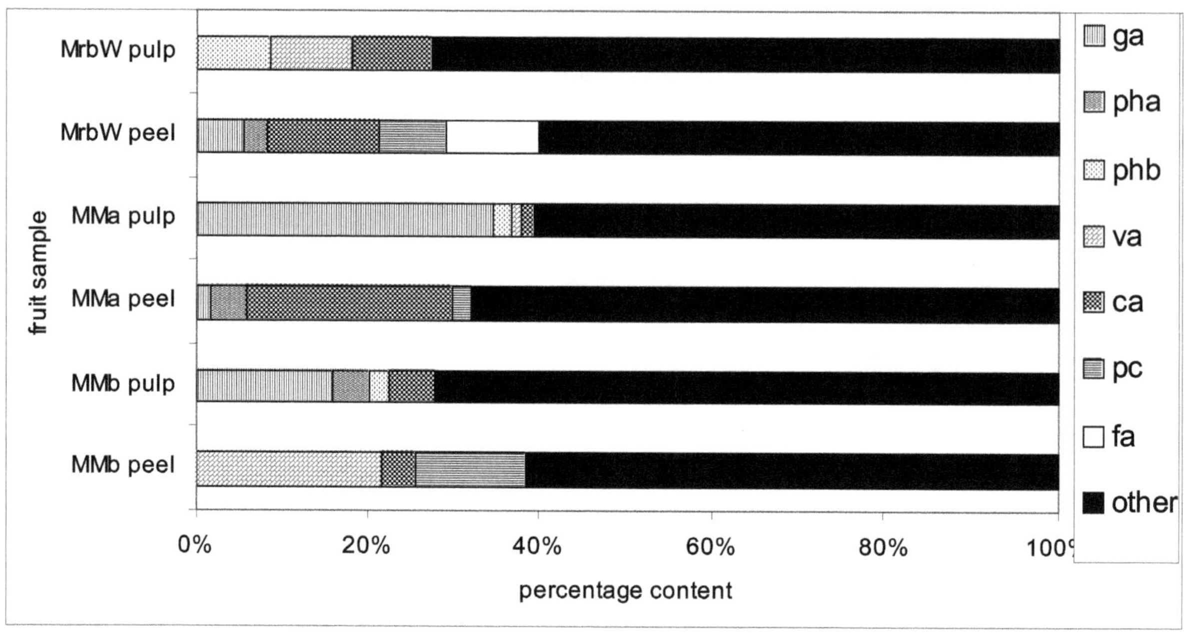

Figure 18.2: The Proportion of Simple Phenolic Compounds in Pear Fruits of Marx Red Bartlett Origin (peel and pulp), Hydrolysed with 2 M HCl for 30 min and Extracted with 50 per cent Methanol (v/v), as Assessed by HPLC at 280 nm. The following compounds were identified: va, ca, pc, pa, fa, pha, phb, ga representing, vanillic, caffeic acid, p-coumaric acid, protocatechuic acid, ferulic acid, p-hydroxybenzaldehyde, p-hydroxybenzoic acid, gallic acid respectively. MMa, Mrb mutant A; MMb, Mrb mutant b; Mrbw, Marx Red Bartlett wild type.

In this study the ant oxidative properties of the methanolic extracts of pear fruits were determined using scavenging effect on DPPH and oxidation of b-carotene model system.

Figure 18.3 shows the scavenging activity of the peel and pulp extracts of ripe common pear fruits to be lower than that of ascorbic acid. Clapp's Favourite peel, as shown in Figure 18.3(a), had the highest activity while wild type Starkrimson peel had the lowest. It would seem that the bud mutant had a higher scavenging activity than the wild type Starkrimson.

The fruit pulp extracts of the cultivars of the Clapp's Favourite lineage in Figure 18.3(b), showed lower scavenging ability compared to ascorbic acid. Marx Red Bartlett wild type fruit peel, as shown in Figure 18.4(a), had the highest scavenging activity while mutant A had the least. There are no noticeable differences in scavenging activities among the pulp extracts of the Marx Red Bartlett cultivar and the bud mutants.

Antioxidant Activity

Figures 18.5 and 18.6 show a fast decline in the concentration of β-carotene as it discolours. The peel extracts of wild type Starkrimson have the highest activity while those of Clapp's Favourite had the least. However, the pulp extracts of Clapp's favourite were slightly lower in activity than that of wild type Starkrimson. The antioxidant activity of the Starkrimson mutant pulp was the lowest and even lower than ascorbic acid.

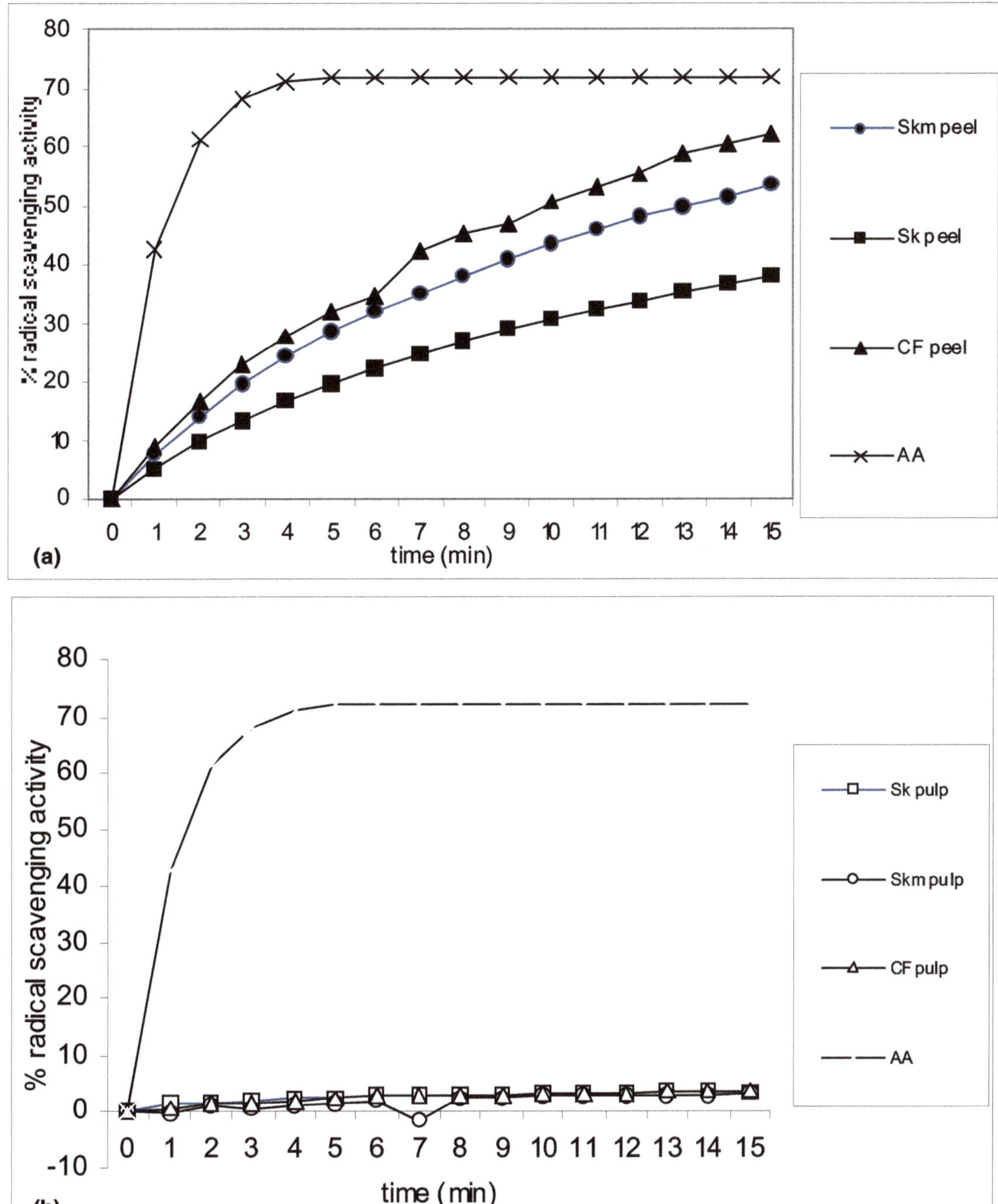

Figure 18.3: Mean Scavenging Effects of Methanolic Extracts from *P. communis* L. (Common Pear) Cultivar and their Mutants, (a) Peel, (b) Pulp. Wild type Starkrimson as compared to Clapp's Favourite and its mutant, as assessed by DPPH stable free radical. Skw, Starkrimson wild type; Skm, Starkrimson mutant; CF, Clapp's favourite. The means are for at least three measurements.

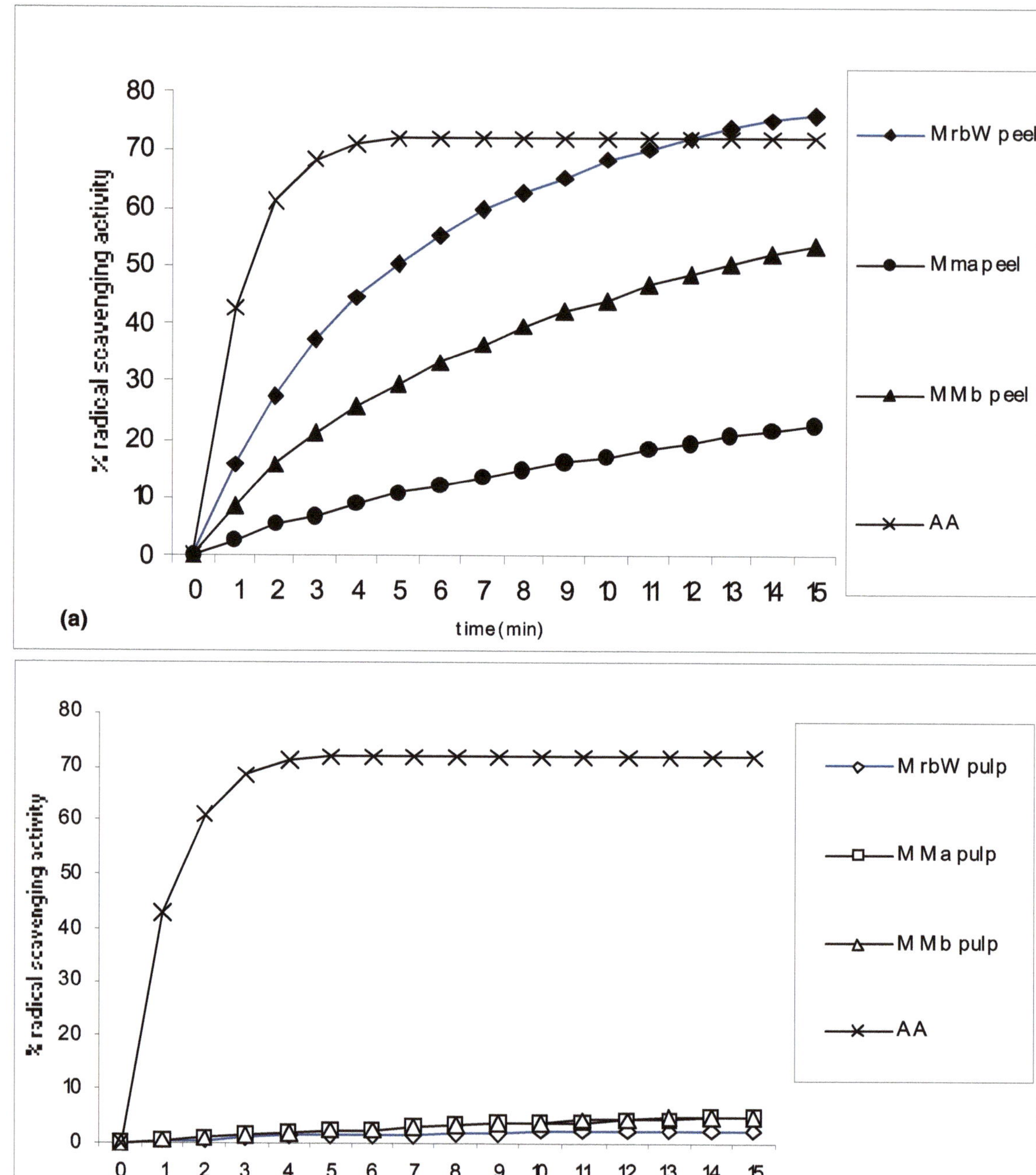

Figure 18.4: Mean Scavenging Effects of Methanolic Extracts from *P. communis* L. (Common Pear) Cultivars and their Reverted Spots, (a) Peel, (b) Pulp. Marx Red Bartlett as compared to its two mutants, as assessed by DPPH stable free radical. MMa, Mrb mutant A; MMb, Mrb mutant b; Mrbw, Marx Red Bartlett wild type. The means are for at least three measurements.

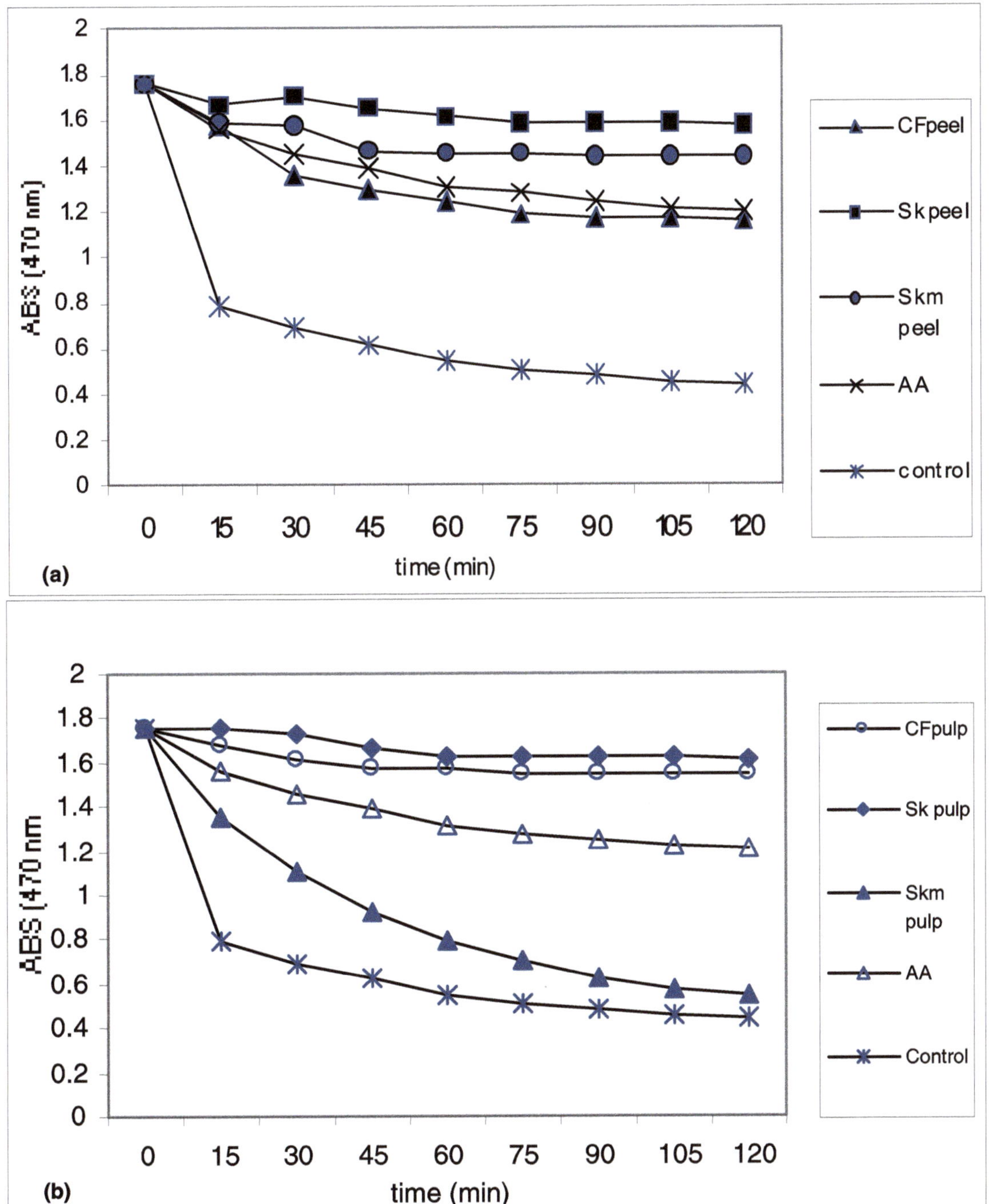

Figure 18.5: Mean Antioxidant Activity of Methanolic Extracts from *P. communis* L. (Common Pear) Cultivars and their Reverted Spots, (a) Peel, (b) Pulp. Wild type Starkrimson compared to Clapp's Favourite and its bud mutant, as assessed by -carotene-linoleic acid model system. Skw, Starkrimson wild type; Skm, Starkrimson mutant; CF, Clapp's favourite. The means are for at least three measurements.

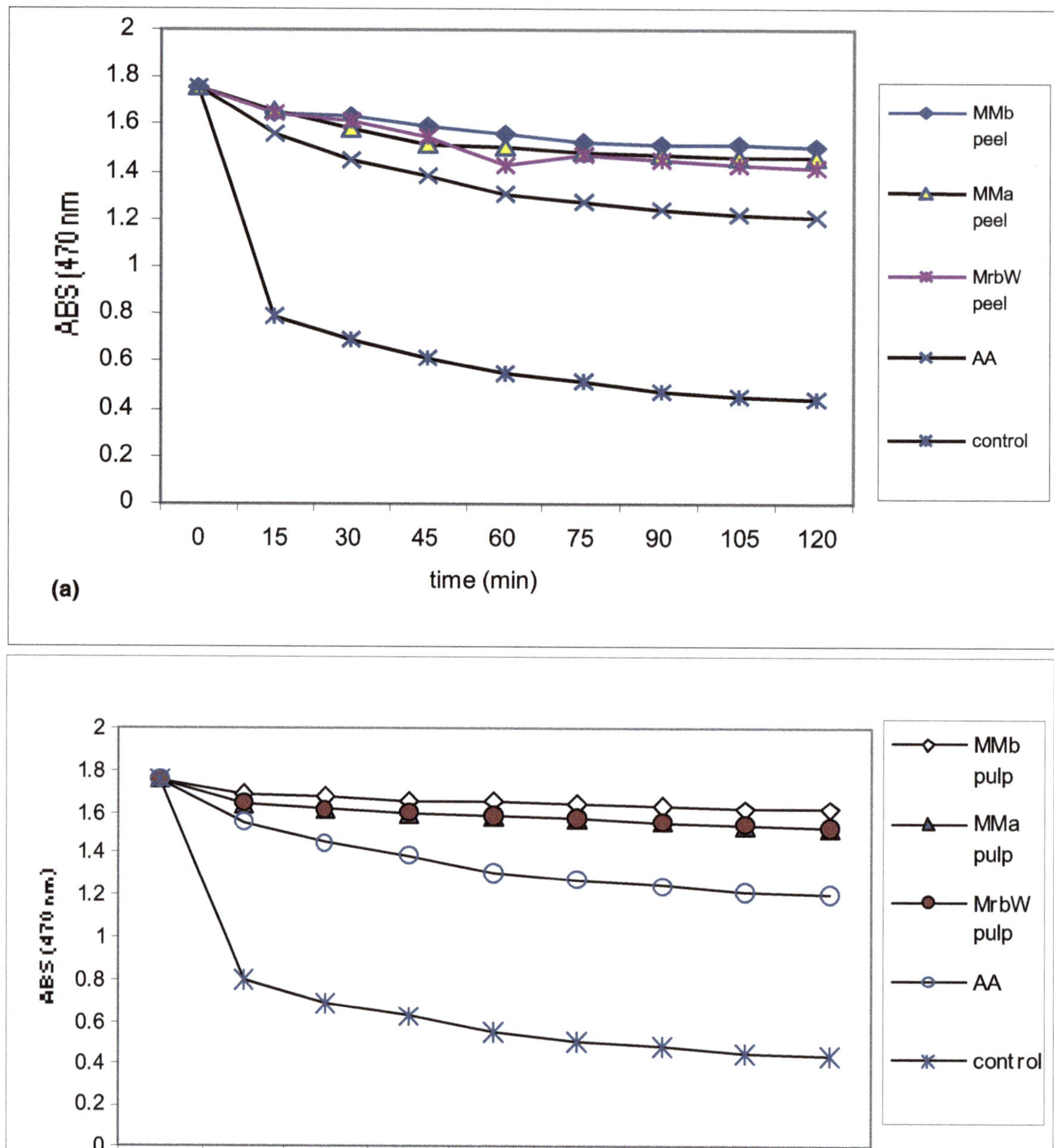

Figure 18.6: Mean Antioxidant Activity of Methanolic Extracts from *P. communis* L. (Common Pear) Cultivars and their Reverted Spots, (a) Peel, (b) Pulp. Marx Red Bartlett as compared to its two mutants, as assessed by b-carotene-linoleic acid model system. MMa, Mrb mutant A; MMb, Mrb mutant b; Mrbw, Marx Red Bartlett wild type. The means are for at least three measurements.

Ascorbic acid reduced the rate of b-carotene discolouring. Figure 18.6 show high activity in peel and pulp extracts of wild type Marx Red Bartlett and its mutants. The peels and pulp extracts of mutant B had the highest activity while those of wild type Marx Red Bartlett and mutant A were almost the same. The activities of the fruit samples were higher than that of ascorbic acid.

The activity of Clapp's Favourite peel extract is lower than ascorbic acid despite having the highest total phenolics. The activity of wild type Starkrimson peel and pulp extracts is relatively high while that of Starkrimson spot is the lowest.

Discussion

Peels of common pear fruits are not normally removed from the fruit during consumption. Thus the nutritional value in the peel is not lost, since both peel and pulp are consumed. The combined peel and pulp total phenolics content is important in determining the nutritional value of fruits and the adaptability of the fruit to field and post harvest handling environment. Green fruits of the Clapp's favourite lineage have been shown to contain more total phenolics than the red Starkrimson wild type fruits.

The total phenolics for Starkrimson peel (0.561 mg/g GAE) do not concur with those obtained by Di Mauro *et al.*, 2003 (3.74 mg/g GAE). These differences are possibly due to varying climatic conditions and extraction procedures, as well as the degree of ripeness, which affects the concentrations and properties of the various phenolic compounds. In this study phenolic compound concentrations were found to be higher in peel compared to the pulp. These results concur with those obtained by Di Mauro *et al.* (2003).

The trend observed in the fruits of Clapp's favourite origin is not entirely the same with the trend observed in fruits from trees of wild type Marx Red Bartlett lineage. Red coloured fruits of the wild type Marx Red Bartlett have been shown to contain the highest total phenolics in comparison with mutant A and mutant B. The green coloured fruits from the bud mutants A and B have been shown to contain different levels of total phenolics. The differences in total phenolics could be explained possibly by the varying positions of fruits within canopy as affected by the sink–source relationship and the uninterrupted ability of the fruit, and leaves supplying nutrients to the fruit, to receive sunlight. It would be expected therefore, that exposed fruits and leaves will be able to intercept sunlight and photosynthesise as well as make and store other secondary metabolites. Fruits with apical dominance will also receive more metabolites compared to those without. The overall fruit number per canopy relative to fruit canopy size and structure affects the total metabolites that a tree canopy will produce; hence few fruits in an open central leader system will be bigger and containing higher levels of metabolites. From this study it has been shown that it is difficult to regard fruit colour as a measure of total phenolics content in common pear fruits. Phenolic content was always higher in the peel compared to the pulp in all the cultivars indicating compatimentation of phenolic compounds in fruits, for defense purposes (Starck, 1997; Macheix *et al.*, 1990; Gorsel *et al.*, 2992). In peach, chlorogenic and caffeic acids concentrations were related to level of resistance to brown rot fungus (*Manilinia fructiccola*) (Hamauzu, 2006). In general plant tissue, flavonoids may also play a role in the first line of defense against insect predation. Another role of phenolics in the defense system of fruit is as filters which protects certain fragile cell structures from UV radiation. These filters consists mainly of flavonoids and are located in the skin of fruits (Hamauzu, 2006), in response to the stressing environment.

The phenolic profiles in Figures 18.1 and 18.2 do not show any down stream products in the anthocyanin biosynthetic pathway. This was mainly because of inadequate standards to identify the respective peaks. Without standards to identify phenolic compounds responsible for the observed colour differences in the fruit peels, the profiles cannot explain the differences in peel colour in the six pear genotypes. Pears, apples and blueberries contain chlorogenic acid (5-caffeoylquinic acid) as a major hydrocynamic acid (Hamauzu, 2006), but this compound could not be detected in this study.

Understanding of the phenolic profile in fruits at a particular physiological stage makes it possible to see the effects of modification of phenolic content and composition by stimulating their biosynthesis. Stimulation of the phenolics by the environmental factors may lead to the creation of a functional fruit that contains high amounts of phenolic compounds (Hamauzu, 2006).

Phenolic content and type of phenolic compounds present in the mixture affect the rate of DPPH discolouring, a chromogenic free radical, by donating H ions. The reducing potential of DPPH relative to the phenolic compounds present in the mixture determine the ease with which H ions can be donated by phenolic compounds to DPPH. The concentration of the phenolic compounds with the ability to donate H ions to DPPH also affects the rate of discolouring. A lower rate of DPPH discolouring indicates lower radical scavenging activity. The free radical scavenging activity was correlated to total phenolic content in all the six genotypes.

Implications for the differences in scavenging activity are that fruits with higher activity have better storage than fruits with lower activity. Fruits with higher activity could also resist/tolerate adverse stress conditions (biotic and abiotic). The edible portion however, did not show much difference in scavenging activity among cultivars. The differences in total phenolics do not seem to explain the similarities in scavenging activities observed in the pulps.

The phenolic compounds identified in Figures 18.1 and 18.2 shows no relationship with the scavenging activity of the methanolic extracts of the fruit portions. The identified compounds do not adequately cover the profile, to be able to explain the differences in scavenging activity of the extracts. Edible portions are important to human diets and their being equally the same means the varieties are nutritionally similar in teams of their polyphenolic free radical scavenging ability.

The differences in scavenging activity could be correlated to the possible health benefits in humans though better assays mimicking the biological systems would give better indications (Goh *et al.*, 2003; Kuti, 2004; Shon *et al.*, 2003)

β-Carotene discolours slowly when fruit extracts are added to the emulsion. The antioxidation is hypothesised to be mainly due to phenolic compounds. Discolouring of β-carotene relates to the donation of H ions from β-carotene (Becker *et al.*, 2004). This does not however relate to the protection of the lipids directly form β-carotene donated H ions as affected by reduction potentials of the existing antioxidants in the mixture. β-carotene may be regenerated or act in regeneration of other high reduction potential compounds. In this reaction b-carotene (b-COH) acts as a chain breaking antioxidant reacting with peroxyl radicals (LOO^-) (Veberic *et al.*, 2005; Becker *et al.*, 2004)

$$(\beta\text{-COH} + LOO^- = \beta\text{-CO}^- + LOOH)$$

The antioxidant and free radical scavenging properties of phenolics can serve as protection against photo-oxidation caused by UV-light (Macheix *et al.*, 1990). The principal phenolics involved in UV–light adsorption are located in the vacuoles, especially in sunlit surfaces. It is suggested that a massive build-up of flavonoids occurs in peel cells located just below the cuticle, resulting in trapping of radiation in a broad spectral range, which plays a dominant role in long-term adaptation of pear fruit to elevated levels of solar radiation (Hamauzu *et al.*, 2006).

Decreasing ascorbic acid levels are accompanied by browning of fruit, owing to the loss of the fruit's capacity to regenerate ascorbic acid, which could prevent oxidative damage (Hamauzu *et al.*,

2006). There is conflicting information on the antioxidative contribution of ascorbic acid to the plant system as assessed by *in vitro* assays. Information from this experiment indicates considerable contribution of ascorbic acid in antioxidative activity, since pulp extracts were observed to have lower activity than ascorbic acid. In such fruit portions where the results show low activity, ascorbic acid may act as the main antioxidant accounting for most of the activity. The results show that phenolic compounds are not the only antioxidant compounds within pear fruit systems.

The presence of a lag phase in the Starkrimson peel and pulp graphs may indicate the presence of a chain breaking antioxidant.

Red fruits or juices have received attention due to their high antioxidant activity, for example, red juices of grape and berries (Gil *et al.*, 2000; Sanchez *et al.*, 2000). Chemical analysis of the fruit portions has shown variation in phenolic compound composition, free radical scavenging and antioxidant activity. The results obtained in this study however, are not in accordance with those obtained by Sanchez *et al.* (2004), and show no relationship with the phenotype of the fruit. It is not clear as to which fruits have higher phenolic content, the green or the red coloured fruits. In this study, wild type Marx Red Bartlett (red peel) has higher phenolic content than its mutants (green peel), while Starkrimson (red peel) had the lowest compared to Clapp's favourite and Starkrimson mutant, both having green peel.

Conclusion

The total phenolics contents obtained in this study were low (1.555 mg GAE/g in Clapp's favourite to 0.424 mg GAE/g in Marx red Bartlett mutant A) (Di Mauro *et al.*, 2003), and showed wide variations in percentage composition of identified phenolic compounds between cultivars and within cultivars. DPPH free radical scavenging activity was correlated to total phenolics, while the antioxidant activity as assessed by the b-carotene-linoleic acid assay model system showed no correlation to total phenolics. The phenolic profiles showed no clear relationship with either activity.

From the nutritional point of view, since most of the phenolics were located in the peel, the consumption of unpeeled pears is recommended to maximize the dietary intake of antioxidant compounds.

As part of a continuing common pear breeding programme, the effect of environmental factors on phenolic changes in fruits and their modification should be investigated. With this knowledge it is possible to enhance the quality of fruit and to produce ideal multifunctional fruits that have good appearance, good taste, high impact on human health, and shelf-life.

Acknowledgements

The authors wish to thank the Kellogg Foundation, UNU-INRA and the University of Zimbabwe Research Board for financial support.

References

Barberan,–T.F.A., J.C. Espin (2001). Phenolic compounds and related enzymes as determinants of quality in fruits and vegetables. *Journal of the Science of Food and Agriculture*, Vol. 81 (9): 853-876

Becker, E.M. and L.R. Nissen, L.H. Skibsted (2004) Antioxidant evaluation protocols: Food quality or health effects. *European Food research and Technology*, 219: 561-571

Cao, G., S.L.Booth, J.A.Sadowski and R.L. (1998). Prior, increase in human plasma antioxidant capacity after consumption of controlled diets high in fruits and vegetables. *American Journal of Clinical Nutrition*, 68: 1081-7

Chun, O.K., D-O. Kim, N. Smith, D. Schroeder, J.T. Han and C.Y. Lee (2005). Daily consumption of phenolics and total antioxidant capacity from fruit and vegetables in the American diet. *Journal of the Science of Food Agriculture*, 85: 1715-1724

Di mauro, A., R. W. Dust, and R. E. Wrolstad (2003). Polyphenolic composition and antioxidant properties of pears. *www.Ift.confex.com* Downloaded 2005.

Escarpa, A., and M.C. Gonnzalez (2001). Total extractable phenolic chromatographic index: an overview of the phenolic class contents from different sources of foods. *European Food Research and Technology*, 212 (4): 439-444

Gil, M.I., F.A.T-Barberan, B.H-Pierce, D.M.Holcroft, and A.A.Kader (2000). Antioxidant activity of Pomegranate juice and its relationship with phenolic composition and processing. J*ournal of Agricultural and Food Chemistry*, 48: 4581-4589

Gorsel, H., C.Li, E. L. Kerbel, M. Simts, and A.A.Kader (1992). Compositional characterization of prune juice. J*ournal of.Agricultural and Food Chemistry*, 40: 784-789

Goh, L.M., P.J. Barlow, and C.S. Yong (2003). Examination of antioxidant activity of *Ginkgo biloba* leaf infissions. *Food chemistry*, 82: 275-282

Hamauzu, Y. (2006). Role and evolution of fruit phenolic compounds during ripening and storage. *Stewart Postharvest review*, 2: 5

Harborne, J.B. (1989). General procedures and measurements of total phenolics. Methods in plant biochemistry. vol. 1. Academic press limited, London

Harborne, J.B, and C.A Williams (1998). Anthocyanins and other flavonoids. *Natural plant products report*, 15: 631–652

Kuti, O.J. (2004). Antioxidant compounds from four *Opuntia cactus* pear fruit varieties. *Food chemistry*, 85: 527-533

Macheix J.–J., J. Billot and A. Fleuriet (1990). Fruit Phenolics. CRC Press, Inc., Boca. Raton, FL, 149–237

Makkar H.P.S. (1999). Quantitation of tannins in tree foliage: A Laboratory manual for the FAO/IAEA coordinated Research project on 'Use of nuclear and Related Techniques to Develop Simple Tannin assay for Predicting and improving the Safety and Efficiency of feeding Ruminants on the Tanniniferous Tree Foliage. Joint FAO/IAEA Division of nuclear Techniques in Food and Agriculture, Vienna, Austria 1-29

Miller, D.D. (1998). Food chemistry: A laboratory manual. John Wiley and Sons, Inc, Canada. p 94-95

Mozetic, B., P. Trebse and J. Hribar (2002). Determination and quantitation of anthocyanins and hydroxycinnamic acids in different cultivars of Sweet Cherries (*Prunus avium* L.) from Nova Gorica region (Slovenia). *Food Technology and Biotechnology*, 40 (3): 207-212

Rehm, S. and G. Espig (1991). The cultivated plants of the tropics and subtropics: Cultivation, economic value, utilisation. *Verlag josef margraf, West Germany*, 205-206.

Rice, R.P., L.W. Rice, and H.D. Tindall (1986). Fruits and vegetables production in Africa. Macmillian, London. p 132

Rooyen, Z. and J.P. Bower (2003). The role of fruits mineral composition, phenolic concentration and polyphenol oxidase activity on mesocarp discolouration in Pinkerton. *South Africa Avocado Growers' Association Yearbook*, 26: 72-75, 77-79, 81-82

Sánchez, A.C.G-, A. G-Izquierdo, M.I. Gil (2000). Comparative study of six pear cultivars in terms of their phenolic and vitamin C contents and antioxidant capacity. *Journal of the Science of Food and Agriculture*, 85: 10, 995–1003

Sanchez, A.C.G, A.M.M.B. Morais, F.X. Malcata, M.I. Gil (2004). Quantification of chlorogenic acid and polyphenol oxidase activity in 'Rocha' pear after CA-long storage. ISHS Acta Horticulture 600: VIII International controlled atmosphere research conference.

Shon, M-Y., T-H. Kim and N-J. Sung (2003). Antioxidants and free radical scavenging activity of *Phellinus baumii* (Phellinus of Hymenochaetaceae) extracts. *Food Chemistry*, 82: 593-597

Singleton, V.L., and E. Trousdale (1983). White wine phenolics: Varietal and processing differences as shown by HPLC. *American Society for Enology and Viticulture*, 34: 1, 27–34.

Strack, D. (1997). Phenolic metabolism, In: P.M. Dey and J. B. Harborne (eds), Plant Biotechnology. Academic Press, San Diego

Vallejo, F., F.A. T-Barberan, and C.G-Viguera (2003). Phenolic compound contents in edible parts of brocolli inflorescence after domestic cooking. *Journal of Science of Food and Agriculture*, 83: 1854–1858.

Veberic, R., M. Trobec, K. Herbinger, M. Hofer, D. Grill, and F. Stampar (2005). Phenolic compounds in some apple (*Malus domestica* Borkh) cultivars on organic and integrated production. *Journal of Science of Food and Agriculture*, 85: 1687-1694.

Yang, C.S., J.M. Landau, M-T. Huang and H.L.Newmark (2001). Inhibition of carcinogenesis by dietary polyphenolic compounds. *Annual Review of Nutrition*, 21: 381-406.

Medicinal Plants: Phytochemistry, Pharmacology and Therapeutics, Vol. 1 *Pages 354–362*
Editors: **V.K. Gupta, G.D. Singh, Surjeet Singh and A. Kaul**
Published by: **DAYA PUBLISHING HOUSE, NEW DELHI**

Chapter 19

Antioxidant Activity of the Methanol Extract of *Hypericum hookerianum* Stem in Ehrlich Ascites Carcinoma Bearing Mice

Santoshkumar H. Dongre, Shrishailappa Badami*, Senthilkumar Natesan and Raghu Chandrashekhar H.
Department of Pharmaceutical Chemistry,
J.S.S. College of Pharmacy, Rock Lands, Ootacamund – 643 001, T.N., India

ABSTRACT

The methanol extract of *H. hookerianum* (MEHH) was studied for *in vitro* antioxidant activity using several standard methods. It exhibited potent activity in ABTS, DPPH and hydrogen peroxide methods. The extract was studied for antioxidant and hepatoprotective properties in Ehrlich ascites carcinoma (EAC) bearing mice. Tumor control animals inoculated with EAC showed a significant alteration in the antioxidant and hepatoprotective parameters. The extract treatment at 100, 200 and 400 mg/kg body weight doses caused a significant reversal of the biochemical changes towards the normal when compared to tumor control animals in serum, liver and kidney indicating the potent antioxidant and hepatoprotective nature of the extract.

Keywords: *Antioxidants, Free radicals, H. hookerianum, Hepatoprotective.*

* Corresponding Author: E-mail: shribadami@rediffmail.com.

Introduction

Reactive oxygen species (ROS) have been implicated in initiating, accompanying or causing pathogenesis of many diseases. Therefore, increased antioxidant concentration at the cellular level could provide considerable protection against ROS (Polidori, 2003). Most of the known antioxidants are derived from the plants, probable due to their increased capacity to defend themselves from various sources of stress (Badami *et al.*, 2005; Natesan *et al.*, 2007; Gupta *et al.*, 2004; Silva *et al.*, 2005; Conforti *et al.*, 2002; Cakir *et al.*, 2003). Strong evidence indicates that ROS plays an important role in the initiation as well as promotion phase of carcinogenesis. Many cancer chemo preventive agents possess antioxidant potentials (Natesan *et al.*, 2007; Gupta *et al.*, 2004). The presence of tumors in the human body or in experimental animals is known to affect many functions of the vital organs specially the liver, even when site of the tumor does not interfere directly with organ functions (De Wys, 1982). High levels of free radicals and malondialdehyde (MDA), the end product of lipid peroxidation were reported in cancer tissues than in non-diseased organs. Hence, currently the reduction of avoidable endogenous and exogenous source of oxidative stress is potentially the most important means of preventive oxygen free radical related cancer (Natesan *et al.*, 2007; Gupta *et al.*, 2004).

The plants of the genus *Hypericum* (Family: Hypericaceae) are widely used in folk medicine. Several species belonging to *Hypericum viz., H. perforatum* (Silva *et al.*, 2005), *H. triquetrifolium* (Conforti *et al.*, 2002), *H. hyssopifolium* (Cakir *et al.*, 2003), etc., are reported to possess potent antioxidant and hepatoprotective activity. Earlier studies carried out in our laboratories have shown strong *in vitro* cytotoxic properties of MEHH (Vijayan *et al.*, 2003). The plant is also reported to possess wound healing and antibacterial properties (Mukherjee *et al.*, 2000; Mukherjee and Suresh, 2001). Strong *in vivo* anticancer properties were observed against EAC induced tumor mice (Dongre *et al.*, 2007). Except these, so far no other biological activities have been carried out on MEHH and no phytoconstituents have been isolated. Hence, in the present study MEHH was evaluated for *in vitro* antioxidant studies using various standard methods and for *in vivo* antioxidant and hepatoprotective nature in EAC tumor bearing mice. High performance liquid chromatography (HPLC) standardized extract containing 0.36 per cent w/w hyperoside was used.

Materials and Methods

Chemicals

5-Flurouracil (5-FU) was obtained from Ranbaxy Ltd., Guregaon, India. DPPH (2,2-diphenyl-1-picryl hydrazyl) and ABTS [2,2′-azino-bis (3-ethylbenzo-thiazoline-6-sulfonic acid) diammonium salt] were obtained from Sigma Aldrich Co, St Louis, USA. HPLC grade solvents and Ecoline diagnostic Kits were obtained from E-Merck Ltd., Mumbai. All chemicals used were of analytical grade.

Plant Material and Extraction

Hypericum hookerianum Weight and Arnot was collected in Ootacamund in July 2004 and authenticated by Dr. S. Rajan, Medicinal Plants Survey and Collection Unit, Ootacamund and retained for future reference. The stem was shade dried, powdered and extracted (190 g) with methanol (1.2 l) in a Soxhlet extractor for 18-20 h. The extract was concentrated to dryness under reduced pressure and controlled temperature (40-50 °C) to yield a dark brown solid weighing 40 g (21.04 per cent). The extract was preserved in a refrigerator at 4 °C till further use.

Animals

Healthy Swiss Albino mice weighing 25±2.0 g were obtained from J. S. S. College of Pharmacy animal house, Ootacamund. The mice were grouped and housed in polyacrylic cages and maintained under standard conditions (temp. 25±2 °C) with 12±1 h dark/light cycle. The animals were fed with rat pellet feed supplied by Hindustan Lever Ltd., Bangalore, India and water *ad libitum*. All procedures were reviewed and approved by CPCSEA, Chennai, India (No. JSSCP/IAEC/PH.D/Ph.Chem/03/2005-2006).

Tumor Cells

EAC cells were supplied by Amala Cancer Research Centre, Thrissur, KL, India. The cells were maintained *in vivo* in Swiss albino mice, by intraperitoneal transplantation. EAC cells aspirated from the peritoneal cavity of mice were washed with saline and given intraperitoneally to develop ascitic tumor.

Preparation of Suspensions and Solutions

MEHH and standard 5-FU were suspended in distilled water using sodium carboxy methyl cellulose (CMC, 0.3 per cent) and administered orally to the animals with the help of an intragastric catheter for *in vivo* activity. MEHH and the standards, ascorbic acid and rutin were dissolved in distilled DMSO separately and used for the *in vitro* antioxidant testing using six different methods. For the hydrogen peroxide method (where DMSO interferes), the extracts and the standards were dissolved in distilled methanol and used. The stock solutions were serially diluted with the respective solvents to obtain the lower dilutions.

In vitro Antioxidant Activity

The *in vitro* antioxidant activity of MEHH was assessed on the basis of scavenging of various radicals like DPPH, ABTS, nitric oxide, superoxide radical by alkaline DMSO and hydrogen peroxide methods (Badami *et al.*, 2005; Natesan *et al.*, 2007).

In vivo Antioxidant Activity

Swiss Albino mice were divided in to six groups (n = 6). All the animals were injected with EAC cells (2 x 10^6 cells/mouse) intraperitoneally except the normal group. This was taken as day zero. Group I was served as normal and group II as tumor control. These two groups were received sodium CMC suspension (0.3 per cent). Group III as a positive control was treated with a suspension of 5-FU at 20 mg/kg body weight. Groups IV, V and VI were treated with MEHH at 100, 200 and 400 mg/kg body weight doses, respectively. All these treatments were given 24 h after the tumor inoculation, once daily for 14 days. After the last dose and 24 h fasting, six mice from each group were sacrificed for the study of biochemical parameters.

Blood was collected from the animals by retro-orbital puncture under mild anesthetic (diethyl ether) condition and the serum was separated by keeping it at 37 °C for half an hour and subjected for the estimation of superoxide dismutase (SOD, Misra and Fridovich, 1972), catalase (CAT, Beers and Sizer, 1952) and thiobarbituric acid reactive substances (TBARS, Ohkawa *et al.*, 1979) and hepatoprotective parameters, aspartate amino transferase (ASAT), alanine amino transaminase (ALAT), alkaline phosphatase (ALP), lactate dehydrogenase (LDH), triglycerides (TGL), creatinine (CR), albumin, total protein (TP), total cholesterol (TC) and total bilirubin (TB) using Ecoline (E Merck Ltd., Mumbai, India) Kits.

After the collection of blood samples, the mice were sacrificed and their liver and kidney were excised, rinsed in ice-cold normal saline followed by cold 0.15 M Tris-HCl (pH 7.4) and blotted dry. A 10 per cent w/v homogenate was prepared in the buffer with Elvenjan homogenizer fitted with teflon plunger and centrifuged at 1500 rpm for 15 min at 4 °C. The supernatants were used for the estimation of the antioxidant parameters.

Statistical Analysis

The significance of the *in vivo* data was analyzed by one-way analysis of variance (ANOVA) followed by Tukey-Kramer multiple comparison tests. $P<0.05$ was considered as statistically significant.

Results

In vitro Antioxidant Activity

MEHH showed potent antioxidant activity in ABTS, DPPH and hydrogen peroxide methods with IC_{50} values of 27.00±0.95, 54.50±0.23 and 84.50±6.67 µg/ml respectively (Table 19.1). However, the activity was found to be less than the standards used. Since the IC_{50} values were found to be high, in the other methods the extract was found to be inactive.

Table 19.1: *In vitro* Antioxidant Activity of *Hypericum hookerianum* Methanol Extract

Extracts/Standard	*DPPH*	*Nitric oxide*	H_2O_2	*ABTS*
H. hookerianum extract	54.50±0.23	>700	84.50±6.67	27.00±0.95
Ascorbic acid	2.69±0.05	–	–	11.25±0.49
Rutin	3.19±0.10	65.40±2.5	36.60±0.2	0.51±0.01

*Average of three determinations.

Biochemical Parameters

The inoculation of EAC cells to tumor control animals significantly increased the levels of ASAT, ALAT, LDH, CR, TP, TC, TB and TBARS and a significant decrease in the levels of ALP and CAT when compared to normal animals in serum (Table 19.2 and Figure 19.1). The treatment with MEHH at all the three dose levels reversed these changes towards the normal except the ALP. The level of ALP in the extract treated groups was found to be further decreased when compared to tumor control animals. However, the treatment with standard 5-FU at 20 mg/kg body weight reversed all the values towards the normal. Most of the values were found to be significant.

A significant increase in the level of TBARS and significant decrease in the levels of SOD and CAT was observed in liver and kidney of animals inoculated EAC when compared with normal animals. MEHH treatment caused a significant reversal of SOD, and TBARS at all the three doses and CAT at 200 and 400 mg/kg doses towards the normal when compared to tumor control animals both in liver and kidney. Among the three doses of MEHH treatment, 100 mg/kg body weight dose was found to be more potent in reversing most of the biochemical parameters towards the normal and no dose dependent results were obtained. However, the standard 5-FU treatment exhibited a reversal of all the biochemical parameters towards the normal.

Table 19.2: Effect of MEHH on Hepatoprotective Parameters of EAC Bearing Mice in Serum on Day 15 of the Experiment

Groups	*ASAT (U/l)*	*ALAT (U/l)*	*ALP (U/l)*	*LDH (U/l)*	*TGL (mg/dl)*	CR *(mg/dl)*	*Albumin (mg/dl)*	*TP (g/dl)*	*TC (U/l)*	*TB (mg/dl)*
Normal	43.33±7.14	43.33±4.94	150.50±14.59	90.66±5.26	21.83±2.15	0.73±0.03	3.33±0.42	2.83±0.47	73.66±6.41	1.00±0.11
Tumor Control	118.33±2.78[b]	73.33±2.47[b]	79.16±2.16[b]	154.00±3.62[b]	21.00±1.73	0.95±0.04[a]	3.00±0.25	5.83±0.74[a]	104.00±2.11[b]	2.67±0.08[b]
5-FU 20 mg/kg	80.00±3.65[d]	38.33±11.69[e]	100.00±3.92	90.16±3.46[e]	24.66±2.23	0.70±0.04[d]	3.33±0.49	3.66±0.55	82.83±1.70[d]	1.26±0.10[e]
MEHH 100mg/kg	56.66±8.02[e]	64.16±0.83[e]	63.75±9.36	88.30±6.42[e]	25.50±2.95	0.80±0.03	3.16±0.30	4.16±0.54	93.00±6.82	1.53±0.05[e]
200 mg/kg	45.00±4.28[e]	50.00±1.29[d]	61.66±4.77	105.00±2.62[e]	38.16±2.02	0.74±0.03[e]	3.16±0.30	3.00±0.36[d]	90.66±3.47	1.13±0.06[e]
400 mg/kg	66.66±7.60[f]	40.00±3.60[e]	72.16±8.72	99.16±4.30[e]	51.66±5.07[e]	0.83±0.05	4.33±0.61[c]	4.00±0.44	86.661.38[c]	1.05±0.06[e]

Values are expressed as mean±SE for six animals in each group.

[a]P <0.01 and [b]P < 0.001 between normal and tumor group values, [c]P < 0.05, [d]P <0.01 and [e]P <0.001 between tumor control and treated groups.

Discussion

Cancer cells are generally more active than normal cells in metabolic ROS generation and are constantly under oxidative stress. The increase in endogenous ROS thus provides a constant stimulus for cell proliferation and most importantly, may cause further damage to DNA, leading to cancer development, genetic instability and disease progression (Kanno *et al.*, 2003). Hence, an anticancer agent with hepatoprotective and antioxidant properties is of much importance in cancer drug discovery.

In the present study, inoculation of EAC induced severe hepatic damage coupled with marked hepatic oxidative stress as represented by markedly elevated and significant levels of ASAT, ALAT, LDH, CR, TP, TC, TB, and TBARS and a significant decrease in the levels of CAT in serum of tumor control animals when compared to normal group. It was also evidenced by the significant increase in the levels of TBARS and significant decrease in the levels of CAT and SOD in liver and kidney. The treatment with MEHH caused a reversal of these changes towards the normal values indicating the potent hepatoprotective and antioxidant nature of the extract. Reduction in the levels of ASAT and ALAT towards the normal values is an indication of stabilization of plasma membrane as well as repair of hepatic and kidney tissue damage caused by EAC tumor cells. Depletion of raised bilirubin

Figure 19.1: Effect of MEHH on (A) SOD; (B) CAT; (C) TBARS in Serum, Liver and Kidney of EAC Bearing Mice on Day 15 of the Experiment. Values are expressed as mean + SE for six animals in each group, $^{a}P < 0.05$, $^{b}P < 0.01$ and $^{c}P < 0.001$ between normal and tumor group values, $^{d}P < 0.05$, $^{e}P < 0.01$ and $^{f}P < 0.001$ between tumor control and treated groups.
Serum; Liver; Kidney

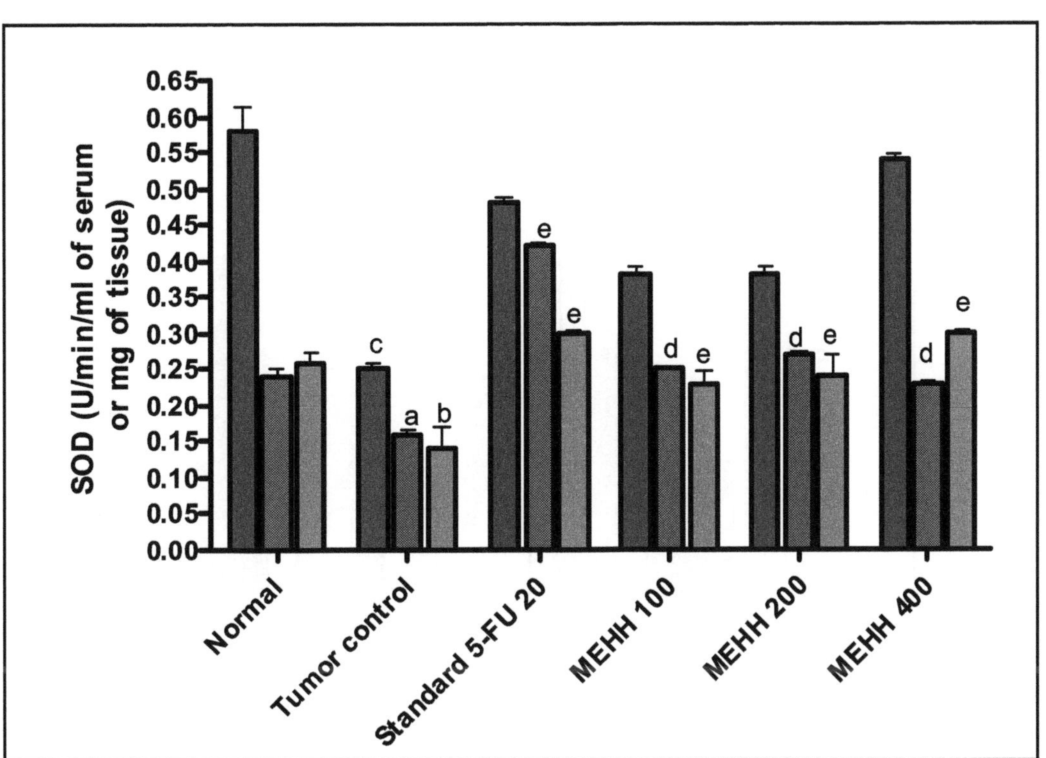

Cotnd...

Figure 19.1–Contd...

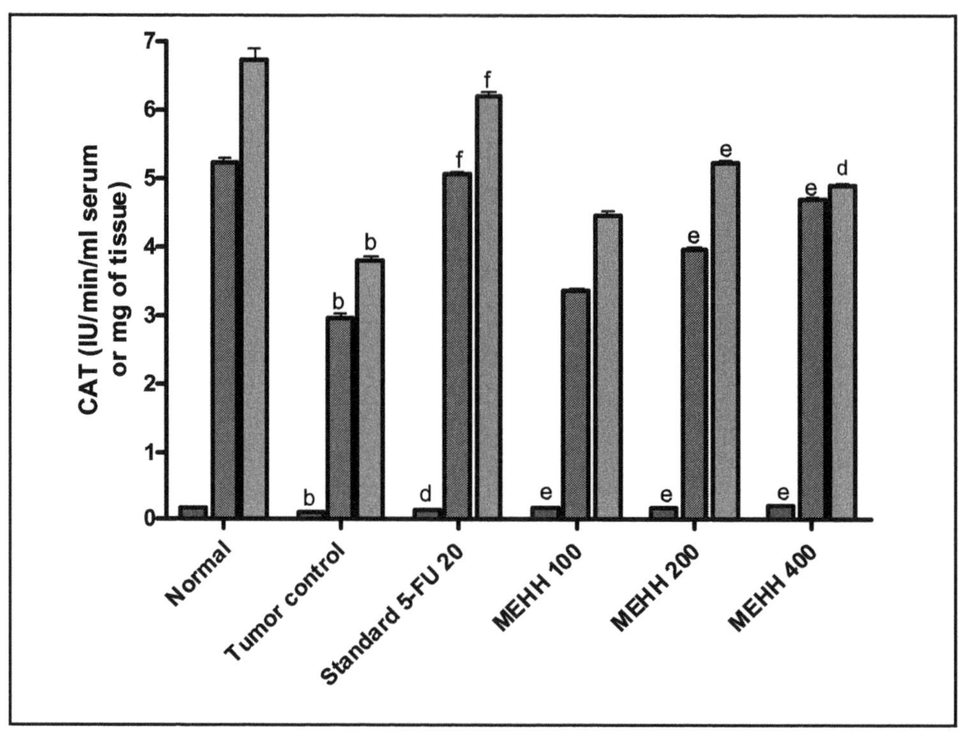

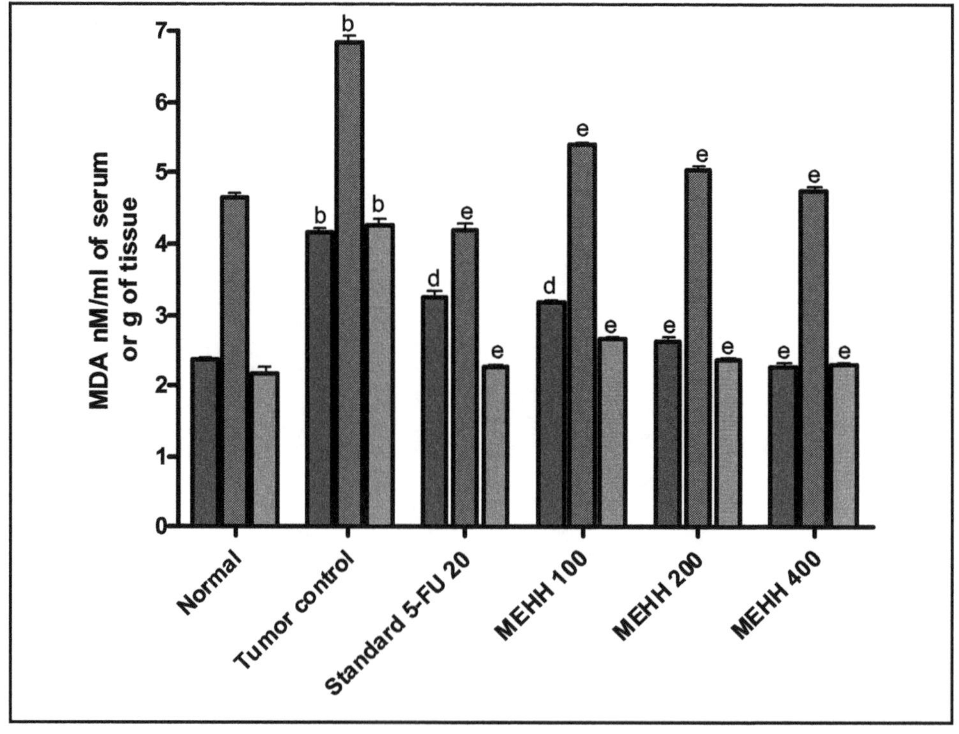

levels suggests the stability of the biliary dysfunction in liver during the extract treatment (Natesan *et al.*, 2007; Gupta *et al.*, 2004; Mukherjee, 2002).

In the recent years, convincing evidence has been accumulated that oxygen free radicals are indeed a relevant class of carcinogens. Cancer development is now commonly recognized as microevolutinary process that requires cumulative action of multiple events. Oxygen free radicals are known to stimulate cancer development at all the three stages, initiation, promotion and progression (Kanno *et al.*, 2003). High levels (up to 5 nM/h/10^6 cells) of hydrogen peroxide are constitutively released from wide variety of human tumors (Szatrowski and Nathan, 1991). SOD and CAT are involved in the clearance of superoxide and H_2O_2. SOD catalyzes the diminution of superoxide into H_2O_2 which has to be eliminated by glutathione peroxidase or CAT (Natesan *et al.*, 2007; Gupta *et al.*, 2004). Further, it has been reported that a decrease in SOD activity in EAC bearing mice may be due to loss of Mn^{2+} containing SOD activity in EAC cells and loss of mitochondria, leading to a decrease in total SOD activity in liver (Rushmore and Picket, 1993).

The Ehrlich tumor growth induces an inhibition of SOD and CAT enzymes which are fundamental in the elimination of free radicals as superoxide and hydrogen peroxide. In Ehrlich tumor bearing mice the antioxidant acts by a mechanism that involves modulating lipid peroxidation and augmenting antioxidant defense system (Gupta *et al.*, 2004). In the *in vitro* studies MEHH exhibited low IC_{50} values in ABTS, DPPH and H_2O_2 methods indicating its potent antioxidant nature. The administration of MEHH at all the three doses *in vivo* significantly increased the levels of SOD and CAT compared to tumor control indicating its antioxidant nature. Several reports demonstrated high levels of TBARS in cancerous tissues than those in normal tissues (Natesan *et al.*, 2007; Gupta *et al.*, 2004). The significant decrease in the levels of TBARS in MEHH treated animals also indicates the reduction in free radical yield and the subsequent decrease in harm and damage to the cell membrane and decrease in MDA production.

Plant derived extracts containing antioxidant phytoconstituents exhibited cytotoxicity towards tumor cells and antitumor activity in experimental animals (Natesan *et al.*, 2007; Gupta *et al.*, 2004). The observed antitumor properties in EAC model (Dongre *et al.*, 2007) may be attributed to the cytotoxic (Vijayan *et al.*, 2003), hepatoprotective and antioxidant effects of MEHH. The preliminary phytochemical studies indicated the presence of flavonoids, saponins, triterpenoids, glycosides and tannins in MEHH. The hepatoprotective and antioxidant properties of the extract observed in the present study may be due to the presence of any of these phytoconstituents. The plant merits further investigation in isolating its active constituents.

Acknowledgements

The authors thank Department of Biotechnology, Ministry of Science and Technology, New Delhi for funding the project. One of the authors (SHD) thanks DBT for awarding Junior and Senior Research fellowships.

References

Badami, S., Om Prakash., Dongre, S.H., and Suresh, B. (2005). *In vitro* antioxidant properties of *Solanum pseudocapsicum* leaf extracts. *Indian Journal of Pharmacology*, 37: 251-252.

Beers, R.F.J., and Sizer, I.W. (1952). A spectrophotometric method for measuring breakdown of hydrogen peroxide by catalase. *Journal of Biological Chemistry*, 195: 133-140.

Cakir, A., Mavi, A., Yildirim, A., Duru, M.E., Harmandar, M., and Kazaz, C. (2003). Isolation and characterization of antioxidant phenolic compounds from the aerial part of *Hypericum hyssopifolium* L. by activity-guided fractionation. *Journal of Ethnopharmacology*, 87: 73-83.

Conforti, F., Statti, G.A., Tundis, R., Menichini, F., and Houghton, P. (2002). Antioxidant activity of methanolic extract of *Hypericum triquetrifolium* Turra aerial part. *Fitoterapia*, 73: 479-483.

De Wys, W.D. (1982). Pathophysiology of cancer cachexia: current understanding and areas for future research. *Cancer Research*, 42: 721-726.

Dongre, S.H., Badami, S., Natesan, S., and Raghu Chandrashekar, H. (2007). Antitumor activity of the methanol extract of *Hypericum hookerianum* stem against *Ehrlich ascites carcinoma* in Swiss albino mice. *Journal of Pharmacological Sciences*, 103: 354-359.

Gupta, M., Mazumder, U.K., Sambath Kumar, R., Sivakumar, T., and Vamsi, M.L.M. (2004). Antitumor activity and antioxidant status of *Caesalpinia bonducella* against Ehrlich ascites carcinoma in Swiss albino mice. *Journal of Pharmacological Science*, 94: 177-184.

Kanno, S., Shouji, A., Asou, K., and Ishikawa, M. (2003). Effects of Naringin on hydrogen peroxide-induced cytotoxicity and apoptosis in P388 cells. *Journal of Pharmacological Sciences*, 92:166-170.

Misra, H.P., and Fridovich, I. (1972). The role of superoxide dismutase anion in the autooxidation of epinephrine and simple assay for superoxide dismutase. *Journal of Biological Chemistry*, 247: 3170-3175.

Mukherjee, P.K. (2002). Quality Control of Herbal Drugs, 1st ed. Business Horizons Pharmaceutical Publication, New Delhi pp. 531.

Mukherjee, P.K., Saritha, G.S., and Suresh, B. (2001). Antibacterial spectrum of *Hypericum hookerianum. Fitoterpia*, 72: 558-560.

Mukherjee, P.K., and Suresh, B. (2000). The evaluation of wound healing potential of *Hypericum hookerianum* leaf and stem extracts. *Journal of Alternative and Complementary Medicine*, 6: 61-69.

Natesan, S., Badami, S., Dongre, S.H., and Godavarthi, A. (2007). Antitumor activity and antioxidant status of the methanol extract of *Careya arborea* bark against DLA induced ascitic and solid tumor in mice. *Journal of Pharmacological Science*, 103:12-23.

Ohkawa, H., Ohishi, N., and Yagi, K. (1979) Assay for lipid peroxides in animal tissue by thiobarbituric acid reaction. *Analytical Biochemistry*, 95: 351-358.

Polidori, M.C. (2003). Antioxidant micronutrients in the prevention of age-related diseases. *Journal of Postgraduate Medicine*, 49: 229-235.

Rushmore, T.H., and Picket, C.B. (1993). Glutathione–S-transferases, structure, regulation and therapeutic implications. *Journal of Biological Chemistry*, 268: 11475–11478.

Silva, B.A., Ferreres, F., Malva, J.O., and Dias, A.C.P. (2005). Phytochemical and antioxidant characterization of *Hypericum perforatum* alcoholic extracts. *Food Chemistry*, 90: 157-167.

Szatrowski, T.P., and Nathan, C.F. (1991). Production of large amounts of hydrogen peroxide by human tumor cells. *Cancer Research*, 51: 794-798.

Vijayan, P., Vinodkumar, S., Badami, S., Mukherjee, P.K., Dhanaraj, S.A., and Suresh, B. (2003). Selective *in-vitro* cytotoxicity of *Hypericum hookerianum* towards cancer cell lines. *Oriental Pharmacy and Experimental Medicine*, 3: 141-146.

Medicinal Plants: Phytochemistry, Pharmacology and Therapeutics, Vol. 1 *Pages 363–377*
Editors: **V.K. Gupta, G.D. Singh, Surjeet Singh and A. Kaul**
Published by: **DAYA PUBLISHING HOUSE, NEW DELHI**

Chapter 20

Antioxidant and Antihypertensive Investigation of Seed Extract of *Parinari curatellifolia*

M.T. Olaleye*, O.O. Adegboye and A.A. Akindahunsi
Department of Biochemistry,
Federal University of Technology, Akure, Ondo State

ABSTRACT

Parinari curatellifolia is used locally in the South Western Part of Nigeria to treat hypertension. Its seed extract was investigated for its antioxidant, antihypertensive potentials as well as its effects on the antioxidant defense system. The extract gave positive tests to alkaloids, terpenoids, steroids flavonoids and saponnins. The antioxidant property results revealed that the per cent DPPH radical scavenge varied from 17.05–68.18 per cent per cent, total phenolic content 12.73mg/g tannic acid equivalent, total flavonoids 22.38mg/g quercertin equivalent, ferric reducing power 13.92mg/g ascorbic acid and the percentage of hydrogen peroxide inhibition 76.38-96.85 per cent. Results of the antihypertensive assays revealed that *Parinari curatellifolia* was able to reduce the force of contraction, heart rate of isolated rabbit heart, caused a dose-dependent reduction in systolic diastolic blood pressure, mean arterial blood pressure and an increase in the percentage change in mean arterial blood pressure as compared with the control in normotensive rats. Equally, the extract reduced both the diastolic, systolic blood pressure in salt induced hypertensive rats. Salt induction increased Nitric Oxide Synthase (NOS) activity as compared to the control, whereas post-treatment with the extract reversed this effect on the NOS activity. Salt induction also resulted in increase production of thiobarbituric acid reactive substances (TBARS) and

* Corresponding Author: E-mail: tolu1967@yahoo.co.uk.

decrease in the catalase, superoxide dismutase and gluthathione peroxidase activities in the liver while the post treatment with the extract abolished these effects. Salt induction brought about a statistically significant elevation in the serum concentrations of creatinine, urea, glucose, triglycerides, low density lipoprotein (LDL) and total cholesterol, reduction in the serum concentration of high density lipoprotein (HDL) as compared with the control. However, post treatment with the extract ameliorated these effects on the biochemical indices. The presence of the phytochemicals coupled with the recorded antioxidant potentials and antihypertensive activity (600mg/Kg), have justified the use of *Parinari curatellifolia* in the treatment of hypertension to a certain extent.

Keywords: *Parinari curatellifolia, Antioxidants, Hypertensive, Normotensive.*

Introduction

Interest in plant research has increased tremendously in recent times all over the world. Results have shown the immense potential of medicinal plants in various traditional systems. These include those that are central nervous system active, antiallergic plants, hypoglycaemic plants, plants acting on the respiratory system and cardioactive plants (Dahanukar *et al.*, 2000). Medicinal plants are generally sources of various phytochemicals some of which are usually responsible for their biological activities. Some antihypertensive plants have been discovered to possess less attendant side effects (Olaleye and Akindahunsi, 2005).

Oxidative stress may play a critical role in the pathogenesis of hypertension, as well as other cardiovascular disorders such as atherosclerosis and myocardial infarction. In the Dahl salt-sensitive (SS) hypertensive rat there is evidence of an elevated number of circulating leukocytes that produce superoxide compared with its normotensive control, the Dahl salt-resistant (SR) rat (Halliwell and Gutteridge, 1989). Also, oxidative stress induced by glutathione depletion in normal rats has been shown to cause and maintain severe hypertension (Shen *et al.*, 1995), consistent with this notion, supplementation with antioxidant substances has been suggested to reduce blood pressure (BP) in hypertensive individuals and provide protection against oxidative cardiovascular injury (Vaziri *et al.*, 2000). Several studies have also reported that levels of some free radical scavengers such as vitamin E and superoxide dismutase are depressed in hypertensive patients (Barbagallo *et al.*, 1999a, 1999b). However, a range of antioxidant defenses have evolved to detoxify reactive oxygen species, a major one of which is the glutathione redox cycle (Yanik *et al.*, 2001). Glutathione is the most abundant nonprotein intracellular thiol with multiple roles as an antioxidant agent (Boegehold, 1992). Reduced glutathione (GSH) acts to scavenge reactive oxygen species as well as to regenerate other antioxidants from their oxidized forms (Halliwell and Gutteridge, 1989). In this process, glutathione is converted to its oxidized form (GSSG), which must be reduced by the combination of glutathione reductase and NADPH. Thus, an index of cellular oxidative events is the ratio of the levels of the reduced and oxidized forms of glutathione. The pathogenesis of hypertension in the SS has also been associated with suppression of nitric oxide (NO) release and impairment of endothelial function (Quyyumi *et al.*, 1995). Reactive oxygen species, such as superoxide radicals may inactivate NO by generating peroxynitrite (Vaziri *et al.*, 2000; Vaziri *et al.*, 1999)

The bark of *Parinari curatellifolia* is used for the treatment of pneumonia, ear troubles, stomach pains, diarrhoea, or dysentery. The root is used in the treatment of cataracts and cough (Bhatt *et al.*, 1988). The seeds are used in the South Western Part of Nigeria for the treatment of hypertension. There is dearth of information in the literature as regards its antihypertensive effects. The present work therefore sought to evaluate the phytochemical constituents, antioxidant and antihypertensive potentials.

Materials and Methods

Plant Materials

Fresh seeds of *Parinari curatellifolia* were collected from a farm on the Federal Polytechnic Staff Quarter, Ado Ekiti, Ekiti State of Nigeria. Sample authentication was done in the Department of Biology, Federal University of Technology, Akure, Nigeria. Authenticated voucher sample was deposited in the herbarium (Code number PC 008) of Biochemistry Department, Federal University of Technology, Akure, Nigeria.

Preparation of Crude Methanolic Extracts

The seeds were air-dried for 28 days at room temperature. The air-dried samples were ground to a mesh size of 1 mm. A 350 g sample of the powdered material was soaked in 1000 ml of a mixture of methanol and water (4:1) for 96 hours. This was filtered and concentrated to a small volume to remove the entire methanol using rotary evaporator. The small volume was later freeze-dried. The extract was kept in the freezer at 4 °C for further studies.

Phytochemical Screening

The methanolic extracts were screened for the presence of alkaloids, saponins, tannins, anthraquinones, cardiac glycosides, flavonoids and phlobatanins according to the methods described by Sofowora (1993).

Antioxidant Activity of Crude Methanol Extract

Free Radical Scavenging Ability

The ability of the sample extract solution to scavenge the DPPH free radicals was measured. (Blois, 1958). Sample stock solution (1mg/ml) was prepared. The sample stock solution was diluted serially to obtain concentrations of 200–1000mg/ml.DPPH ethanol solution (0.2mM) was prepared by dissolving 0.03g of DPPH in 250ml of ethanol.About1ml of DPPH ethanol solution was added to 2.5 ml of each of the concentrations and allowed to react at room temperature. The absorbance was read after 30mins at 519nm against absorbance of control.

The per cent of DPPH scavenged was calculated as:

$$\text{Per cent DPPH scavenged} = \frac{(A_{control} - A_{test})}{A_{control}} \times 100$$

Total Phenol

0.5ml of (1mg/ml) aqueous ethanolic extract was mixed with 1ml of folin colcateau reagent (v/v) and 2.5ml of 20 per cent Na_2CO_3 was added and the reaction mixture was shaken thoroughly. The reaction mixture was incubated at 40°C for 20mins and the absorbance was read at 760nm. Tannic acid was used as standard phenolic compound (Mc Donald *et al.*, 2001).

Ferric Reducing Antioxidant Property

2.5ml of 1mg/ml of the aqueous methanolic extract was mixed with 2.5ml of 200mm sodium phosphate (pH 6.6) and 2.5ml of 1 per cent potassium ferricyanide. The reaction mixture was incubated at 50°C for 20mins 2.5ml of Trichloroacetic acid was added and centrifuged at 650 rpm for 10mins, 5ml of the supernantant was mixed with 5ml of water and 0.1 per cent $FeCl_3$ was added. The absorbance was read at 700nm (Pullido *et al.*, 2000).

Total Flavonoid

Aluminium chloride colorimetric method was used for flavonoids determination (Cheng *et al.*, 2002). Each plant extract (0.5ml of 1:10g/ml) in methanol were separately mixed with 1.5ml 955methanol, 0.1ml of 10 per cent aluminium 2.8ml of distilled water. It was allowed to stand for 30min; the absorbance of the reaction mixture was measured at 415nm with double Perkin Elmer UV/ Visible Spectrophotometer (USA). The calibration curve was prepared by preparing quercetin solution at concentrations at 12.5 to 100µg/ml in methanol.

H_2O_2 Radical Scavenging Activity

The ability of extract to scavenge H_2O_2 was determined according to the method of Ruch *et al.* (1989) with slight modifications of solutions of H_2O_2 was prepared in phosphate buffer (PH7.4) extracts (5-40mg/ml) of the aqueous ethanolic extract were added to 0.6ml of 40mm H_2O_2 solution. Absorbance of H_2O_2 was measured at 230nm after 10mins against a blank solution containing phosphate buffer without H_2O_2 solution. per cent of H_2O_2 scavenging was calculated as follows:

$$\text{per cent } H_2O_2 \text{ scavenged} = \frac{(A_{control} - A_{test})}{A_{control}} \times 100$$

Hypotensive Activities of Crude Methanol Extract

Wister albino rats (150–200 g), bred at the animal house of the Department of Physiology, Lagos University Teaching Hospital (LUTH), Lagos Nigeria were used. They were all clinically healthy and maintained in standard environmental conditions of temperature (27.0±0.5°C), relative humidity (73.0±15 per cent) and 12 hrs darkness and12 hrs light cycle. They were fed a standard diet and water *ad libitum*. The hypotensive activity was investigated according to the method of Adeboye *et al.* (1999). The Wistar albino rats were divided into 7 groups of 5 rats each. Groups 2-7 received varying doses (0.05-200mg/kg) of *Parinari curatellifolia* extract while group 1 (control) received an equivalent volume of distilled water. One hour after the administration of extract, they were anaesthetized with urethane (1.75 mg/kg). As soon as the animals reached the state of surgical anaesthesia, each of them was placed on its back and pinned on a rat dissecting board. Splitting the muscle in front using a forceps and scissors exposed the trachea of the rats. The trachea cannula for rat was dissected pointing to the thorax and tied firmly in place using a soft thread. The femoral artery was located and exposed carefully and a bulldog clip was placed on the artery and it was then cannulated. The bulldog clip was removed and the cannula was pushed in further and then tied securely using a disposable syringe and the cannula was filled with heparinized saline to prevent blood clotting. The femoral vein was also located and exposed carefully and a bull dog clip was put on the vein and then cannulated at one end. Heparinized saline was filled into a three-way tap and the cannula. The other end of the tap was connected to the transducer for blood pressure recording. After the stabilization period of 30 min, the initial blood pressure was taken followed by the administration of extract in volume not exceeding 1 ml/kg body weight. The extract was injected intravenously into the femoral artery and the blood pressure was recorded using a Glass polygraph Model 7D, calibration 1cm = 50 mm Hg. The mean arterial blood pressure (MABP) was calculated using

$$MABP = DP + {}^{1}/_{3}\,(DP{-}SP)$$

where,

SP: Systolic pressure.

DP: Diastolic pressure.

Effect of Crude Extract on Isolated Rabbit Hearts Preparations

The animals were anaesthetized with urethane (1.75 mg/kg). The chest was cut open and the heart exposed and the aorta was freed from its attachment to the pulmonary artery. It was then quickly transferred into a basin containing Ringer Locke solution and squeezed gently to remove as much blood as possible from the aorta (Burande *et al.*, 1983). The heart was then tied to the Langendorff's set up with the aorta tied to the cannula connected to the tube leading from the reservoir of the Ringer Locke solution (temperature 37 °C, flow rate of 7-8 ml/min, pH 7.4). The Ringer Locke solution was continuously bubbled with oxygen. After the stabilization period of 5 minutes, extract was administered at concentration 10 mg/ml (stock) through the side arm of the cannula at various volumes of 0.1, 0.2 and 0.3 ml. The contractility of the heart was recorded on the Glass polygraph model 7D by means of a planar clip placed at the apex of the heart connected through a lever to the transducer for recording (calibration, 2.0 cm = 1.0 g).

Effect of Crude Extract on Salt-Induced Hypertension

Wister albino rats (150–200 g), bred at the animal house of the Department of Physiology, Lagos University Teaching Hospital (LUTH), Lagos Nigeria, were used. They were all clinically healthy and maintained in standard environmental conditions of temperature (27.0±0.5°C), relative humidity (73.0±15 per cent) and 12 hrs darkness and12 hrs light cycle for two weeks before inducing hypertension. The Wistar albino rats were divided into 6 groups of 4 rats each. Groups 3-6 were fed with 8 per cent salt diet for six weeks after which varying doses (200-800mg/kg) of *Parinari curatellifolia* extract were administered for two weeks. Group 2 was given 8 per cent salt diet alone for six weeks while group 1(control) received an equivalent volume of distilled water throughout the experimentation period. They were all anaesthetized with 5ml/kg urethane-chloralose (25 per cent urethane and 1 per cent chloralose). As soon as the animals reached the state of surgical anaesthesia, each of them was placed on its back and pinned on a rat dissecting board. Splitting the muscle in front using a forceps and scissors exposed the trachea of the rats. The trachea was cannulated. The carotid artery was located and exposed carefully and a bulldog clip was placed on the two ends of the artery and it was then cannulated towards the heart (1 per cent heparin in 9 per cent NaCl). The bulldog clip was removed and the cannula was pushed in further and then tied securely using a disposable syringe and the cannula was filled with heparinized saline to prevent blood clotting. Heparinized saline was filled into a three-way tap and the cannula. The other end of the tap was connected to the transducer for blood pressure recording. After the stabilization period of 30 min, the blood pressure was taken and recorded using a Glass polygraph Model 7D, calibration 1cm = 40 mm Hg. The mean arterial blood pressure (MABP) was calculated using:

$$MABP = DP + {}^{1}/_{3}\,PP$$

where, PP = Pulse.

Effect of Crude Extract on Serum Biochemical Indices

Creatinine was measured by Heinegard and Tiderstrom (1973) using jafe reaction (Slot, 1965).Urea was measured by an enzymatic method of Jansen *et al.*, 1970.

Cholesterol was estimated according to Katayama *et al.* (1999).

Triglycerides was estimated using the Hantzchcondensation reaction method outlined in tietz

Lipid Peroxidation Assay

Thiobarbituric acid reactive species (TBARS) production was determined as described by Ohkawa *et al.*(1979).

Superoxide Dismutase Activity (SOD)

The liver homogenate was adequately diluted by NaCl 0.9 per cent to a factor of 20 for the estimation of superoxide dismutase (SOD) assay according to the method described by Misra and Firdovich, 1972. Briefly, epinephrine undergoes autooxidation rapidly at pH 10.0 to produce adrenochrome, a pink colored product that will be detected at 480 nm in kinetic mode using UV/VIS spectrophotometer. The amount of enzyme required to produce 50 per cent inhibition is defined as one unit of enzyme activity. The SOD is expressed as per cent control.

Catalase Activity (CAT)

Catalase (CAT) activity was measured by the method of Aebi (1974). An aliquot of liver and kidney supernatants (10 µL) was added to a quartz cuvette and the reaction was started by the addition of freshly prepared H_2O_2 (30 mM) in phosphate buffer (50 mM, pH 7.0). The rate of H_2O_2 decomposition was measured spectrophotometrically at 240nm during 120 seconds.

Glutathione Peroxidase Activity (GPx)

GPx activity estimation is based on the following principle: GPx catalyses the oxidation of glutathione by cumen hydroperoxide (Chance, 1951). In the presence of hydrogen peroxide, glutathione is immediately converted to the reduced form. The decrease in absorbance at 340 nm is measured.

Results

Phytochemical Constituents

Phytochemical screening revealed the presence of alkaloids, terpenes, glycosides and flavonoids (Table 20.1).

In vitro Antioxidants Activities

The results revealed that the percentage of DPPH radical scavenge varied from (17.05 per cent) to (68.18 per cent) (600mg/ml–1000mg/ml), total phenolic content (12.73mg/g tannic acid equivalent), total flavonoids (22.38mg/g Quercertin), ferric reducing power (13.92mg/g ascorbic acid) and the percentage of hydrogen peroxide inhibition 76.38-96.85 per cent (5-40mg/ml) (Table 20.2).

Effect on Blood Pressure of Normotensive Albino Rats and Isolated Rabbit Heart Preparation

Parinari curatellifolia seed extract produced a dose dependent (0.05–200mg/kg) statistically significant ($P<0.05$) reduction in systolic blood pressure (120.84–45.30), diastolic blood pressure (98.4.19-19.63), mean arterial blood pressure (111.74–15.10) and an increase in the percentage change in mean arterial blood pressure (0-39 per cent) as compared with the control (Table 20.3). Equally the extract produced dose dependent (4-12 mg/kg) statistically significant ($P<0.05$) decreases in the force of contraction of isolated rabbit heart preparation (8-3g) and heart rate (708-350 beats/min) (Table 20.4).

Table 20.1: The Phytochemical Constituents of *Parinari curatellifolia*

Phytochemical Constituents	*Results*
Alkaloid	present
Saponin	present
Tannins	present
Phlobatanins	present
Anthraquinones	absent
Cardiac Glycosides	absent
Flavonoids	present
Terpenoids	present
Steroids	present

Table 20.2: Antioxidant Properties of *Parinari curatellifolia*

Property	*Level*
Free Radical Scavenging (600–1000mg/ml)	17.05–68.18 per cent
Total phenol	12.7mg/g tannic acid
H_2O_2 inhibition (5–40 mg/ml)	73.0–96.4 per cent
Ferric Reducing Property	13.92mg/g ascorbic acid
Total Flavonoids	22.38mg/g quercertin equvalent

Table 20.3: Effect of *Parinari curatellifolia* on Blood Pressure of Bormotensive Albino Rats

Dosage (mg/kg)	*Systolic (BP mmHg)*	*Diastolic (BP mmHg)*	*MABP* in MABP*	*Per cent Change*	*Duration (sec.)*
Control	$120.84^{c}\pm0.00$	$98.4.19^{b}\pm0.00$	$111.74^{c}\pm0.00$	0.0	0
0.05	$123.90^{c}\pm0.00$	$97.39^{b}\pm11.80$	$111.3^{c}\pm7.99$	6.1	30
0.50	$119.41^{c}\pm5.23$	$90.49^{b}\pm11.99$	$110.26^{c}\pm9.71$	5.7	32
5.0	$91.37^{bc}\pm7.85$	84.56 ± 20.76	$96.08^{c}\pm16.33$	1.1	30
50.0	$80.33^{b}\pm5.23$	$40.77^{b}\pm23.25$	$53.86^{bc}\pm17.17$	-9.0	25
100.0	$67.95^{ab}\pm9.43$	$19.63^{ba}\pm2.9$	$35.74^{b}\pm2.23$	-19.0	25
200.0	$45.30^{a}\pm3.40$	$11.14^{a}\pm3.67$	$15.10^{a}\pm1.53$	–39.0	30

*MABP, Mean Arterial Blood Pressure; Values are mean±SD; n = 5; Values with the same superscript

Letter (s) down a column are not stastically significantly ($P>0.05$) different.

Table 20.4: Effects of *Parinari curatellifolia* on the Isolated Rabbit Heart Preparation

Dose mg/kg [Force of contraction (g)]	*Response Beats/min*	*Heart Rate*
0.0	$8.0^{b}\pm0.3$	708
4.0	$3.0^{a}\pm0.1$	686
8.0	$3.0^{a}\pm0.2$	504
12.0	$3.0^{a}\pm0.2$	350

Effect on Blood Pressure of Salt Induced Hypertensive Albino Rats

There was a statistically significant increase in the systolic blood pressure, diastolic and pulse pressure of the animals fed salt diet as compared with the control (Table 20.5).

Table 20.5: Effect of *Parinari curatellifolia* on Blood Pressure of Salt Induced Hypertensive Albino Rats

Groups	*SYS*	*DIA*	*PP*	*MABP*	*HR*	*NOS (μM)*
Control	83.5 ± 7.00^{a}	69 ± 6.83^{a}	19.5 ± 3.42^{a}	75.4 ± 8.05^{a}	414.5±11.7	43
Induced	174 ± 19.77^{b}	129.75 ± 65^{c}	42.5 ± 22.23^{b}	145.9±5.10c	362.0±37.3	93
Induced+ 200mg/Kg	155.0 ± 3.83^{c}	132.0 ± 8.16^{c}	25.5 ± 8.54^{a}	140.48 ± 5.88^{b}	408.00±0.00	20.4
Induced+ 600mg/Kg	105.0 ± 5.74^{c}	94.0 ± 4.00^{d}	11.5 ± 1.91^{a}	97.73 ± 4.40^{d}	384.0±0.00	46
Induced+ 800mg/Kg	66.25 ± 5.36^{d}	52.0 ± 3.27^{c}	14.25 ± 2.06^{a}	56.73 ± 3.82^{d}	432.0±0.00	43
Induced+ Nifedipine	93.00 ± 12.70^{a}	75.75 ± 9.95^{b}	15.75 ± 5.19^{a}	82.00 ± 12.62^{a}	400.0±11.31	33

* SYS: Systolic Blood Pressure; DIA: Diastolic Blood Pressure; PP: Pulse pressure; MABP: Mean Arterial Blood Pressure; HR: Heart rate. Values are mean±SD; n = 5; Values with the same superscript letter(s) down a column are not stastically significantly (P>0.05) different.

Post treatment with the extract brought about a statistically significant reduction in the blood pressure of the animals treated with *Parinari curatellifolia* as compared with the induced group. The reduction in the blood pressure was dose dependent (200-800mg/kg).

Equally, post treatment with Nifedipine (0.67mg/kg) was able to return the blood pressure to the control. Nitric Oxide Synthase activity was significantly increased in the salt induced hypertensive rats as compared with the control (Figure 20.1). Treatment with the *parinari* extract caused a dose dependent statistically significant decrease in the Nitric Oxide Synthase activity as compared with the group treated with salt alone.

Effect of Crude Extract on Serum Biochemical Indices of Salt Induced Hypertensive Rats

Salt induction brought about a statistically significant elevation in the serum concentration of creatinine, urea, glucose, Triglycerides, low density lipoprotein (LDL) and total cholesterol (Table 20.6). Salt induction also produced a statistical significant (P<0.05) reduction in the serum concentration

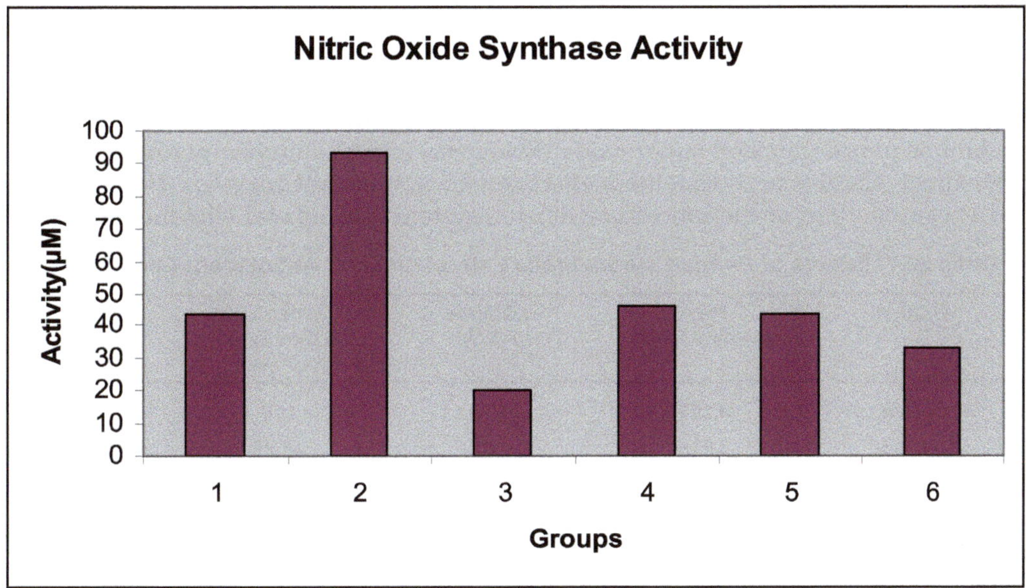

Groups: 1: Control; 2: Salt Induced; 3: Salt induced +nifedipine;
4: Salt induced+200mg/Kg *Parinari curatellifolia*; 5: Salt induced+600mg/kg *Parinari curatellifolia*;
6: Salt induced+800mg/kg *Parinari curatellifolia*

Figure 20.1: The Effect of *Parinari curatellifolia* on Plasma Activity of Nitric Oxide Synthase

of high density lipoprotein (HDL) as compared with the control. However, post treatment with the extract ameliorated these effects on the biochemical indices.

Table 20.6: Effect of *Parinari curatellifolia* on Plasma Biochemical Indices of Salt Induced Hypertensive Albino Rats

Group	*CREATINE*	*UREA*	*GLUCOSE*	*TRIGLY*	*HDL*	*LDL*	*T.CHOL.*
Control	15.11±1.41[a]	6.93±1.78[b]	0.43±0.09[a]	0.33±0.06[b]	0.8±0.08[a]	0.18±0.10[a]	1.37±0.19[a]
Induced	44.49±2.20[d]	14.32±1.37[a]	6.8±1.49[e]	1.51±0.44[d]	0.35±0.26[b]	0.9±0.08[b]	2.39±0.43[d]
Induced+ 200mg/kg	20.24±1.33[a]	1.40±0.29[c]	0.45±0.26[a]	0.06±0.03[a]	0.25±0.1[b]	0.32±0.04[a]	0.29±0.07[e]
Induced+ 600mg/kg	21.01±1.03[c]	1.33±0.32[c]	1.18±0.17[b]	0.21±0.07[b]	0.23±0.19[b]	0.25±0.13[a]	1.72±0.07[b]
Induced+ 800mg/kg	23.53±1.91[b]	1.68±0.10[d]	0.09±0.01[c]	0.44±0.05[b]	0.68±0.10[a]	0.25±0.13[a]	1.41±0.39[b]
Induced+ Nifedipine	56.33±7.68[e]	13.80±1.75[a]	1.18±0.22[d]	0.22±0.09[b]	0.73±0.13[a]	0.28±0.21[a]	1.24±0.38[c]

CREATI: Creatinine; TRIGLY: Triglycerides; HDL: High Density Lipoprotein; LDL: Low Density Lipoprotein; T. CHOL: Total Cholesterol. Values are mean±SD; n = 5; Values with the same superscript letter(s) down a column are not stastically significantly (P>0.05) different.

Effects of the Extract on the Antioxidant Defence System of Salt Induced Hypertensive Rats

Salt induction resulted in a statistically significant increase the production of thiobarbituric acid reactive substances (TBARS) in the liver, statistically significant decrease in the liver activities of the antioxidant enzymes (catalase, super oxide dismutase, and glutathione peroxidase) (Table 20.7). *Parinari* extract was able to abolish these effects on the antioxidant enzymes. However, Nifedipine exerted a negative effect on the antioxidant defense system as compared with the control.

Table 20.7: Effects of *Parinari curatellifolia* Extract on Liver Antioxidant Defense System

Groups	*MDA µmole/g tissue*	*Catalase (mg/dl)*	*Superoxide Dismutase (per cent)*	*Glutathione Peroxidase*
Control	0.123	0.23	100	0.605
Induced	0.618	0.06	43.75	0.670
Induced+Nifedipine	0.283	0.14	18.75	0.000
Induced+200mg/Kg	0.080	0.10	62.50	0.167
Induced+600mg/Kg	0.075	0.25	87.50	0.955
Induced+800mg/Kg	0.052	0.22	78.10	2.319

Discussion

The presence of alkaloids, terpenes and flavonoids in the seed extract stands some pharmacological potential. Flavonoids decrease capillary fragility and exert a cortisone-like effect on tissues (González *et al.*, 2001). Red wine polyphenols (RWPs) have been reported to exert beneficial effects in preventing cardiovascular diseases, such as hypertension and vascular dysfunction (Jimeneze *et al.*, 2007).

Phenolics are found in large quantities in the plant kingdom, and they have been shown to have multiple biological functions, including antioxidant activity (Kaplan and Aviram, 2004). The phenolic content of *Parinari curatellifolia* was 12.7mg/g tannic acid. This implies that *Parinari curatellifolia* extract contains a higher amount of phenolics than the bark and heartwood extracts of *Acacia confusa* (Chang *et al.*, 2001). Therefore, *Parinari curatellifolia* is a significant source of phenolics. The results in this study suggest that the antioxidant activity of *Parinari curatellifolia* extract is probably related to the high contents of phenolics, and the observed antioxidant activities of the extract may be due to the hydroxyl groups in phenolics (Hatano *et al.*, 1989). A similar finding has been demonstrated in the plant extracts of *Eucommia ulmoides* (Du-zhong) and *Acacia confusa* in which enriched phenolics correlated well with their antioxidant activities (Chang *et al.*, 2001; Yen and Hsieh, 1998). Flavonoids have been said to decrease capillary fragility and exert a cortisone-like effect on tissues (González *et al.*, 2001). It therefore implies that the high flavonoids content in *Parinari curatellifolia* extract is responsible for the therapeutic effect (antihypertensive). *Parinari curatellifolia* reported in this study may be due the presence of flavonoids and other phytochemicals in it. DPPH is a stable radical at room temperature and accepts electron or hydrogen radical to become a stable diamagnetic molecule (Soares *et al.*, 1997) and has been used widely to evaluate the antioxidant activity of various natural products (Hu and Kitts, 2000). In this study, DPPH scavenging activity has been found in *Parinari curatellifolia* extract. The maximum inhibition of *Parinari curatellifolia*, is about 68 per cent in this study. The inhibitory curve of DPPH scavenging activity of *Parinari curatellifolia* is similar to that of *Acacia confusa* (Chang *et al.*, 2001), Cat's claw (*Uncaria tomentosa*) (Sandoval *et al.*, 2000), and *Anthriscus cerefolium* (Fejes *et al.*, 2000). *Parinari curatellifolia* extract may be a potential source of natural antioxidant. The maximum per cent inhibition of hydrogen peroxide radicals is about 96 per cent at 40mg/ml while the minimum is 73 per cent at 5mg/ml. Hydrogen peroxide itself is not very reactive, but sometimes may give rise to hydroxyl radicals in the cells (Halliwell, 1991). The cellular damage resulting from hydroxyl radicals is strongest among free radicals. Hydroxyl radicals can be generated by biochemical reactions. Superoxide radical is converted by superoxide dismutase to hydrogen peroxide, which subsequently can produce extremely reactive hydroxyl radicals in the presence of transition metal ions, such as iron and copper or by UV photolysis. Hydroxyl radicals can attack DNA to cause strand scission.

High dietary salt has long been associated with hypertension, evidences point to a link between dietary salt, kidney function and hypertension. Oxidative stress seems to be directly involved in the renal dysfunction in Dahl Salt-sensitive rats (Trolliet *et al.*, 2001). The result of the lipid peroxidation indicated that their was about 5 fold increase in the lipid peroxidation of the induced group as compared with control and group treated with nifedipine. *Parinari curatellifolia* caused a dose dependent reduction (about 50 per cent) as compared with control. There were also significant reductions in the levels of catalase, glutathione peroxidase and superoxide dismutase of the induced compared with the control and *Parinari curatellifolia* was able to return the level of antioxidant enzymes back to the level in the control.

There is an elevation in the serum concentration of creatinine, urea, glucose, Triglycerides, LDL and total cholesterol and reduction in the serum concentration of HDL in the induced group as compared with the control. Creatinine and urea are markers used in evaluating kidney functions, there were significant increases in the serum concentrations of creatinine and urea in the induced group as compared with the control, equally there was significant reduction in the group treated with *Parinari curatellifolia* as compared to the induced group. High dietary salt has been discovered to have a link with kidney function and hypertension. The results of Dobrian *et al.* (2003) indicated that high-salt diet accelerated the development of hypertension and increased oxidative stress in the vasculature and kidney and induced kidney glomeruloscleross is and microalbuminuria. One important contributor to hypertension in salt-sensitive animal models and humans seems to be the endothelial dysfunction, in particular the altered vascular reactivity due to impairment in nitric oxide (NO) production (Hayakawa *et al.*, 1997; Nishida *et al.*, 1998). Inducible nitric oxide synthase (NOS II) is important in salt-induced hypertension (Audrey Rudd *et al.*, 1999). Data from the work of Donald *et al.* (1983) supported the hypothesis that a neurogenic component, possibly mediated via central epinephrine containing neurons, contributes to the blood pressure (BP) elevation induced by salt excess. There was increase in plasma level of nitric oxide synthase of the induced as compared with the control, it has been discovered that the leakage of NOS from the endothelium might be due to free radicals attack to the endothelium (Duarte *et al.*, 2002). NOS is an enzyme that catalyses the formation of nitric oxide, a potent vasodilator in the endothelium. Dietary sodium may inhibit L-arginine transport in the renal medulla and thereby inhibiting renal NO production and medullary flow (Zewde *et al.*, 2004). High salt diet may also increase renal medullary, osmolality and decrease NOs activity is associated with salt-sensitive hypertension.

There was an increase in the plasma levels of glucose of the induced group as compared with the control and also a dose dependent reduction in the group treated with *Parinari curatellifolia* as compared with the induced group. However, 200mg/kg of *Parinari curatellifolia* was able to return plasma glucose back to control. Hyperglycemia results in glucose auto-oxidation, non enzymic glycation and monocyte dysfunction which lead to increase in production of free radicals (Brownlee *et al.*, 1994), this further leads to decrease in the level of antioxidants and oxidative damage (Dandona *et al.*, 1996). West *et al.* (2004) discovered that increase in carbohydrate diet causes hypertension and also increase in blood glucose of hypertensive patient's worsened hypertension.

The plasma cholesterol, low density lipoprotein and triglycerides of the induced group were significantly higher than that of control. *Parinari curatellifolia* had a dose dependent reduction as compared with the induced group. The plasma concentration of the induced group reduced significantly as compared with the control. There was significant increase in the treated group and the group treated with nifedipine as compared with the induced.

According to Mohammed *et al.* (2004) salt induced hypertension is associated with oxidative stress and it has been shown that Dahl salt sensitive rat has a compromised antioxidant status, defined by significantly decrease in the antioxidant enzymes compared with salt sensitive rats.

Also, plasma levels of isoprostane, a recognized marker of oxidative stress were elevated in both strains when placed on high salt diet. These observations suggest that OS and the maladaptive changes may occur due to increase in the formation of MDA is attributed to increase in the formation of MDA.

Conclusion

It was discovered that salt induced hypertension can be linked with oxidative stress and hyperglycemias. Salt induced hypertension increases the level of serum nitric oxide synthase. *Parinari curatellifolia* was able to effectively protect the oxidative damage done in salt induced hypertension.

Acknowledgements

We wish to acknowledge Dr. C.N. Anigbogu and Mr. A.K. Oloyo of the Department of Physiology, University of Lagos for their technical assistance.

References

Adeboye, J.O., Fajonyomi, M.O., Makinde, J. M and Taiwo, O.B (1999). A preliminary study on the hypotensive activity of Persea americana leaf extracts in anaesthetized normotensive rats. *Fitoterapia*, 70: 15-20.

Aebi, H (1974). Catalase. In: Bergmeyer, H.U. (Ed.), Methods of Enzymatic Analysis, Chemie Weinheim, pp. 673-677.

Audrey Rudd, M., Maria, T, Susan, H, Anne, W.S., Geraldine D., George T., Timothy C., and Joseph L. (1999). Salt-induced hypertension in Dahl salt-resistant and salt-sensitive rats with NOS II inhibition. *Am J Physiol Heart Circ Physiol.*, 277: H732-H739.

Barbagallo, M., Dominguez, L. J., Tagliamonte, M. R., Resnick, L. M. and Paolisso, G. (1999a). Effects of glutathione on red blood cell intracellular magnesium: relation to glucose metabolism. *Hypertension*, 34: 76–82.

Barbagallo, M., Dominguez, L. J., Tagliamonte, M. R., Resnick, L. M. and Paolisso, G. (1999b). Effects of vitamin E and glutathione on glucose metabolism: role of magnesium. *Hypertension*. 34: 1002–1006.

Bhatt, J.D, Panchakshari, U.D, Itemavati, KG and Guati, O.D (1998). Effect of Abana, an Ayurevedic preparation of ethinyl estradiol-induced hypertension in rats. *Ind.J. Pharmacol.*, 30:339.

Boegehold, M. A. (1992). Reduced influence of nitric oxide on arteriolar tone in hypertensive Dahl rats. *Hypertension,* 19: 290–295.

Blois, M.S (1958). Antioxidant determination by the use of stable free radical. *Nature,* 181: 1199-1200.

Brownlee, M. (1994). Glycation and diabetic complications. *Diabetes,* 43: 836-841

Burande, M. D., Goyal, B. K. and Verma, S. C. (1983). Studies on the Mechanism of Cardiotonic effects on radio calcium movement. *Acta Isohop.,* 7: 271–279.

Chance, B. (1951), The Iron-Containing Enzymes. C. The Enzyme–Substrate Compounds and Mechanisms of Action o.f Hydroperoxideases. The Enzymes, II, Pt 1(Summer J., and Myback, K., eds), Academic Press, NY

Chang, C., Yang, M., Wen, H., Chern, J. (2002). Estimation of total flavonoid content in propolis by two complementary colorimetric methods. *J. Food Drug Analaysis,* 10: 178-182

Chang, S.T, Wu, J.H, Wang, S.Y, Kang, P.L, Yang, N.S, Shyur, L.F (2001) Antioxidant activity of extracts from *Acacia confuse* bark and heartwood. *J Agric Food Chem.,* 49: 3420-3424

Dahanukar, S.A., Kulkarni, R.A and Rege, N.(2000). Pharmacology of medicinal and natural products. *Indian Journal of Pharmacology,* 32:581-5118

Dandona, P., Thusu, K., Cook, S. and Nicotera, T. (1996). Oxidative damage to DNA in Diabetes mellitus. *Lancet,* 347: 444-447

Demacker,, P.N, Hijmans, A.G, van Sommeren-Zondag, D.F, Jansen, A.P. (1982). Stability of frozen liquid control sera for assay of cholesterol in high-density lipoprotein. *Clin Chem.,* 28:155-157.

Dobrian Anca, D., Suzanne, D. Schriver, T. L, and Russell L. P. (2003). Effect of salt on hypertension and oxidative stress in a rat model of diet-induced obesity. *Am J Physiol Renal Physiol* 285: F619–F628.

Donald, D., Bernard, W., Ladislaw, V., Pauline, C., Irene, G., Haralambos, G. and Hans, B. (1983). Salt-induced hypertension in chronic renal failure: Evidence for a neurogenic mechanism. Life SciencesVolume 32, Issue 7, 14 February, Pages 733-740

Duarte, J., Perez-Palencia, R., Vargas, F., Ocete,M. A., Perez-Vizcaino, F., Zarzuelo, A., Tamargo, J. (2001). *Br. J. Pharmacol.,* 133, 117–124.

Fejes, S, Blázovics, A, Lugasi, A, Lemberkovics, E, Petri, G, Kéry, A (2000) *In vitro* antioxidant activity of *Anthriscus cerefolium* L. (Hoffm.) extracts. *J Ethnopharmacol.,* 69: 259-265

González, B. M, Yslas, N, Reyes, E, Ouiroz, V, Santana, J, Jiménez, G (2001) Clinical effect of a Mexican Sanguinaria extract (*Polygonum aviculare* L.) on gingivitis. *J Ethnopharmacol.,* 74: 45-51

Halliwell, B. (1991). Reactive oxygen species in living system: Source, biochemistry and role of human disease. *Am J Med.,* 91: 14-22.

Halliwell, B. and Gutteridge, J. M. (1989). Protection against oxidants in biological systems: the superoxide theory of oxygen toxicity, in Oxford Science Publications (ed): Free Radicals in Biology and Medicine, 2nd ed. Oxford, UK, Clarendon. 87–187.

Hatano, T, Edamatsu, R, Hiramatsu, M, Mori, A, Fujita, Y, Yasuhara, T, Yoshida, T, Okuda, T (1989) Effects of interaction of tannins with co-existing substances. VI. Effects of tannins and related polyphenols on superoxide anion radical and on DPPH radical. *Chem Pharm Bull.,* 37: 2016-202

Hayakawa, H, Coffee, K, and Raij, L. (1997). Endothelial dysfunction and cardiorenal injury in experimental salt-sensitive hypertension: effects of antihypertensive therapy. *Circulation*, 96: 2407–2413.

Heinegard, D and Tiderstrom, G. ((1973) Determination of serum creatinine by direct colorimetric method. *Clinica chemical Acta.*, 43: 305-310

Hu, C, and Kitts, D.D (2000) Studies on the antioxidant activity of *Echinacea* root extract. *J Agric Food Chem.*, 48: 1466-1472

Jansen, A.P, Peters, KA, Zelders, T (1970). Modifications and improvements of a continuous flow system for colorimetric analysis. *Clin Chim Acta.*, 27(1): 125-132.

Jiménez, R, López-Sepúlveda, R, Kadmiri,, M, Romero, M, Vera, R, Sánchez, M, Vargas, F, O'Valle, F, Zarzuelo, A, Dueñas, M, Santos-Buelga, C, Duarte, J. (2007) Polyphenols restore endothelial function in DOCA-salt hypertension: role of endothelin-1 and NADPH oxidase. *Free Radic Biol Med.*, 43(3):462-73.

Kaplan, M and Aviram, M (2004). Red wine administration to apolipoprotein E-deficient mice reduces their macrophage-derived extracellular matrix atherogenic properties. *Biol Res.*, 37: 239-245

Kayamori, Y., Hatsuyama H., Tsujioka T., Nasu, M., and Katayama, Y. (1999). Endpoint Colorimetric Method for Assaying Total Cholesterol in Serum with Cholesterol Dehydrogenase. *Clin. Chem.*, 45: 2158-2163.

Kitiyakara, C, Chabrashvili, T, Chen, Y, Blau, J, Karber, A, Aslam, S, Welch, W.J, and Wilcox, C.S. (2003) Salt intake, oxidative stress, and renal expression of NADPH oxidase and superoxide dismutase. *J Am Soc Nephrol.*, 14: 2775–2782.

Knekt, P., Jarvinen, R., Reunanen, A. and Maatela, J. (1996). Flavonoid intake and coronary mortality in Finland: a cohort study. *Biomedical Journal*, 312: 478-481.

Levinson, S.S (1978). Kinetic centrifugal analyzer and manual determination of serum urea nitrogen, with use of *o*phthaldialdehyde reagent. Clin Chem. 24(12): 2199–2202.

McDonald, S, Prenzler, P.D, Autolovich, M, K (2001) Phenolic content and antioxidant activity of olive extracts. *Food Chemistry*,73:73-84

Misra, H.P, Fridovich, I. (1972) The role of superoxide anion in the autoxidation of epinephrine and simple assay for superoxide dismutase. *Journal of Biological Chemistry*, 247: 3170–3175.

Mohamed, A. B., Agaba, A. G., Robin, R. S, Natalia, S., Imad, K. A. (2004); The role of Oxidative Stress in Salt-Induced Hypertension. *Am J Hypertens.*, 17: 31–36

Nishida, Y, Ding, J, Zhou, M.S., Chen, Q.H, Murakami, H, Wu, X.Z., and Kosaka, H. (1998). Role of nitric oxide in vascular hyperresponsiveness to norepinephrine in hypertensive Dahl rats. *J Hypertens* 16: 1611–1618.

Northam, B.E, Smith, J.H, Fitzgerald, M.G, Nattrass, M, Wright, A.D (1982). Value of serum glucose assay as part of the biochemical profile in screening for diabetes. *Ann Clin Biochem.*, 19: 412-415.

Ohkawa, H., Ohishi, H., Yagi, K. (1979). Assay for lipid peroxide in animal tissues by thiobarbituric acid reaction. *Anal. Biochem.* 95:351-358

Olaleye, M.T and Akindahunsi, A.A (2005). Hypotensive activity of methanolic extract of the calyces of *Hibiscus sabdariffa* L on Normotensive rats. Recent Progress in Medicinal plants, In Plant Bioactives in Traditional Medicine,USA Vol IX pg461.

Pulido R, Bravo L, Saura-Calixto F (2000). Antioxidant activity of dietary polyphenols as determined by a modified ferric reducing/antioxidant power assay. *J.Agric Food Chem.*, 48: 3396-3402

Quyyumi, A. A., Dakak, N., Andrews, N. P., Husain, S., Arora, S., Gilligan, D. M., Panza, J. A. and Cannon, R. O. III (1995). Nitric oxide activity in the human coronary circulation. *J Clin Invest.* 95: 1747–1755.

Ruch, R.J, Cheng, S.J, Klaunig, J.E.(1989) Prevention of cytotoxity and inhibition of intercellular communication by antioxidant catechins isolated from Chinese tea. *Carcinogen.*, 10: 1003-1008.

Sandoval, M, Charbonnet, R.M, Okuhama, N.N, Roberts, J, Krenova, Z, Trentacosti, A.M, Miller, M.J (2000) Cat's claw inhibits TNFalpha production and scavenges free radicals: Role in cytoprotection. *Free Radical Biol Med.*, 29: 71-78

Shen, K., DeLano, F. A., Zweifach, B. W. and Schimd-Schonbein, G. W. (1995). Circulating leukocyte counts, activation, and degranulation in Dahl hypertensive rats. *Circ Res.* 76: 276–283.

Slot, C. (1965). Plasma Creatinine Determination. A new and specifiv jaffe reaction method. *Scand. J. clin. Lab. Invest.*, 17:381-387.

Soares, J R., Dins, T.C.P., Cunha, A.P. (1997). Antioxidant activity of some extracts of *Thymus zygis*. *Free Radical Research.*, 26: 469-478.

Sofowora, A. (1993). Phytochemical screening of medicinal plants and traditional medicine in Africa, 2nd Edition. Spectrum Books Ltd Nigeria, pp. 150–156.

Trolliet, M.R, Rudd, M.A, and Loscalzo, J. (2001). Oxidative stress andrenal dysfunction in salt-sensitive hypertension. *Kidney Blood Press Res.*, 24: 116–123.

Vaziri, N. D., Liang, K. and Ding, Y. (1999). Increased nitric oxide inactivation by reactive oxygen species in lead-induced hypertension. *Kidney Int.*, 56: 1492–1498.

Vaziri, N. D., Wang, X. Q., Oveisi, F. and Rad, B. (2000). Induction of oxidative stress by glutathione depletion causes severe hypertension in normal rats. *Hypertension*, 36: 142–146.

West, J, Logan, R.F, Card, T.R, Smith, C, Hubbard, R. (2004). Risk of vascular disease in adults with diagnosed coeliac disease: a population-based study. *Aliment Pharmacol Ther.*, 20: 73-9.

Yanik, F. F., Amanvermez, R., Kocak, I., Yanik, A. and Celik, C. (2001). Serum nitric oxide and glutathione levels in preeclamptic and normotensive women during labor. *Gynecol Obstet Invest.*, 1: 110–115.

Yen, G.C and Hsieh, C.L (1998) Antioxidant activity of extracts from Du-zhong (*Eucommia ulmoides*) toward various lipid peroxidation models *in vitro*. *J Agric Food Chem.*, 46: 3952-3957

Zewde, T, Wu, F, and Mattson, D.L. (2004) Influence of dietary NaCl on L-arginine transport in the renal medulla. *Am J Physiol Regul Integr Comp Physiol.*, 286: R89–R93.

Medicinal Plants: Phytochemistry, Pharmacology and Therapeutics, Vol. 1 *Pages 378–383*
Editors: V.K. Gupta, G.D. Singh, Surjeet Singh and A. Kaul
Published by: DAYA PUBLISHING HOUSE, NEW DELHI

Chapter 21

Studies on the Analgesic and Antipyretic Activities of Ethanolic Extract of *Carica papaya* Leaves in Rats

B.V. Owoyele*, A.O. Soladoye and O.A. Omopariola
Department of Physiology, Faculty of Basic Medical Sciences
College of Health Sciences, University of Ilorin, P.M.B. 1515, Ilorin, Nigeria

ABSTRACT

An ethanolic extract of the dried leaves of *Carica papaya* was investigated for analgesic and antipyretic activities in male Wistar rats using three laboratory models which include hotplate latency assays, formalin induced paw licking test and brewers yeast induced hyperpyrexia test. The extract (50–200 mg/Kg, orally) significantly ($p < 0.05$) increased the reaction from 4.4±0.6 to 11.1±0.7s in the hot plate model. Like wise the extract at the same doses demonstrated analgesic activity by significantly ($p < 0.05$) reducing the early and late phases of the formalin test. The extract also produced dose related reduction of pyrexia. The result from the study confirms the analgesic and antipyretic activities of *Carica papaya* leaves.

Keywords: *Analgesic activity, Antipyretic, Brewer's yeast, Ethanolic, Reaction time, Rats.*

Introduction

Carica papaya (family caricaceae) is a tree indigenous to south and Central America where it is found both in the wild and in farms. It is now cultivated throughout the tropical and subtropical

* Corresponding Author: E-mail: deleyele@yahoo.com.

regions of the world for its edible fruits, leaves and flowers (Duke, 1984). The leaves, fruits, seeds, latex and roots of *Carica papaya* are used medicinally in the treatment of many ailments (Gill, 1992). The fallen dry leaves of *carica papaya* along with some other leaves like *A. indica, C. citratus* are used for the treatment of malaria fever. Likewise, the fallen dry leaves with *R.vomitoria* and *A. leiocarpus* is used locally in the western part of Nigeria to reduce body temperature (Gill, 1992). Other medicinal uses of the leaves include treatment of syphilis, amoebic dysentery, asthma, inflammation and also as a purgative (Gill, 1992; Akah *et al.*, 1997; Oloyede, 2005). The ripe and unripe fruits are used as laxative and as a diuretic. The ripe fruit is eaten fresh or cooked. The roots and leaves are used as abortifacient agents (Gill, 1992).

There have been some speculations in literature about the analgesic and antipyretic activities of the leaves of this plant (Gill, 1992, Gupta *et al.*, 1990; Oloyede, 2005). Some of the reports (Gupta *et al.*, 1990) show that the leaves are sedative while we could not find any scientific paper that clearly reports the analgesic activity of this plant. Our decision to conduct this study was based on the practice of using dried and powdered leaves of *Carica papaya* as snuff for the induction of euphoria, and the consumption and bathing of the decoction of the dried leaves for the treatment of pain and fever by some indigenes of the western parts of Nigeria.

Materials and Methods

Plant Material

Carica papaya leaves used for this study were collected in May, 2004 from a herbal garden along Ajase Ipo road, Ilorin, Nigeria. A voucher specimen (FHI 106933) of the plant was deposited in the herbarium of the forestry research institute of Nigeria, Ibadan.

Ethanolic Extract

Shade dried leaves of *carica papaya* were reduced to a powder form and 400g of the powder was extracted with 2 L of ethanol for 48h. The macerated mixture was filtered and evaporated in a carefully regulated water bath maintained at 50°C to yield a dark green, oily and semi solid extract weighing 27.2 g. The extract was stored in a refrigerator at 4°C and dilutions of the extract were made in normal saline with the aid of an organic solvent (Tween 80, 2.5 per cent) before oral administration to animals.

Animals

Male Wistar rats weighing 206.7g±6.4g were used for this study. They were housed and bred in the animal house of the Faculty of Basic Medical Sciences, College of Health Sciences, University of Ilorin. The animal house was well ventilated with adequate humidity and light (12 h dark/light cycles). The rats were fed with mouse cubes (Bendel feeds, Ilorin) and provided with water *ad libitum*.

Analgesic Test Using Hotplate Model

The hotplate test was carried out by slightly modifying the method described by Woolfe and MacDonald, (1944). The rats were placed on a hotplate maintained at 55°C±1°C and the time taken for the rat to respond to the thermal stimulus (Usually by jumping) was noted as the latency or the reaction time (in seconds).

For this study, the rats were divided into five groups, A–E, each made up five rats. Rats in groups B, C and D were given extracts of *Carica papaya* orally after 12 h fasting. The dosages were 50, 100 and 200 mg/kg for the rats in groups B, C and D respectively representing low, medium and high doses. The rats in groups A and E were given equivalent doses of normal saline (10ml/kg) and indomethacin (5 mg/kg, p.o.) respectively. Each of the five rats was placed on the hotplate following which the latency were recorded and the mean latency for each group was also determined. The short lasting stimulus elicited from the hotplate surface causes little or no damage at all to paw tissues, so the test can be followed immediately by the formalin test according to the method used by Back-Rojecky, (2003).

Analgesic Test Using the Formalin Induced Paw Licking Model

The formalin test was carried out according to the method of Hunskaar and Hole (1987). Immediately after the hotplate test (Back-Rojecky, 2003) 100 µl of 3 per cent formalin was injected subcutaneously into the plantar surface of the right front paw of the rats one hour after oral administration of the extract, indomethacin or saline. The time spent by the rats in licking the injected paw as soon as the injection was given (early phase, 0–5 min post injection) and in the late phase (20–30 min post injection) were recorded and the mean licking time for each group was determined.

Pyrexia Test Using Brewer's Yeast Induced Pyrexia Model

The pyrexia test was carried out by slightly modifying the method described by Adams *et al.* (1968). Male Wistar rats were fasted overnight with water provided *ad libitum* before the experiment. The rats were randomly divided into four groups, A–D, each made up of five rats. Pyrexia was induced by subcutaneous injection of 20 per cent w/v brewer's yeast suspension (10 ml/kg) into the dorsum of the rats. Seventeen hours after injection, the rectal temperature of each of the rats was measured using a Clinical thermometer (UNESCO international, Michigan 48197, USA). Only the rats that showed an increase in temperature of at least 0.7°C compared to the rectal temperatures taken immediately before the injection of brewer's yeast were used for this test. The rats in groups A to C were given (orally) 50, 100 and 200 mg/kg of the extract respectively. The rats in group D were given indomethacin (5 mg/kg). The initial rectal temperatures of the rats served as the control temperatures. The temperatures were then measured at 60, 90 and 120 min after each administration and the mean temperature in each of the groups were recorded.

Statistical Analysis

In this study, values are recorded as Mean±S.E.M. Statistical analysis was carried out using the student's t–test. P values < 0.05 were accepted as significant

Results

Hotplate Antinociceptive Test

The results from this study shows that the reaction time increased significantly ($p<0.05$) from 4.4±0.6 to 11.1±0.7 sec after 1 h of *Carica papaya* extract administration. This increase was dose dependent (Table 21.1).

Formalin Induced Paw Licking Test

In this study, oral doses of the extract significantly ($p<0.05$) decreased licking time from 30.6±1.2 to 10.6±1.4 sec in the early phase. Similarly, in the late phase, licking time was significantly ($p<0.05$) reduced from 140.2±4.6 to 40±1.4 sec (Table 21.2).

Brewer's Yeast Induced Pyrexia Test

In this test, the rectal temperatures of the fevered rats were significantly ($p<0.05$) reduced from 39.1±0.3 °C to 37.3±0.5 °C after 60 min of extract administration. Significant ($p<0.05$) reductions of rectal temperatures were also observed after 90 and 120 min of extract administration (Table 21.3).

Table 21.1: Effects of the Ethanolic Extract of *Carica papaya* Leaves on Rats in the Hotplate Test

Groups	*Doses (mg/kg)*	*Reaction Time (sec)*[a]
A. Control	–	4.4±0.6
B. *C. papaya*	50	6.1±0.7**
C. *C. papaya*	100	8.3±0.7**
D. *C. papaya*	200	11.1±0.7**
E. Indomethacin	5	7.2±0.5**

[a] Each value is the mean±S.E.M. for 5 rats.

* P < 0.05; **P < 0.01; *** P < 0.001 compared with control; Students t-test.

Table 21.2: Effects of the Ethanolic Extract of *Carica papaya* Leaves on Rats in the Formalin Test

Groups	*Dose (mg/kg)*	*Licking Time (sec)*[a]	
		Early Phase	*Late Phase*
A. Control	---	30.6±1.2**	140.2±4.6**
B. *C. papaya*	50	22.2±0.7**	65.2±1.6**
C. *C. papaya*	100	18.4±3.1**	53.6±3.9**
D. *C. papaya*	200	10.6±1.4**	40.0±1.4**
E. Indomethacin	5	24.2±1.5**	63.1±2.3**

[a] Each value is the mean±S.E.M. for 5 rats.

* P < 0.05; **P < 0.01; *** P < 0.001 compared with control; Students t-test.

Table 21.3: Effects of the Ethanolic Extract of *Carica papaya* Leaves on Pyrexia Test in Rats[a]

Groups	*Dose (mg/kg)*	*Pre drug Temp °C*	*Post Drug Temperature °C*		
			60 min	*90 min*	*120 min*
A) *C. papaya*	50	39.1±0.3	37.3±0.5**	37.3±0.5**	37.3±0.4*
B) *C. papaya*	100	38.9±0.1	37.4±0.4**	37.2±0.5*	37.1±0.4*
C) *C. papaya*	200	38.4±0.2	37.0±0.3*	36.7±0.4*	36.5±0.2*
D) Indomethacin	5	39.2±0.3	37.6±0.3*	37.3±0.2**	37.1±0.2**

[a] Each value is the mean±S.E.M. for 5 rats.

* P < 0.05; **P < 0.01; *** P < 0.001 compared with control; Students t-test.

Discussion and Conclusion

The analgesic and antipyretic properties of the ethanolic extract of *Carica papaya* leaves were investigated in this study based on the claims of folk medicine practitioners. The analgesic properties were studied using models that could provide different grades of noxious stimuli *i.e.* thermal stimulus using the hotplate test and clinically induced tissue damage using formalin induced paw licking test (Eddy *et al.*, 1950; Hunskaar and Hole, 1987; Tjolsen *et al.*, 1992). The hotplate test was selected for use in this study because of several advantages including sensitivity to strong analgesics and very limited tissue damage (Back-Rojecky, 2003; Prado *et al.*, 1990; Tjolsen *et al.*, 1992; Santos *et al.*, 1997; Hunskaar and Hole, 1987). Furthermore, it utilizes phasic stimulus of high intensities mimicking responses in conditions that involve high threshold pain of short duration. However, a disadvantage of this model is that since it is short lasting, it does not assess modulatory mechanisms that may be triggered by the stimulus itself (Tjolsen *et al.*, 1992). The formalin test is different from most other models of pain in that it is possible to assess the way the animal responds to moderate and continuous pain generated by the injured tissue. Because of its connection to tissue injury, it is believed that the formalin test provides a more valid model for clinical pain than the tests with phasic stimulus (Dubuisson and Dennis, 1971; Eaton, 2003). The results of the present study show that the ethanolic extract of *Carica papaya* leaves can significantly inhibit responses to thermal stimuli and formalin induced pain. The inhibition in both models was dose dependent, thus showing that the extract, at the doses administered, had strong analgesic activities.

In the pyrexia test, brewer's yeast was used to induce pyrexia. Brewer's yeast is commonly used to induce pyrexia in rats and mice (Santos *et al.*, 1997; Olajide *et al.*, 2000; Gupta *et al.*, 2003). The pyrexia results from the activity of brewer's yeast such as its ability to cause infections, tissue damage, inflammation etc. The infections serves as a pyrogenic stimulus and the pyrogens are phagocytized by the Kupffer cells, monocytes, macrophages etc. leading to the release of cytokines. Cytokines have the capacity raise the set point of normal body temperature. The results from this study shows that the extract at doses of 50, 100 and 200 mg/Kg p.o. significantly reduced the brewer's yeast induced hyperthermia in the rats at 60, 90 and 120 min post extract administration.

In general, it was observed that the groups of animals administered with the extract appeared to be inactive and drowsy, thus showing some degree of sedation. Previous reports have shown that *Carica papaya* leaves contain alkaloids, saponins, tannins and nicotinic acid (Gill, 1992). The observed analgesic and antipyretic activities in this study may be due to the flavonoids, saponins and alkaloids contents of the extract since these agents have been linked with analgesic and antiinflammatory effects (Bittar *et al.*, 2002; Gupta *et al.*, 2003). The basic mechanism by which *Carica papaya* produces analgesic and antipyretic effects is not clear yet and this could be the focus of further studies. In conclusion, the present study has established the analgesic and antipyretic activities of *Carica papaya* thus justifying the traditional uses of the plant for the treatment of pain and fever.

Acknowledgements

The authors are grateful to Mr J.L Fwangle, Mr A.U Akapa, (Department of Physiology, University of Ilorin) and Mr Adeleke (Department of Pharmacognosy, College of Medicine, University of Lagos) for their technical assistance.

References

Akah, P. A., Oli, A. N., Enwere, N.M. and Gamaliel, K. (1997). Preliminary studies on purgative effect of *Carica papaya* root extract. *Fitoterapia*, 68: 327–331.

Adams, S. S., Hebborn, P. and Nicholas, J. S. (1968). Some aspect of the pharmacology of ibufenac a non-steroidal antiinflammatory agent. *Journal of Pharmacy and Pharmacology*, 20: 305–312.

Back-Rojecky, L. (2003). Analgesic effect of caffeine and clomipramine: A possible interaction between adenosine and serotonin system. *Acta Pharmaceutica*, 53: 33–39.

Bittar, M., de Souza, M. M., Yunes, R. A., Lento, R., Delle Monache, F., Cechinel Filho, V. (2000). Antinociceptive activity of I3, II8-binaringenin, a bioflavonoid present in plants of the guttiferae. *Planta Medica*, 66: 84–86.

Dubuisson, D. and Dennis, S. G. (1997). The formalin test: a quantitative study of the analgesic effects of morphine, meperidine, and brain stem stimulation in rats and cats. *Pain*, 4: 161–174.

Duke J.A. (1984). Borderline herbs. CRC Press. Boca Raton, FL.

Eaton M. (2003). Common animal models for spasticity and pain. *Journal of Rehabilitation Research and Development*, 40: 41-54.

Eddy, N.B. Touchberry, C.F and Lieberman, *I.E.* (1950). Synthetic analgesics, a methadone isomers and derivatives. *Journal of Pharmacology and Experimental Therapeutics*, 98: 121–137.

Gill, L. S. (1992). Ethnomedical Uses of Plants in Nigeria, Uniben Press. Benin, Nigeria. Pp 51–54.

Gupta, A., Wambebe, C. O. and Parsons, D. L. (1990). Central and cardiovascular effects of alcoholic extract of the leaves of *Carica papaya*. *International Journal of Crude Drug Research*, 28: 257-266.

Gupta, M., Mazumder, U. K., Kumar, R. S. and Kumar, T. S. (2003). Studies on antiinflammatory, analgesic and antipyretic properties of methanol extract of *Caesalpinia bonducella* leaves in experimental animal models. *Iranian Journal of Pharmacology and Therapeutics*, 2: 30-34.

Hunskaar, S., Hole, K. (1997). The formalin test in mice-dissociation between inflammatory and non inflammatory pain. *Pain*, 30: 103–114.

Olajide, O.A., Awe, S.O., Makinde, J.O., Ekhelar, A.I., Olusola, A., Morebise, O. and Okpako D.T. (2000). Studies on the antiinflammatory, antipyretic and analgesic properties of *Alstonia boonei* stem bark. *Journal of Ethnopharmacology*, 71:179–186.

Oloyede, O. I. (2005). Chemical profile of unripe pulp of *Carica papaya*. *Pakistan Journal of Nutrition*, 4: 379–381.

Prado, W.A. Tonussi, C.R., Rego, E.M. and Corrado, A.P. (1990). Anti nociception induced by intraperitoneal injection of gentamicin in rats and mice. *Pain*, 41: 365–37.

Santos, F.A., Rao, V.S.N., Silveira, E.R. (1997). Antiinflammatory and analgesic activites of the essential oil of *Psidium guianense*. *Fitotererapia*, 68: 65–68.

Tjølsen, A., Berge, O., Hunskaar, S., Rosland, J. H. and Hole, K. (1992). The formalin test; an evaluation of the method. *Pain*, 51: 5–17.

Woolfe, G. and MacDonald, A. D. (1944). The evaluation of the analgesic action of pethidine hydrochloride (Demerol). *Journal of Pharmacology and experimental Therapeutics*, 80: 300–307.

Medicinal Plants: Phytochemistry, Pharmacology and Therapeutics, Vol. 1 *Pages 384–389*
Editors: **V.K. Gupta, G.D. Singh, Surjeet Singh and A. Kaul**
Published by: **DAYA PUBLISHING HOUSE, NEW DELHI**

Chapter 22

Degradation Kinetics Studies of the Powdered Leaves, Extracts and Formulations of *Loranthus micranthus* Parasitic on *Kola acuminata*

I.C. Uzochukwu[1] and P.O. Osadebe[2]*
[1]Department of Pharmaceutical and Medicinal Chemistry,
Faculty of Pharmaceutical Sciences,
Nnamdi Azikwe University, Awka, Anambra State, Nigeria
[2]Department of Pharmaceutical and Medicinal Chemistry,
Faculty of Pharmaceutical Sciences,
University of Nigeria, Nsukka, Enugu State, Nigeria.

ABSTRACT

The degradation kinetics of the powdered leaves, aqueous and alcoholic extracts, aqueous and alcoholic formulations of *L. micranthus* parasitic on *Kola acuminata* were studied. Ethanolic and aqueous extract of the leaves were formulated. The pH and organoleptic properties of the formulations were determined. Accelerated stability tests of the powdered leaves, aqueous and alcoholic extracts, aqueous and alcoholic formulations were done at 40, 50 and 60 °C respectively. Samples were withdrawn at intervals and analysed using a validated ultraviolet spectrophotometric method. The ethanolic extract formulation was pale yellow and had a sweet alcoholic taste. The aqueous extract formulation was also pale yellow and had a sweet taste. Mean pH of 5.58±0.11 and 4.79±0.20 were obtained for the ethanolic and aqueous extracts

* Corresponding Author: E-mail: icuzochukwu@yahoo.com.

formulations respectively. While the powdered leaves degraded by zero order kinetics, the ethanolic extract, aqueous extract, ethanolic extract formulation and aqueous extract formulation degraded by first order kinetics. Shelf lives of 21, 19, 15, 18 and 17 days were predicted for powdered leaves, ethanolic and aqueous extracts, ethanolic and aqueous liquid formulations respectively. The employment of heat stress in the prediction of shelf life of *Loranthus micranthus* herbal products is not recommended.

Keywords: *Degradation kinetics, Formulation, Loranthus micranthus, Phytomedicine, Shelf-life, Spectrophotometry.*

Introduction

Loranthus micranthus Linn (African mistletoe) is a semi-parasitic plant traditionally employed in the management of diabetes mellitus and respiratory infections. Its safety, antidiabetic, antimotility and antimicrobial activities have been scientifically validated (Osadebe *et al.*, 2004; Osadebe and Ukwueze, 2004; Osadebe and Uzochukwu, 2006; Osadebe and Akabogu, 2005). Medicinal products including phytomedicines are subject to degradation over time and the consumption of such degraded medicinal product may be deleterious to health. The raw materials for a phytomedicine such as leaves and extracts may be stored for some time before the actual formulation. Knowledge of the degradation kinetics will help us to use such raw materials within their shelf life, prevent formulation of substandard products and ensure consistent batches of the phytomedicine. It is therefore necessary that the stability of medicines during the storage period is ascertained and their shelf lives predicted based on the obtained stability data. High temperature accelerated stability studies are usually employed in order to predict the shelf life of a drug in a considerable short time (Onunkwo, 2005). The Arrhenius plot is used as a basis for predicting the time required for a drug to decompose to 90 per cent of its original concentration at room temperature (shelf life).

Materials and Methods

Preparation of 0.05 M Aluminum Nitrate Solution

Aluminum nitrate (3.7513 g) was weighed and dissolved with about 80 ml of distilled water in a volumetric flask. The resulting solution was made up to 100 ml mark with distilled water (0.1 M). Ten milliliter of the prepared 0.1 M aluminum nitrate solution was added to 10 ml of absolute methanol.

Plant Material

Loranthus micranthus (Linn) leaves parasitic on *Kola acuminata* were collected from Akwaeze, Eastern Nigeria in January 2005. Mr Ekekwe, J. M. C., a plant kingdom scientific analyst, formerly at the Botany Department of the University of Nigeria, Nsukka, identified the plants. The leaves were dried under the shade to a constant weight and pulverized with a Corona ® grinder. The powder was sieved with a 1 mm sieve.

Preparation and Formulation of Ethanolic and Aqueous Extracts of *L. micranthus* Leaves

Thirty gram each of dry powdered leaves of *L. micranthus* parasitic on *Kola acuminata* was macerated with 100 ml each of 48.5 per cent aqueous ethanol and hot distilled water respectively for 24 hours with intermittent shaking. The alcoholic and aqueous extracts were filtered through a Whatman filter paper no 1. Ten millilitre of each of the filtrate was evaporated to dryness in a tarred flat-bottomed dish and dried in a hot air oven at 105 °C to a constant weight. The percentage weight of water-soluble extractive per ml of the extract was calculated. The resulting filtrate was stored in the refrigerator until used.

Sodium benzoate (2 g) and saccharin were dissolved in hot distilled water with stirring and added to the mixing tank. The aqueous extracts required to prepare a 0.1 per cent formulation was added to the mixing tank. The mixture was blended and allowed to cool to about 40 °C. Pineapple flavour was added, the mixture made up to the 2 litre mark with distilled water and blended.

Similarly, saccharin was dissolved in 48.5 per cent aqueous ethanol with stirring and added to the mixing tank. The ethanolic extracts required to prepare a 0.1 per cent formulation was added to the mixing tank. The mixture was blended and allowed to cool to about 40 °C. Pineapple flavour was added, the mixture made up to the 2 litre mark with aqueous ethanol and blended.

The resulting formulations were filtered through a funnel stocked with cotton wool. Formulations were packed in 60 ml amber coloured bottles, and labelled. Two other batches of the alcoholic and aqueous extracts formulations were similarly prepared.

Determination of pH and Organoleptic Properties of Ethanolic and Aqueous Liquid Formulations of *L. micranthus*

The pH values of the ethanolic and aqueous formulations were determined using a digital pH meter (Haach® Singapore, C105). The colours of the formulations were also assessed visually in bright light. The samples of the two formulations were also tasted orally in order to determine the palatability of the formulations.

Determination of Order of Degradation Reaction and Activation Energy of Powdered Leaves, Ethanolic and Aqueous Extracts Alcoholic and Aqueous Liquid Formulations

Powdered leaves of *L. micranthus* was stored in hot air ovens set at 40, 50, and 60 °C±1 °C respectively for 7 days. Five hundred milligrams each of the samples were weighed out daily, macerated in test-tubes with 10 ml each of 90 per cent aqueous methanol for exactly 1 h. The extract (E_1) was filtered through a Whatmann filter paper No 1. One ml of the extract (E_1) was diluted with 49 ml of 90 per cent aqueous methanol (E_2). One ml of E_2 was mixed with 2 ml methanolic aluminum nitrate and 2 ml of acetate buffer (pH, 6.0) and the absorbance of the resulting complex determined at 300 nm using UNICO® 2102 UV-Vis PC spectrophotometer.

Similarly, 60 ml each of crude ethanol and crude aqueous extracts of *L. micranthus* were stored in hot air ovens set at 40, 50, and 60 °C±1 °C respectively for 7 days. One milliliter each of crude ethanol and crude aqueous extracts of *L. micranthus* were withdrawn daily and each diluted with 49 ml of 90 per cent aqueous methanol. One millimeter of the diluted extract was mixed with 2 ml methanolic aluminum nitrate and 2 ml of acetate buffer (pH, 6.0) and the absorbance of the resulting complex determined at 300 nm using UNICO® 2102 UV-Vis PC spectrophotometer.

One sample of the ethanolic and aqueous formulations were stored in hot air ovens set at 40, 50, and 60 °C±1 °C respectively for 7 days. The aqueous or alcoholic extract formulation (2 ml) was withdrawn, mixed with 2 ml of buffer (pH, 6.0) and 2 ml of methanolic aluminum nitrate solution. The absorbance value of the resulting complex was determined using UV–Vis PC spectrophotometer at 300 nm.

The percentage amount of the drug that remained in the samples for each of the temperature storage condition at the different time intervals were plotted against time. Also a graphical plot of the logarithm of the percentage amount of drug remaining was plotted against time. The graph that yielded a straight-line plot (based on higher regression coefficient) was noted as representative of the order of reaction. The degradation rate constants for the tested samples were derived from the slope of graphical plots. The activation energy of the samples were calculated from the graphical plot of the logarithm of the degradation constant against the inverse (Arrhenius plot) of the absolute temperature.

Determination of Degradation Rate Constants of Powdered Leaves, Ethanolic and Aqueous Extracts, Alcoholic and Aqueous Liquid Formulations at Room Temperature

The degradation rate constants of powdered leaves, ethanolic and aqueous extracts, alcoholic and aqueous liquid formulations of *L. micranthus* at room temperature were determined mathematically by employing the equation below:

$$\text{Log}K_2/K_1 = Ea/2.303R \times (T_2 - T_1/T_1T_2) \qquad \text{Equation 1}$$

where,

- Ea: Activation energy
- R: Gas constant
- T_1: Temperature of the experiment of known rate constant, K_1
- T_2: Room temperature at which the rate constant, K_2 is to be determined
- K_1: Known rate constant at T1
- K_2: Rate constant at the room temperature

Estimation of Shelf Life of Powdered Leaves, Ethanolic and Aqueous Extracts, Alcoholic and Aqueous Liquid Formulations at Room Temperature

The shelf life of powdered leaves, ethanolic and aqueous extracts, alcoholic and aqueous liquid formulations of *L. micranthus* at room temperature was determined by substituting into the first order equation shown below:

$$t_{0.9} = 2.303/K \times \log a/a\text{-}x \qquad \text{Equation 2}$$

where,

- $t_{0.9}$: Time at which 90 per cent of the initial concentration of the drug remains.
- K: Degradation rate constant of the formulation at room temperature
- A: initial concentration of the formulation
- X: 90 per cent of the initial concentration of the formulation

Results and Discussion

The results of pH and the organoleptic properties of the ethanolic and aqueous formulations are shown in Table 22.1. Both formulations are palatable, a condition that will favour acceptance and hence compliance by patients. The aqueous extract formulation was more acidic than the ethanolic extract formulation. The absorption of the formulations into the body will vary from one region of gastrointestinal tract to the other. The drug is most likely to be absorbed in the stomach (pH, 1-3), since in this region the drug will be largely unionized.

In the stability studies of the powdered leaves, extracts and liquid formulations of *L. micranthus*, we employed the developed and validated spectrophotometic assay for flavonoids present in the plant products. This approach was adopted because the material under investigation is a herbal drug and constituent of known therapeutic activity is not known (EMEA, 2001).

Table 1: Result of determination of pH and organoleptic properties of formulations

Formulation	Batch	Colour	Taste	pH	Mean pH±SD
Ethanolic	Batch 1	Pale yellow	Sweet alcoholic taste	5.64	5.58±0.11
	Batch 2	Pale yellow	Sweet alcoholic taste	5.60	
	Batch 3	Pale yellow	Sweet alcoholic taste	5.49	
Aqueous	Batch 1	Pale yellow	Sweet taste	4.66	4.79±0.20
	Batch 2	Pale yellow	Sweet taste	4.78	
	Batch 3	Pale yellow	Sweet taste	4.94	

As recommended by the European Agency for the Evaluation of Medicinal Products, the mere determination of the stability of constituents of a herbal preparation is not enough (EMEA, 2001).There is need to show, as far as possible *e.g.* by means of appropriate fingerprint chromatograms, that other substances present in the herbal drug or preparation are likewise stable and that their proportional content remains constant. The European Agency for the Evaluation of Medicinal Products recommends an overall method of assay that regards the herbal drug preparation in its entirety as the active ingredient (EMEA, 2001). We have therefore adopted the overall assay of the flavonoids-rich extract based on the UV-Vis spectroscopic fingerprint of the methanolic aluminum nitrate complex.

The result of determination of order of degradation reaction, degradation rate constants and shelf life of powdered leaves, ethanol and aqueous extracts, ethanol and aqueous liquid formulations are shown in Table 22.2. While the extracts and formulations degraded by first order kinetics, the powdered leaves degraded by zero order kinetics. These findings are consistent with previous studies that showed that solid state degradation reactions generally follow zero order kinetics, while liquid phase degradation reactions follow first order kinetics (Florence and Attwood, 1981). The predicted shelf lives were short. This raises the question of suitability of heat stress as means of assessing the stability of this herbal product. The employment of heat stress in the prediction of shelf life of *Loranthus micranthus* herbal products is not recommended. It is therefore suggested that the shelf storage of *L. micranthus* herbal products at room temperature for prolonged period should be used for the prediction of their shelf life.

Table 22.2: Result of Determination of Order of Degradation Reaction, Degradation Rate Constants and Shelf Life of Powdered Leaves, Ethanolic and Aqueous Extracts, Ethanolic and Aqueous Liquid Formulations

Sample	Order of Degradation	Degradation Rate Constant at Room Temp	Activation Energy (KJ/mol)	Shelf Life (Days)
Powdered Leaves	Zero order	-0.111 mol/day	3181.87	21
Ethanolic extract	First order	-0.121/day	3975.80	19
Aqueous extracts	First order	-0.156/day	3211.53	15
Ethanolic liquid formulation	First order	-0.128/day	7457.71	18
Aqueous liquid formulation	First order	-0.134/day	4835.81	17

Acknowledgements

The authors appreciate the contribution of Ibeme, Anthonia towards the realization of this work.

References

EMEA (2001). Note for Guidance on Quality of Herbal Medicinal Products. The European

Agency for the Evaluation of Medicinal Products, London, UK, pp.1-7.

Florence, A. T. and Attwood, D. (1981). Chemical stability of drugs: In *Physio-chemical Principles of Pharmacy*. Macmillan Press Ltd, London, 483.

Onunkwo, G. C. (2005). Quality assurance and stability testing of herbal medicine. *Journal of Medical and Pharmaceutical Sciences*, 1(1): 21-27.

Osadebe, P. O., Okide, G. B. and Akabogu, I. C. (2004). Study on antidiabetic activities of crude methanolic extracts of *Loranthus micranthus* Linn sourced from five different host trees. *Journal of Ethnopharmacology*, 95:133-138.

Osadebe, P.O. and Ukwueze, S.E. (2004). Comparative study of the antimicrobial and phytochemical properties of mistletoe leaves sourced from six host trees, *Journal of Biolog. Res. and Biotech.*, 2(1): 18-23.

Osadebe, P.O. and Akabogu, I.C. (2005). Antimicrobial activity of *Loranthus micranthus* harvested from kola nut tree. *Phytotherapia*, 77: 54-56.

Osadebe, P. O. and Uzochukwu, I. C. (2006). Chromatographic and antimotility studies on the extracts of *Loranthus micranthus*. *Journal of Pharmaceutical and Allied Sciences*, 3(1): 263-268.

Medicinal Plants: Phytochemistry, Pharmacology and Therapeutics, Vol. 1 *Pages 390–396*
Editors: V.K. Gupta, G.D. Singh, Surjeet Singh and A. Kaul
Published by: DAYA PUBLISHING HOUSE, NEW DELHI

Chapter 23

Phytochemical Analysis and Antimicrobial Activity of *Hyptis suaveolens*

R.A.U. Nwobu[1], I.C. Uzochukwu[2*] and E.L. Okoye[3]
[1]Department of Applied Microbiology and Brewing, Faculty of Natural Sciences, Nnamdi Azikiwe University, Awka, Anambra State, Nigeria
[2]Department of Pharmaceutical and Medicinal Chemistry, Faculty of Pharmaceutical Sciences, Nnamdi Azikiwe University, Awka, Anambra State, Nigeria
[3]Department of Parasitology and Entomology, Faculty of Natural Sciences, Nnamdi Azikiwe University, Awka, Anambra State, Nigeria

ABSTRACT

The antimicrobial activities and phytochemical analysis of the leaves and root of *Hyptis sauveolens* were investigated. The agar-well diffusion method was used for the antimicrobial analysis. The minimum inhibitory concentrations (MIC) and the minimum bactericidal concentrations (MBC) of the extracts were determined using two-fold serial dilution method. The results showed that the methanolic and chloroform extracts were active against Gram positive bacteria but not against Gram negative bacteria and fungi. The phytochemical analysis of the crude extracts showed the presence of alkaloids, flavonoids, saponins, tannins, resins, reducing sugars, terpenoids, steroids, glycosides and carbohydrates. Thin layer chromatography of the methanolic extracts of the leaves and roots of *H. sauveolens* gave six fractions. The fractions

* Corresponding Author: E-mail: icuzochukwu@yahoo.com.

that showed antibacterial activity were found to contain steroids, terpenoids and glycosides. Hence, the antimicribial activities of *H. sauveolens* may be attributed to the presence of these secondary plant metabolites.

Keywords: *Antimicrobial activity, Chloroform extract, Hyptis sauveolens, Methanolic extract, Phytochemical analysis, Thin layer chromatography.*

Introduction

The relationship between man and plants has been very close throughout all civilizations. Historically, natural products provide the oldest source of medicines. Competition and natural selection during evolution between species have produced powerful biologically active natural products lying in the 'heart of our rain forest flora and waiting to be harnessed for human welfare (Farn-Sworth, 1990). Today's world is plagued by a catalogue of chronic, incurable or barely manageable ailments, and hence the need to research into medicinal plants and medicinal recipes for the discovery of novel drugs against the chain of ailments tormenting the world.

Hyptis sauveolens Poit is an obnoxious weed distributed throughout the tropics and sub-tropics (Mandal *et al.*, 2007). *H. sauveolens* plant is used mainly as decoctions in traditional medicine for the treatment of various illnesses such as wound infections, eye infections etc (Kuhnt *et al.*, 1995). It has been reported to possess anticancerous properties (Mudgal *et al.*, 1997) and tumorigenic properties (Peerzada, 1997). Among the Ibos in Nigeria, the leaves are used as mosquito repellant.

This study aims at establishing the antimicrobial potentials of *Hyptis sauveolens* and identifying the phyto-constituents responsible for the antimicrobial activities.

Materials and Methods

Plant Material

The fresh leaves and roots of *H. sauveolens* were collected in the flowering stage at Awka, Nigeria. The plant was identified by Dr. C. Okeke of the Department of Botany, Nnamdi Azikiwe University, Awka, Nigeria.

Micro Organisms

Stock cultures of seven clinical isolates of *Staphylococcus aureus,* and *Bacillus subtilis* (Gram positives), *Escherichia coli, Pseudomonas aeruginosa* and *Salmonella paratyphi* (Gram negatives), *Aspergillus niger* and *Candida albicans* (fungi) were obtained from the Pharmaceutical Microbiology Unit of the Department of Pharmaceutics, Faculty of Pharmaceutical Sciences, University of Nigeria, Nsukka.

Extraction Procedure

The leaves and roots of *H. sauveolens* were dried under shade at room temperature for 14 days and pulverized using a mechanical grinder. A 40 g portion of the leaves and roots powder were each extracted by maceration in methanol and chloroform (400 ml) respectively for 72 hours. The resulting extracts were subsequently filtered using Whatman No 1 filter paper. The methanolic and chloroform extracts were each evaporated to dryness at room temperature in a steady air current.

Phytochemical Studies

The phytochemical constituents of the methanolic and chloroform extracts of the leaves and roots of *H. sauveolens* were investigated following the methods as described by Trease and Evans (Trease and Evans, 1989). Preliminary phytochemical tests were carried out on the extracts to detect the presence of steroids, alkaloids, saponins, resins, proteins, carbohydrate, fats and oil, glycosides, reducing sugars, flavonoids and terpenoids.

Antimicrobial Screening of *H. sauveolens* Extracts

The methanolic and chloroform extracts of the leaves and roots of *H. sauveolens* were screened for antimicrobial activity using the agar-well diffusion method. Broth culture (0.1 ml) containing 1×10^5 cells per ml of the required micro-organism was introduced into a sterile petri dish and 20 ml of molten nutrient agar added. The content was thoroughly mixed and then allowed to set. After solidification, uniform and equidistant wells (6 mm, diameter) were cut in the agar using a sterile cork borer. Two drops of each extracts were placed in each cup, allowed to diffuse and then incubated at 37 °C for 24 hours (for bacteria) and for 48 hours (for fungi). The diameters of the zone of inhibition were measured using a transparent meter rule.

Determination of the Minimum Inhibitory Concentration (MIC) and Minimum Bactericidal Concentration (MBC) of the Leaves and Roots Extracts of *H. sauveolens*

The minimum inhibitory concentration (MIC) and minimum bactericidal concentration (MBC) of each plant extract were determined using broth dilution method. A total of eleven sterile test tubes were placed on a test tube rack. For each of the plant extract, 1 ml was placed in the first test tube while 4.5 ml of nutrient broth was added to each of the remaining ten tubes using a sterile pipette. The plant extract was then serially diluted two fold. Extract (0.5 ml) was pipetted from the first into the second test tube, thoroughly shaken and 0.5 ml transferred from the second to the third test tube. This transfer was repeated until the last test tube. The eleventh test tube served as the negative control tube. Each test tube was then inoculated with 20 ml of the standardized inoculum of each test organisms and then incubated at 37 °C for 24 hours. Similar dilutions were also made with gentamycin and nystatin which served as the positive and negative control respectively. The MIC of the methanolic and chloroform extracts were determined. This was the lowest concentration of the extract at which no visible growth was observed as compared with the growth in the positive control tube. Subsequently those tubes showing no growth (without turbidity) were inoculated for 24 hours. The MBC of the methanolic and chloroform extracts were also determined. This was the concentration of the extracts in the tubes with the highest dilution that gave no growth on the agar plates after incubation.

Thin Layer Chromatography of the Leaves and Roots Extracts *H. sauveolens*

The methanolic extracts of the leaves and roots of *H. sauveolens* were separated into different constituents by thin layer chromatography (TLC) using aluminum oxide (GF 254 type E) coated plates in a solvent system of diethyl ether and chloroform (2:1) for the leaf extract and toluene/ethyl acetate (2:1) with 10 drops of glacial acetic acid for the root extract. Each extract gave six fractions. The fractions were aseptically scrapped with a sterile spatula, extracted with methanol and tested for antibacterial activities against *S. aureus* and *B. subtilis* by the agar-well diffusion method.

Results and Discussion

The result of the phytochemical analysis of the extracts indicated the presence of flavonoids, terpenoids, tannins, saponins, resins, glycosides, reducing sugars and carbohydrates. Proteins, fats and oil were absent from the methanolic and chloroform extracts. Tannins and flavonoids (polyphenols) were detected in the leaf extracts but absent in the root extracts. The phytochemical tests of the methanolic extract of both leaves and roots showed higher quantities of tepernoids, glycosides and reducing sugars. The result of the phytochemical analysis of the TLC bands suggests that the major constituents of the plant responsible for antimicrobial activities are terpenoids, steroids and glycosides.

Table 23.1: Results of Phytochemical Screening of the Crude Root and Leaf extracts of *H. suaveolens*

Test	*Root*		*Leaves*	
	Methanolic Extract	*Chloroform Extract*	*Methanolic Extract*	*Chloroform Extract*
Saponins	+++	–	+++	–
Acidity	–	–	–	–
Protein	–	–	–	–
Tannins	–	–	+++	–
Carbohydrate	+++	+++	+++	+++
Resins	++	++	+	+++
Fats and Oil	–	–	–	–
Glycosides	++	–	+++	–
Reducing Sugar	+++	–	+++	–
Flavonoids	–	–	+++	++
Alkaloids	+	–	–	–
Terpenoids	+++	++	+++	++
Steroids	+++	++	++	++

–: Not detected; +: Low concentration; ++: Medium concentration; +++: High concentration.

Table 23.2: Results of Phytochemical Screening of TLC Fractions of the Crude Root and Leaf Methanolic Extracts of *H. suaveolens*

Test	*Root*						*Leaves*					
	F1	*F2*	*F3*	*F4*	*F5*	*F6*	*F1*	*F2*	*F3*	*F4*	*F5*	*F6*
Saponins	–	–	–	–	–	–	–	–	–	–	–	–
Tannins	–	–	–	–	–	–	–	–	–	–	–	–
Carbohydrate	+	++	++	+	++	+	++	+	++	+	+	+
Resins	–	–	–	–	–	–	–	–	–	–	–	–
Glycosides	++	++	++	++	+++	++	++	+	+++	++	–	++
Reducing Sugar	++	+	++	+	++	+	+	+	++	+	+	++
Flavonoids	–	–	–	–	–	–	–	–	–	–	–	–
Terpenoids	++	+++	+++	+++	+	+	++	++	+++	++	+	+++
Steroids	++	+++	+++	++	++	+	++	++	++	++	+	++

–: Not detected; +: Low concentration; ++: Medium concentration; +++: High concentration.

Table 23.3: Result of Antimicrobial Activity of Root and Leaf Extract (inhibition zone diameter in mm) of *H. sauveolens*

Test	*Inhibition Zone Diameter in mm*						
	Bacteria					*Fungi*	
	S. aureus	*B. subtilis*	*P. aeruginosa*	*E. coli*	*S. paratyphi*	*C. albicans*	*A. niger*
Methanolic extract(root)	26.00	16.00	8.00	–	–	–	–
Methanolic extract (leaves)	22.00	12.00	4.00	–	–	–	–
Chloroform extract (root)	24.00	20.00	6.00	–	–	–	–
Chloroform extract (leaves)	18.00	14.00	6.00	–	–	–	–
Gentamicin	32.00	30.00	20.00	18.00	6.00	–	–
Nystatin	–	–	–	–	–	24.00	27.00
Distilled water	–	–	–	–	–	–	–

The results obtained from this investigation provide direct evidence of the antibacterial activity of *H. suaveolens*. The methanolic and chloroform extracts exhibited different degrees of antibacterial activities against the bacteria isolates but exhibited no activity against the fungi. The antimicrobial screening of *H. suaveolens* has shown that both the plant leaves and roots possess antimicrobial activity against the tested Gram-positive bacteria. Either or both the leaves and roots of *H. suaveolens* can be used in the management of bacterial infections. However, the antimicrobial activities of the root extracts were more pronounced than those of the leaf extracts. The traditional use of both the leaves and roots of the plant for administration to sick people is supported by our studies.

The extracts were active against the two Gram-positive bacteria used (*S. aureus* and *B. subtilis*). The methanolic and chloroform extracts were not active against Gram-negative bacteria (*E. coli*, and *S. paratyphi*) except *P. aeruginosa* where the extracts showed minimal inhibition. These results are consistent with the pattern of *in vitro* inhibition emerging from other studies in which it was also found that plant extracts readily inhibit Gram-positive rather than Gram-negative bacteria (Grosvenor *et al.*, 1995). The antimicrobial activity of the extracts against *S. aureus* is of great interest. There is an increasing resistance of *S. aureus* to conventional antibiotics. Plant extracts possessing antimicrobial activity against *S. aureus* will be of great benefit in the management of drug resistant staphylococcus infections. The use of the plant extracts of *H. suaveolens* is therefore recommended for the treatment of wounds, eye infections and other diseases in which *S. aureus* is incriminated as a causative agent.

Table 23.4: Result of Inhibition Zone Diameter in mm of Fractions from the Root and Leaves Methanolic Extracts of *H. sauveolens*

Organism	*Root*						*Leaves*					
	F1	*F2*	*F3*	*F4*	*F5*	*F6*	*F1*	*F2*	*F3*	*F4*	*F5*	*F6*
S. aureus	12.00	14.00	15.00	13.00	16.00	11.00	11.00	13.00	12.00	14.00	–	16.00
B. subtilis	8.00	10.00	9.00	8.00	–	–	–	10.00	9.00	8.00	–	10.00

Table 23.5: Result of MIC and MBC of Leaf and Root Extract of *H. suaveolens*

Organism	*MIC (mg/ml)*					*MBC (mg/ml)*				
	Methanolic Extract (Root)	*Methanolic Extract (Leaves)*	*Chloroform Extract (Root)*	*Chloroform Extract (Leaves)*	*Gentamicin*	*Methanolic Extract (Root)*	*Methanolic Extract (Leaves)*	*Chloroform Extract (Root)*	*Chloroform Extract (Leaves)*	*Gentamicin*
S. aureus	0.78	1.56	0.78	3.13	0.19	1.56	6.25	3.13	12.50	0.39
B. subtilis	3.13	6.25	1.56	3.13	0.19	12.50	25.00	6.25	12.50	0.78
P. aeruginosa	25.00	100.00	50.00	50.00	1.56	100.00	–	–	–	3.13
E. coli	–	–	–	–	3.13	–	–	–	–	12.50
S. paratyphi	–	–	–	–	50.00	–	–	–	–	100

The crude extracts of the leaves and roots showed greater inhibition zone diameter than the TLC fractions against the two Gram-positive bacteria used for the TLC fractions bioassay. This agrees with the findings made by Kafaru (1994) that crude preparations of whole plant parts (containing both the active and non-active components) possess higher efficacy than semi-crude or pure plant substances. Antimicrobial activity of the plant may not be due to just one chemical species. A number of constituents may contribute to bioactivity. The pooling of more than one fraction or the use of the crude extract of the plant is therefore recommended for maximal antimicrobial activity.

The results of the MIC and MBC show that the methanolic extracts, especially the root extract, of *H. suaveolens* possess reasonable antimicrobial activity against *S. aureus.* The methanolic extracts generally showed better antimicrobial activity than the chloroform extracts suggesting the major contribution polar plant constituents to the antimicrobial activities of the plant.

Further research involving *in vivo* assays would be needed to establish the relationship between the MICs, MBCs obtained in this study and the effective doses at which the herbs should be applied in ethno-medical practice. Also further purification of the extracts should be done extensively to determine the main active constituents using more analytical processes and instruments. Studies aimed as the standardization of the extract using identified biomarker will also be needed.

The whole extract or fractions of H. *suaveolens* is recommended for used in alternative medicine to control and treat infections of bacteria origin especially in cases where *S. aureus* has been implicated.

References

Farn-Sworth, N.R (1990). The role of ethnopharmocology in drug development. In bioactive compounds from plants. Eds.Chichester Ciba Foundation Symposium 154: 2-20.

Grosvenor, P. W; Supriono, A. S and Grey, D.O (1995). Medicinal plants from Riau province, Sumatra, Indonesia. Part 2: Antibacterial and antifungal activity. *J. Ethnopharmacol,* 45: 97–111.

Kafaru, E (1994). Immense Help from nature's workshop Lagos. Elikat Health Services, Nigeria, pp. 31–210.

Kuhnt M, Probstle A, Rimpler H, Baver R and Heinrich M (1995). Biological and pharmacological activities and further constituents of *Hyptis verticillata. Planta Medica,* 61 (03): 227-232.

Mandal, S.M, Mondal, K.C, Dey, S, Pati, B.R (2007). Antimicrobial activity of the leaf extracts of *Hyptis suaveolens* (L) Poit. *Indian J. Pharm. Sci.,* 69: 568-9.

Mudgal V, Khanna KK and Hazra PK (1997). Flora of Madhya Pradesh 11 Botanical Survey of India, pp. 403–404.

Peerzada N (1997). Chemical composition of the essential oil of *Hyptis suaveolens*. *Molecules*, 2: 165–168.

Trease, E.G and Evans, W.C (1989). Pharmacognosy 13th edition, Braillere Tindall, London, pp. 167–188.

Medicinal Plants: Phytochemistry, Pharmacology and Therapeutics, Vol. 1 *Pages 397–405*
Editors: V.K. Gupta, G.D. Singh, Surjeet Singh and A. Kaul
Published by: DAYA PUBLISHING HOUSE, NEW DELHI

Chapter 24

Pharmacognostical and Preclinical Studies on Stembark of *Gmelina arborea*: An Ayurvedic Medicinal Plant

K. Yogesh and A. Veeranjaneyulu*
Department of Pharmacology,
School of Pharmacy and Technology Management,
NMIMS University, V.L. Mehta road, Vile Parle (W)
Mumbai – 400 056, Maharashtra, India

ABSTRACT

Gmelina arborea locally known as Gamhar is an ayurvedic plant having many medicinal properties. Pharmacognostical studies of bark with respect to its macroscopy, microscopy, powder characteristics and fluorescence characteristics have been carried out. The important identifying characteristic of the bark is presence of belt of lignified sclereids and laminated fracture. The physicochemical parameters like different ash values, extractive values and loss on drying were determined. Preliminary phytochemical analysis of aqueous and methanolic extracts indicated presence of phenolics, saponins and alkaloids. These two extracts were used for the preclinical studies. Acute oral toxicity studies were performed according to OECD guidelines. The extracts do not produced any behavioral changes in animals. The extracts are safe upto the dose of

* Corresponding Author: E-mail: add_bits@yahoo.com.

5g/kg. Antidiabetic potential of the two extracts were tested in alloxan induced diabetic rats. Aqueous and methanolic extracts used in the study significantly lowered the plasma glucose.

Keywords: *Acute toxicity, Antidiabetic, Gmelina arborea, Pharmacognostical.*

Introduction

Diabetes mellitus is a metabolic disorder characterized by hyperglycemia and alterations in carbohydrate, fat, and protein metabolism. The condition is associated with several complications such as atherosclerosis, neuropathy, and cataract formation (Xiang-Yang Qia *et al.*, 2008). Diabetes is currently growing at a rapid rate throughout the world, and it is the 16th leading cause of global mortality (Murray and Lopez, 1997).

According to a widely accepted estimation, the number of diabetic patients would reach 366 million by the year 2030 (Wild *et al.*, 2004).

India now has the world's largest diabetic population, encompassing an estimated 35 million people out of an overall population of 1 billion. Another 79 million people have impaired glucose tolerance. The country will have almost 200 million people (approximately 15 per cent of the population) affected by diabetes or its precursor upto year 2025 (Kaushik *et al.*, 2008).

In recent years, because many current oral hypoglycemic agents are synthetic drugs with certain adverse side effects, interest in alternative therapeutic approaches has become very popular (Holman and Turner, 1991). For several thousands of years, the plant kingdom has been a source of a wide variety of potentially beneficial natural effective oral hypoglycemic agents that have lower toxicity and fewer side effects compared to synthetic drugs (Pari *et al.*, 2000).

Gmelina arborea (Family: Verbanaceae) locally known as Gamhar is a beautiful fast growing deciduous tree occurring naturally throughout greater part of India up to 1500 m.The root and bark of *Gmelina arborea* are used as stomachic, galactagogue, laxative and anthelmintic, improve appetite, useful in hallucination, piles, abdominal pains, burning sensations, fevers, 'tridosha' and urinary discharge (Nadkarni, 2000). Leaf paste is applied to relieve headache and juice is used as wash for ulcers (Chopra, 1956). Flowers are sweet, cooling, bitter, acrid and astringent. They are useful in leprosy and blood diseases. In ayurveda it has been observed that Gamhar fruit is acrid, sour, bitter, sweet, cooling, diuretic tonic, aphrodisiac, alternative astringent to the bowels, promote growth of hairs, useful in 'vata', thirst, neuropathy causing peripheral burning sensation, anaemia, leprosy, ulcers and vaginal discharge. The plant is recommended in combination with other drugs for the treatment of snake bite and scorpion–sting. In snake bite a decoction of the root and bark is given internally (Kirtikar and Basu, 1984).

Gmelina arborea is a traditional medicinal plant used in antidiabetic formulations. There is no detailed pharmacognostical and pharmacological work reported on the bark of the plant. Recent studies indicated that the other species from the same genus have significant antidiabetic properties (Kasiviswanath and Ramesh, 2005). However, antidiabetic activity of the bark of *Gmelina arborea* have not been reported, therefore in order to establish scientific basis for ethnomedicinal uses of the stembark of the plant, we planned to study its effect diabetes.

Materials and Methods

Plant Material

The stembark of the *Gmelina arborea* was collected from Jawhar (Dist.Thane), Maharashtra. The sample of stembark was identified and authenticated by the scientists of Botanical Survey of India, Pune.

Pharmacognostical Studies and Determination of Physico-chemical Parameters

Fresh bark of medium size was selected for the microscopical studies. Sections were cut on a microtome and by free hand sectioning. The microchemical tests for histological zones were performed according to methods given by Kay (1938), Trease and Evans (1972) and Wallis (1967). Fluorescence characteristics of the powdered drug were studied as per Kokoski (1958). Physicochemical parameters like ash values, extractive values and loss on drying were determined as per methods described in Indian Pharmacopoeia. Fluorescence characteristics of powdered bark with different chemical reagents and powder were observed under UV (254nm, 365nm), visible light (Kokoski *et.al.,*).

Preliminary Phytochemical Screening

Preliminary phytochemical investigations were carried out according to methods in Harborne (1973).

Preparation of Aqueous Extract (AE)

Five hundred grams of powdered bark was macerated with one liter of chloroform water for seven days, with frequent shaking. After seven days, the aqueous extract was filtered and the marc was again kept for maceration with chloroform water for complete extraction. After filtration the aqueous extracts were combined and concentrated with the help of rotary vacuum evaporator at 60° C. The extract was freeze-dried at –20°C (yield 20 per cent, w/w, dry weight basis) and stored at 4°C until use.

Preparation of Methanolic Extract (ME)

1 Kg of powdered bark of *Gmelina arborea* was extracted with methanol in several batches by using soxhlet apparatus. The extract was filtered and the filtrate was evaporated to dryness under reduced pressure at 50°C (yield 28 per cent, w/w, dry weight basis) and stored at 4°C until use.

Animals

Experimental animals consisted of albino mice (25–35 g) and Wistar rats (180–230 g), housed in standard environmental conditions (21°C, 60–70 per cent humidity) under a 12-h light:12-h dark cycle. Animals were given free access to water and normal diet.

Mice were used for acute toxicity evaluation and rats were used for antidiabetic studies. The experimental study was approved by the Institutional Animal Ethics Committee of NMIMS University.

Acute Toxicity Studies

The acute toxicity of the aqueous and methanolic extract of *Gmelina arborea* was evaluated in mice using fixed dose procedure (OECD, 2001b). Mice of either sex (three females and three males, age: 6–8 weeks) received aqueous and methanolic extract starting at 300 mg/kg upto 5000 mg/kg, orally by gavage. The animals were observed for toxic symptoms continuously for the first 4 h after dosing. Finally, the number of survivors was noted after 24 h and these animals were then maintained for further 14 days with observations made daily.

Induction of Diabetes in Rats

Diabetes was induced in 24 h fasted male adult rats of Wistar strain by a single i.p. injection of alloxan, at a dose of 120 mg/kg b.w. in cold saline. The diabetic rats, after confirmation of stable hyperglycemia, were then divided into five groups of six rats each. Group I animals receiving vehicle served as control, Group II to Group V received ME (250 mg/kg), ME (500 mg/kg), AE (250 mg/kg) and AE (500 mg/kg) respectively. The groups received the various extracts, as mentioned above, once a day, for 28 days. From these animals, glucose level was determined on day 0, day 7, day 14, day 21 and day 28. The changes in body weight, feed and water intake were also recorded.

Statistical Analysis of Results

The variability of results is expressed as mean±S.E.M. The significance of differences between mean values was determined by the student's *t*-test.

Results and Discussion

Pharmacognostical Studies

Organoleptic Characteristics (Figure 24.1)

- ☆ Size: 10-12 cm × 5-6 cm
- ☆ Shape: Curved and Flat.

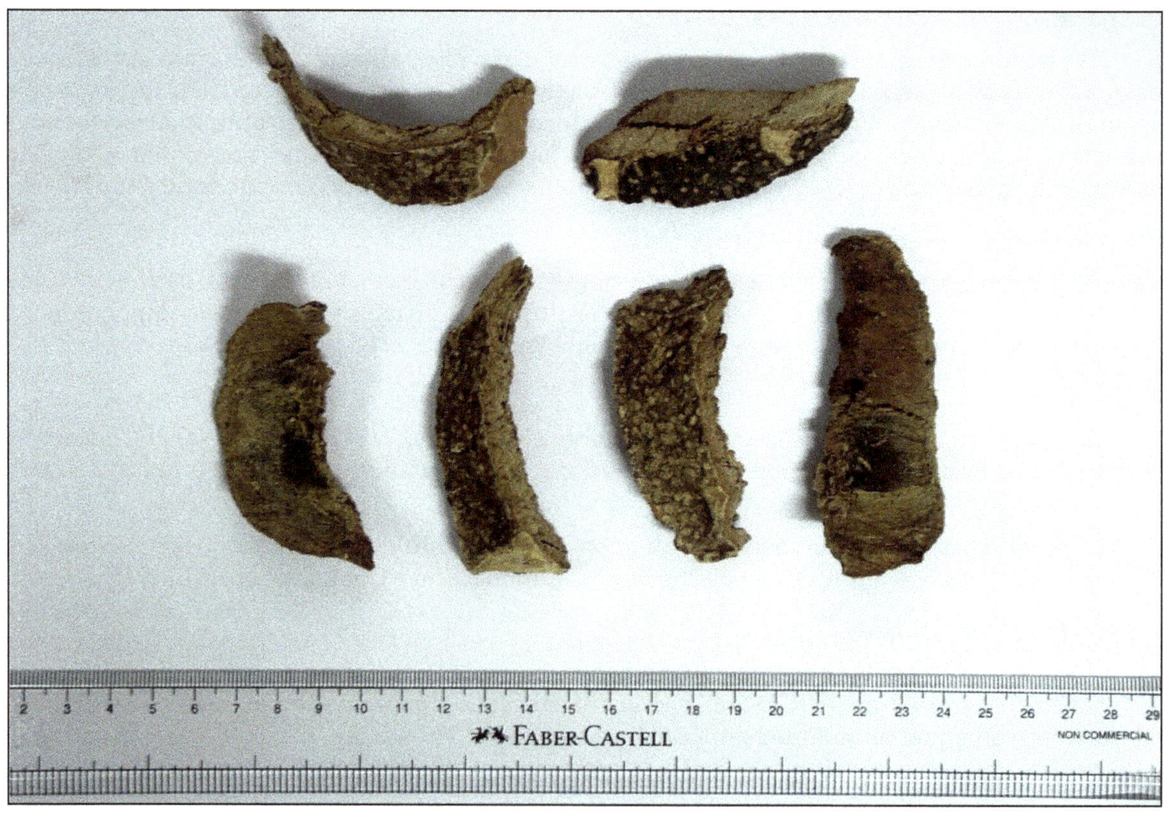

Figure 24.1: Stembark of *Gmelina arborea*

- ✰ Colour: Internally buff coloured, externally slightly brown.
- ✰ Fracture: Laminated and granular
- ✰ Taste: Tasteless
- ✰ Odour: Characteristic
- ✰ Special characters: Shows patches of adhered lichens.

Microscopy (Figure 24.2)

Transverse section of bark showed broadly four parts–periderm, cortex, a band of sclerenchyma and secondary phloem.

Periderm is composed of cork, phellogen and phelloderm. Cork is lignified and stratified It consists of several layers of radially arranged rows of thin walled, elongated cells. Cortex is composed of six to nine layers of parenchymatous cells, encircling either single isolated or groups of scattered sclereids.

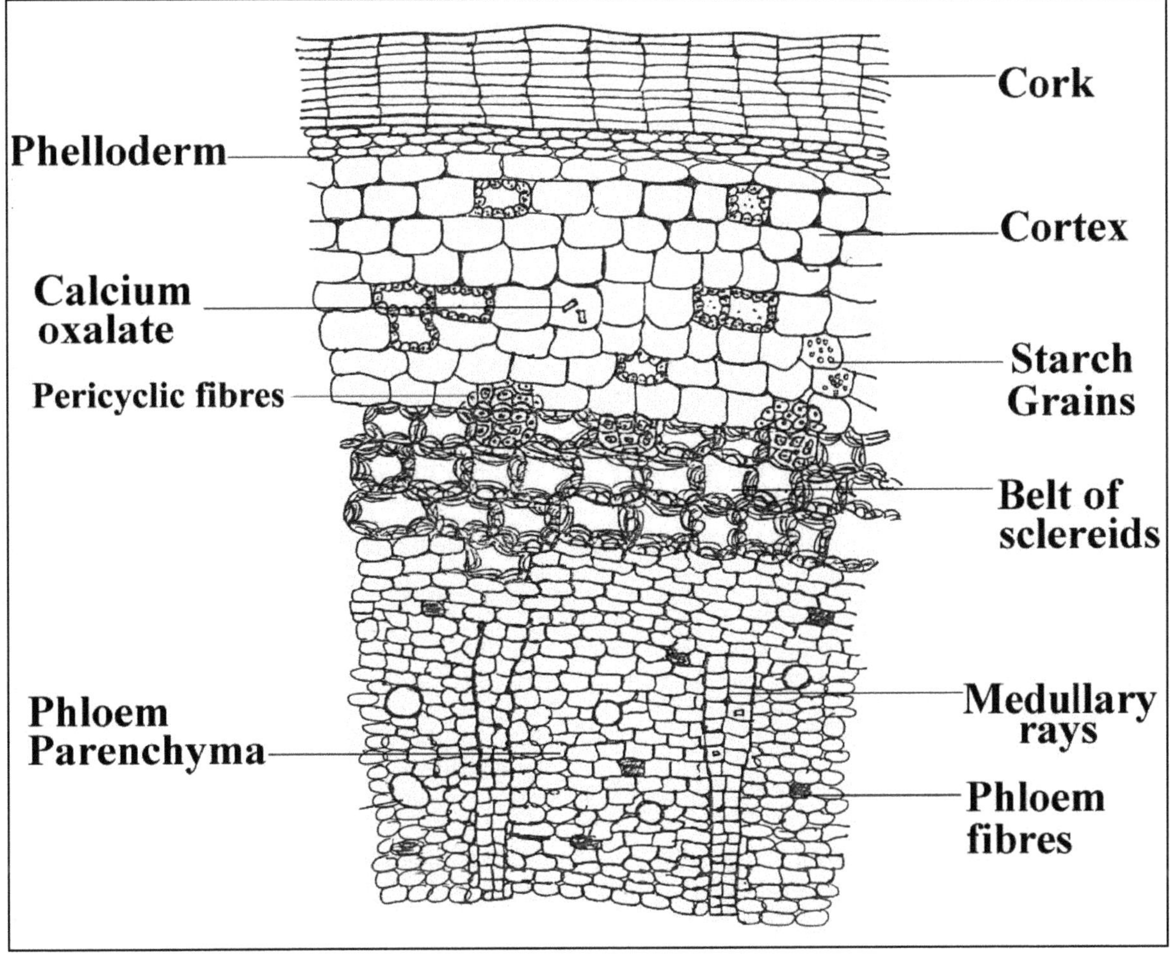

Figure 24.2: T.S. of *Gmelina arborea* Stembark (x100)

Some of parenchymatous cells contain minute prismatic, microsphenoidal calcium oxalate crystals, and simple starch grains.

Table 24.1: Physico-chemical Parameters of *Gmelina arborea* Bark

Parameter	*% w/w (Mean a± SEM)*
Total ash	12.1±0.17
Acid insoluble ash	0.89±0.02
Water soluble ash	3.05±0.10
Petroleum ether extractive	0.61±0.01
Chloroform extractive	1.0±0.11
Ethyl acetate extractive	12.6±0.26
Methanol extractive	27.86±0.27
Ethanol extractive	20.01±0.08
Water extractive	20.04±0.22
Loss on drying	6.2±0.15

a: Mean value of three readings.

A continuous, well-developed layer of sclereids (sclerenchymatous band) occurs in between the primary cortex and secondary phloem region. Groups of small pericyclic fibres are found on the outer side of sclerenchymatous band.

Secondary phloem region is comprised of phloem parenchyma, phloem fibres and medullary rays. Phloem parenchyma consists of thin walled cells containing starch grains and calcium oxalate crystals. Phloem fibres occur mostly single and isolated or in group of 2-3, embedded in phloem parenchyma. Medullary rays divide radially several times the phloem parenchyma, which are generally 1-3 cells wide.

Histochemical colour reactions on the transverse section of the stembark showed the presence of starch, lignin, alkaloids, and phenolics.

Fluorescence analysis failed to indicate fluorescence characteristic of the bark

Powder Analysis

Preliminary Examination

- ☆ Colour : Brown.
- ☆ Odour : Characteristic.
- ☆ Taste : Tasteless
- ☆ Texture : Smooth.

1. After addition of small quantity of water, a mucilagenous mass was not formed which indicates absence of considerable amount of mucilage.
2. After pressing a little amount of powder between filter paper, no greasy stain was found, indicating absence of fatty oils.
3. After shaking the powder with water in a test tube, persistent froth was formed indicating presence of saponins.

Microscopical Examination (Figure 24.3)

- ✰ Cork cells-hexagonal in shape
- ✰ Stone cells-lignified
- ✰ Calcium oxalate crystals–prismatic
- ✰ Starch grains
- ✰ Fibres-nonlignified, rare

Preliminary Phytochemical Screening

It indicated presence of phenolics, saponins and alkaloids in aqueous and methanolic extracts.

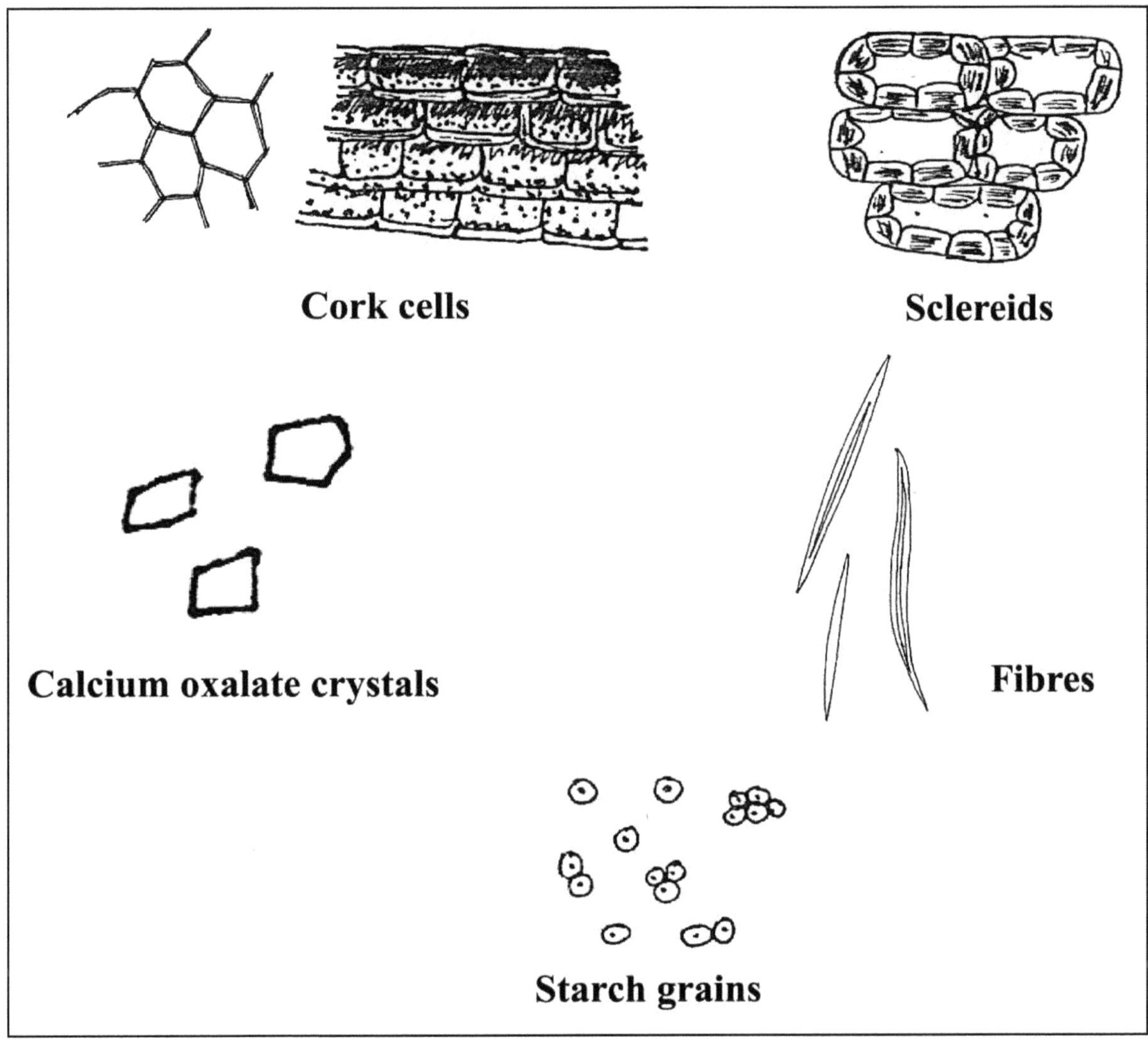

Figure 24.3: Power Characteristics of *Gmelina arborea* Stembark

Acute Toxicity Studies

Acute toxicity studies revealed that all extracts were practically nontoxic when administered orally; the LD_{50} value was higher than 5 g/kg. No mortality or any toxic reactions were found up to the end of the study. Even at this high dose there were no gross behavioral changes.

Alloxan Induced Diabetes

Figure 24.4 reported the antidiabetic effects of the extracts on fasting plasma glucose levels in alloxan-induced diabetic rats treated for 28 days. The antidiabetic effects induced by the extracts, as observed, were dose-related. It is well established that alloxan administration to experimental rats selectively causes pancreatic beta cell-membrane disruption and ultimately cytotoxicity after its intracellular accumulation. Based on the observed blood glucose lowering activities of both tested extracts, our results, therefore, suggest increased peripheral utilization of glucose as the likely mechanism of lowering the blood glucose. Treatment with the two extracts also decreased loss of body weight and water and feed intake.

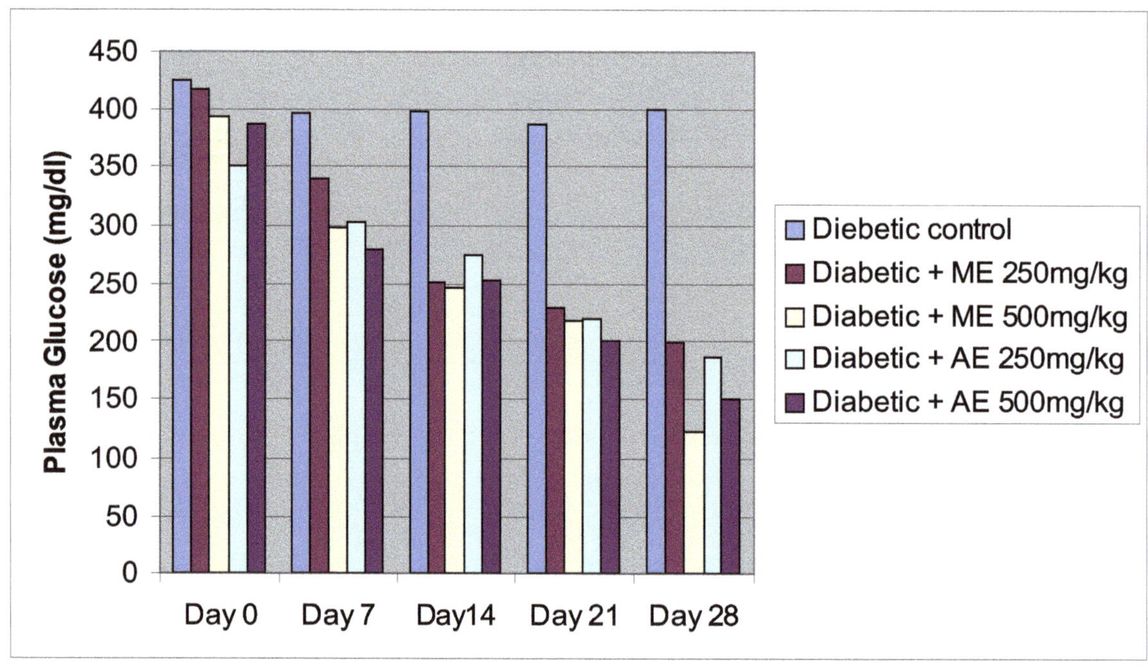

Figure 24.4: Antidiabetic Effect of Various Extracts of *Gmelina arborea* Bark

The present pharmacognostical study may be useful to supplement information with regards to its identification and standardization.

The results have shown that two extracts of *Gmelina arborea* possess blood glucose lowering effect in alloxan-induced hyperglycemic rats.

Acknowledgements

Authors are thankful to Dr.R.S.Gaud, Dean, School of Pharmacy and Technology Management, NMIMS University, Mumbai for providing necessary facilities to carry out this research work. We are also grateful to Prof. S.B.Gokhale, Principal, SVKM's College of Diploma in Pharmacy and Dr. Meena C. HOD, Clinical Pharmacology for technical assistance.

References

Anonymous (1996). Pharmacopoeia of India (2nd Ed.)Govt. of India publication, New Delhi.

Chopra, R.N., Nayar, S.L., Chopra, I.C. (1956). Glossary of Indian Medicinal Plants. CSIR, New Delhi.

Harborne, J.B. (1973). Phytochemical methods. Chapman and Hall, London.

Holman, R.R., Turner, R.C. (1991). Diabetes. In: Pickup JC, Williams G, editors. Oral agents and insulin in the treatment of NIDDM. Oxford: Book of Blackwell; pp. 467-9.

Kasiviswanath, R., Ramesh, A. (2005). Hypoglycemic and antihyperglycemic effect of *Gmelina asiatica* LINN. in normal and in alloxan induced diabetic rats. *Biol Pharm Bull.*, 28: 729-32.

Kaushik,G., Satya, S., Khandelwal, R., Naik, S.N. (2008). Commonly consumed Indian plant food materials in the management of diabetes mellitus. *Clin Res and Rev.*, Article in Press.

Kay, L.A. (1938). The microscopic studies of drugs. Bailliere Tindall and Cox, London.

Kirtikar, K.R., Basu, B.D. (1984) Indian Medicinal Plants. 2nd ed. Vol.II, International Book Distributors, Dehradun.

Kokoski, J., Kokoski, R., and Salma, F.J. (1958). Fluorescence of powdered vegetable drugs under ultraviolet radiation. *J Am Pharm Assoc.*, 47:715.

Murray, C.J., Lopez A.,D. (1997). Mortality by cause for eight regions of theworld: global burden of disease study. *Lancet*, 349: 1269-76.

Nadkarni K.M. (2000). Indian Materia Medica. Vol: 1, Popular Prakashan, Mumbai.

Pari, L., Umamaheswari, J. (2000). Antihyperglycaemic activity of *Musa sapientum* flowers: effect on lipid peroxidation in alloxan diabetic rats. *Phytother Res.*, 14:1-3.

The Organization of Economic Co-operation Development (OECD), (2001b). The OECD Guideline for Testing of Chemical: Acute Oral Toxicity. OECD, Paris, pp. 1–14.

Trease, G.E. and Evans, W.C. (1972). Pharmacognosy, 10th Ed., Bailliere Tindall, London.

Vogel, G.,H, (2002). Drug discovery and evaluation: Pharmacological assays. Berlin, Heidelberg, New York, Springer.

Wallis, T.E. (1967). Textbook of Pharmacognosy, 5th Edition, J. and A. Churchill Ltd., London.

Wild, S., Roglic, G., Green, A., Sicree, R., King, H. (2004). Global prevalence of diabetes: estimates for the year 2000 and projections for 2030. *Diabetes Care.*, 27:1047-53.

Xiang-Yang, Qia,, Wei-Jun, Chen, Li-Qin Zhang, Bi-Jun, Xie. (2008). Mogrosides extract from *Siraitia grosvenori* scavenges free radicals *in vitro* and lowers oxidative stress, serum glucose, and lipid levels in alloxan-induced diabetic mice. *Nutr Res.*, 28: 278–284.

Medicinal Plants: Phytochemistry, Pharmacology and Therapeutics, Vol. 1 *Pages* ***406–412***
Editors: **V.K. Gupta, G.D. Singh, Surjeet Singh and A. Kaul**
Published by: **DAYA PUBLISHING HOUSE, NEW DELHI**

Chapter 25

Clinical Evaluation of *Anacardium occidentale*

Verônica S. Lopes[1,2*], Zélia M.S. Assis[1], Vanusia S. Galdino[1], Iaperi S. Araújo[1], Carlos L. Camacho[3], Dámaso P. Chacon[3], Tereza N.C. Dantas[2] and Maria Aparecida M. Maciel[2]**

[1]Maternidade Escola Januário Cicco (MEJC), Universidade Federal do Rio Grande do Norte, Campus Universitário, 59012-300, Natal, RN, Brazil

[2]Departamento de Química, Universidade Federal do Rio Grande do Norte, Campus Universitário, 59078-970, Natal, RN, Brazil

[3]Hospital Universitário Onofre Lopes (HUOL), Universidade Federal do Rio Grande do Norte, Campus Universitário, 59012-300, Natal, RN, Brazil

ABSTRACT

This study has the aim of identifying clinical action of antiinflammatory, analgesic and cicatrizing effects of an aqueous extract obtained from the steam bark of *Anacardium occidentale* (AE). Clinical evaluation of AE was performed to 1384 patients infected with skin (SL, caused by injury or disease) or mucous membrane lesions (MML, aphta, vulva erosion, uterus inflammation and body ulceration). The assisted patients were randomly separated in two groups, *e.g.* A (GA with 834 adult persons) and B (GB with 550 adult persons, corresponding to a control group receiving allopathic medication) and were attended at the Maternidade Escola Januário Cicco (MEJC) and Hospital Universitário Onofre Lopes (HUOL) medical centers. AE was administered

* Corresponding Author: E-mail: veronicalopes@ufrnnet.br.
** Corresponding Author for the submission process: E-mail: mammaciel@hotmail.com.

in two different formulations DF and EF [aqueous diluted AE formulation (DF) and emulsified-AE, in which 1 per cent of AE, 3.5 per cent of stearic acid, 2.5 per cent of monostearoyl glycerol, 0.5 per cent of tryethanolamine and 92.5 per cent of distilled water, corresponding to EF-formulation] and then prescribed to GA to treat and cure SL and MML. In the treatment of aphta the aqueous extract AE (in the DF-formulation) was prescribed twice or tree times/day (during a period of tree days). Meanwhile, EF-formulation indicated in the treatment of vulva erosion uterus inflammations (in dose of 2 g/day). The whole period of treatment ranged from 2 to 60 days, depending of each inflammation process. Several GA-patients showed scarification in their MML, which improve the cicatrizing process. The safe use of AE was proved by the reductions of the characteristic lesions symptoms growing to the total lesions cure, without any single registration of side effects or adverse reactions.

Keywords: *Anacardium occidentale, Aqueous extract, Cicatrizing effects, Clinical evaluation.*

Introduction

It seems paradoxical that, at a time when modern scientific medicine appears to be making such giant strides and enjoying unparalleled prestige, so much interest should be taken in traditional medicine, in both developed and developing countries (Bannerman, 1982). This statement is valid when one considers *Anacardium occidentale* a tropical specimen largely used in the Brazilian traditional health care. Generally, medicinal plants had long been used around the world without any medical recommendation or control. A Brazilian typical example could be cited for the street market called *Ver-o-peso* in Belém (capital of Pará State), which is part of the centuries-old folk medicine culture of Brazilian Amazon region. According to Prance (1992), Van Den Berg correlated 1,200 different medicinal Amazonian plants available for sale at *Ver-o-peso* representing the strong cultural Amazon belief. Moreover, in other regions of Brazil the use of extracts from Brazilian medicinal plants in the treatment of human disease is a common practice, which has increased greatly in recent years. However, many vegetal extracts are used by Brazilian people without knowledge of the side effects they can have upon their health.

Concerning to *Anacardium occidentale* L. (Anacardiacea) popularly known as 'cajueiro' (cashew), which occurs widely in all parts of Brazil and has a history of safe use in folk medicine, its leaves, stem bark, and nut/seed are largely used in the northeast region. *Anacardium occidentale* stem bark has popular indication to treat diabetes, diarrhoea, stomachache, and inflammation (Mota, 1985). Actually, this plant is extensively cultivated in India and east Africa. Additionally, has worldwide pharmacological uses, *e.g.*, cytotoxic (Africa, Mexico, Turkey and Guatemala) and tattoo (Africa), against caries, toothache, wart, stomach, diabetes and sore (Haiti, Venezuela, Turkey, Mexico, Malaya). *Anacardium occidentale* ethnobotanical importance consisting in treatment of several diseases such as hypertension, inflammatory diseases, asthmas, and bronchitis, gastric (peptic ulcers) and intestinal disturbances (Corrêa, 1984).

Previously pharmacological results obtained with the anacardic acid isolated from this species, showed antiinflammatory, antibacterial and febrifuge action (Eichbaum, 1949), been the antiinflammatory activity correlated to *Anacardium occidentale* methanolic and ethanolic extracts, and also to the tannin constituents isolated from those extracts (Akinpelu, 2000, Mota *et al.*, 1985). Its action against leishmania was also published (FranCa, 1993). The stem-bark is astringent because it is rich in tannin, then the possible validity of the popular indication as healing. In fact, previously studies conducted by Mota *et al.* (1985) have demonstrated that tannins isolated from the stem-bark of *Anacardium occidentale* possess analgesic and antiinflammatory effects. This antiinflammatory activity of the plant's stem-bark have been recently described, in two different models of inflammation, it reduced the rat paw oedema induced by fresh egg albumin (Ojewole, 2004) and produced inhibition in the leakage of dye in the mouse skin after subcutaneous injection of LPS (Olajide *et al.*, 2004).

In this work an aqueous extract obtained from stem bark of *Anacardium occidentale* (AE) was prescribed in both diluted (DF) and emulsion (EF) formulations, to a large amount of patients located at Rio Grande do Norte, a northeast State of Brazil. The present study has benefited from the involvement of chemistry, pharmacology and medical professionals, and summarizes clinical action of antiinflammatory, analgesic and cicatrizing effects.

Materials and Methods

Plant Material

Plant material was collected in January, May and September during all period of the present search (northeast of Brazil) and were identified by Maria Iracema Bezerra Loiola. A voucher specimen has been deposited in Herbarium of Universidade Federal do Rio Grande do Norte (Natal, Brazil) and a voucher specimen (number 1782) has been deposited in Herbarium of the Universidade Federal do Rio Grande do Norte (Natal, Brazil).

Phytochemical Approach

The adopted method in the phytochemical investigation involved the extraction of the powdered bark (1.3 kg) with water in a Soxhlet apparatus, affording 58 g the aqueous extract (AE) of AE, which was submitted to chromatography procedure over silica gel column giving three different chemical-type fractions F1 a non-polar fraction (eluted with hexane) corresponding to fixed oil constituents (hydrocarbon substances), F2 (eluted with CH_2Cl_2) a very poor chemical constituents fraction, and F3 a polar tannin fraction [eluted with $MeOH:H_2O$ (7:3)]. These fractions were analyzed using spectroscopic data (IV and NMR). The whole phytochemical methodology was previously described (Barcelos *et al.*, 2007). In this work only the AE was biologically examined.

Emulsion Formulation and Medical Treatment Approach

Several aqueous extraction of the powdered stem bark (each one using 400 g) of *Anacardium occidentale* afforded 12 L of an aqueous extract (AE), which was obtained by boiling water. After evaporation of the solvent the reduced volume of AE (10 l) was correlated to a diluted formula DF [DF + H_20 (1:1)], which was ingested in doses of by the selected patients. The emulsion formulation (EF) was performed with 1 per cent of the AE and 3.5 per cent of stearic acid, 2.5 per cent of monostearoyl glycerol, 0.5 per cent of tryethanolamine and 92.5 per cent of distilled water. Each patient received a tube with 200 g of AE in the EF and other ones if necessary. The conservation of both DF and EF was obtained by 0.05 per cent of EDTA (ethylenediaminetetraacetic), 0.1 per cent of methyl paraben and 0.1 per cent of propyl paraben, in addition 0.5 per cent of glycerin as an emollient agent. A total of 1384 patients were randomly separated into two groups. The group A (GA, a number of 834, in which 47 per cent were females) received AE in the both formulation DF and EF and to the control group B (GB, a number of 550, 47 per cent were females) was prescribed allopathic medication (antiinflammatory, analgesic and cicatrizing remedies). The assisted patients were from Natal (the capital city of Rio Grande do Norte) and also from a local community called Murici. The AE in both DF and EF formulations were prescribed by the medical team (V. S. Lopes, Z. M. S. Assis, V. S. Galdino, I. S. Araújo, C. L. Camacho, and D. P. Chacon).

Results and Discussion

The choice to study this specific medicinal plant *Anacardium occidentale* L. based on its ethnopharmacological data. This species may found in different countries around the world, resulting in possible chemical changes which may take place due to different environmental factors such as fertility, humidity, solar radiation, wind temperature, herbivores, air/soil pollution, and seasonality. According to Maciel *et al.* (2000, 2002, 2005) these variations may account for different results in the pharmacological action of the plant. Other factors such as the plants age and time for gathering may also bring changes into the chemical components contents as well as pharmacological results. Since secondary metabolites represent a chemical interface between plants and surrounding environment, their biosyntheses are frequently affected by environmental conditions. Thus, variations in the total content and/or of the relative proportions of secondary metabolites in plants can take place. Recently, Maciel *et al.* (2000, 2002, 2005), Munné-Bosch *et al.* (2000), Raffo *et al.* (2006), Gobbo-Neto and Lopes (2007), and also Kowalski (2007) have shown how environmental conditions influenced on the content of bioactive secondary metabolites. This statement justifying the phytochemical investigation performed in this work to the evaluated specimen *Anacardium occidentale*. This present work links phytochemistry and clinical investigations of the specimen *Anacardium occidentale* L. collected in Natal (Brazil) in order to improve its safe biological importance. The phytochemical investigation confirmed the presence of tannins that was correlated to the medicinal effectiveness of this plant.

Recently we developed new pharmacological investigations with *Anacardium occidentale* stem bark in order to prove its antioxidant and antimutagenicity efficacy. In that, two different microemulsions systems (SME) were obtained, in order to optimize the uses of due to the poor solubility in biological solvents of its stem bark tannin fraction. Those SME were used as solubilizing systems on the evaluation of the antioxidant potential of this plant. The SME were obtained using a mixture of Tween 80 and Span 20 (3:1) as surfactant, isopropyl myristate as oil phase and bidistilled water, consisting on two different systems (SME-1 and SME-4)]. In one of these systems ethanol was included as cosurfactant (SME-1) and for SME-4 ethanol-free. The antioxidant activity of a methanolic extract (MeOH, obtained from stem bark of this plant) and its tannin fraction (FT) after its solubilization in both SME-1 and SME-4, were evaluated in DPPH-method. The obtained results showed high antioxidant activity for both MeOH-extract (CE_{50} = 42.47±0.14 mg/mL) and FT (CE_{50} = 39.27±1.07 mg/mL for FT-SME-1, and CE_{50} = 42.20±5.20 mg/mL for FT-SME-4). These results indicated that the antioxidant activity of the MeOH-extract corresponded to the presence of tannins constituents. The tested microemulsions systems do not caused any significant interference in the antioxidant activity results evidenced on those tested fractions (Gomes *et al.*, 2006).

The mutagenicity and antimutagenicity of cashew stem bark methanolic extract (MeOH extract) on cell cultures of Chinese hamster lung fibroblasts (V79) were also evaluated. The cultures were treated with different concentrations of this MeOH-extract (500; 1000 and 2000 µg/ml) or the extract associated with doxorubicin (DXR) during the cell cycle phases G1, S, and G2 and throughout continuous treatment. Apart from these treatments, the cell cultures were also treated with PBS (negative-control) and DXR (positive-control). The data obtained in the chromosomal aberration (CA) test showed a significant reduction in CA frequency in the cultures treated with DXR extract and in comparison with those that received only DXR during the cell cycle phases G1 and S and throughout the entire cycle, as well as the absence of mutagenicity in all the treatments realized. The antimutagenic effect observed in this work reinforces the presence of the previously described therapeutic properties of cashew and indicates the safe use of this extract (Barcelos *et al.*, 2007). Moreover, the pharmacological evaluation of the analgesic, antioedematogenic and inhibitory leukocytes migration effects of *Anacardium occidentale* stem bark AE extract involves oral administration of mice (0.1, 0.3 and 1g/kg) or positive control indomethacin (10 mg/kg) inhibited the acetic acid-induced writhing at 18.9, 35.9, 62.9, and 68.9 per cent respectively (ID_{50} = 530 mg/kg). The higher dose of AE also was able to inhibited croton oil-induced ear oedema formation in 56.8 per cent (indomethacin at 10 mg/kg, *p.o.*; 57.6 per cent inhibition). When submitted to the carrageenan-induced peritonitis test AE (0.1, 0.3, and 1 g/kg, *p.o.*) impaired the leukocyte migration into the peritoneal cavity in 24.8, 40.5, and 49.6 per cent respectively. Dexamethasone (2 mg/kg, *s.c.*), the positive control, inhibited the leukocyte migration by 66.9 per cent (Vanderlinde *et al.*, 2008).

Those results jointed with previous pharmacological evidences such as antiinflammatory properties of this plant encourage us to report a clinical research developed at the Maternidade Escola Januário Cicco (MEJC) and Hospital Universitário Onofre Lopes of the Universidade Federal of Rio Grande do Norte (Natal, Brazil). The patients were assisted in a whole period of seventeen years (1986 to 2003). The assisted patients came to those medical centers infected with skin lesions (SL) caused by injury or disease or mucous membrane lesions (MML) such as aphta, vulva erosion, uterus inflammation and body ulceration.

In the treatment of aphta the AE were prescribed in the DF formulation twice or tree times/day (during a period of tree days) and the EF formulation was indicated in the treatment of vulva erosion uterus inflammations (in dose of 2 g/day). The observed reduction of the characteristic symptoms such as pain and redness, in the vulva erosion lesion, was detected from the second day of the beginning treatment and the total cure was observed in the period of the 8th to 15th day. Concerning to uterus inflammations in the same cited above dose, the reduction of the clinical symptoms came in the period of 8th to 20th days. From these results the total period of treatment was enlarged to 30-60 days (depending on the patient lesion response). The SL was treated using the EF formulation by topic skin use (2 to 3 times/day) in the whole period of 3 to 60 days, depending of the patient lesion. In all of the situations, the patients were previously submitted to an asepsis with PVPI (polyvinylpolypyrrolidone) or an aqueous solution of permanganato de potássio (1:10000). It was observed that several GA-patients (that had chronic lesions) showed scarification in their MML, this clinical result improve the cicatrisation process. Meanwhile the GB-patients did not show this cure process. In this case (GB-patients) the scarification was forced by surgical procedure leading to the total cure.

Conclusion

In Brazil the use of extracts from Brazilian medicinal plants in the treatment of human disease is a common practice, which has increased greatly in recent years. However, many vegetal extracts are used by people without knowledge of the side effects they can have upon their health. In this context the medicinal specimen *Anacardium occidentale* has a safe folk history of uses and are included in the whole of Brazilian medicinal plants scientific researches. In this work, the clinic effect of AE obtained from the stem bark of the *Anacardium occidentale* was confirmed by the analgesic, antiinflammatory and cicatrisation action of AE prescribed in the both tested formulations DF and EF, on skin and mucous lesions of 834 patients. The safe use of DF and EF was proved by the reductions of the characteristic lesions symptoms (pain, redness, flame, craving and oedema) growing to the total lesions cure without any single registration of side effects or adverse reactions. Taking into account the total amount (1384) of the treated patients (550 of them as a control group) the potential medicinal value of the *Anacardium occidentale* is undeniable. The pre-clinical research reported data against pain and inflammatory diseases jointed to these clinical results support the renowned folk medicinal use of *Anacardium occidentale*.

Acknowledgements

The authors thank Professor Dr. Maria Iracema Bezerra Loiola (UFRN) for the botanic identification and CNPq for scholarship support.

References

Akinpelu, D.A. (2000). Antimicrobial activity of *Anacardium occidentale*. *Fitoterapia*, 72: 286-287.

Bannerman, R.H. (1982). Traditional medicine in modern health care, *World Health Forum*, 3: 8-26.

Barcelos, G.R.M., Shimabukuro, F., Mori, M.P., Maciel, M.A.M., Cólus, I.M.S. (2007). Evaluation of mutagenicity and antimutagenicity of cashew stem bark methanolic extract *in vivo*. *Journal of Ethopharmacology*, 114: 268-273.

Corrêa, P.M. (1984). Dicionário das Plantas Úteis do Brasil. Rio de Janeiro, Imprensa Nacional, p. 402.

Eichbaum, F. W. (1949). Biological properties of anacardic acid (O-penta-decadienyl-salicylic acid and related compounds. *Memorias do Instituto Butantã*, 19: 119-133.

FranCa, F., Cuba, C.A., Moreira, E.A., Miguel, O., Almeida, M., Das Virgens, M.L., Maarsden, P.D. (1993). An evaluation of the effect of a bark extract from the cashew (*Anacardium occidentale* L.) on infection by Leishmania (Viannnia) brasiliensis. *Revista da Sociedade Brasileira de Medicina Tropical*, 26: 151-155.

Gobbo-Neto, L., and Lopes, N. P. (2007) Medicinal Plants: factors of influence on the content of secondary metabolites. *Química Nova*, 30: 374-381.

Gomes FES, Anjos GC, Dantas TNC, Maciel, MAM, Esteves A, Echevarria A (2006): ObtenCão de NanoformulaCões do Tipo Microemulsão Objetivando a BiodisponibilizaCão de *Anacardium occidentale* e sua Eficiência como Agente Antioxidante. *Revista Fitos*, *2*(3): 82-88.

Kowalski, R. (2007). Studies of selected plant raw materials as alternative sources of triterpenes of oleanolic and ursolic acid types. *Journal of Agricultural and Food Chemistry*, 55: 656-662.

Maciel, M.A.M., Pinto, A.C., Arruda, A.C., Pamplona, S.G.S.R., Vanderline, F.A., Lapa, A.J., Echevarria, A., Grynberg, N.F., Côlus, I.M.S., Farias, R.A.F., Luna Costa, A.M., and Rao, V.S.N. (2000). Ethnopharmacology, phytochemistry and pharmacology: a successful combination in the study of *Croton cajucara*. *Journal of Ethnopharmacology*, 70: 41-55.

Maciel, M.A.M., Pinto, A.C., and Veiga JR., V.F. (2002). Plantas Medicinais: a necessidade de estudos multidisciplinares. *Química Nova*, 25: 429-438.

Maciel, M. A. M., Dantas, T. N. C., Pinto, A.C., Veiga Jr., V. F., Grymberg, N. F., and Echevarria, A. (2005). Medicinal Plants: the need for multidisciplinary scientific studies. Part II. *Current Topics in Phytochemictry*, 7: 73-88.

Mota, M.L., Thomas, G., and Barbosa Filho, J.M. (1985). Antiinflammatory actions of tannins isolated from the bark of *Anacardium occidentale* L. *Journal of Ethnopharmacology*, 13: 289-300.

Munné-Bosch, S., Alegre, L., and Schwarz, K. (2000). The formation of phenolic diterpenes in *Rosmarinus officinalis* L. under Mediterranean climate. *European Food Research Technology*, 210: 263-267.

Ojewole, J.A. (2004). Potentiation of the antiinflammatory effect of *Anacardium occidentale* L. stem-bark aqueous extract by grapefruit juice. *Methods and Findings Experimental Clinical Pharmacology*, 26:183-188.

Olajide, O.A., Aderogba, M.A., Adedapo, A.D., Makinde, J.M. (2004). Effects of *Anacardium occidentale* stem bark extract on *in vivo* inflammatory models. *Journal of Ethnopharmacology*, 95: 139-142.

Prance, G.T. (1992). Out of the Amazon. London: HMSO Publicatins Centres. p.87.

Raffo. A., La Malfa, G., Fogliano, V., Maiani, G., and Quaglia, G. (2006) Seasonal variations in antioxidant components of cherry tomatoes (*Lycopersicon esculentum* cv. Naomi F1). *Journal of Food Composition Analysis*, 19: 11-19.

Vanderlinde, F.A., Landim, H.F., Costa, E.A., Matos, L.G., Maciel, M.A.M., Anjos, G. C., Dants, T.N.C., Côrtes, W.S., Rocha, F.F. (2008) Antinociceptive, antioedematogenic and inhibitory leukocytes migration effects produced by an acetonic extract (AE) from *Anacardium occidentale*, Anacardiaceae. *Journal of Psychology*, (submitted).

Medicinal Plants: Phytochemistry, Pharmacology and Therapeutics, Vol. 1 *Pages* ***413–420***
Editors: **V.K. Gupta, G.D. Singh, Surjeet Singh and A. Kaul**
Published by: **DAYA PUBLISHING HOUSE, NEW DELHI**

Chapter 26

Effect of *Emblica officinalis* Diet in Streptozotocin Diabetic Mice

Richa Shri* and Disha Arora
Department of Pharmaceutical Sciences and Drug Research,
Punjabi University, Patiala, Punjab, India

ABSTRACT

The popular and commonly used fruit–amla (*Emblica officinalis*), is called a maharasaayana in the Ayurveda and is traditionally used for the management of diabetes. Diet plays a major role in the management of diabetes. Hence in the present study diet containing various doses of amla fruit powder (5, 10 and 15 per cent) was fed to normal and diabetic mice (Blood glucose levels ? 250mg/dl induced by STZ 200mg/kg IP) for 21 days. Results show that amla diet showed hypoglycemic effect that was most significant with diet containing 20 per cent amla *i.e.* there was a 6 per cent reduction in the blood glucose level as compared to the basal value. After induction of diabetes amla diets were continued in one set of animals and significant antihyperglycemic effect was observed. Feeding 5, 10 and 20 per cent diet produced a reduction in blood glucose by 20.7, 31 and 38.9 per cent respectively when compared with diabetic control on day 32 of the study. In another set of experimental animals after pretreatment with amla diets, there was induction of diabetes following which animals were fed normal diet. In this group negligible antihyperglycemic effect (4 per cent reduction of blood glucose was observed in group which had pretreatment with 20 per cent amla diet) was observed. Also serum TBARS levels among the groups treated with amla diet were lower with respect to diabetic control. This shows that diet containing *Emblica officinalis* has hypoglycemic and antihyperglycemic effect and reduces the oxidative stress in experimental diabetes.

Keywords: *Emblica officinalis, Diet, Antioxidant, Diabetes, Streptozotocin.*

* Corresponding Author: E-mail: rshri587@hotmail.com.

Introduction

Diabetes mellitus is one of the most common endocrine disorders that affect more than 100 million people worldwide (6 per cent of the population) and in the next 10 years it may affect about five times more population (King *et al.*, 1998; Grover *et al.*, 2002). The effects of diabetes are devastating and well documented. Diet, exercise and medical intervention with drugs like insulin, thiazolidinediones etc are used for the management of diabetes mellitus (White and Campbell, 1996; Tripathi, 2003).

Oxidative stress is involved in the pathogenesis of diabetes and its complications. Use of antioxidants reduces oxidative stress and alleviates diabetic complications (Sabu and Kuttan, 2002). Antioxidants, vitamins C and E have been shown to reduce the oxidative stress in experimental diabetes (Madhu and Devi, 2000; Rahimi *et al.*, 2005). Antioxidant-enriched dietary strategy using specific traditional plant food combinations can generate a whole food profile that has the potential to reduce hyperglycemia-induced pathogenesis and also associated complications (Ruhe and McDonald, 2001). Hence dietary supplementation with antioxidant nutrients may be a safe and simple complement to traditional therapies for preventing and treating diabetic complications (Tapsell *et al.*, 2006; Kwon *et al.*, 2007).

Emblica officinalis (family Euphorbiaceae) which is used traditionally to manage diabetes (Kirtikar and Basu, 1993; Ghosal *et al.*, 1996), possesses potent antioxidant activity because of its rich vitamin C and polyphenol contents (Ghosal *et al.*, 1996; Bhattacharya *et al.*, 1999; Prakash *et al.*, 2000; Khopde *et al.*, 2001; Sabu and Kuttan, 2002; Jain and Khurdiya, 2004; Rao *et al.*, 2005) but so far its role in diabetes has not been investigated. Hence the present study has been designed to investigate the effect of pretreatment with amla (*Emblica officinalis*) diet on blood glucose levels, body weight and TBARS (Thiobarbituric acid reactive substances) levels of normal and diabetic mice.

Materials and Methods

Plant Material

Fruits of *Emblica officinalis* were purchased from the local market (Patiala, Punjab, India) in the month of March and April, 2007 and were authenticated by Dr. H. B. Singh, National Institute of Science Communication and Information Resources, New Delhi, India (vide voucher number NISCAIR/ RHM/F-3/2006/Conslt/662/143).

Chemicals

Thiobarbituric acid; streptozotocin; 1,1,3,3-tetraethoxypropane were obtained from Sigma Chemicals; solvents (petroleum ether, methanol, chloroform) were of analytical reagent grade and purchased from Loba Chem. All the other reagents were of analytical reagent grade.

Animals

Swiss albino mice weighing 20-30g of either sex were employed in the present study. Animals were housed in the institutional animal house under standard conditions, with 12 hour light and 12 hour dark cycle and they had free access to food (Kisan feeds Ltd., New Delhi, India) and tap water *ad libitum*.

Preparation of Treatment Diet

The authenticated fruits of *Emblica officinalis* were dried under shade at room temperature (<30 °C). After complete drying, the fruits were grounded into a fine powder using a domestic electric grinder and mixed thoroughly with the already grounded standard chow diet. Binder in the form of 1 per cent starch solution was added to the mixture and kneaded into a dough, with a semisolid consistency. The dough was then spread on a tray and cut into pieces of suitable size. Different dose diets were prepared by mixing fruit powder with chow powder in the ratio of 5 per cent, 10 per cent and 20 per cent separately.

Sample Collection

Blood samples were collected retro-orbitally from inner canthus of eyes using Micro Hematocrit Capillaries from overnight fasted animals.

Induction of Experimental Diabetes

Administration of streptozotocin (200 mg/kg, i.p.) produced hyperglycemia. Three days after administration of the diabetogenic agent fasting blood glucose was determined and mice with blood glucose level more than 250mg/dl were included in the study.

Parameters Studied

- *Fasting blood glucose*: Blood glucose was estimated by commercially available glucose kit based on glucose oxidase method (Trinder, 1969).
- *Body weight*: Gravimetrically
- *TBARS*: Malondialdehyde concentration was measured by estimating thiobarbituric acid reactive substances (TBARS) (Liu *et al.*, 1995).

Experimental Protocol

The experimental animals were divided into five groups:

Normal Control (Group I, n = 5)

Blood samples of the overnight fasted mice were collected retro-orbitally on day 0, just prior to the initiation of various treatment schedules, for the estimation of the three parameters.

Diabetic Control (Group II, n = 5)

Three weeks after the administration of streptozotocin (200 mg/kg, i.p.) *i.e.* 21st day, blood samples of the overnight fasted mice were collected retro-orbitally for the experimental parameters.

Treated Groups (Group III-V, n = 30)

Three different dose diets containing *Emblica officinalis* fruit powder (5 per cent, 10 per cent and 20 per cent) were fed to normal mice *i.e.*, groups III–V (each group consisted of 10 animals) for ten days.

On the 10th day, the experimental parameters were determined. This was done to assess the hypoglycemic effect of *Emblica officinalis.*

On 11th day, the treated groups were rendered diabetic by single streptozotocin injection (200 mg/kg, i.p.). After induction of diabetes, groups III-V were subdivided as:

Group III divided into III_a (n = 5) and III_b (n = 5)

Group IV divided into IV_a (n = 5) and IV_b (n = 5)

Group V divided into V_a (n = 5) and V_b (n = 5)

Groups III_a, IV_a and V_a were continued on the amla diet (5 per cent,10 per cent and 20 per cent, respectively) for 21 days to assess the antihyperglycemic effect of amla diet.

While groups III_b, IV_b and V_b were fed normal chow diet for 21 days in order to observe prophylactic effect of pretreatment with amla diet.

After 3 weeks of the treatment, blood samples from the overnight fasted mice were collected retro-orbitally from both the subgroups for the estimation of the different parameters.

Statistical Analysis

The data for blood glucose, body weight and thiobarbituric acid reactive substances (TBARS) was expressed as mean±S.D. Data was analysed using one way ANOVA. Multiple range Tukey's test was employed as post-hoc test for comparison between various groups and with control group. p? 0.05 was considered to be statistically significant.

Results and Discussion

Single dose of streptozotocin (STZ) is well reported to induce insulin dependent diabetes mellitus (IDDM) in mice (200 mg/kg, i.p.) (Anjaneyulu and Chopra, 2003) and in rats (65 mg/kg, i.p.) (Malcangio and Tomlinson, 1998; Utugol *et al.*, 2002). STZ selectively destroys pancreatic β cells, induces uniform hyperglycemia due to fragmentation of DNA in pancreatic b cells (Yamamoto *et al.*, 1981; Morgan *et al.*, 1994; Delaney *et al.*, 1995; Elsner *et al.*, 2000).

Diabetes mellitus of long duration is associated with several complications such as atherosclerosis, myocardial infarction, neuropathy, nephropathy etc. These complications are related to chronically elevated glucose levels and subsequent oxidative stress. Oxidative stress in diabetes may partially be reduced by antioxidants and hence antioxidants have been prescribed to reduce the long term complications seen in diabetes (Sabu and Kuttan, 2002).

In this study, *Emblica officinalis* a known antioxidant was incorporated in the diet of the experimental animals and effect on blood glucose levels, body weight and serum TBARS level was observed.

Effect of *Emblica officinalis* Diet on Blood Glucose Levels

The results of *Emblica Officinalis* diet treatments on blood glucose levels are reported in Table 26.1. Basal blood glucose levels of normal control (NC) as well as treated groups were well matched (86-89mg/dl). In normal mice, after 10 days of treatment with amla diets (5, 10, 20 per cent), a dose dependent hypoglycemic effect was observed. The lowering of blood glucose in normal animals was most significant with diet containing 20 per cent amla.

The study was continued by dividing these animals which had received pretreatment with amla diets into two groups–in first group animals amla diet was continued and in second group animals normal diet was given to the animals. Results show that *Emblica officinalis* produces significant inhibition of STZ induced diabetes in mice. The blood glucose levels among the groups treated with amla diet were lower with respect to diabetic control (most significant in amla 20 per cent) indicating antihyperglycemic effect of amla diet. When the effect of amla diet was compared with normal diet, the blood glucose lowering effect was significantly more with amla diet. In addition to this, the blood glucose levels among the groups pretreated with amla diet and followed by normal diet were lower with respect to diabetic control (most significant in amla 20 per cent). This shows that amla diet has prophylactic antihyperglycemic effect.

Table 26.1: Effect of Feeding Various Diets of *Emblica officinalis* on Blood Glucose Levels (mg/dl)

Groups	*Blood Glucose (mg/dl) Day 0*		*Blood Glucose (mg/dl) Day 32*	
NC	89.2±2.02		90.3±4.22	
DC	89.2±2.02		251.1±9.24*	
Groups	*Basal Blood Glucose (mg/dl) Day 0*	*Blood Glucose Before STZ treatment Amla Diet Day 10*	*Blood Glucose After STZ treatment Day 32*	
			Amla Diet	*Normal Diet*
Amla 5 per cent	86.6±7.24	84.6±8.54	198.3±5.22**#	246.5±14.60**
Amla 10 per cent	86.7±8.86	82.8±6.42•	173.2±14.61**#	243.2±9.24**
Amla 20 per cent	86.1±7.43	80.6±5.45•	153.5±6.10**#	240.1±6.41**

The results were expressed as mean±SD (n = 5).

**p<0.05 as compared to diabetic control. # p<0.05 as compared to the effect produced by respective standard chow diet.

• p<0.05 as compared to the basal blood glucose level.

Effect of *Emblica officinalis* Diet on Body Weight

The following body weight observations were recorded in the experimental animals (Table 26.2).

Table 26.2: Effect of Feeding Various Diets of *Emblica officinalis* on Body Weight (g)

Groups	*Blood Glucose (mg/dl) Day 0*		*Blood Glucose (mg/dl) Day 32*	
NC	22.0±1.32		23.0±1.58	
DC	22.0±1.32		15.8±1.92*	
Groups	*Basal Blood Glucose (mg/dl) Day 0*	*Blood Glucose Before STZ treatment Amla Diet Day 10*	*Blood Glucose After STZ treatment Day 32*	
			Amla Diet	*Normal Diet*
Amla 5 per cent	22.6±1.94	21.2±2.10	17.8±2.16	17.2±2.16
Amla 10 per cent	22.6±1.81	21.5±1.9	17.4±1.51	16.6±1.81
Amla 20 per cent	23.4±1.51	23.4±1.51	19.6±1.51**	18.4±1.14**

The results were expressed as mean±SD (n = 5).

**p<0.05 as compared to diabetic control.

A reduction in body weight was observed in mice with STZ induced diabetes. Loss of weight is due to excessive breakdown of tissue proteins (Chatterjea and Shinde, 2002). Hakim *et al.* (1997) have stated that decreased body weight in diabetic rodents could be due to dehydration and catabolism of fats and proteins. Increased catabolic reactions leading to muscle wasting might also be the cause for the reduced weight gain by diabetic rodents (Rajkumar *et al.*, 1991). Body weight in diabetic control showed continuous decrease throughout the experimental period and remained significantly less than the normal control. When the amla diet was given to diabetic groups, the decrease in body weight was minimized as compared to the diabetic groups treated with standard diet. This may be due to decreased dehydration, catabolism of fats and proteins.

Effect of *Emblica officinalis* Diet on TBARS Levels

The results also show a strong antioxidant activity of *Emblica officinalis* which may be due to the presence of vitamin C which has potent antioxidant effect (Khopde *et al.*, 2001) or due to the presence of several gallic acid derivatives including epigallocatechin gallate (Sabu and Kuttan, 2002). Reactive oxygen species (ROS) produce malondialdehyde (MDA), an end product of lipid peroxidation. MDA reacts with thiobarbituric acid (TBA) and is thus estimated as thiobarbituric acid reactive substances (TBARS) (Dib *et al.*, 2002).

The respective serum TBARS levels among the groups treated with amla diet were lower with respect to diabetic control (significant in amla 20 per cent) as compared with the groups treated with standard chow diet. Also, when the effect of amla diet was compared with the normal diet, the reduction in TBARS levels was significantly more with amla diet. This shows that *Emblica officinalis* diet reduces the oxidative stress in experimental diabetes.

Table 26.3: Effect of Feeding Various Diets of *Emblica officinalis* on TBARS Levels (nM)

Groups	*TBARS Levels (nM) Day 0*	*TBARS Levels (nM) Day 21*		
NC	20.0±3.4	20.0±3.4		
DC	20.0±3.4	60.0±4.0*		
Groups	*Basal TBARS Levels Day 0*	*TBARS Levels Before STZ treatment Amla Diet Day 10*	*TBARS Levels After STZ treatment Day 32*	
			Amla Diet	*Normal Diet*
Amla 5 per cent	10.0±2.0	19.0±1.0*	35.3±1.0**#	50.0±30.0**
Amla 10 per cent	11.0±1.0	18.0±1.0*	32.2±1.0**#	48.0±4.0**
Amla 20 per cent	20.0±1.0	16.0±1.0*	25.9±2.0**#	47.0±4.0**

The results were expressed as mean±SD (n = 5).

p<0.05 as compared to normal control. **p<0.05 as compared to diabetic control.

# p<0.05 as compared to the effect produced by respective standard chow diet.

Conclusion

In Ayurveda, two forms of diabetes have been described–one based on genetic causes and second as a result of dietary indiscretion. Hence diet is the cornerstone in the management of diabetes.

In the present study, we have investigated the efficacy of feeding amla (*Emblica officinalis*) as a dietary constituent in the management of diabetes. *Emblica officinalis* exerted hypoglycemic and antihyperglycemic effect as diet containing higher proportion of *Emblica officinalis* (*i.e.* 20 per cent) significantly prevented the rise in blood glucose as well as reduced the TBARS levels in normal and STZ diabetic mice. *Emblica officinalis* prevented loss in body weight due to diabetes. This shows that diet containing *Emblica officinalis* has hypoglycemic and antihyperglycemic effect and reduces the oxidative stress in experimental diabetes.

The fruit is safe in long-term use as it has been consumed through ages as a dietary constituent and no toxic effects have been reported. Thus, in conclusion of the above mentioned facts, the present study suggests that *Emblica officinalis* if incorporated in diet can play an important role in the prophylaxis and management of mild diabetes.

References

Anjaneyulu, M. and Chopra, K. (2003). Quercetin, a bioflavonoid, attenuates thermal hyperalgesia in a mouse model of diabetic neuropathic pain. *Neuro. Psychopharmc.*, 27:1001-1050.

Bhattacharya, A., Chatterjee, A., Ghosal, S. and Bhattacharya, S.K. (1999). Antioxidant activity of active tannoid principles of *Emblica officinalis* (amla). *Indian J. Exp. Biol.*, 37: 676-680.

Chatterjea, M.N. and Shinde, R. (2002). In: *Textbook of medical biochemistry*. Jaypee Brothers, Medical Publishers Pvt. Ltd., New Delhi, p.317.

Delaney, C.A., Dunger, A., Di Matteo, M., Cunningham, J.M., Green, M.H. and Green, I.C. (1995). Comparison of inhibition of glucose-stimulated insulin secretion in rat islets of Langerhans by STZ and methyl and ethyl nitrosoureas and methane sulphonates. Lack of correlation with nitric oxide-releasing or O6-alkylating ability. *Biochem. Pharmacol.*, 50: 2015-2020.

Dib, M., Garrel,C., Favier, A., Robin, V., Desnuelle,C. (2002) Can malondialdehyde be used as a biological marker of progression in neurodegenerative disease? *J. Neurol.*, 249:367.

Elsner, M., Guldbackke, B., Tiedge, M., Munday, R. and Lenzen, S. (2000). Relative importance of transport and alkylation for pancreatic beta-cell toxicity of STZ. *Diabetologia*, 43: 1528-1533.

Ghosal, S., Tripathi, V.K. and Chauhan, S. (1996). Active constituents of *Emblica officinalis*: Part 1–The chemistry and antioxidative effects of two new hydrolysable tannins, Emblicanin A and B. *Indian J. Chem.*, 35B:941-948.

Grover, J.K., Yadav, S. and Vats, V. (2002). Medicinal plants of India with antidiabetic potential. *J. Ethnopharmacol.*, 81: 81-100.

Hakim, Z.S., Patel, B.K. and Goyal, R.K. (1997). Effects of chronic ramipril treatment in streptozotocin-induced diabetic rats. *Indian J. Physiol. Pharmacol.*, 41: 353-360.

Jain, S.K. and Khurdiya, D.S. (2004). Vitamin C enrichment of fruit juice based ready-to-serve beverages through blending of Indian gooseberry (*Emblica officinalis* Gaertn.) juice. *Plant Foods for Human Nutrition*, 59: 63-66.

Khopde, S.M., Priyadarsini, K.I., Mohan, H., Gawandi, V.B., Satav, J.G., Yakhmi, J.V., Banavaliker, M.M., Biyani, M.K. and Mittal, J.P. (2001). Characterizing the antioxidant activity of amla (*Phyllanthus emblica*) extracts. *Curr. Sci.*, 82(2): 185-190.

King, H., Aubert, R.E. and Herman, W.H. (1998). Global burden of diabetes, 1995-2025: prevalence numerical estimates and projections. *Diabetes Care*, 21: 1414-1431.

Kirtikar, K.R. and Basu, B.D. (1993). *Phyllanthus* Linn. In: *Indian Medicinal Plants*, 2nd Edition, III, Blatter, E., Caius, J.F. and Mhaskar, K.S. (eds.), Basu, L.M., Allahabad, India, pp. 2219-2227.

Kwon YI, Apostolidis E, Kim YC, Shetty K. (2007) Health benefits of traditional corn, beans and pumpkin: *in vitro* studies for hyperglycemia and hypertension management. *J Med Food.*,10(2):266-75.

Liu J, Edamatsu R, Kabuto H, Mori A. (1990) Antioxidant action of guilingji in the brain of rats with $FeCl_3$-induced epilepsy. *Free Radic Biol Med.*, 9(5): 451-454.

Madhu, C.G. and Devi, D.B. (2000). Protective antioxidant effect of vitamins C and E in streptozotocin induced diabetic rats. *Indian J. Exp. Biol.*, 38: 101-104.

Malcangio, M. and Tomlinson, D.R. (1998). A pharmacologic analysis of mechanical hyperalgesia in STZ/diabetic rats. *Pain*, 76:151-157.

Morgan, N.G., Cable, H.C., Newcombe, N.R. and Williams, G.T. (1994). Treatment of cultured pancreatic b-cells with STZ induced cell death by apoptosis. *Biosci. Rep.*, 14: 243-250.

Prakash, D., Niranjan, A. and Tewari, S.K. (2000). Vitamin C in *Emblica officinalis* (amla) and its products. *JMAPS.*, 22: 237-241.

Rahimi R, Nikfar S, Larijani B, Abdollahi M. (2005) A review on the role of antioxidants in the management of diabetes and its complications. *Biomed Pharmacother.*, 59(7):365-73.

Rajkumar, L., Srinivasan, N., Balasubramanian, K. and Govindarajulu, P. (1991). Increased degradation of dermal collagen in diabetic rats. *Indian J. Exp. Biol.*, 29: 1081-1083.

Rao, T.P., Sakaguchi, N., Juneja, L.R., Wada, E. and Yokozawa, T. (2005). Amla (*Emblica officinalis* Gaertn.) extracts reduce oxidative stress in streptozotocin-induced diabetic rats. *J. Med. Food.*, 8(3): 362-368.

Ruhe RC, McDonald RB.(2001) Use of antioxidant nutrients in the prevention and treatment of type 2 diabetes. *J Am Coll Nutr.*, (5 Suppl):363S-369S

Sabu, M.C. and Kuttan, R. (2002). Antidiabetic activity of medicinal plants and its relationship with their antioxidant property. *J Ethnopharmacol.*, 81: 155-160.

Tapsell LC, Hemphill I, Cobiac L, Patch CS, Sullivan DR, Fenech M, Roodenrys S, Keogh JB, Clifton PM, Williams PG, Fazio VA, Inge KE.(2006) Health benefits of herbs and spices: the past, the present, the future. *Med J Aust..*, 185(4 Suppl):S4-24.

Trinder, P. (1969) Determination of glucose in blood using glucose oxidase with an alternative oxygen receptor, Ann. Clin. Biochem. 6: 24-27

Tripathi, K.D. (2003). Insulin, Oral hypoglycemic drugs and glucagon In: *Essentials of Medical Pharmacology*, 5th edition, Tripathi K.D. (ed.), Jaypee Brothers, Medical Publishers (P)Ltd., New Delhi, pp. 235-253.

White, J.R. and Campbell, R.K. (1996). Diabetes mellitus In: *Textbook of therapeutics: Drug disease and management*. 6th Edition. Herfindal, E.T. and Gourley, D.R. (eds.), Williams and Wilkins A Waverly Company, pp. 357-386.

Yamamoto, H., Uchigata, Y. and Okamoto, H. (1981). STZ and alloxan induce DNA strand breaks and poly (ADP-ribose) synthetase in pancreatic islets. *Nature*, 294: 284-286.

Medicinal Plants: Phytochemistry, Pharmacology and Therapeutics, Vol. 1 *Pages* **421–429**
Editors: **V.K. Gupta, G.D. Singh, Surjeet Singh and A. Kaul**
Published by: **DAYA PUBLISHING HOUSE, NEW DELHI**

Chapter 27

Investigation into the Folkloric Antimicrobial and Antiinflammatory Properties of *Nauclea latifolia* Leaves and Stem Bark Extracts and Fractions

P.O. Osadebe*, U. Ajali, F.B.C. Okoye and C. Diara
Department of Pharmaceutical and Medicinal Chemistry,
Faculty of Pharmaceutical Sciences, University of Nigeria,
Nsukka, Enugu State, Nigeria

ABSTRACT

Nauclea latifolia leaves and stem bark are used traditionally as tonic and fever medicine, and in the management of toothache, dental caries, septic mouth and malaria. The antimicrobial and antiinflammatory properties of these plant materials are investigated. The crude methanolic extracts and its various solvent fractions L1-L5 for leaves and S1-S4 for stem bark were screened for antimicrobial activities against selected clinical strains of microorganisms. The crude extracts were also subjected to antiinflammatory screening using egg-albumen-induced rat paw edema as a model of inflammation. At 200 mg/kg, the crude methanolic extracts of *Nauclea latifolia* leaves and stem bark showed mild antiinflammatory activity with edema inhibitions of 33.3 and 13.3 per cent at 4 h respectively. The crude extracts showed antimicrobial activity against *Bacillus subtilis, Eschericia coli* and *Salmonella parathyphi.* All the fractions showed activity against *Eschericia coli.* Only fractions L4, S2 and S4 have activity against *Salmonella parathyphi,* fractions L1 and L2 have activity against *Bacillus subtilis,* while fractions L4, S2 and S3 have activity against

* Corresponding Author: E-mail: mkemamaka@yahoo.com.

Staphylococcus aureus. The antimicrobial activity of S2 against *Staphylococcus aureus*, *Escherichia coli* and *Salmonella parathyphi* is comparable to that of standard drug, Gentamicin. Phytochemical tests revealed the presence of alkaloids, terpens, flavonoids, saponins and tannins in the crude extracts and in the fractions. S2 contains only flavonoids, which were found on UV analysis to lack free hydroxyl groups at positions 7, 3^1 and 4^1 of the flavonoid nucleus. In conclusion, the antimicrobial activity of the leaves may be due to the flavonoids and tannins found in L4 while that of the stem bark may be due the flavonoids in S2. The mild antiinflammatory effect could be an added advantage in management of toothache, which is normally associated with microbial inversion and mild inflammation.

Keywords: *Antiinflammatory, Antimicrobial, Folkloric, Nauclea latifolia.*

Introduction

Infectious disease is the number one cause of death accounting for approximately one-half of all deaths in tropical countries (Iwu, 1999). Several efforts towards combating the menace of infectious disease are yet to achieve the desired goals. The situation even becomes worrisome with the emergence of newer forms of respiratory tract infections, HIV/AIDS, and increase in antibiotic resistance in nosocomial and community acquired infections. Plant derived products have shown great promise in the treatment of intractable infectious diseases including opportunistic AIDS infections. Numerous and diverse classes of plants metabolites have been isolated and their structures characterized in the past century (Kirkpatrick, 2002). Efforts are still directed in current times towards generating novel lead antiinfective agents from plants.

Nauclea latifolia Smith (Rubiaceae) is a shrub or small spreading tree widely distributed in Savanna. It is found in forests and fringe tropical forests. The plant has been used traditionally as a tonic and fever medicine, as a chewing stick, and in the management of toothache, dental caries, septic mouth, malaria, diarrhoea and dysentery (Lamidi *et al.*, 1995). Owing to these rich folkloric uses, several attentions have been directed in recent times towards investigating some pharmacological activities of the plant with the view of validating the claimed ethnomedicinal uses. Some of these studies are: hepatoprotective effects of the leaf extract (Akpanabiatu *et al.*, 2005a, 2005b), effects of the leaf and root extract on purinergic neurotransmission in rat bladder and on cardiovascular systems (Udoh, 1995, 1998) and effect of leaf extracts on blood glucose levels (Gidado *et al.*, 2005). Other studies include anthelminthic effect of the stem bark extract (Onyeliyi *et al.*, 2001), amoebicidal activity (Moundipat *et al.*, 2005), trypanosomidal activity of the root bark extract (Madubuenyi, 1996) antimalarial activity (Iwu, 1993). Recently, Otimenyi and Uguru (2006) investigated the acute toxicity, antiinflammatory and analgesic activities of the methanolic extracts of the stem bark. The key phytoconstituents which have been isolated from the plant are indole-quinolizidine alkaloids, glycolalkaloids, monoterpene indole alkaloids and saponins (Iwu *et al.*, 1999; Shigemiri *et al.*, 2003).

In spite of the numerous attentions directed to this plant in the recent times, there is yet no scientific report on the antimicrobial properties of the leaf and stem bark extracts. In the present study, the antimicrobial activity of the extracts and fractions of *Nauclea latifolia* leaves and stem bark is reported. Since the plant is used traditionally in the management of septic mouth, toothache and dental caries, disease conditions which are usually associated with microbial inversion and inflammatory response, we also investigated the antiinflammatory effect of the leaf and stem bark extracts.

Materials and Methods

Plant Material

The leaves and stem bark of *Nauclea latifolia* were collected an identified by Mr Ozioko Alfred of BDCP, Nsukka. The materials were cleaned, air-dried and reduced to course powder.

Chemicals

Analytical grades n-hexane, chloroform, ethylacetate, acetone and methanol (BDH) were used. Other materials used are silica gel (70-230) (May and Baker), Sabouraud's Dextrose Agar (SDA), Nutrient Agar (Merck). Freshly distilled water was used when required. Phytochemical reagents were freshly prepared.

Test Microorganisms

Clinical strains of *Salmonella paratyphi, Bacillus subtilis, Klebsiella pneumonia, Pseudomonas aeruginosa, Escherichia coli, Staphylococcus aureus, Candida albicans, Aspergillus niger* obtained from the pharmaceutical microbiology unit of the Department of Pharmaceutics, University of Nigeris were used.

Animals

Wistar rats weighing 100±20 g were purchased from the laboratory animal house of Department of Pharmacology and Toxicology.

Extraction and Fractionatin

The powder leaves and stem bark (100 g each) were extracted for 48 h by cold maceration in methanol. Another 100 g portions were extracted by soxhlet for 4 h in methanol. All the crude extracts were subjected to antimicrobial studies.

A 15–g portion of the soxhlet methanol extract of the leave (LS) was adsorbed onto silica gel and eluted successively with hexane, chloroform, ethylacetae, acetone and methanol to yield hexane (L1), chloroform (L2), ethylacetate (L3), acetone (L4) and methanol (L5) fractions. Similarly 13 g of the soxhlet methanolic extract of the stem bark (SS) was adsorbed onto silica gel and eluted in succession with chloroform, ethyl acetate, acetone and methanol to yield chloroform (S1), ethyl acetate (S2), acetone (S3) and methanol (S4) fractions. All the fractions were subjected to antimicrobial screening

Antimicrobial Screening

The sensitivity of the extracts and fractions were determined by Agar well diffusion method (Lovian, 1991). The minimum inhibitory concentration (MIC) of the active fractions was determined by 2–fold serial dilution according to reported procedure (Esimone et al, 1999).

Antiinflammatory Tests

The antiinflammatory activity of the leave and stem bark extracts of *Nauclea latifolia* was determined using a variation of egg-albumen induced rat paw edema as a model of inflammation as previously described (Osadebe and Okoye, 2003).

Phytochemical Tests

The phytochemical constituents of the extracts and fractions were determined using standard procedure (Harbourne, 1998). In each case a small quantity of the extracts or fractions is dissolved in appropriate solvent and the required reagent added. Colour changes or precipitate were observed to indicate the presence or absence of alkaloids, tannins, flavonoids, terpens, steroids etc.

UV/Visible Spectral Analysis of the Active Flavonoid Fraction (S2)

UV/VIS Scan of S2 was determined in Ethanol and Methanol. The effect of addition of drops of 2 M NaOH on the spectrum of S2 in Ethanol was investigated. The effects of the addition of Sodium acetate and Boric acid in succession on the spectrum of S2 in Ethanol were also investigated.

Statistical Analysis

Data were analyzed using student's *t*-test and expressed as mean±SEM. Differences between means were considered significant at $p<0.05$.

Results and Discussion

The result of the preliminary antimicrobial screening of the crude extracts of *Nauclea latifolia* leaves and stem bark is shown in Table 27.2. For both the stem bark and leaves, the soxhlet extracts (LS and SS) showed better antimicrobial activity than the extracts obtained by cold maceration (LC and SC). Soxhlet erxtraction usually gives better yield of plant secondary metabolites than cold maceration. This might account for the observed better antimicrobial activity of LS and SS. It is possible that higher quantities of the antimicrobial constituents are extracted using soxhlet. It is also possible that the antimicrobial constituents are not thermolabile or volatile else the soxhlet extracts would have given very poor activity.

Table 27.1: Crude extracts and their phytochemical constituents

Extract	*Yield % (w/w)*	*Alkaloids*	*Flavonoids*	*Terpenoids*	*Steroids*	*Tannins*	*Saponins*	*Glycosides*
LC	14	–	++	++		++	++	+
LS	20	–	++	+++		++	++	+
SC	12	++	++	–		+++	++	++
SS	15	++	+++	–		+++	++	++

–: Absent; +: Present. Multiple pluses indicate the degree of abundance.

We therefore investigated the antimicrobial activity of different solvent fractions of the leaf and stem bark Soxhlet extracts. The result as shown in Table 27.3 indicates that all the fractions showed antimicrobial activity against *E. coli*. Only L4, S2 and S4 had activity against *Salmonella paratyphi*. L1 and L2 had activity against *B. subtillis* while L4, S2 and S4 had activity *Staphylococcus aureus*. This results showed that L4 (acetone fraction of leaf extract) and S2 (ethyl acetate fraction of stem bark extract) are the most active of all the fractions from the leaf and stem bark extracts respectively. The activity of S2 is quite high and comparable to the standard antibiotic, gentamycin. Phytochemical investigation revealed the presence of tannins and flavonoids in L4 but only flavonoids in S2. Tannins and flavonoids have been shown in several studies to be responsible for the antimicrobial activities of some medicinal plants of traditional use (Geissman, 1963; Scalbert, 1991; Haslem, 1996). The antimicrobial activity of the flavones, isoflavones, flavonols, etc has been reported in previous studies (Wachter *et al.*, 1999; Waage and Hedin, 1985; Bojase *et al.*, 2002).

Table 27.2. Different Solvent Fractions and their Phytochemical Constituents

Fractions	*Yield % (w/w)*	*Alkaloids*	*Flavonoids*	*Terpenoids*	*Steroids*	*Tannins*	*Saponins*	*Glycosides*
L1	13.3*		–	++	–	–	–	–
L2	11.3*		–	+	–	–	–	–
L3	16.67*		++	–	–	–	–	–
L4	30.67*		+	–	–	++	–	–
L5	27.3*		–	–	++	–	+++	+
S1	14.62**	+	+	–	–	–	–	–
S2	18.46**		+++	–	–	–	–	–
S3	33.85**		–	–	–	–	+	–
S4	31.54**		–	–	+	+++	++	+

–: Absent; +: Present. Multiple pluses indicate the degree of abundance.

*Percent yield calculated with 15 g of starting material

**Percent yield calculated with 13 g of starting material

Table 27.3: Results of Preliminary Antimicrobial Screening IZD (Mean±SEM)

Extracts	*Bacillus subtilis*	*Staph. aureus*	*Pseudo-monas aerigunosa*	*Escheri-chia coli*	*Salmo-llena paratyphi*	*Klebsiella pnemonia*	*Candida albican*	*Aspergillus niger*
LC	–	–	–	9.67±0.58	–	–	–	–
LS	5.33±0.58	–	–	9.67±0.53	–	–	–	–
SC	3.67±0.58	–	–	7.33±2.1	9.67±0.58	–	–	–
SS	6.67±0.58	–	–	8.67±1.15	9.67±1.15	–	–	–

In our preliminary chemical investigation of–we found on UV analysis that the fraction in ethanol exhibited two prominent peaks at 249 and 275 nm (Figure 27.1). These peaks are characteristic of flavonoids (Finar, 1975). In methanol, the first shift showed a hypsochromic shift to 236 nm while the second exhibited a hypochromic effects (Figure 27.2). These peaks showed bathochromic shift on addition of 2 drops of 2 M NaOH further confirming the presence of flavonoid nucleus (Figure 27.3). However, the peaks did not show any shift on sequential addition of sodium acetate and boric acid powder in the ethanol solution. This suggests the presence of flavones, which may not contain free hydroxyl groups at positions 7, 3^1 and 4^1 of the flavonoid nucleus (Scott, 1964; Harboune, 1998). Studies to confirm the real chemical identities of these flavonoids are in process.

Our results seem to justify the ethnomedicinal uses of the plant materials in the management of toothache, dental caries, septic mouth, diarrhea and dysentery. The extracts and fractions showed activity against some groups of microorganism, which have been implicated as causes of these diseases. Apart from microbial inversion, some of these diseases are also known to involve inflammatory responses. This led to our investigation of the antiinflammatory effect of the extracts of *Naulea latifolia* leaves and stem bark. The result as shown in Table 27.4 indicates that both the extracts of leaves and

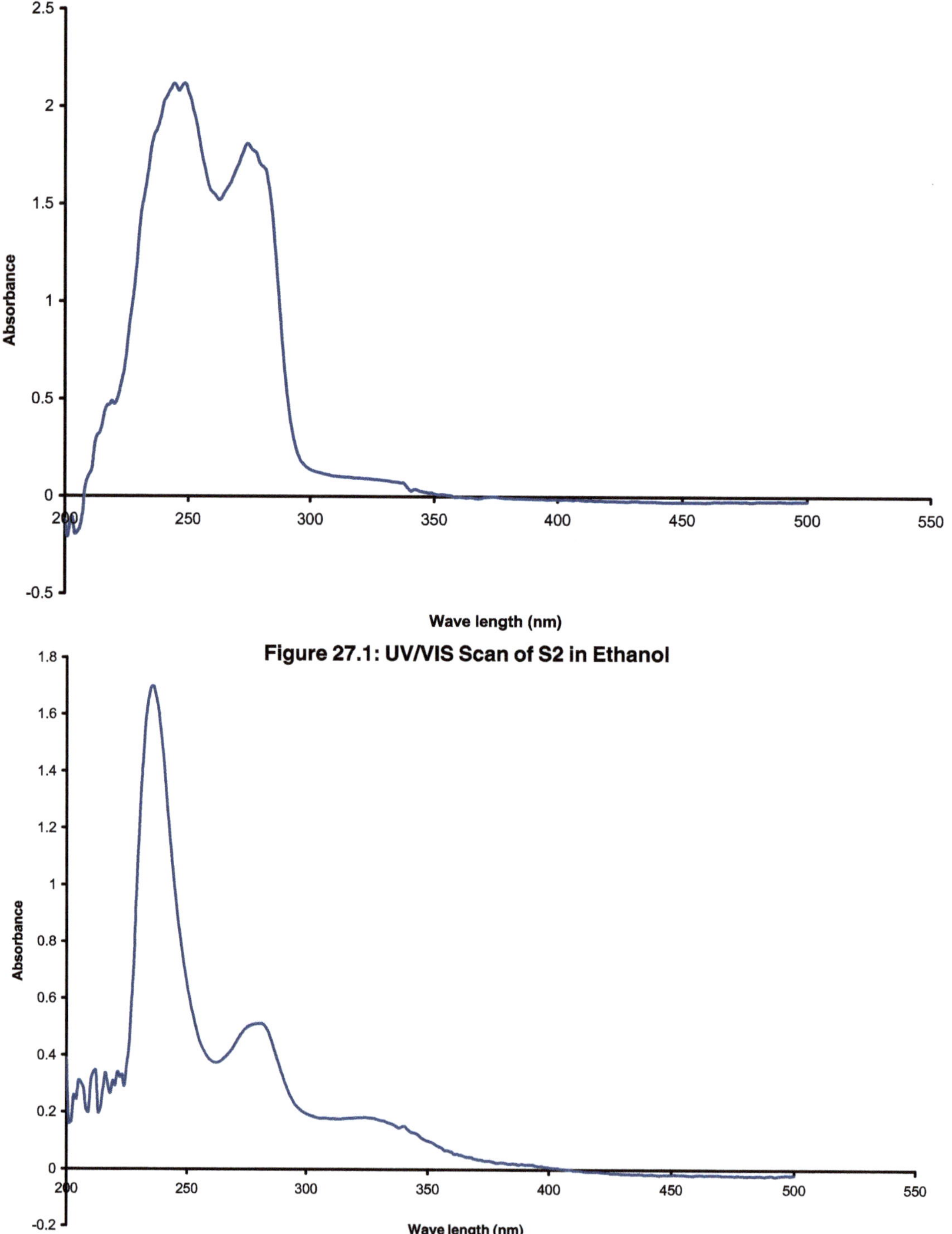

Figure 27.1: UV/VIS Scan of S2 in Ethanol

Figure 27.2: UV/VIS Scan of S2 in Methanol

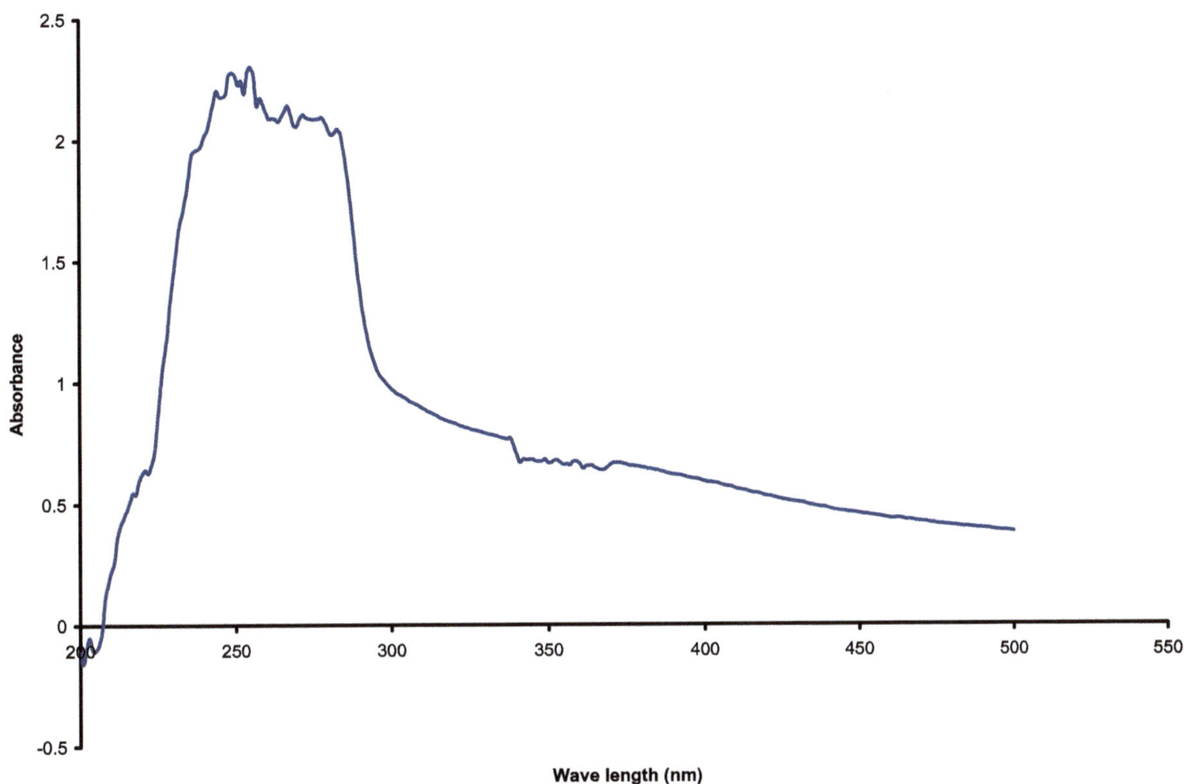

Figure 27.3: UV/VIS Scan of S2 in Ethanol Plus Drops of 2 M NaOH Solution

Table 27.4 Result of the Minimum Inhibitory Concentration of the Active Fractions MIC mg/ml (Mean±SEM)

Fractions/ Sts Drug	*Bacillus subtilis*	*Staph aureus*	*Psedomonas aerigunosa*	*Escherichia coli*	*Salmollena paratyphi*	*Klebsiella pnemonia*
L1	4.183±0.032	ND	ND	4.039±0.031	ND	ND
L2	ND	"	"	3.899±0.006	"	"
L3	"	"	"	3.398±0.0.005	"	"
L4	"	4.249±0.005	"	4.346±0.009	"	"
L5	"	ND	"	ND	"	"
S1	"	"	"	3.405±0.009	"	"
S2	"	1.210±0.006	"	1.55±0.0.01	1.226±0.008	"
S3	"	ND	"	ND	ND	"
S4	"	"	"	"	"	"
Gentamycin	0.629±0.039	"	0.623±0.007	0.78±0.006	0.752±0.002	0.489±0.004

stem bark exhibited mild ant-inflammatory activity at 200 mg/kg in egg albumen–induced rat paw edema. This observation is in agreement with a previous study on the stem bark by Otumenyi and Uguru (2006). However, this mild activity could be beneficial in the management of toothache since this disease involves only mild inflammation.

Table 27.5: Antiinflammatory Effects of the Extracts of *Nauclea latifolia* Leaves and Stem Bark

Extract	*Dose (mg/kg)*	*Edema volume ml (mean±SEM)*			
		1 h	*2 h*	*3h*	*4 h*
SL	200	0.88±0.12 (22.0)	0.75±0.1 (27.2)	0.70±0.08 (24.7)	0.60±0.15* (33.3)
SS	200	1.10±0.11 (2.0)	0.98±0.16 (4.9)	0.88±0.13 (5.4)	0.78±0.13* (13.3)
ASA	100	1.0±0.1 (11.5)	0.63±0.12 (38.8)	0.50±0.12* (46.2)	0.43±0.1* (52.2)
10 per cent Tween 80	0.4 ml	1.13±0.09	1.03±0.14	0.93±0.14	0.90±0.14

* $p<0.05$, n = 5, values significantly different compared with the control.

Values in parenthesis represent percent inhibition of edema.

ASA: Acetyl salycilic acid; SL: Soxhlet methanolic extract of leave; SS: Soxhlet methanolic extract of stem.

In conclusion, our results seem to justify the ethnomedicinal uses of *Nauclea latifolia* in the management of a wide range of infectious disease. Tannins and flavonoids may be responsible for the observed antimicrobial activity of the plant materials.

References

Akpanabiatu MI, Umoh IB, Uddosen EO, Udoh AE, Edet EE. (2005). Rat serum electrolyte, lipid profile and cardiovascular activity of Nauclea latifolia leaves extracts administration. *Indian Journal of Clinical Biochemistry*, 20(2): 29–34.

Akpanabiatu MI, Umoh IB, Eyong EU, Udoh FV.(2005). Influence of *Nauclea latifolia* leaf extracts on some Hepatic enzymes of Rats fed on coconut oil and non-coconut oil meals. *Pharmaceutical Biology*, 43(2): 153–157.

Bojase G, Majinda R, Gashe B, Wanjada C. (2002).Antimicrobial flavonoids from *Bolusanthus speciosus*. *Planta Medica*, 68: 615-620.

Esimone, CO., Adikwu, MU., Uzuegbu, DB and Udeogaranya, PO. (1999). The effect of ethylenediaminetetraacetic aid on the antimicrobial properties of Benzoic acid and Cetrimide. *J. Pharm. Res. and Development*, 4(1): 1–8.

Finar IL. (1975). Organic Chemistry Volume 2: Stereochemistry and the Chemistry of Natural Products, 5th edition. Longman, Singapore.

Geissman, T. A. (1963). Flavonoid compounds, tannins, lignins and relatedcompounds, p. 265. *In* M. Florkin and E. H. Stotz (ed.), Pyrrole pigments, isoprenoid compounds and phenolic plant constituents, vol. 9. Elsevier, New York, N.Y.

Gidado A, Ameh DA, Atawodi SE. (2005). Effect of *Nauclea latifolia* leaves aqueous extracts on blood glucose levels of normal and alloxan-induced diabetic rats. *African Journal of Biotechnology*, 4(1): 91–93.

Harbourne, J.B. (1998). Phytochemical Methods: A guide to Modern Techniques of Plant Analysis, 2nd ed. Chapman and Hall, London.

Haslam, E. (1996). Natural polyphenols (vegetable tannins) as drugs: possible modes of action. *J. Nat. Prod.,* 59:205–215.

Iwu MW, Duncan AR, Okunji CO. (1999). New antimicrobials of plant origin. In: J. Janick (ed), Perspectives on New Crops and New Uses. ASHS Press, Alexandria, VA, pp. 457–462.

Kirkpatrick P. (2002). Antibacterial drugs: stitching together naturally. Nature Review Drug Discovery 1: 748.

Lamidi M, Ollivia E, Faere R, Debrauwer L, Nze-Ekekang L, Balansard G. (1995). Quinovic acid glycosides from Nauclea diderichie. *Planta Medica,*61: 280–281.

Lovian, I. (1980). Antibiotics in laboratory medicine. Williams and Williams, Baltimore, London pp. 7-22.

Madubunyi II.(1996). Antihepatotoxic and trypanocomidal activities of the ethanolic extracts of Nauclea latifolia root bark. *Journal of Herbs, Spices and Medicinal Plants,* 3(2): 23–35.

Moundipa PF, Kamini G, Melanie F, Charles FBB, Iris B. (2005). In vitro amoebicidal activity of some medicinal plants of the Bamum Region (Cameroon). African *Journal of Traditional, Complementary and Alternative Medicine,* 2(2): 113–121.

Otimenyin SO, Uguru MO. (2006). Acute toxicity studies, antiinflammatory and analgesic activities of the methanolic extracts of the stem bark of Enantia chlorantha and *Nauclea latifolia*. *Journal of Pharmacy and Bioresources,* 3(2): 111 –115.

Onyeyili PA, Nwosu CO, Amin JD, Jibike JI. (2001). Anthelmintic activity of crude aqueous extract of *Nauclea latifolia* stem bark against ovine nematodes. *Fitoterapia,* 72(1): 12–21.

Osadebe, P.O., Okoye, F.B.C. (2003). AntiInflammatory Effects of Crude Methanolic Extract and Fractions of *Alchornea cordifolia* leaves. *Journal of Ethnopharmacology,* 89: 19-24.

Scalbert, A. (1991). Antimicrobial properties of tannins. *Phytochemistry,* 30: 3875–3883.

Scott AI. (1964). Interpretation of the ultraviolet spectra of Natural Products. Pergammon Press, London.

Shigemori H, Kagata T, Ishiyama H, Morah F, Ohsaki A Kobayashi J. (2003). Naucleamides A–E, New Monoterpene Indole Alkaloids from *Nauclea latifolia Chemical and Pharmaceutical Bulletin,* 51(1): 58

Udoh FV. (1995). Effects of leaf and root extracts of Naeclea latifolia on purinergic neurotransmission in rat bladder. *Phytotherapy Research,* 9: 239–234.

Udoh FV. (1998). Effects of leaf and root extracts of Naeclea latifolia on cardiovascular system. *Fitoterapia,* 69(2): 141–146.

Waage SK, Hedin PA. (1985) Quercetin 3-O-galactosyl-(1Æ6)-glucoside, a compound from narrowleaf vetch with antibacterial activity. *Phytochemistry,* 24:243-5.

Wachter GA, Hoffmann JJ, Furbacher T, Blake ME, Timmermann BN. (1999)Antibacterial and antifungal flavonones from *Eysenhardtia texana. Phytochemistry,* 52:1469-1471.

Medicinal Plants: Phytochemistry, Pharmacology and Therapeutics, Vol. 1 *Pages* ***430–440***
Editors: **V.K. Gupta, G.D. Singh, Surjeet Singh and A. Kaul**
Published by: **DAYA PUBLISHING HOUSE, NEW DELHI**

Chapter 28

Herbal Drug Therapy: A Promising Solution for Helminthes Parasites

J.K. Chamuah, C.C. Barua*, A.G. Barua[1] and D. Lahkar
Department of Pharmacology and Toxicology, [1]Public Health and Hygiene
College of Veterinary Science, Khanapara, Guwahati – 781 022, Assam, India

ABSTRACT

Parasitic diseases is one of the constraints for profitable animal production in terms of meat and milk. Though treatment with chemical compound is the right solution, but it leads to development of resistance with frequent use. In recent times, the bio-prospection of natural resources has gained unprecedented impetus all over the world for search of new and novel molecules as therapeutic agents. Consequently, a number of clinically useful drugs have been discovered and many complex physiological and biochemical pathways have been defined and are now well understood. Many studies carried out in the last few years have also demonstrated that plants represent an unparallel source of molecular diversity for drug development. Research based pharmaceutical companies of developed countries like USA, UK, Japan, France, Germany and Switzerland are the major global players in the area of drug discovery. India's contribution has been insignificant, but has attained some global visibility with respect to its self-reliant technological status. The prioritization of disease related search for new therapeutic agents may be different for developed and developing countries. Future studies on plant based anthelmintic in account of their suitable dosage regiments, effective formulation with other standard drugs will be one of the promising solution for development of anthelmintic resistance problem. This

* Corresponding Author: E-mail: chanacin@satyam.net.in; Phone: (R) 0361-2361485 , (M) 098640-13231.

review article is intended to highlight the significant achievement of drug development from plant sources as anthelmintic and identification of Indian emerging medicinal plants for lead generation and development of novel herbal anthelmintic.

Keywords: *Herbal drug therapy, Helminthes parasites, Parasitic diseases.*

Introduction

The subcontinent of India possesses the largest livestock population in the world which comprises 7 per cent of its national income. India has a population of 185181 thousand cattle, 97922 thousand buffaloes, 124358 thousand goats, 61469 thousand sheep, 13518 thousand pigs, 751 thousand horses, 632 thousand camels, 65 thousand yaks, 278 thousand mithuns and 2489012 thousand poultry (17th livestock census, 2003.) The productivity of domesticated animals is poor due to complex factors which are many and varied, compounded by sub clinical or clinical often with multiple infections. An understanding of the epidemiology of parasites is crucial for development and implementation of effective management practices.

The hot and humid tropical climate is very much conducive for development and survival of pre-parasitic stages of the parasites. Owing to favorable climatic conditions for development and survival of pre-parasitic stages and in absence of alternate control strategies, control of parasitic problem in livestock is primarily attempted by the frequent use of anthelmintic at short intervals particularly in intensive and semi-intensive management system which has been shown to result in the emergence of anthelmintic resistance. Efforts are now being made to develop and use alternatives to chemotherapy *viz.* grazing, management, biological control and worm vaccine. However, use of commonly used anthelmintic not only induces resistance but also its residues produce toxicity in the host.

To overcome this problem, herbal remedies are considered to be one of the promising solution for control of parasites. Hence, efforts are now being made to develop herbal drugs by screening medicinal plants and their validation in clinical cases through *in vitro* and *in vivo* clinical trials. India has huge source of medicinal plants and enjoys a good place in terms of ayurvedic formulations from time immemorial. Herbal medicine is a practice that is as old as mankind and certainly older than agriculture or writing; every human culture in every continent on earth has practiced herbal medicine of one form or the other. Quite possibly the earliest form of herbal medicine was marshallow root, which is a common grass chewed for setting an upset stomach and has been eaten for presumably that reason by our closest evolutionary cousins, chimpanzee and baboons. In India, the herbalist tradition was ayurvedic, focusing on the use of metals, herbs and parts of animal generally considered inedible.

Modern herbal medicine takes a synergetic approach, trying to cross reference the benefits of various herbs and treatments from different traditions and find the best combination of herbal remedies. Most traditional herbs are aromatics–the compounds we use to treat illness are an effect of plants conducting chemical warfare on each other and fend off herbivores. The same compounds that make many herbs bitter or smell strongly are the one used in herbal medicine and clinical trials.

Among the plant based remedies, use of medicinal plant against parasitic disease in livestock is a great step towards the sustainable parasite control programme in India. The search for safe and efficacious herbal anthelmintic may overcome some of problems associated with synthetic drugs. In this paper, recent studies on anthelmintic evaluation of some indigenous plants against parasites have been reviewed.

Helminth Parasites

Helminth parasites from all three major groups have been utilized as experimental models to evaluate the anthelmintic activity of different plants. Different parasites namely *Strongylus, Ascaris, Oesophagostomum, Ascaridia, Heterakis, Setaria, Haemonchus, Bunostomum, Dipylidium, Taenia, Moneizia, Hymenolepis, Raielletina, Fasciola* and other flukes have been employed *in vitro* and *in vivo* studies in naturally infected animals.

Koko *et al.* (2000) evaluated the oral dose of 9g/kg body weight of *Albizzia anthelmintica* Brong. Mimoseae stem bark water extract and 9g/kg body weight. of *B. aegyptica* fruit mesocarp water extract which are traditionally used as an anthelmintic in Sudan and compared with 20 mg/kg body weight of albendazole against *Fasciola gigantica*. Based on percentage reduction in fluke count from the liver post mortem 2 weeks after treatment, the efficacy of mentioned therapeutic was 95.5, 93.2 and 97.7 per cent.

To control fascioliasis, extract from indigenous plants *viz. Carica papaya, Mallotous philippinensis* (Kamala), *A. indica* were screened against *F. gigantica in vitro* to develop safer, cheaper and more effective remedy for fascioliasis in ruminants. The *in vitro* activity of root-tuber peel extract of *Flemingia vestita*, an indigenous plant consumed by the natives of north east India was tested against *Paramphistomum* sp.by Tandon *et al.* (1997) from Shillong, Meghalaya. We have found encouraging result using crude, methanolic, hexane and chloroform extract of AAU-EVM-NW-3 on *in vitro* trial of *F. gigantica.*

With a view to clarify the induction of the "Crabtree consequence" in liver cells of *Schistosoma mansoni* infected mice, the curative effect of oil extract of *C. longa* was tested and compared to praziquantel (PZQ) the effective drug against all schistosome species occurring in man. Protein, glucose, glucose-6-phopsphatase, AMP-deaminase, adensoine deaminase, urea concentration, pyruvate kinase (PK), phosphorenol pyruvate carboxykinase (PEPCK) and PK/PEPCK ratio were estimated. In addition, worm burden and ova count in mice infected with *S. mansoni* were elucidated. The result showed that *C. longa* normalized the concentration of protein, glucose, AMP-deaminase and adenosine deaminase, which were changed by infection. Moreover, it lowered pyruvate kinase level, while PZQ-treatment induced more elevation of this enzyme. PZQ was more effective in lowering worm burden while *C. longa* extract was more potent in reducing egg count (El-Ansary *et al.*, 2007).

The anthelmintic properties of tanniferous plants and of their secondary metabolites represent one possible alternative to chemotherapy that is currently being explored as a means of achieving sustainable control of gastrointestinal nematodes in ruminants. Previous *in vivo* and *in vitro* results suggest that tanniferous plants can have direct antiparasitic effect against different stages of nematodes. However, the mode of action of the bioactive plant compounds remains obscure. To examine the hypothesis that extracts of tanniferous plants might interfere with the exsheathment of third-stage infective larvae (L3) and to assess the role of tannins in the process by examining the consequence of adding an inhibitor of tannins (polyethylene glycol: PEG) to extracts, the effects of 4 tanniferous plant extracts on exsheathment have been examined on L3 of *Haemonchus contortus* and *Trichostrongylus colubriformis*.

Artificial exsheathment was induced *in vitro* by adding hypochloride solution to larval suspension. The evolution of exsheathment with time was measured by repeated observations at 10-min interval for 60 min. The selected plants were: genista (*Sarothamnus scoparius*), heather (*Erica erigena*), pine tree (*Pinus sylvestris*) and chestnut tree (*Castanea sativa*), with tannin contents ranging from 1.5 to

24.7 per cent of DM. Extracts of a non-tanniferous plant (rye grass, tannin content: 0.3 per cent of DM) were included in the assay as negative controls. The extracts were tested at the concentration of 600 µg/ml and the effects were compared to the rate of exsheathment of control larvae in PBS.

No statistical differences in the pattern of exsheathment was observed after addition of rye grass or genista extracts for both nematode species and with heather extracts for *T. colubriformis*. In contrast, pine tree extracts on larvae of both species and heather extracts with *H. contortus* induced a significant delay in exsheathment. Last, contact with chest nut extracts led to a total inhibition of the process for both nematodes. These results suggest that extracts of tanniferous plants might affect a key process in the very early stages of larval invasion of the host. In most cases, the addition of PEG led to a total or partial restoration towards control values. This suggests that tannins are largely involved in the inhibitory process. However, other secondary metabolites may also interfere with the process that would help to explain some of differences between two nematode species (Bahuaud *et al.*, 2006).

Anthelmintic activity of *Azadirachta indica* and *A. juss* against sheep gastrointestinal nematodes was reviewed by Costa *et al.* (2006). The anthelmintic activity of *A. indica* was investigatedafter feeding sheep with the dried leaves. In this experiment, 40 sheep were allotted into four treatment groups. Group I received a treatment of *A. indica* dry leaves mixed in a concentrate at a rate of 0.1 g/kg dose for 3 months. Group II was treated with double the dose of Group I. Group III was treated with closantel (Diantel) at the manufacturer-recommended dose once at the beginning of the study and Group IV was not treated. To compare treatment effects, the following parameters were evaluated: egg count per gram of feces (EPG), worm burden, weight gain and haematocrit. EPG and worm burden results were statistically evaluated using the Kruskal-Wallis test. Haematocrit and live weight gain were submitted to analysis of variance (ANOVA) and the means evaluated by Tukey's test with 95 per cent probability. None of the evaluated parameters of the treatment groups were statistically different when compared to the control group, demonstrating that, with the protocol used, *A. indica* has no anthelmintic effect.

Anthelmintic activity of *Spigelia anthelmia* extract against gastrointestinal nematodes of sheep using *in vitro* (larval development assay) and *in vivo* studies were conducted to determine possible direct anthelmintic effect of ethanolic and aqueous extracts of *S. anthelmia* towards different ovine gastrointestinal nematodes (Ademola *et al.*, 2007). The effect of extracts on development and survival of infective larvae stage L(3)) was assessed. Best-fit LC (50) values were computed by global model of non-linear regression curve fitting (95 per cent confidence interval). Therapeutic efficacy of the ethanolic extracts administered orally at a dose rate of 125, 250, and 500 mg/kg, relative to a non-medicated control group of sheep harboring naturally acquired infection of gastrointestinal nematodes, was evaluated *in vivo*. The presence of *S. anthelmia* extracts in the cultures decreased the survival of L (3) larvae. The LC (50) of aqueous extract (0.714 mg/ml) differ significantly from the LC(50) of the ethanolic extract (0.628 mg/ml) against the strongyles ($P < 0.05$, paired t-test). Faecal egg counts on day 12 after treatment showed that the extract is effective, relative to control (one-way analysis of variance [ANOVA], Dunnett's multiple comparison test) at 500 mg/kg against *Strongyloides* spp. ($P<0.01$), 250 mg/kg against *Oesophagostomum* spp., *Trichuris* spp. ($P < 0.05$), and 125 mg/kg against *Haemonchus* spp. and *Trichostrongylus* spp. ($P < 0.01$). The effect of the doses is significant in all cases, the day after treatment is also extremely significant in most cases, whereas interaction between dose and day after treatment is significant (two-way ANOVA). *S. anthelmia* extract could, therefore, find application in the control helminth in livestock by ethno veterinary approach.

The anthelmintic efficacy of five plant products against gastrointestinal trichostrongylids in artificially infected lambs was studied by Hordegen *et al.* (2003). During his study, Forty eight helminth-free lambs were divided into eight groups (A-H) of six animals. Groups A-G were infected artificially with 10,000 third stage larvae of *Haemonchus contortus* and 20,000 third stage larvae of *Trichostrongylus colubriformis*, whereas group H remained uninfected. Thirty days post-infection, the lambs were treated orally with a single dosage of one of the following products: group A with 3 mg/kg body weight (BW) of an aqueous ethanol extract (70 per cent,v/v) of the seeds of *Azadirachta* indica *A. Juss* syn. *Melia azedarach* L. (Meliaceae); group B with 1 g/kg BW of a raw powder of the leaves of *Ananas comosus* (L.) Merr. (Bromeliaceae); group C with 0.3 mg/kg BW of an aqueous ethanol extract of a 1:1 mixture (g/g) of *Vernonia anthelmintica* (L.) Willd. (Asteraceae) seeds and *Embelia ribes* Burm (Myrsinaceae) fruits; group D with 183 mg/kg BW of an aqueous ethanol extract of the whole plants of *Fumaria parviflora* Lam. (Fumariaceae); group E with 28 mg/kg BW of an aqueous ethanol extract of the seeds of *Caesalpinia crista* L. (Caesalpiniaceae); group F with 25 mg/kg BW of pyrantel tartrate and group G with 50 per cent ethanol. Group H remained untreated. Only the ethanol extract of *F. parviflora* caused a strong reduction of the faecal egg counts (100 per cent) and a 78.2 and 88.8 per cent reduction of adult *H. contortus* and *T. colubriformis* on day 13 post-treatment. The extract was as effective as the reference compound pyrantel tartrate. Therefore, the ethanol extract itself or single constituents of *F. parviflora* could be a promising alternative source of anthelmintic for the treatment of gastrointestinal trichostrongylids in small ruminants.

On the basis of eggs per gram of faeces, Raje *et al.* (2003) evaluated anthelmintic activity *in vivo* against the parasite of *Hemonchus contortus, Oesophagostomum columbianum* and *Paramphistomum cervi* using the combined the equal proportion of powdered *A. indica* (bark), *Burea frondosa* (Seeds) and *Piper longum* (fruits). In the same way, Sharathkumar *et al.* (2004) studied anthelmintic properties of eight medicinal plant against gastrointestinal parasite of cattle. The selected medicinal plants were *Tinospora cordifolia, Vitex trifolia, Artemisia nilagrica, Arundo donax, Melia azaderach, Dicrocephala sp., Asclepius curassaica, Sesbanis sebana* and treated plants showed 40-58 per cent efficacy rate against gastrointestinal parasite. Among the medicinal plants, *T. cordifolia* and *A. curassavica* had the highest and lowest anthelmintic properties. *Ascaris* and *Paramphistomum* were the most and least affected group.

Anthelmintic activity of extracts of *Spondias mombin* against gastrointestinal nematodes of sheep was studied *in vivo* by Ademola *et al.* (2005). This study was carried out to validate the efficacy of *Spondias mombin,* used locally as an anthelmintic and to standardize the effective dose of the plant extract required for worm control in livestock. *In vitro* and *in vivo* studies were conducted to determine the direct anthelmintic effect of ethanolic and aqueous extracts of *S. mombin* towards different ovine gastrointestinal nematodes. A larval development assay (LDA) was used to investigate the *in vitro* effect of extracts on strongyle larvae. Another study was conducted *in vivo* to evaluate the therapeutic efficacy of the extracts administered orally at dose rates of 125, 250, 500 mg/kg to sheep naturally infected with gastrointestinal nematodes. Twenty sheep were selected on the basis of positive faecal egg counts (750 EPG). The sheep were allocated randomly to a non-medicated control group (A) or to groups given 125 mg/kg (B), 250 mg/kg (C) or 500 mg/kg (D) of extract, respectively. Sheep in groups B-D were given extracts orally on two days. Individual faecal egg counts were performed on days 0, 3, 6, 9 and 12. The presence of *S. mombin* extracts in *in vitro* cultures of larvae decreased the survival of L3 larvae. The LC50 of the aqueous extract of *S. mombin* was 0.907 mg/ml, while the LC50 of the ethanolic extract was 0.456 mg/ml. This difference in LC50 was statistically significant ($P > 0.05$). The mean percentage faecal egg reduction of sheep drenched with 500 mg/kg *S. mombin* extracts was 15.0 per cent, 27.5 per cent, 65.0 per cent, 65.0 per cent, 100.0 per cent against *Haenmonchus* spp., *Trichostrongylus* spp., *Oesophagostomunm* spp., *Strongyloides* spp. and *Trichuris* spp. respectively, on day 12. Extracts of *S. mombin* could find application to control the helminth parasites

Sericea lespedeza hay as a natural deworming agent against gastrointestinal nematode infection in goats was reported by Sharik *et al.* (2006). A study was designed to test the efficacy of a high condensed tannin (CT) legume, sericea lespedeza [SL, *Lespedeza cuneata* (Dum.-Cours. G. Don)] against GIN of goats fed in confinement. The goats were given a infection of 500 *H. contortus* larvae/animal three times per week during the trial to simulate natural infection. Twenty bucks (6-8 months old) were fed Bermuda grass [BG, *Cynodon dactylon* (L.) Pers.] hay plus concentrate for 5 weeks in confinement and then 10 animals were switched to SL hay for an additional 7 weeks. Throughout the trial, feces and blood were collected weekly from individual animals to determine fecal egg count (FEC) and blood packed cell volume (PCV). Fecal cultures were made weekly from pooled samples to determine treatment effects on GIN larval development. All goats were slaughtered at the end of the trial, with adult worms in the abomasum and small intestine of each goat recovered, counted, and identified to species. Feeding SL hay to goats significantly ($P<0.01$) reduced FEC and increased PCV compared with BG hay. In addition, a lower percentage of ova in feces from SL-fed goats developed into infective (L3) larvae. There was a direct effect of SL hay on adult worms, with significantly ($P<0.01$) lower numbers of both abomasal (*H. contortus, Teladorsagia circumcincta*) and small intestinal (*Trichostrongylus colubiformis*) nematodes compared with goats fed BG hay. Feeding SL hay to goats is an effective means of controlling parasitic nematodes and may be a potential supplement for chemical anthelmintic.

In vitro and *in vivo* anthelmintic efficacy of plant cysteine proteinases against the rodent gastrointestinal nematode, *Trichuris muris* was studied (Stepek *et al.*, 2006). Extracts of plants, such as papaya, pineapple and fig, are known to be effective at killing intestinal nematodes that inhabit anterior sites in the small intestine, such as *Heligmosomoides polygyrus*. They demonstrated that similar *in vitro* efficacy also occurs against a rodent nematode of the large intestine, *Trichuris muris* and confirmed that the cysteine proteinases present in the plant extracts are the active principles. The mechanism of action of these enzymes involved an attack on the structural proteins of the nematode cuticle, which was similar to that observed with *H. polygyrus*. However, not all plant cysteine proteinases were equally efficacious because actinidain, from the juice of kiwi fruit, had no detrimental effect on either the motility of the worms or the nematode cuticle. Papaya latex was also shown to significantly reduce both worm burden and egg output of mice infected with adult *T. muris*, demonstrating that enzyme activity survived passage to the caecum and was not completely inactivated by the acidity of the host's stomach or destroyed by the gastric or pancreatic proteinases. Thus, the cysteine proteinases from plants may be a much-needed alternative to currently available anthelmintic drugs due to their efficacy and novel mode of action against gastrointestinal nematode species.

Haemonchosis is one of the important cause of calfhood mortality of ruminants. To overcome their mortality, different workers have reviewed *in vitro* anthelmintic activity of different medicinal plants. The hot and cold aqueous, methanol, di-ethyl ether, hexane and chloroform extract residues prepared from *Embelia ribes*, *Psoralea coryfolia* and *Verononis anthelmintica* were evaluated against *H. contortus*. In another study conducted by Raje and Jangde (2003) concluded that *Nicotiana tabacum* have good anthelmintic action against *H. contortus*. However, *N. tobacum* is also effective in treatment of swine ascariasis and stephanofilarial dermatitis.

Ovicidal and larvicidal activity of *Melia azedarach* extracts on *Haemonchus contortus* was studied by Maciel *et al.* (2006). The ovicidal and larvicidal activity of *M. azedarach* extracts on *H. contortus* was evaluated through egg hatching and larval development tests. Hexane and ethanol extracts of seeds and chloroform and ethanol extracts of leaves of *M. azedarach* were used in the tests. To perform the larval development test, feces of an animal free from parasites were mixed with third instar *H. contortus* larvae and extracts in several concentrations. The coprocultures were incubated for 7 days at 30° C, then the larvae were recovered and counted. LC_{50} was calculated by probits using the SPSS 8.0 program. The seed ethanol extract was the most active on eggs (LC50=0.36mgmL(-1)) and the leaf ethanol extract showed the best inhibition of larval development (LC50=9.18mgmL (-1). Phytochemical analysis of the most active extracts revealed the presence of condensed tannins, triterpenes and alkaloids.

In vitro screening of six anthelmintic plant products against larval *H. contortus* with a modified methyl-thiazolyl-tetrazolium reduction assay was done by (Hordegen *et al.*, 2006). Because of the increasing anthelmintic resistance and the impact of conventional anthelmintic on the environment, it is important to look for alternative strategies against gastrointestinal nematodes. Phytotherapy could be one of the major options to control these pathologies. Extracts or ingredients of six different plant species were tested against exsheathed infective larvae of *Haemonchus contortus* using a modified methyl-thiazolyl-tetrazolium (MTT) reduction assay. Pyrantel tartrate was used as reference anthelmintic. Bromelain, the enzyme complex of the stem of *Ananas comosus* (Bromeliaceae), the ethanolic extracts of seeds of *Azadirachta indica* (Meliaceae), *Caesalpinia crista* (Caesalpiniaceae) and *Vernonia anthelmintica* (Asteraceae), and the ethanolic extracts of the whole plant of *Fumaria parviflora* (Papaveraceae) and of the fruit of *Embelia ribes* (Myrsinaceae) showed an anthelmintic efficacy of up to 93 per cent, relative to pyrantel tartrate. Based on these results obtained with larval *H.contortus*, the modified MTT reduction assay could be a possible method for testing plant products with anthelmintic properties.

In vitro and *in vivo* anthelmintic activity of crude extracts of *Coriandrum sativum* against *H. contortus* was reported by Eugale, (2007). *In vitro* anthelmintic activities of crude aqueous and hydro-alcoholic extracts of the seeds of *C. sativum* (Apiaceae) were investigated on the egg and adult nematode parasite *H. contortus*. The aqueous extract of *C. sativum* was also investigated for *in vivo* anthelmintic activity in sheep infected with *Haemonchus contortus*. Both extract types of *Coriandrum sativum* inhibited hatching of eggs completely at a concentration less than 0.5 mg/ml. ED(50) of aqueous extract of *C. sativum* was 0.12 mg/ml while that of hydro-alcoholic extract was 0.18 mg/ml. There was no statistically significant difference between aqueous and hydro-alcoholic extracts ($P>0.05$). The hydro-alcoholic extract showed better *in vitro* activity against adult parasites than the aqueous one. For *in vivo* study, 24 sheep artificially infected with *H. contortus* were randomly divided into four groups of six animals each. The first two groups were treated with crude aqueous extract of *C. sativum* at 0.45 and 0.9 g/kg dose levels, the third group with albendazole at 3.8 mg/kg and the last group was left untreated. Efficacy was tested by faecal egg count reduction (FECR) and total worm count reduction (TWCR). On day 2 post treatment, significant FECR was detected in groups treated with higher dose of *C. sativum* ($p<0.05$) and albendazole ($p<0.001$). On days 7 and 14 post treatment, significant FECR was not detected for both doses of *C. sativum* ($P>0.05$). Significant ($P<0.05$) TWCR was detected only for higher dose of *C. sativum* compared to the untreated group. Reduction in male worms was higher than female worms. Treatment with both doses of *C. sativum* did not help the animals improve or maintain their PCV while those treated with albendazole showed significant increase in PCV.

The root extract of *Artemisia maritima* and seed extract of *B. frondosa* individually and in combination was found to cause cessation of mortality and death of *H.contortus* at different hours when exposed to the conc. of 25, 50 and 75 mg/ml of Tyrode solution in their *in vitro* trial (Jangde *et al*, 2001). Taeniasis is one of the significant zoonotic problems faced by people in world wide. In an attempt to treat by plant based drugs, Rasfen (1991) used breadfruit tree (*Artocarpus tonkinensis*), is used in Laotian folk medicine for the treatment of taeniasis. Breadfruit tree preparation impair the *in vitro* motility of the cestodes *Hymenolepis nana*, causing their motor excitation and death where as Chung and Ko (1976) used mixture of areca nuts and pumpkin seeds in the treatment of taeniasis. Likewise efficacy of *Commiphora molmol* (Mirazid) against sheep naturally infected with *Monieizia expansa* also studied by Haridy *et al.* (2004). The essential oil in pure state and at various dilution from the seeds of *Nigella sativa* has been screened *in vitro* against tapeworms and earthworms which was comparable with that of Piperazine phosphate in 1979.

In vitro nematodicidal effects of medicinal plants from the Sierra de Huautla, Biosphere Reserve, Morelos, Mexico against *Haemonchus contortus* infective larvae was reported by Lopez *et al.* (2007). Twenty extracts from plants from Sierra de Huautla Biosphere Reserve, Morelos, Mexico were evaluated against *Haemonchus contortus* infective larvae in an *in vitro* assay. The plant species evaluated were *Bursera copallifera, B. grandifolia, Lippia graveolens, Passiflora mexicana, Prosopis laevigata, Randia echinocarpa* and *Urtica dioica*. The plants were separated into their parts and macerated with different solvents (n-hexane, acetone, ethanol and methanol). An *in vitro* assay was used to evaluate the anthelmintic activity against unsheathed third stage *H. contortus* infective larvae. The experiment was carried out in 24-well cell culture plates at room temperature with three replicates per treatment and using a concentration of 20 mg ml^{-1}. Ten 5 µl aliquots were taken from the corresponding wells and deposited on a slide for microscopical observation at 24, 48, 72 and 96 h post-exposure. The evaluation criteria were based on the average numbers of live and/or dead larvae in the different treatments. Alive and dead larval numbers were statistically analysed through the ANOVA test ($P>0.01$). The Tukey test was used as a complementary tool to determine which treatment was different from the other treatments ($P>0.05$). The highest mortality was observed with *P. laevigata* hexanic extract from stem and leaves combined, which produced 51 per cent, 81 per cent and 86 per cent larval mortality at 24, 48 and 72 h post-exposure, respectively. On the other hand, *B. copallifera* stem acetonic extract exhibited 18 per cent, 59 per cent and 66 per cent nematicidal activity after 24, 48 and 72 h of exposure, respectively.

In view of the lack of an effective pharmacological treatment against human anisakiosis, a disease produced by L(3) larvae of the genus Anisakis present in raw fish, *in vivo* larvicidal effect of certain monoterpenic derivatives against L (3) of *A. simplex* was studied by Hierro *et al.* (2006).The aldehydic monoterpene citral and the alcoholic citronellol, when they are administered together to the larvae of the nematode at the concentration of 46.90 mg/0.5 ml in olive oil, achieve 85.90 per cent and 67.53 per cent dead L (3), respectively, and also stop rats suffering gastrointestinal hemorrhages produced by the larvae

Effect of *Nigella sativa* and *Allium cepa* oils on *Trichinella spiralis* in experimentally infected rats was extensively studied by Abu El (2005). Prophylactic and therapeutic effect of two oils had been carried out either prior to infection or post infection respectively in rats. Each rat in either case was orally administered with *N. sativa* oil or *A. cepa* oil in a dose 5 mg/kg body weight/day for 2 weeks. Assessment of results was by: (1) adult worm count in the intestine on 7th and 20th day post infection. (2) larval count in the muscles on the 60th day post infection. (3) Index of reproductive capacity. (4) Detection of antibodies against *T. spiralis* larvae by using ELISA. The results showed that, *N. sativa* oil as prophylactic treatment prior to *T. spiralis* infection is more effective than *A. cepa* oil on both adult worms and muscle larval count. While, *A. cepa* oil was showed more effectiveness than *N. sativa* on decline number of adult worms and muscle larvae when used as therapeutic treatment post infection. The level of antibody was recorded early in the groups that treated with *N. sativa* oil. So, *N. sativa* and *A. cepa* oils have anthelmintic effect in the rats infected with *T. spiralis* infection and increased the production of antibodies generated during the life cycle of the parasites.

Efficacy of aqueous and butanolic fractions of *Albizzia anthelmintica* against experimental *Hymenolepis diminuta* infestation in rats was reported by Galal *et al.* (1991).The aqueous extract of *A. anthelmintica* bark at 10-15 mg/kg orally showed no toxicity and high anthelmintic activity against experimental *H. diminuta* infection.

Now a day's herbal formulation containing different plant constituents and combined with standard drugs enjoys a good marketable place in treating different parasitic infection. Some of the herbal products are as follows (Kumar *et al.*, 2005).

1. Helminta (Phenothiazine, Piperazine, Stannons oxide, *Vernonia anthelmintica, Senna* leaves and embelin)–Effective against *Ascaridia galli, Raillietina* sp.
2. Liv-52: Useful in fasciolasis
3. Triphala (*Terminalia chebula, Terminalia belerica* and *Emblica myrobalans*) Helminth parasites.
4. Wopell(*Mallotous philippinensis, Butrea frondosa, Embelica ribes, Acacia cat*echu and *Droypteris felix* in man)–Use extensively in the treatment of *Ascaridia galli infestation.*
5. Sonex (Nicotine sulphate, *Embelia ribes* and *Punica granatum*) Helminth parasites.
6. Krimos (Herbal preparation): *Ascaridia galli* and *Heterakis gallinarum.*
7. Janata (*Artemisia maritima, Brassica nigra, Cassia lanceolata, Vernonia anthelmintica* and *Embelia ribes*) Effective against *Trichostrongylus* sp., *H. contortus, Strongylus* and *Nematodirrus* sp.

Conclusion

In the twenty first century of world, plant derived anthelmintic could play a major role in protecting man and animals from different parasitic infection due to its ecofriendly nature and easy biodegradability. Due to development of anthelmintic resistance, there is need for alternative solution which have different modes of mechanism. Future studies on plant based anthelmintic on account of their suitable dosage regiment, effective formulation with other standard drugs will be one of the promising solution for development of anthelmintic resistance problem. Biotechnological involvement with gene manipulation may be a golden era in future for production of plant based anthelmintic.

References

Abu, El Ezz N.M. (2005). Effect of Nigella sativa and Allium cepa oils on Trichinella spiralis in experimentally infected rats. *J Egypt Soc Parasitol.*, 35(2):511-523.

Ademola,I.O., Fagbemi, B.O. and Idowu, S.O. (2005). Anthelmintic activity of extracts of *Spondias mombin* against gastrointestinal nematodes of sheep: studies in vitro and in vivo. *Trop Anim Health Prod.*, 37(3):223-235.

Ademola, I.O., Fagbemi, B.O. and Idowu, S.O. (2007). Anthelmintic activity of *Spigelia anthelmia* extract against gastrointestinal nematodes of sheep. *Parasitol Res.*, 101(1):63-69.

Bahuaud, D., Martinez-Ortiz, de Montellano C., Chauveau, S., Prevot, F., Torres-Acosta, F., Fouraste, I. and Hoste, H. (2006). Effects of four tanniferous plant extracts on the *in vitro* ex sheathment of third-stage larvae of parasitic nematodes. *Parasitology*, 2(Pt 4):545-554.

Chung, W.C. and Ko, B.C. (1976). Treatment of *Taenia saginata* infection with mixture of areca nuts and pumpkin seeds. *Zhonghua Min Guo wei sheng wu xue Za Zhi.*, 9(1-2): 31-35

Costa, C.T., Bevilaqua, C.M., Maciel, M.V., CamurCa-Vasconcelos, A.L., Morais. S.M., Monteiro, M.V., Farias, V.M., da Silva, M.V., Souza, M.M. (2006). Anthelmintic activity of *Azadirachta indica A. Juss* against sheep gastrointestinal nematodes. *Vet Parasitol.*, 137(3-4):306-310.

Eguale, T., Tilahun, G., Debella, A., Feleke, A., Makonnen, E. (2007). *In vitro* and *in vivo* anthelmintic activity of crude extracts of *Coriandrum sativum* against *Haemonchus contortus. J Ethnopharmacol.*, 110(3): 428-433.

El-Ansary, A.K., Ahmed, S.A., Aly, S.A.(2007).Antischistosomal and liver protective effects of *Curcuma longa* extract in *Schistosoma mansoni* infected mice. *Indian J Exp Biol.*,45 (9):791-801.

Galal, M., Bashir, A.K., Salih, A.M. and Adam, S.E. (1991). Efficacy of aqueous and butanolic fractions of *Albizzia anthelmintica* against experimental *Hymenolepis diminuta* infestation in rats. *Vet Hum Toxicol.*, 33 (6):537-539.

Haridy, F.M., Dawoud, H.A and Morsy, T.A.(2004). Efficacy of *Coumiphora molmol* (Mirazid) against sheep naturally infected *Monieizia expansa* in Al-Santa center, Gharbia Governorate, Egypt. *J. Egypt Soc. Parasitol.*, 34 (3): 775-782.

Hierro, I., Valero, A., Navarro, M.C. (2006). *In vivo* larvicidal activity of monoterpenic derivatives from aromatic plants against L3 larvae of Anisakis simplex *Phytomedicine,* 13 (7):527-531.

Hördegen, P., Hertzberg, H., Heilmann, J., Langhans, W. and Maurer, V. (2003). The anthelmintic efficacy of five plant products against gastrointestinal trichostrongylids in artificially infected lambs. *Vet Parasitol.*, 117(1-2):51-60.

Hördegen, P., Cabaret, J., Hertzberg, H., Langhans, W. and Maurer, V. (2006). *In vitro* screening of six anthelmintic plant products against larval *Haemonchus contortus* with a modified methyl-thiazolyl-tetrazolium reduction assay. *J Ethnopharmacol.*, 108 (1):85-89.

Koko, W.S., Galal, M. and Khalid, H.S.(2000). Fasciolicidal efficacy of *Albizia anthelmintica* and *Balanites aegyptica* compared with albendazole. *J. Ethnopharmacol.*, 71 (1-2): 247-252

Kumar, D. Rao, G.S. Raviprakash,V. Tripathi, H.C. Tandan, S.K. Lal, J. and Malik, J.K. (2005). Indigenous plants active against helminth infection of domestic animals in India : An overview. *In* : Infectious diseases of domestic animals and zoonoses in India. 75(B). special issue: 287-298

López-Aroche, U., Salinas-Sánchez, D.O., Mendoza, de Gives P, López-Arellano, M.E., Liébano-Hernández, E., Valladares-Cisneros, G., Arias-Ataide, D.M. and Hernández-Velázquez, V. (2007). *In vitro* nematodicidal effects of medicinal plants from the Sierra de Huautla, Biosphere Reserve, Morelos, Mexico against *Haemonchus contortus* infective larvae. *J Helminthol.*, 6:1-7.

Maciel, M.V., Morais, S.M., Bevilaqua, C.M., CamurCa-Vasconcelos, A.L., Costa, C.T. and Castro, C.M. (2006). Ovicidal and larvicidal activity of *Melia azedarach* extracts on *Haemonchus contortus. Vet Parasitol.*, 140 (1-2): 98-104.

Massoud, A., Morsy T.A. and Haridy, F.M. (2003). Treatment of Egyptian dicrocoeliasis in man and animals with Mirazid. *J Egypt Soc Parasitol.*, 33 (2):437-442.

Raje, A.A. and Jangde, C.R (2003). *In vitro* anthelmintic activity of *Nicotiana tabacum* against *H.contortus* of goats. *Indian Vet. J.*, 80: 364-365.

Raje, A.A., Jangde,C.R and Kolte, S.W. (2003).Evaluation of anthelmintic activity of mixture of indigenous plants in cow calves. *J. Vet. Parasitol.*, 17 (2):97-99.

Rasfon, K (1991). The anticestodal activity of preparations made from the breadfruit. *Med. Parazitol (Mosk).*, 5: 49-52.

Shaik, S.A., Terrill, T.H., Miller, J,E., Kouakou, B., Kannan, G., Kaplan, R.M., Burke, J.M. and Mosjidis, J.A. (2006). *Sericea lespedeza* hay as a natural deworming agent against gastrointestinal nematode infection in goats. *Vet Parasitol,* 139 (1-3):150-157.

Stepek, G., Lowe, A.E., Buttle, D.J., Duce, I.R. and Behnke, J.M. (2006). *In vitro* and *in vivo* anthelmintic efficacy of plant cysteine proteinases against the rodent gastrointestinal nematode, *Trichuris muris*. *Parasitology,* 132(Pt 5):681-689.

Tandon,V., Pal, P., Roy, B., Rao, HS., Reddy, KS.(1997). *In vitro* anthelmintic activity of root-tuber extract of *Flemingia vestita,* an indigenous plant in shillong, India. *Parasitol Res.*, 83(5): 492-498.

Medicinal Plants: Phytochemistry, Pharmacology and Therapeutics, Vol. 1 *Pages* **441–447**
Editors: **V.K. Gupta, G.D. Singh, Surjeet Singh and A. Kaul**
Published by: **DAYA PUBLISHING HOUSE, NEW DELHI**

Chapter 29

Antimalarial Bioactivity of *Enantia chlorantha* Stem Bark

Ayoade A. Adesokan* and Musbau A. Akanji
Department of Biochemistry, University of Ilorin, Ilorin, Nigeria

ABSTRACT

The antimalarial bioactivity of aqueous extract of stem back of *Enantia chlorantha* was investigated in *Plasmodium berghei* infected mice. Stem bark of *Enantia chlorantha* was analysed for its phytochemicals. Twenty five (25) albino mice were infected by intraperitoneal injection of standard inoculum of chloroquine sensitive *Plasmodium berghei* (NK 65 strain). The animals were randomly divided into 5 groups of 5 mice each. Group A served as the control while groups B and C were administered 1.75 and 5 mg/kg body weight of artesunate and chloroquine respectively. Groups D and E received 100 and 400 mg/kg of extract of *E. chlorantha* orally. The results showed the presence of alkaloids saponins, phenolics, flavonoids and glycosides. There was 100 per cent parasite clearance in the 400mg/kg extract and chloroquine groups, and 98.6 per cent clearance in the group that received 100mg/kg body weight of extract. There was no parasite clearance in the artesunate group. There was 100 per cent mortality in the negative control group; 40 per cent mortality in the artesunate, chloroquine and 100mg/kg body weight extract group and 60 per cent mortality in the 400mg/kg extract group. The Mean Survival Time for the control group was 9.0 days; artesunate 22 and chloroquine 19.8 days, while the groups that received 100 and 400 mg/kg body weight of extract recorded 19.6 and 17.0 days respectively.

* Corresponding Author: E-mail: adesokan_ayoade@yahoo.com.

The results showed that aqueous extract of *Enantia chlorantha* possess potent antimalarial activities comparable to that of chloroquine and may be ascribed to the significant presence of alkaloids and phenolics.

Keywords: *Antimalarial bioactivity, Enantia chlorantha, Stem bark, Plasmodium berghei, Mice.*

Introduction

Malaria remains the major cause of morbidity and mortality in the tropical regions of the world with over 300 million new cases reported annually (WHO, 2005). Almost 90 per cent of the deaths from malaria occur in sub-Saharan Africa, where the vulnerable groups are children under 5 years and the pregnant women (WHO, 1999).

WHO experts say that the number of people infected with malaria is still increasing at the rate of about 5 per cent annually, and this has been attributed largely to increasing incidence of resistance to antimalarial drugs formerly effective against the pathogen. Antimalarial drug resistance has become one of the greatest challenges against malaria control. There is widespread multi-drug resistance to common antimalarial drugs (Muregi *et al.*, 2003; WHO, 2005).

In Africa, more than 80 per cent of the people use traditional herbal remedies for the treatment of many ailments including malaria (Akerele, 1984; Wright and Phillipson, 1990).

Rodent plasmodia such as *Plasmodium yoeli* and *Plasmodium berghei* are commonly used as malaria models in mice and have tremendous impact on the investigation of antimalarial activity of plant extracts.

The need to search and develop more effective antimalarial drugs that are inexpensive and readily available to people in the developing countries like Nigeria has necessitated this study.

Materials and Methods

Plant Materials

The stem bark of *Enantia chlorantha* [family–Annonaceae], was harvested in the month of April at *Ifetedo* along Ife–Ondo road, and was authenticated at the Department of Botany, Obafemi Awolowo University, Ile-Ife, Nigeria with voucher number: oliv. IFE No 13968.

Aqueous Extraction

Stem bark of the plant was air-dried to constant weight and ground into powdered form with an electric blender (Blender/Miller III, model MS 223) Taiwan, China. Aqueous extract was prepared as described previously (Akanji and Adesokan, 2005).

Phytochemical Analysis

A portion of the stem powder was subjected to phytochemical analysis, using standard chemical tests as described earlier (Odebiyi and Sofowora, 1978; Trease and Evans, 1989).

Experimental Animals

Albino mice, weighing 20-25g, were obtained from the small Animal Holding Unit of the Department of Pharmacology, College of Health Sciences, University of Ilorin, Ilorin, Nigeria. The animals were housed in wire mesh cages under standard conditions, and the study conducted in accordance with the recommendations from the declaration of Helsinki on guiding principles in the care and use of animals.

Drugs and Reagents

Artesunate used in this study was manufactured by Mekopharm Chemical Pharmaceutical Joint Stock Company, Vietnam, while the chloroquine was from Mayer and Baker Pharmaceutical Company Limited. Nigeria. Other reagents were of analytical grade.

Malaria Parasite

Plasmodium berghei (chloroquine sensitive NK 65 strain) was obtained from the Institute for Advanced Medical Research and Training (IMRAT), College of Medicine, University of Ibadan, Ibadan, Nigeria.

Inoculation of Experimental Mice

Albino mice were infected by intraperitoneal injection of standard inoculum (0.2 ml of 1×10^7 infected erythrocytes) from a single donor mouse previously infected with *Plasmodium berghei* (29.8 per cent parasitaemia).

Animal Groupings

The animals were randomly divided into 5 groups of 5 mice each, after confirmation of parasitaemia 72 h post-inoculation. Group A, (control) was left untreated but administered appropriate volume of distilled water. Group B received artesunate orally at a dose of 1.75mg/kg body weight daily for 4 days and group C 5mg/kg body weight of chloroquine base for the same period. Groups D and E were administered aqueous extract of *Enantia chlorantha* through oropharyngeal canula at the doses of 100 and 400mg/kg body weight respectively.

Estimation of Percentage Parasitaemia

Percentage parasitaemia was estimated at the end of the observational period of 28 days using the formula:

$$\frac{\text{Parasitized RBC}}{\text{Parasitized RBC + Non-parasitized RBC}} \times 100$$

Estimation of Percentage Mortality

The number of deaths was recorded for the animals in each group for the experimental period and the percentage mortality calculated thus:

$$\frac{\text{Number of dead animals in a group}}{\text{Total number of animals in the group}} \times 100$$

Estimation of Mean Survival Time (MST)

The number of days each animal survived was recorded for the animals in each group and the mean survival time calculated using the formula:

$$\frac{\text{Sum of days of survival of animals/group}}{\text{Total number of animals in the group}}$$

Results

Phytochemical analysis

Qualitative and quantitative screening of the components of the plant stem bark yielded the phytochemicals shown in Table 29.1. The phytochemicals that were present included Alkaloids (46.26 per cent), Saponins (26.82 per cent), Phenolics (18.77), Flavonoids (6.71 per cent) and Glycosides (1.44 per cent).

Table 29.1: Qualitative and Quantitative Phytochemical Analysis of *Enantia chlorantha*

Phytochemical	*Qualitative*	*Quantitative Mg*	*Percentage*
Phenolics	++	1.12±0.00	18.77
Flavonoids	+	0.40±0.02	6.71
Alkaloids	++	2.76±0.02	46.26
Glycosides	±	0.086±0.01	1.44
Saponins	++	1.60±0.02	26.82
Tannins	Nd	0.00	0.00
Phlebotanins	Nd	0.00	0.00
Steroids	Nd	0.00	0.00

++: Strongly positive; +: Positive; ±: Weakly positive; nd: Not detected.

Percentage Parasitaemia

Estimation of percentage parasitaemia at the end of 28 days showed the results in Table 29.2. There was no parasitaemia in the blood of mice in the chloroquine group and the group that received 400mg/kg body weight of extract of *Enantia chlorantha*. Less than 2 per cent parasitaemia was found in the blood of mice that received 100mg/kg body weight of the extract. There was high parasitaemia of 55 per cent in the artesunate group.

Table 29.2: Percentage Parasitaemia (Day 28) in Experimental Groups Following Administration of Standard Antimalarial Drugs and Extracts of *Enantia chlorantha*

Treatment Groups	*Percentage Parasitaemia*
Artesunate (1.75mg/kg)	55
Chloroquine (5mg/kg)	0
E. chlorantha (100mg/kg)	<2
E. chlorantha (400mg/kg)	0

Percentage Mortality

At the end of the observational period, 100 per cent mortality was recorded for the untreated control group (Table 29.3). Forty percent (40 per cent) mortality was recorded for the artesunate and chloroquine groups and the extract group that received 100mg/kg body weight dose, but 60 per cent in the group that received 400mg/kg body weight of the extract.

Table 29.3: Percentage Mortality (Day 28) in Experimental Groups Following Administration of Standard Antimalarial Drugs and Extracts of *Enantia chlorantha*

Treatment Groups	*Percentage Mortality*
Control	100
Artesunate (1.75mg/kg)	40
Chloroquine (5mg/kg)	40
E. chlorantha (100mg/kg)	40
E. chlorantha (400mg/kg)	60

Mean Survival Time (MST)

Table 29.4 showed the mean survival time for the animals in each group. The least MST of 9 days was recorded for the control group that was left untreated. The mice in the artesunate group recorded the highest MST of 22 days. The MST of 19.8 and 19.6 days were recorded respectively for the chloroquine and the group that received 100mg/kg body weight of the extract, while the group that received 400mg/kg body weight of the extract recorded 17 days.

Table 29.4: Mean Survival Time (MST) of Animals in Each Experimental Group

Treatment Groups	*MST (Days)*
Control	9.0±0.8
Artesunate (1.75mg/kg)	22.0±2.1
Chloroquine (5mg/kg)	19.8±1.8
E. chlorantha (100mg/kg)	19.6±1.6
E. chlorantha (400mg/kg)	17.0±1.3

Discussion

Results from this study showed that aqueous extract of *Enantia chlorantha* possess potent antimalarial activities that were comparable to that of chloroquine, while the observed antimalarial activities were not dose dependent.

The stem bark of *E. chlorantha* consisted of preponderant alkaloids and phenolics, both of which may be responsible for the pharmacologic activity of the extract. Earlier workers have shown that isolated alkaloid, 9-methoxycanthin-6-one displayed higher antimalarial activity against *Plasmodium falciparum* Gombak A isolate, when compared with chloroquine (Chan *et al.*, 2004). In addition, potent antimalarial agents, raphidecurperoxin and polysyphorin, were isolated from the Vietnamese medicinal plants, *Rhaphidophora decursiva* (Zhang *et al.*, 2001). The extracts of *Nigella sativa* (Black seed), contained different classes of alkaloids that were believed to block protein synthesis in *Plasmodium falciparum* (Abdulelah and Zainal-Abidin, 2007).

In addition, phenolics, which are known to possess antiparasitic, anticarcinogenic, antiinflammatory and immunomodulatory effects, may also play a significant role in the antimalarial activity of the extract (Abdulelah and Zainal-Abidin, 2007).

Consistent with this concept, different extracts of *Enantia chlorantha* have been reported to exert antimicrobial activities, including antibacterial (Agbaje and Onabanjo, 1991; Adesokan *et al.*, 2007).

The antioxidant effect of plant alkaloids may represent another mechanism that contributed to its antimalarial activity. Antioxidant components might inhibit nitric oxide (NO) production in macrophages which will lead to increased degradation of tryptophan and thereby starve the parasite of an essential amino acid leading to its death (Daubener, 1999; Mahmoud *et al.*, 2003).

The antimalarial activity as demonstrated by the percentage parasitaemia in the groups that received the extracts compared favourably with that of chloroquine. The percentage mortality of the animals in the group that received 100mg/kg body weight of the extract was similar to those of the artesunate and chloroquine groups and better than the negative control group.

Further more, the mean survival time of 19.6 days in the group that received 100mg/kg body weight was similar to 19.8 days for the chloroquine group and compared well with 22 days of the group that received artesunate. Even MST of 17 days in the group that was administered 400mg/kg body weight of the extract has proven that the extract possess potent antimalarial activity. Survival of experimental animals beyond 12 days is regarded as significant activity (Peters, 1980; Obih and Makinde, 1985; Abosi and Raseroka, 2003; Ajaiyeoba *et al.*, 2006).

The active principles responsible for these antimalarial activities are yet to be identified but the results from this study have largely justified its use in folklore medicine for malaria treatment in Africa.

References

Abdulelah, H. A. A and Zainal-Abidin, B. A. H (2007). *In vivo* Antimalarial tests of *Nigella sativa* (Black Seed) different extracts. *Amer. J. Pharmacol. Toxicol.*, 2 (2): 46–50.

Abosi, A. O. and Raseroka, B. H (2003). *In vivo* antimalarial activity of *Vernonia amygdalina*. *Brit. J. Biomed. Sci.*, 5: 1–3.

Adesokan, A. A., Akanji, M. A and Yakubu, M. T (2007). Antibacterial potentials of aqueous extract of *Enantia chlorantha* stem bark. *Afr. J. Biotechnol.*, 6(22): 2502–2505.

Agbaje, E. O and Onabanjo A. O (1991). The effects of extracts of *Enantia chlorantha* in malaria. *Ann. Trop. Med. Parasitol.*, 85 (6): 585–590.

Ajaiyeoba, E., Falade, M., Ogbole, O., Okpako, L and Akinboye, D (2006). *In Vivo* antimalarial and cytotoxic properties of *Annona senegalensis* extract.*Afri. J. Trad. CAM.*,3(1): 137–141.

Akanji, M. A and Adesokan, A. A (2005). Effects of repeated administration of aqueous extract of *Enantia chlorantha* stem bark on some selected enzyme activities of rat liver. *Biokemistri*, 17(1): 13–18.

Akerele O (1984). WHO's traditional medicine programme: progress and perspectives. *WHO Chronicle*, 38: 76–81.

Chan, K., Choo, C., Abdullah, N. R and Ismail, Z (2004). Antiplasmodial studies of *Eurycoma longifolia Jack* using the lactate dehydrogenase assay of *Plasmodium falciparum*. *J. Ethnopharmacol.*, 92: 223–227.

Daubener, W (1999). Interleukin-1 inhibit gamma interferon-induced bacteriostasis in human uroepithelial cells. *Infection and Immunity*, 67: 5615–5620.

Mahmoud, M. S., Gilani, A. H and Khwaja *et al.* (2003). The *in vitro* effect of aqueous extract of *Nigella sativa* seeds on nitric oxide production. *Phytother. Res.*, 17: 921–924.

Muregi, F. W., Chhabra, S. C., and Njagi, E. N. M *et al.* (2003). *In vitro* antiplasmodial activity of some plants used in Kisii, Kenya against malaria and their chloroquine potentiation effects. *J. Ethnopharmacol.*, 84: 235–239.

Obih, P. O and Makinde, J. M (1985). Effect of *Azadirachta indica* on *Plasmodium berghei* in mice. *Afr. J. Med. Sci.*, 14: 51–54.

Peters, W. (1980). In: The chemotherapy of malaria in: (Kreler J. ed.) Vol. 1 Academic Press New York, pp 145–283.

WHO (1999). Making a difference: Rolling Back Malaria: The World Health Report; pp 49–61.

WHO (2005). The World Malaria Report from WHO and UNICEF. World Health Organisation, Geneva.

Wright, C. W and Philipson, J. D (1990). Natural products and the development of selective antiprotozoal. *Phytother. Res.*, 4: 127–139.

Zhang, H. J., Tamez, P. A., Floang, V. D., Tan, G. T and van Hung, N (2001). Antimalarial compounds from *Rhaphidophora decursiva*. *J. Nat. Products*, 64: 777–782.

Index

B

N

O

P

Q

R

S

U

V

W

X

Y

Z

www.ingramcontent.com/pod-product-compliance
Ingram Content Group UK Ltd.
Pitfield, Milton Keynes, MK11 3LW, UK
UKHW051504310726
14059UKWH00009BB/106

9 789351 241058